AN ILLUSTRATED GUIDE TO GASTROINTESTINAL MOTILITY

AN ILLUSTRATED GUIDE TO GASTROINTESTINAL MOTILITY

Edited by

DEVINDER KUMAR

Surgical and Gastrointestinal Science Research Unit, London Hospital Medical College, London, UK

and

SVEN GUSTAVSSON

Department of Surgery, University Hospital, Uppsala, Sweden

JOHN WILEY & SONS

Chichester · New York · Brisbane · Toronto · Singapore

Library of Congress Cataloging-in-Publication Data:
An Illustrated guide to gastrointestinal motility/edited by
    Devinder Kumar and Sven Gustavsson.
        p.   cm.
    Includes index.
    ISBN 0 471 91949 7
    1. Gastrointestinal system—Motility—Disorders.
    2. Gastrointestinal system—Motility.   I. Kumar, Devinder.
    II. Gustavsson, Sven.
    RC811.I45   1988
    616.3—dc19   88–2435 CIP

British Library Cataloguing in Publication Data:
An illustrated guide to gastrointestinal motility.
    1. Gastrointestinal tract. Motility
    I. Title   II. Kumar, Devinder
    III. Gustavsson, Sven
    612'.32

    ISBN 0 471 91949 7

Printed in Great Britain by Butler & Tanner Ltd,
Frome and London

CONTENTS

v

PREFACE

Gastrointestinal motility encompasses a very wide area of medicine ranging from the structure and function of single muscle cells to complex brain–gut interactions. The subject is sufficiently broad that even a specialist cannot cover more than a limited number of sub-sets. It has been the focus for basic as well as clinical research for almost a century, and has generated a large body of information. In recent decades the clinical application of these findings has increased such that many gastroenterology units are establishing diagnostic and/or research facilities for the study of patients with disorders of gastrointestinal motility. We, therefore, thought that a practical guide to the understanding, diagnosis and management of such problems would be helpful. In this book, we outline a practical approach to gastrointestinal motility problems. Subjects range from 'making your own manometry tube' to the interpretation of complex motility problems. All available methods for the study of motility, and their possible application to patients, have been discussed. Motor physiology of the oesophagus, stomach, duodenum, biliary tree, small and large intestine, anorectum as well as the sphincteric regions has been described and discussed. We have attempted to define areas where motility studies are of established value and those in which they still have only investigational merit. Effects on gastrointestinal motility of various pharmacological agents, psychological stress, and postsurgical states have been identified. We believe that this work will assist all those who may want a comprehensive and practical guide to this subject.

DEVINDER KUMAR
SVEN GUSTAVSSON
March 1988

CONTRIBUTORS

Hasse Abrahamsson *Division of Gastroenterology, Department of Internal Medicine II, Sahlgren's Hospital, Gothenberg, Sweden*

T. F. Burks *Department of Pharmacology, University of Arizona, Health Sciences Center, Tucson, Arizona 85724, USA*

James Christensen *Division of Gastroenterology–Hepatology, Department of Internal Medicine, University of Iowa College of Medicine, Iowa City, Iowa 52242, USA*

Enrico Corazziari *Cattedra di Gastroenterologia I, Clinica Medica II, Universitá 'La Sapienza', Rome, Italy*

Roberto Corinaldesi *Institute of Clinical Medicine and Gastroenterology, University of Bologna, Bologna, Italy*

S. S. Davis *Department of Pharmacy, University of Nottingham, University Park, Nottingham, UK*

Tom R. DeMeester *Department of Surgery, Creighton University School of Medicine, 601 North 30th Street, Omaha, Nebraska 68131, USA*

Ghislain Devroede *University Hospital, University of Sherbrooke, Sherbrooke, Quebec, Canada*

Andre Dubois *Digestive Disease Division, Department of Internal Medicine, Uniformed Services University of Health Sciences, 4301 Jones Bridge Road, Bethesda, Maryland 20814, USA*

Giorgio Gabella *Department of Anatomy, University College London, London WC1E 6BT, UK*

Sven Gustavsson *Department of Surgery, University Hospital, S 75185 Uppsala, Sweden*

J. G. Hardy *Department of Medical Physics, Queen's Medical Centre, Nottingham, UK*

R. C. Heading *Department of Internal Medicine, Edinburgh Royal Infirmary, Edinburgh, UK*

J. Janssens *Department of Internal Medicine, AZ St Rafael, University Hospital Leuven, B-3000 Leuven, Belgium*

Michael Karaus *University Hospital, Division of Gastroenterology, Department of Medicine, Moorenstrasse 5, D-4000 Dusseldorf 1, West Germany*

K. A. Kelly *Department of Surgery, Mayo Clinic, Rochester, Minnesota 55905, USA*

Chung H. Kim *Gastroenterology Division, Mayo Clinic, Rochester, Minnesota 55905, USA*

Peter M. King *Department of Internal Medicine, Edinburgh Royal Infirmary, Edinburgh, UK*

Devinder Kumar *Surgical and Gastrointestinal Science Research Unit, London Hospital Medical College, Whitechapel, London E1 2AJ, UK*

Susan Mathers *Department of Anorectal Physiology, St Mark's Hospital, London E1, UK*

Sidney F. Phillips   *Gastroenterology Unit, Mayo Clinic, Rochester, Minnesota 55905, USA*

Harry M. Richter   *Division of Surgery, Cook County Hospital, 1835 West Harrison Street, Chicago, Illinois 60612, USA*

Michael G. Sarr   *Department of Surgery, Mayo Medical School, Rochester, Minnesota 55905, USA*

Michael D. Schuffler   *Department of Medicine, Division of Gastroenterology, Seattle Public Health Hospital, Seattle, Washington 98114, USA*

K. Schulze-Delrieu   *Division of Gastroenterology-Hepatology, Department of Internal Medicine, University of Iowa Hospitals and Clinics, Iowa City, Iowa 52242, USA*

Nathaniel J. Soper   *Department of Surgery, Mayo Medical School, Rochester, Minnesota 55905, USA*

V. Stanghellini   *Institute of Clinical Medicine and Gastroenterology, University of Bologna, Bologna, Italy*

Robert W. Summers   *Center for Digestive Diseases, Department of Internal Medicine, University of Iowa Hospitals and Clinics, Iowa City, Iowa 52242, USA*

J. A. Sutton   *Roussel Laboratories Limited, Kingfisher Drive, Covingham, Swindon, Wiltshire SN3 5BZ, UK*

Michael Swash   *Department of Anorectal Physiology, St Mark's Hospital, London E1, UK*

Aldo Torsoli   *Cattedra di Gastroenterologia, Universitá 'La Sapienza', Rome, Italy*

Richard Tucker   *Gastroenterology Unit, St Mary's Hospital, Rochester, Minnesota 55902, USA*

Roland Valori   *Division of Medicine, Selly Oak Hospital, Selly Oak, Birmingham, UK*

G. Vantrappen   *Department of Internal Medicine, AZ St Rafael, University Hospital Leuven, B-3000 Leuven, Belgium*

Martin Wienbeck   *University Hospital, Division of Gastroenterology, Department of Medicine, Moorenstrasse 5, D-4000 Dusseldorf 1, West Germany*

N. S. Williams   *Surgical Unit, The London Hospital, Whitechapel, London E1, UK*

D. L. Wingate   *Gastrointestinal Science Research Unit, The London Hospital Medical College, 26 Ashfield Street, London E1 2AJ, UK*

N. R. Womack   *Surgical Unit, The London Hospital, Whitechapel, London E1, UK*

Giovanni Zaninotto   *Department of Surgery, Creighton University School of Medicine, 601 North 30th Street, Omaha, Nebraska 68131, USA*

I
MORPHOPHYSIOLOGY

1
GROSS MORPHOLOGY OF THE GASTROINTESTINAL TRACT

Devinder Kumar
London Hospital Medical College, London, UK

An adequate knowledge of morphology of the gastrointestinal tract is necessary for successful planning and performance of motility studies. The alimentary tract is a muscular tube extending from the mouth to the anus. It shows a similar structure throughout its entire length, consisting of serosa, muscle layer, submucosa and mucosa. The muscle layer consists of an inner circular and outer longitudinal layer of smooth muscle. The upper third of the oesophagus consists of striated muscle. There are striated muscle sphincters at either end; the upper oesophageal sphincter above and the anal sphincter below.

Innervation of the Gut

Detailed morphophysiology of the enteric nervous system will be discussed in Chapter 2. Broadly speaking, the nerve supply of the gastrointestinal tract comprises extrinsic and intrinsic components. The extrinsic component is provided by the autonomic nervous system (parasympathetic and sympathetic). The oesophagus, stomach, small intestine and the proximal colon derive their parasympathetic supply from the vagus nerve. The colon is also innervated by the sacral spinal nerves. The sympathetic supply to the gut is through the lower thoracic and lumbar spinal nerves. The intrinsic innervation is through the submucosal and myenteric plexuses which contain intercommunicating ganglia (Figure 1).

Oesophagus

In the adult, the oesophagus measures approximately 25 cm, the oesophagogastric junction being 40 cm from the incisor teeth. In the supine posture with the head fully extended, the distance between the lower incisors and the xiphisternum provides a fairly accurate estimate of the length of the oesophagus. This may be important in studies on the lower oesophageal sphincter.

The lower oesophagus and the diaphragmatic hiatus have intrigued investigators for many years and it is, therefore, not surprising that many terminologies and subdivisions of this region are encountered. Figure 2 shows a schematic representation of the lower oesophagus and surrounding structures. The oesophagus passes from a low pressure area (thoracic cavity) to a high pressure area (abdominal cavity). The pressure differential between the two cavities is maintained by loose areolar tissue which fills the hiatus around the oesophagus. This is further helped by the presence of the phreno-oesophageal ligament which is inserted into the oesophagus approximately 3 cm above the diaphragmatic opening.

The presence of an anatomical equivalent of the lower oesophageal sphincter has been disputed by

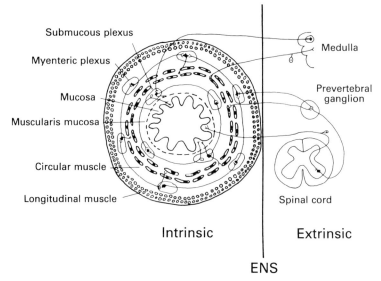

Submucous plexus

Myenteric plexus

Mucosa

Muscularis mucosa

Circular muscle

Longitudinal muscle

Medulla

Prevertebral ganglion

Spinal cord

Intrinsic   Extrinsic

ENS

Figure 1. Transverse section of the gut showing the intrinsic plexuses, the extrinsic enteric nervous system (ENS) and some intrinsic and extrinsic interconnections.

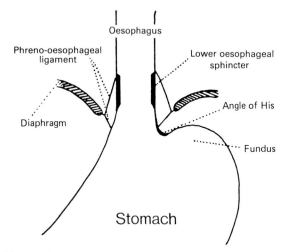

Oesophagus

Phreno-oesophageal ligament

Lower oesophageal sphincter

Angle of His

Diaphragm

Fundus

Stomach

Figure 2. Schematic representation of the anatomy of the lower oesophagus.

(Waldeck et al, 1973). It is therefore possible that both anatomical as well as sphincteric factors contribute towards maintaining competence at the gastro-oesophageal junction.

The oesophagus derives its motor nerve supply from the dorsal motor nucleus of the vagus nerve

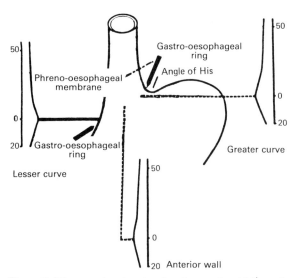

Gastro-oesophageal ring

Angle of His

Phreno-oesophageal membrane

Greater curve

Lesser curve

Gastro-oesophageal ring

Anterior wall

Figure 3. Diagram showing the site of muscular thickness in the lower oesophagus. Adapted from Liebermann-Meffert et al. 1979.

most workers. Liebermann-Meffert et al (1979) demonstrated the presence of an asymmetrical thickening of the circular muscle just above the angle of His in the lower oesophagus (Figure 3). It is not certain whether this area of asymmetrical thickening coincides precisely with the lower oesophageal sphincter but the highest pressure is found in the area of greatest muscle thickening and the nucleus of the spinal accessory nerve which supplies the cervical portion of the oesophagus. The vagus nerve also carries afferent fibres; however, precise details of the afferent supply of the oesophagus are not known. The sympathetic innervation of the oesophagus is derived from the cervical sympathetic ganglia and the thoracic sympathetic chain.

Stomach

The stomach is the most dilated portion of the gastrointestinal tract. It is J-shaped (Figure 4) in most individuals and has a capacity of approximately 1500 ml in adults. It is located in the upper part of the abdomen and is relatively fixed at its upper and lower ends where it joins the oesophagus and the duodenum respectively. However, its shape and position vary with the degree of distension and body posture. This is important, particularly when carrying out noninvasive studies of gastric emptying, for example epigastric impedance, as change in position during the test can give rise to erroneous results.

The stomach has been divided into various anatomical regions (Figure 4). It consists of the cardia, fundus, body, antrum, and the pylorus. There is a notch-like indentation, known as the incisura

angularis, on the lesser curve. The portion of the stomach distal to the incisura angularis is the antrum. Moore et al (1986) have demonstrated the presence of a gastric transverse band representing an anatomical separation between the body and the antrum (Figures 5 and 6). It has been suggested that this band of separation may play a role in the regulation of emptying from the gastric body into the antrum. Manometrically, the antrum is the most commonly studied part of the stomach as the majority of contractions in this region tend to be occlusive in nature. In contrast, contractions in the body and fundus of the stomach tend to be non-occlusive and can therefore be easily missed by intraluminal manometric assemblies. The pylorus is the most distal part of

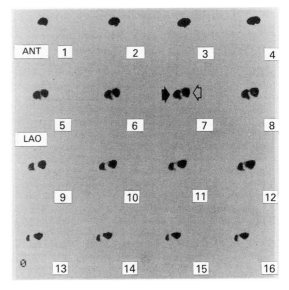

Figure 5. Single photon emission computed tomography images of the stomach in a healthy subject after ingesting an unhomogenized 900 g meal labelled with ^{99m}Tc-chicken liver. Each 60 sec image is acquired every 5.6° throughout 360° rotation of the scintillation camera around the abdomen with the subject in the supine position. Only the first 16 images of a total of 64 are shown, representing the anterior (ANT) and left anterior oblique (LAO) positions, or through 90° of rotation counter-clockwise around the abdomen. Note the persistence of the transverse band in frames 5–15. As illustrated here, the band is observed most clearly in the LAO position and is poorly defined in the anterior-posterior position (frames 1–4). The gastric body lies to the right (open arrow, frame 7) and the gastric antrum to the left (closed arrow, frame 7) of the radiopenic region representing the band. Reproduced with permission from Moore et al, 1986.

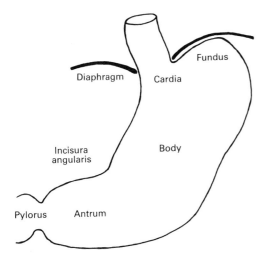

Figure 4. Diagrammatic sketch showing anatomic regions of the stomach.

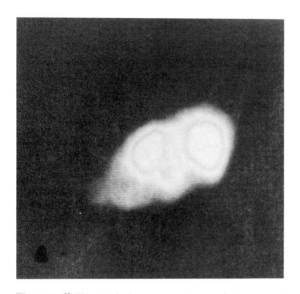

Figure 6. ^{99m}Tc gastric images in a human following solid labelled meal. The scintiphoto was taken 10 minutes after ingestion of the meal. Gastric antrum lies to the left and gastric body-fundus to the right of the midgastric band. Reproduced with permission from Moore et al, 1986.

the stomach and has a thick muscular wall (Figure 7). It is approximately 1 in long and is usually located 1 in to the right of the midline at the level of the first lumbar vertebra. It is an important landmark as it helps in the placement of manometric assemblies at or across the pylorus. It can

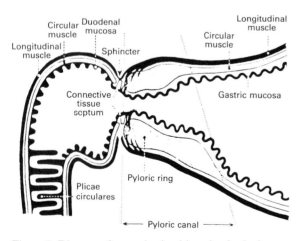

Figure 7. Diagram of gastroduodenal junction in the human being. Reproduced with permission from Edwards and Rowlands, 1963.

also be identified on manometric tracings because it shows a dual frequency of contractions.

The parasympathetic nerve supply of the stomach is from the right and left vagus nerves. The sympathetic innervation is derived from the coeliac plexus and contains the afferent pain transmitting nerve fibres.

Small Intestine

The adult human small intestine measures 4–6 m in length. The length seems to vary both with the tone of the muscle wall and the method of measurement. This can be important when placing electrodes on the surface of the intestine under general anaesthetic because the actual distance between electrodes may be totally different when the effect of the anaesthetic has worn off and the muscles have regained their normal tone. Therefore the data obtained from such studies have to be interpreted with caution especially with regard to propagation velocity of various motor events. Except for the duodenum, the small intestine is suspended by a mesentery and has considerable mobility within the abdominal cavity. There is an acute bend at the junction of the duodenum and jejunum, known as the duodeno–jejunal flexure. It is a useful anatomical landmark in upper small bowel studies and helps to anchor manometric assemblies and stops them from pulling back into the stomach. The diameter of the proximal jejunum is approximately twice that of the distal ileum. The wall of the jejunum is considerably thicker than that of the ileum. The division of the small bowel into jejunum and ileum is somewhat arbitrary; the proximal two fifths is generally referred to as the jejunum and the distal three fifths is called the ileum. The ileum occupies the lower abdomen and a portion of the pelvis.

The distal few inches of the terminal ileum are closely applied to the caecum by the superior and inferior ileocaecal ligaments (Figure 8) (Kumar and Phillips, 1987) and is therefore the least mobile. The mesentery of the ileum is thicker and contains more fat. This feature may be important in identification of the ileum on fluoroscopy or X-

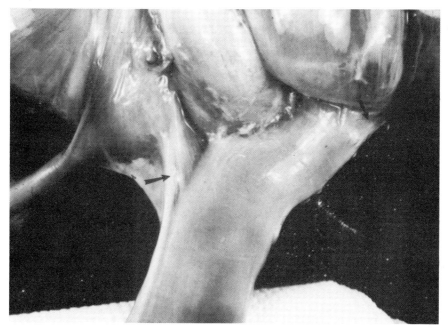

Figure 8. Close-up of the ileocaecal junction showing the superior and inferior ileocaecal ligaments (arrows). Reproduced with permission from Kumar and Phillips, 1987.

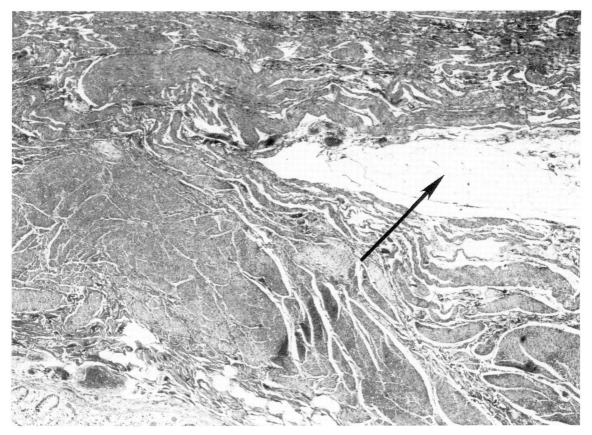

Figure 9. Longitudinal section of the ileocaecal junction showing separation of the ileal and caecal muscle by loose areolar tissue (arrow).

ray films during the placement of long tubes in the distal small bowel.

The ileocaecal junction has generally been thought to be a sphincter. Anatomically, it consists of an upper and lower lip. There is no easily identifiable anatomical equivalent of a sphincter at the ileocaecal junction. In fact, the ileal and caecal circular muscle is separated by loose areolar tissue (Figure 9) and the apparent thickening at the junction is due to the superimposition of the ileal muscle on the caecal circular muscle. Kumar and Phillips (1987), in a recent study, have shown that continence at the ileocaecal junction is maintained at least in part by the anatomical configuration of the junction. Division of the ileocaecal ligaments renders the junction incompetent.

Large Intestine

The caecum is the widest part of the large intestine (Figure 10). The rest of the colon is divided into ascending, transverse, descending and sigmoid

colon segments. The bulk of the longitudinal muscle in the colon is arranged in three longitudinal bundles called taeniae. A thin layer of intertaeniae longitudinal muscle surrounds the colonic circular muscle layer. The taeniae extend from the base of the appendix to the rectosigmoid junction where they blend with the longitudinal muscle of the rectum. Unlike the ascending and descending colon, the transverse and sigmoid colon have a mesentery and are therefore mobile. In between the tacniae, the colon forms haustra which allow segmental movements. Different regions of the large intestine are functionally different and it is therefore important that data obtained from one segment of the large intestine should be discussed with respect to that individual segment and not taken to be representative of the entire colon.

The rectum is the most distal part of the large intestine. It follows the curve of the sacrum and does not have a great degree of mobility. The terminal 3–4 cm form the anal canal. The internal anal sphincter is part of the smooth muscle of the rectum and should be studied in combination with the rectum.

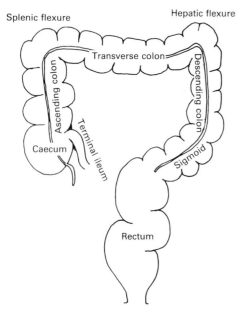

Figure 10. Diagram showing anatomical regions of the large bowel.

References

Edwards, D. A. W. and Rowlands, E. N. (1968), Physiology of the gastroduodenal junction. In: *Handbook of Physiology*. (Eds Code, C. F. and Heidel, W.) Section 6, Volume 4: 1985–2000

Kumar, D. and Phillips, S. F. (1987), The contribution of external ligamentous attachments to function of the ileocaecal junction. *Dis. Colon Rectum*, **30**: 410–16

Liebermann-Meffert, D., Allgower, M., Schmid, P. and Blum, A. L. (1979), Muscular equivalent of the lower esophageal sphincter. *Gastroenterology*, **76**: 31

Moore, J. G., Dubois, A., Christian, P. E., Elgin, D. and Alazraki, N. (1986), Evidence for a midgastric transverse band in humans. *Gastroenterology*, **91**: 540–5

Waldeck, F., Jennewein, H. M. and Siewert, R. (1973), The continuous withdrawal method for the quantitative analysis of the lower esophageal sphincter (LES) in humans. *Eur. J. Chir. Invest.*, **3**: 331–7

2
THE ENTERIC NERVOUS SYSTEM

James Christensen

University of Iowa College of Medicine, Iowa, USA

Introduction

The apparent self-determination of the motor behaviour of the gut is based partly in the autonomy of the smooth muscle and partly in the autonomy of the enteric nerves. The nerves of the gut are not, however, wholly autonomous. Custom dictates that they be treated as 'autonomic', an approach which tends to lead us to forget that they function as a part of the whole nervous system.

The operation of the gut requires constant modulation in normal function. Some of this input is central, though independent of the consciousness. Most of the input, however, comes from sensory nerves in the gut. Such modulation is necessary because the gut is never in a steady state.

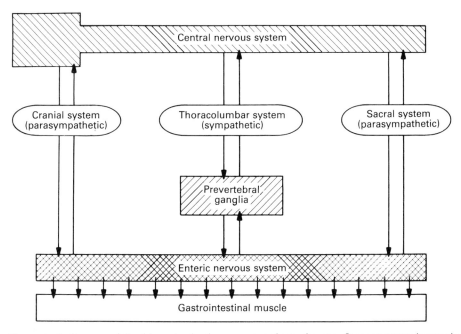

Figure 1. A diagram of the hierarchy in the nerve supply to the gut. Sensory-motor integration (reflexes) can occur at three levels, in the central nervous system, in the prevertebral ganglia, and in the intramural plexuses. From Davison (1983), with permission.

Some sensory inputs to motor nerves prompt widespread effects, while others require local responses. Thus, the sensory inputs occur at various different levels in the nervous system. Figure 1 shows the hierarchy of the extrinsic enteric nerves. Sensory–motor integration occurs in the *central nervous system*, in the *prevertebral ganglia* and in the *intramural plexuses*.

The Extrinsic Nerves to the Gut: Gross Arrangement (Davison, 1983)

General Arrangement

The nerves to the gut pass from the central nervous system at many levels between the hindbrain and the spinal cord. The nerves are segregated into two groups, the *thoracolumbar* and *craniosacral* systems. The nerves from the cranial and sacral cord regions are physiologically similar, while those from the thoracic and lumbar segments of the cord are physiologically similar, but different from the craniosacral nerves. The thoracolumbar nerves are commonly called *sympathetic*, and the craniosacral nerves *parasympathetic*. These divisions are shown in Figures 1 and 2.

Craniosacral Pathways (Figure 2)

The *cranial pathways* are the ninth (glossopharyngeal) and tenth (vagus) cranial nerves. The ninth nerve is distributed along the gut as far as the upper oesophageal sphincter. The domain of the tenth nerve extends to the right colon. These cranial nerves arise from nuclei in the region of the fourth ventricle. Each tenth nerve contains a ganglion just beneath the skull, the *nodose ganglion*, which contains sensory nerve cell bodies. The tenth nerve forms a plexus about the distal oesophagus, the oesophageal plexus, branches from which supply the oesophagus. The bundles of the oesophageal plexus fuse above the diaphragm to form the *vagal trunks* which supply the abdominal gastrointestinal viscera.

The *sacral pathways* arise from sacral segments 1 to 4, forming the pelvic nerves and the pudendal

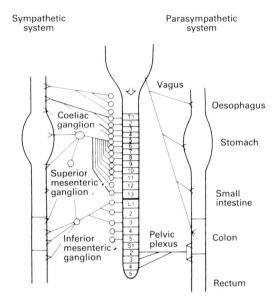

Figure 2. A diagram of the extrinsic innervation of the gut. Central nervous system structures are not shown. From Davison (1983), with permission.

nerves. The pelvic nerves form the *pelvic plexus*. The *colonic nerves* pass from the pelvic plexus to the upper rectum where they penetrate the longitudinal muscle layer, to continue within the plane of the myenteric plexus all along the colon. The pudendal nerves supply the striated muscle of the pelvic floor and, to some extent, the colon.

Thoracolumbar Pathways (Figure 2)

The *thoracolumbar pathways* arise from the thoracic and lumbar segments of the cord, traverse the paravertebral ganglia and pass through the splanchnic nerves to the prevertebral ganglia, the *coeliac*, *superior mesenteric* and *inferior mesenteric* ganglia. From these ganglia, nerves pass alongside mesenteric vessels to reach the gut.

The Intramural Nerves of the Gut: Morphology (Gabella, 1979, 1987)

The General Arrangement of Intramural Nerves

Intramural nerve cell bodies are located in ganglia in two planes in the gut wall, the submucosa and the intermuscular plane between the two major muscle layers. These layers of ganglia are the *submucous* and *myenteric plexuses* (Figure 3). Other less-complex nerve plexuses that contain no ganglia lie just beneath the serosa, deep within the circular muscle layer (only in the intestine), between the circular and oblique muscle layers (only in the stomach), at the interface between circular muscle layer and submucosa (only in the colon), and in the lamina propria throughout the gut.

The Histology of the Intramural Nerves

Within the collagen sheath of a ganglion, the nerve cell bodies lie in a stroma of Schwann cells and convoluted neurites (the *neuropil*). The neurites form synaptic arrangements ('baskets') around ganglion cell bodies. The neuropil and Schwann cells constitute about half of the mass of a ganglion. Bundles of neurites, which may contain occasional isolated nerve cell bodies, join adjacent ganglia. These are the interganglionic fascicles. A 'typical' ganglion is shown in Figure 4.

The network formed by the ganglia and interganglionic fascicles of the myenteric plexus is called the *primary plexus*. Small branches from the interganglionic fascicles form a *secondary plexus*, devoid of ganglia, that fills the spaces in the primary plexus. In turn, the spaces of the sec-

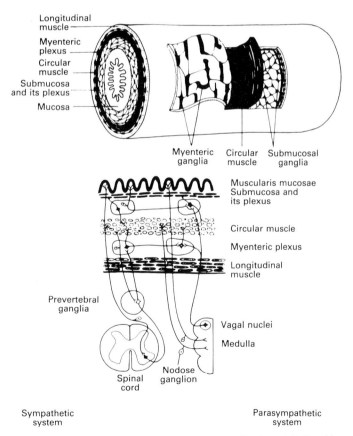

Figure 3. The intramural nerves of the gut. From Davison (1983), with permission.

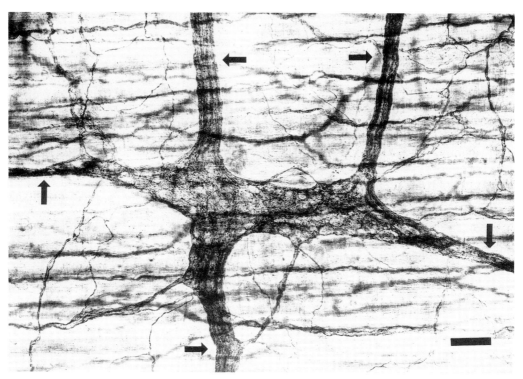

Figure 4. A ganglion of the myenteric plexus of the cat small intestine. Neurites appear as linear beaded black lines which fill the ganglion (the neuropil), the interganglionic bundles (arrows) and their branches. Ganglion cell bodies are poorly stained so that they appear as rounded unstained spaces in the ganglion. The finer branches from the interganglionic bundles are the secondary plexus. The tertiary plexus cannot be seen in this photograph. The bar indicates 50 μm. Osmic acid-zinc iodide stain.

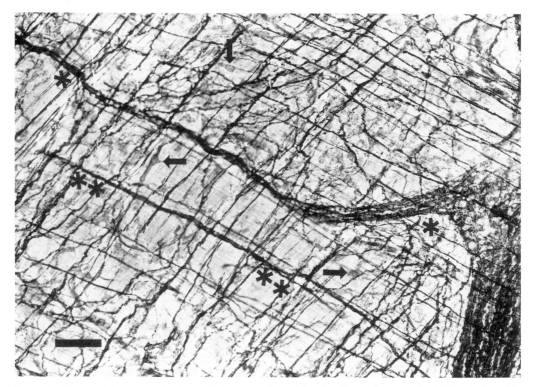

Figure 5. An area of the myenteric plexus of the cat small intestine showing an interganglionic bundle (asterisk), smaller branches forming the secondary plexus (double asterisks) and the finest branches which form the tertiary plexus. Pleomorphic stellate cells stained grey (arrows) are interstitial cells of Cajal. The bar indicates 100 μm. Osmic acid-zinc iodide stain.

ondary plexus are filled with still smaller fascicles and single neurites that branch from the secondary plexus. This is the *tertiary plexus* (Figure 5). This tertiary plexus is intimately related to special cells that resemble fibroblasts, the *interstitial cells of Cajal*. The secondary and tertiary plexuses are fully formed in the gastric antrum, small intestine and abdominal colon. They are rudimentary or absent in the oesophagus, gastric fundus and rectum.

The submucous plexus consists of a primary plexus only. It varies greatly in its structure among organs.

The Interstitial Cells of Cajal (Thuneberg, 1982; Rumessen and Thuneberg, 1982; Rumessen et al, 1982)

The interstitial cells of Cajal are pleomorphic branching cells intimately associated with the terminal branches of the intrinsic nerves throughout much of the gut (Figure 6). They are abundant in the tertiary plexus of the myenteric plexus, and in the terminal innervation of the muscle in some locations. They have a synaptic relationship to neurites, and form gap junctions with smooth muscle cells. Thus, they are intercalated between nerve and muscle, forming a pathway from nerve to muscle that is parallel to the pathway of the direct innervation of the muscle. The interstitial cells of Cajal may be modified fibroblasts or other connective tissue cells, modified nerve cells, or modified Schwann cells. In some locations, they are pacemaking cells, generating the electrical slow waves that pace rhythmic contractions. They are thought, also, to be involved in nerve-to-muscle communication or in electrotonic links among muscle cells.

The Intramural Nerves of the Oesophagus (Christensen and Robison, 1982)

The *submucous plexus* of the oesophagus is nearly

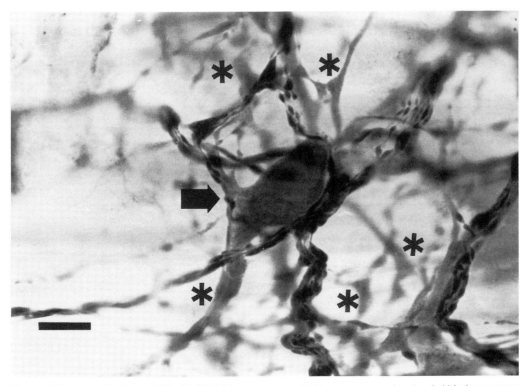

Figure 6. The soma of an interstitial cell of Cajal (arrow) surrounded by varicose neurites, beaded black structures, from the cat stomach. Many flat broad branching processes of interstitial cells extend throughout the field (asterisks). The bar indicates 10 μm. Osmic acid-zinc iodide stain.

devoid of ganglia in most species (Table 1). For that reason, ganglion cells of the myenteric plexus are probably the source of the abundant nerves found in the relatively thick muscularis mucosae of the oesophagus, and of the sensory nerves in the squamous epithelium (Rodrigo et al, 1975).

The *myenteric plexus* of the oesophagus contains comparatively few ganglion cells (Table 2). It con-

sists mainly of thick fascicles of neurites running cephalocaudad and connected by thinner lateral bundles (Figure 7). The secondary and tertiary plexuses are rudimentary. Ganglia are highly variable in size and shape. Many fascicle branch-points are devoid of ganglia. Many ganglia lie a little away from major fascicles (Figure 8). These are called *parafascicular ganglia*. The density of

Table 1. Submucous plexus. Numbers of ganglia per unit surface area and numbers of perikarya per ganglion throughout the gut of cat and opossum. From Christensen and Rick (1985b), with permission.

	Cat		Opossum	
Organ	Ganglia per cm^2	Perikarya per ganglion	Ganglia per cm^2	Perikarya per ganglion
Proximal oesophagus	0	0	4.5 ± 1.3	8.1 ± 1.6
Midoesophagus	0	0	5.5 ± 1.8	9.4 ± 0.9
Distal oesophagus	0	0	9.7 ± 1.9	8.7 ± 1.0
Fundus	7.1 ± 1.0	11.8 ± 1.0	not determined	not determined
Antrum	2.8 ± 0.8	6.4 ± 0.6	not determined	not determined
Duodenum	188.7 ± 14.4	30.9 ± 1.8	161.8 ± 21.2	11.2 ± 0.6
Jejunum	148.0 ± 13.1	31.3 ± 1.7	214.8 ± 15.1	10.4 ± 0.6
Ileum	90.4 ± 6.8	35.3 ± 2.1	148.8 ± 9.0	10.0 ± 0.6
Proximal colon	41.4 ± 3.6	30.8 ± 1.9	13.3 ± 2.7	15.5 ± 1.2
Midcolon	26.4 ± 1.2	26.1 ± 1.6	11.4 ± 1.3	17.3 ± 1.7
Distal colon	17.0 ± 1.3	21.1 ± 1.4	8.3 ± 1.1	14.6 ± 1.7
Rectum	10.5 ± 1.8	13.7 ± 1.0	5.4 ± 1.9	11.3 ± 1.4

Table 2. Myenteric plexus. Ganglion and perikaryon density per unit mass of muscle throughout the opossum gut. From Christensen et al (1983), with permission.

Region	Ganglia/gram	Perikarya/gram
Smooth-muscled oesophagus (uniform thirds, proximal to distal)	12×10^2	27×10^3
	17×10^2	20×10^3
	10×10^2	8×10^3
Lower oesophageal sphincter	4.2×10^2	2.6×10^3
Ventral fundus	12×10^2	53×10^3
Dorsal fundus	13×10^2	55×10^3
Antrum	8×10^2	37×10^4
	7.6×10^2	34×10^3
Small intestine (uniform fifths, proximal to distal)	8×10^2	35×10^3
	10×10^2	38×10^3
	12×10^2	46×10^3
	17×10^2	39×10^3
Caecum	5.4×10^2	16×10^3
	9.2×10^2	35×10^3
Abdominal colon (uniform fifths, proximal to distal)	8.9×10^2	34×10^3
	5.6×10^2	22×10^3
	5.9×10^2	23×10^3
	1.9×10^2	10×10^3
Rectum	1.1×10^2	1.5×10^3

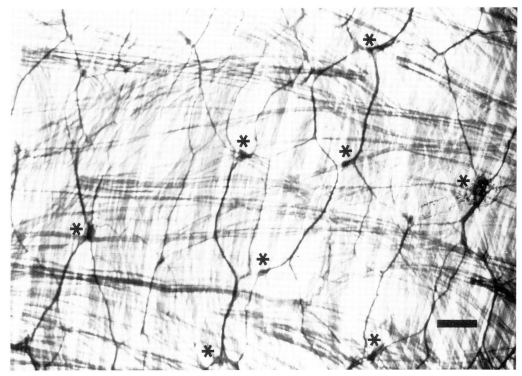

Figure 7. A low-power view of the myenteric plexus of the distal oesophagus of the opossum showing the general pattern. The major bundles run cephalocaudad (top to bottom) with thinner lateral branches. Ganglia (asterisks) are sparse and small, and many branch-points in the bundles are devoid of ganglia. The faint broad striations are muscle bundles. The bar indicates 1 mm. Silver stain.

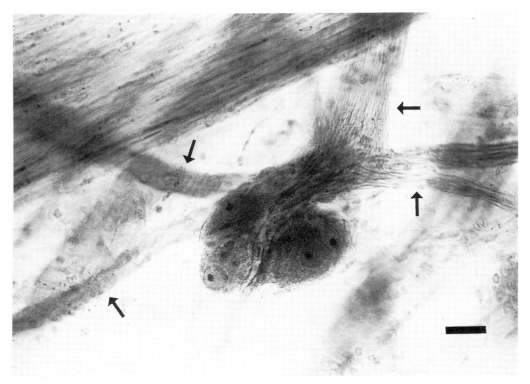

Figure 8. A parafascicular ganglion of the opossum oesophageal myenteric plexus. There are four ganglion cells in this ganglion, recognizable by their round nuclei with peripheral chromatin and a single large nucleolus. This is called a parafascicular ganglion because the cell bodies lie outside the major nerve bundles (arrows). The bar indicates 25 μm. Silver stain.

ganglion cells declines along the smooth muscle segment, to reach a nadir at the oesophagogastric sphincter. Ganglia are present in the myenteric plexus of the striated muscle part of the oesophagus. Their function there is not clear.

In the oesophageal muscularis mucosae and the longitudinal muscle layer, the terminal innervation consists of small bundles of neurites and single neurites lying between the muscle bundles. In the circular muscle layer, the neurites branch and spread more widely, because they must supply *intramuscular interstitial cells*, confined to the circular muscle layer (Christensen et al, 1987; Daniel and Posey-Daniel, 1984). These abundant cells have a sparse cytoplasm surrounding an elliptical nucleus. Broad processes extend from the poles of the elliptical somas of these cells to branch and extend between muscle bundles (Figure 9). These cells lie in chains with their processes entangled. Neurites run along these chains, contacting the

processes and somas of the interstitial cells. The interstitial cells form gap junctions with the smooth muscle cells. They contain many mitochondria, an extensive endoplasmic reticulum, a conspicuous Golgi apparatus and a plethora of caveolae (Figure 10), suggesting that they are metabolically very active (Daniel and Posey-Daniel, 1984).

The Intramural Nerves of the Stomach
(Christensen and Rick, 1985a, 1985b)

The *submucous plexus* of the stomach is comparatively sparse, the distribution density of ganglion cells being considerably less than that in the small intestine (Table 1).

In the fundus, the *myenteric plexus* ganglia are comparatively sparse, and the secondary and tertiary plexuses are not well developed. In the antrum, the ganglia are larger and more closely

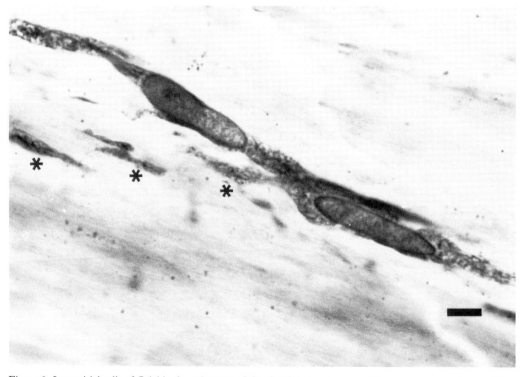

Figure 9. Interstitial cells of Cajal in the substance of the circular muscle layer of the opossum oesophagus. There are two oval nuclei with rims of cytoplasm which give broad flat branches. Sections through these convoluted branches are marked with asterisks. The branches interdigitate. The bar indicates 5 μm. Osmic acid-zinc iodide stain.

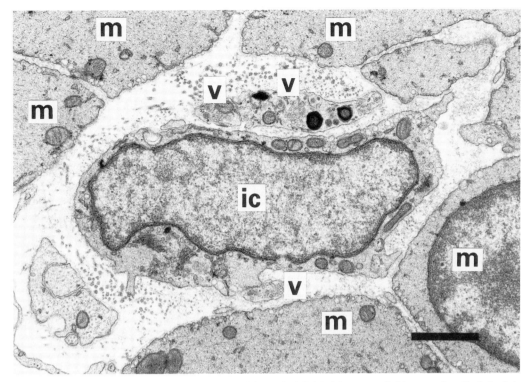

Figure 10. Electron photomicrograph of an interstitial cell of Cajal (ic) surrounded by muscle cells (m) of the circular layer of the opossum oesophagus. The cytoplasm of the interstitial cell is packed with organelles and it branches extensively. Axonal varicosities (v) encased in Schwann cells lie nearby. The bar indicates 1 μm.

spaced, and the secondary and tertiary plexuses are very dense. The tertiary plexus contains many interstitial cells, each such cell having long processes branching from a small soma about a round or ovoid nucleus. The processes intersect to form a mat, over and within which the neurites lie. Interstitial cells are much more prominent in the myenteric plexus of the antrum than they are in that of the fundus.

The myenteric plexus of the stomach contains many coarse nerve bundles, called *shunt fascicles*, that enter from the oesophagus and branch extensively to spread towards the greater curvature (Figure 11). They give off branches to ganglia (Figure 12), but they do not enter into or pass through ganglia. They disappear into the ganglionated plexus in the distal stomach and along the greater curvature. These shunt fascicles have the structure of extramural autonomic nerves, with a perineurium, a collagen stroma and a central capillary. They contain myelinated fibres. They

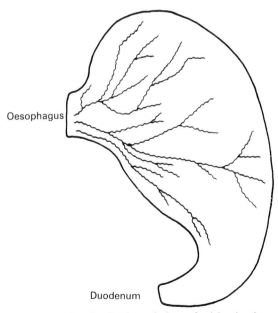

Figure 11. The distribution of shunt fascicles in the cat stomach. Only the anterior surface is shown. From Christensen and Rick (1985a), with permission.

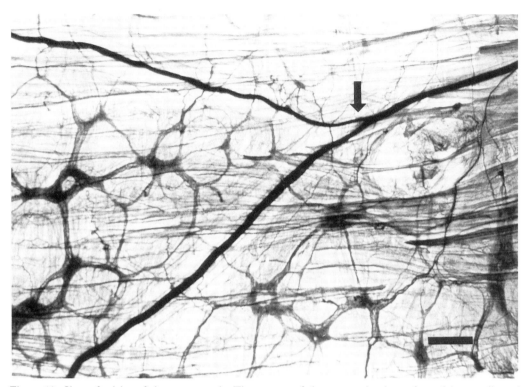

Figure 12. Shunt fascicles of the cat stomach. The pattern of the myenteric plexus formed by ganglia and interganglionic fascicles is overlaid by a thick branching fascicle (arrow) which gives branches to the ganglionated plexus. The bar indicates 1 mm. Silver stain.

may be a second pathway for vagal fibres to the stomach, parallel to the direct gastric innervation of the stomach from the gastric branches of the vagus.

In the proximal part of the stomach, there is a third layer of muscle (the oblique layer) between the circular muscle layer and the submucosa. The space between the oblique and circular layers contains an aganglionic plexus of branching and intersecting nerve bundles, probably derived from the myenteric plexus. There are no secondary or tertiary plexuses, and interstitial cells are sparse in this space.

The Intramural Nerves of the Small Intestine (Gabella, 1987)

The *submucous plexus* in the small intestine is denser than it is in the other viscera (Table 1). The ganglia are arranged in two strata, one just beneath the muscularis mucosae (*Meissner's plexus*) and the other adjacent to the circular muscle layer (*Henle's* or *Schabadasch's plexus*). The term 'Meissner's plexus' is also used for the whole of the submucous plexus. To avoid ambiguity, the more luminal plane of ganglia is also called the *plexus internus*, and the more serosal plane the *plexus externus* (Stach, 1972). The ganglia are small, densely distributed, and interconnected by interganglionic fascicles. There are a few interstitial cells in the submucous plexus.

The *myenteric plexus* in the small intestine is dense (Table 2). Its large ganglia are uniformly spaced, and there are well-developed secondary and tertiary plexuses. There are no major differences in the plexus along the intestine. The tertiary plexus contains many interstitial cells, like those of the gastric antrum.

Nonganglionated plexuses of neurite bundles lie in planes beneath the serosa, in the lamina propria, and deep in the circular muscle layer (the *plexus muscularis profundus*). This latter plexus lies closer to the luminal border of that muscle layer than to the serosal border. It is a dense network of neurites with abundant interstitial cells.

The Intramural Nerves of the Colon
(Christensen et al, 1984; Christensen and Rick, 1987b; Stach, 1972)

The *submucous plexus* is less dense than that of the intestine (Table 1). It constitutes two strata of ganglia, as in the intestine, the *plexus internus* (*Meissner's* plexus) and the *plexus externus* (*Henle's* or *Schabadasch's* plexus). A unique feature of the colon is a third plane of the submucous plexus, a dense nonganglionated bed of neurites and interstitial cells on the submucosal surface of the circular muscle layer (Figures 13, 14). This is called the *plexus externus extremus* (Stach, 1972).

The *myenteric plexus* in the colon resembles that of the small intestine, with large uniformly-spaced ganglia and well-developed secondary and tertiary plexuses. Interstitial cells abound in the tertiary plexus. In the distal colon, many *shunt fascicles* (the *ascending nerves of the colon*) lie among the ganglia (Figure 15). These are extensions of the colonic nerves from the pelvic plexus, and they have the structure of peripheral nerves. They contain myelinated nerve fibres. They give branches to ganglia, disappearing into the ganglionated plexus about half-way up the colon. Ganglion cell density declines along the colon to reach a nadir in the rectum (Table 1). The rectal plexus consists of coarse nerve bundles with small, sparse ganglia and poorly-developed secondary and tertiary plexuses. This plexus closely resembles that of the smooth-muscled part of the oesophagus.

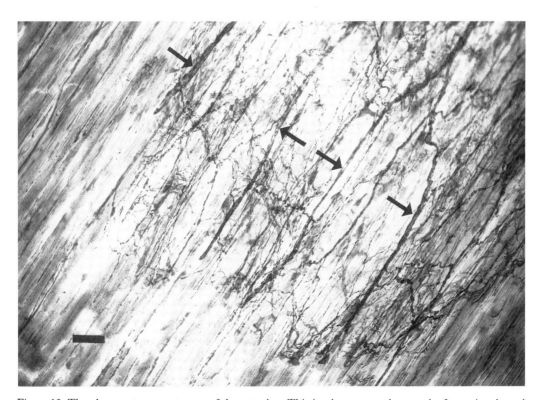

Figure 13. The plexus externus extremus of the cat colon. This is a low-power photograph of a section through the circular muscle layer. The section lies deep in the circular muscle layer to the left and bottom of the picture, but to the right and top of the picture it lies at the submucosal surface of the circular muscle layer. In this region there is a dense plexus of neurites branching from thick neurite bundles (arrows). Interstitial cells of Cajal can be seen as abundant stellate grey cells among the neurites. The bar indicates 50 μm. Osmic acid-zinc iodide stain.

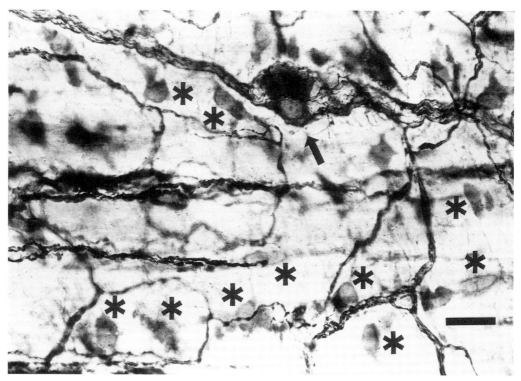

Figure 14. The plexus externus extremus of the cat colon. A single ganglion cell (arrow) lies in a thick bundle of neurites, and other varicose neurites fill the field. Many interstitial cells of Cajal (asterisks) are present, just out of the focal plane, which was set on the neurites. The interstitial cells form a mat on the submucosal surface of the circular muscle layer just below the plane of the neurite plexus. The bar indicates 25 μm. Osmic acid-zinc iodide stain.

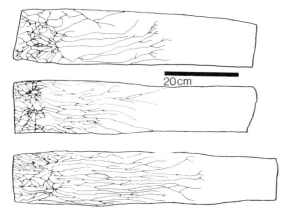

Figure 15. The distribution of the ascending nerves of the cat colon (shunt fascicles). From Christensen and Rick (1987), with permission.

The Intramural Nerves of the Biliary Tract

The biliary tract and gallbladder are relatively sparsely innervated. The innervation is a scanty plexus of small ganglia with a loose net of nerve fascicles that lie mostly on the outer surfaces of the walls.

Sensory Functions in the Gut (Wood, 1987)

The only established sensory structures in the gut are *intraganglionic laminar endings* found in certain ganglia of the myenteric plexus of the oesophagus and stomach (Rodrigo et al, 1982). They have not been seen in ganglia of the myenteric plexus elsewhere. These are leafy structures often clustered in the part of a ganglion that is devoid of nerve cell bodies (Figure 16).

The morphologically undifferentiated neurites in the gut wall are presumed to be responsive to local stimuli that can excite pain and reflexes. Undifferentiated neurites are abundant in the

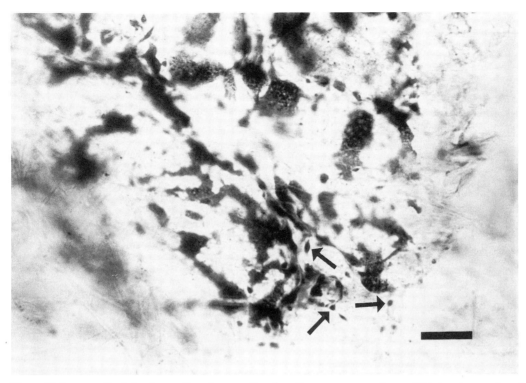

Figure 16. Intraganglionic laminar endings in a ganglion from the opossum oesophagus. This is only one edge of the ganglion, and no ganglion cell bodies are present in the field. Some neurite varicosities appear as black spots (arrows). The intraganglionic laminar endings are the black, flat granular structures with spike-like projections, which fill the field. These are found only in some ganglia in the oesophagus and in the cardiac portion of the stomach. The bar indicates 10 μm. Osmic acid-zinc iodide stain.

lamina propria of the glandular epithelia, as well as in the other layers of the wall.

Reflex motor responses can be demonstrated in response to both mechanical and chemical stimuli. Some of the best known of these reflexes are the following:

1. *Reflex oesophageal peristalsis after oesophageal distension.* Localized distension of the distal oesophagus evokes peristalsis in the oesophagus and relaxation of the lower oesophageal sphincter. This response can be excited both *in vitro* and *in situ*. It is mediated by both central and local pathways.

2. *Reflex relaxation of the stomach in response to an increase in gastric volume.* The expansion of the stomach in eating to accommodate the ingested volume represents reflex neurogenic inhibition of the proximal stomach. This reflex is mediated by both vago-vagal and intramural pathways.

3. *Reflex control of gastric emptying.* Acids, fats and hypertonic solutions in the duodenum all slow gastric emptying. This is the main mechanism for the regulation of the delivery of gastric contents to the intestine. The effect is so profound, so sensitive and so finely modulated that it seems likely to be a reflex. The pathways are unknown.

4. *The peristaltic reflex of the intestine.* Distension of the intestine enhances contractions above the distension and inhibits contractions below it. The pathways are intramural.

5. *Reflex relaxation of the internal anal sphincter by rectal distension.* Distension of the rectum relaxes the internal anal sphincter. The pathways of the reflex are presumably intramural.

The Morphology of Enteric Neurons and their Processes

Rapid long-distance transmission in nerves requires long cell processes, *axons* which transmit away from the cell soma, and *dendrites* which transmit towards the soma. Axons are relatively thick and long and arise from a swelling in the soma, the *axon hillock*, while dendrites are relatively thin and short and lack a swelling at their somal attachment.

Neurons in the intramural plexuses have been classified into five classes on the basis of axon and dendrite morphology, the classification of Dogiel (1899) as extended by Stach (1980, 1981, 1982a, 1982b, 1985). This classification has found use only in description, but the variety of cell shapes is striking. One common cell lacks dendrites but has multiple (usually two to four) axons. This,

Dogiel's Type II cell, supplies both main muscle layers. The other four types of cells have many dendrites and only one axon. They are distinguished on the basis of dendrite length, breadth or shape, and position on the cell soma. The different types of cells occupy different positions in the ganglion. The features of these five types of neurons (as described by Stach) are listed in Table 3. These descriptions come only from study of the myenteric plexus of the intestine of rodents and the pig. There may well be differences among species and among organs in their forms and distributions.

Axon terminals have a varicose appearance. The *varicosities* are nodules containing packets of neural transmitters, stored in the varicosities as *vesicles*. Vesicles can be classified according to size and to the appearance of their core material in electron microscopy. Cholinergic nerves generally

Table 3. The morphological features of the five types of neurons in the myenteric plexus (descriptions from Stach, 1980, 1981, 1982a, 1982b, 1985).

Type of cell	Number of dendrites	Shape of dendrites	Position of dendrites	Number of axons	Destination of axons	Position in ganglion
Type I	Many	Short, flat, broad	Radiating from whole cell soma	One	Mostly orad in the plexus	Orad and peripheral parts
Type II	None	—	—	Two to five	Muscle layers	Peripheral parts
Type III	Many	Long, thin, tapering	Radiating from whole cell soma	One	Mostly aborad in the plexus	Central and aborad parts
Type IV	Many	Long, thin, tapering	Mainly at only one pole or part of soma	One	Submucosal plexus	Not specific
Type V	Many	Short to very long, thin, tapering	Radiating from whole cell soma	One	Mostly aborad in the plexus	In aggregates in central and aborad parts

Table 4. Types of vesicles found in autonomic neuromuscular junctions of nerve–nerve synapses. From Davison (1983), with permission.

Transmitter	Size of vesicles	Appearance
Cholinergic	35–60 nm 80–110 nm	Small agranular vesicles and some large granular vesicles
Adrenergic	50–90 nm 90–130 nm	Small vesicles with intensely osmiophilic granules, mixed with small agranular and large granular vesicles
Unknown	80–200 nm	Large opaque vesicles (medium electron-dense granule not clearly separated from vesicle membrane) Some small agranular vesicles

contain small agranular and large granular vesicles. Adrenergic nerves generally contain small vesicles with very dense granules, some small agranular and some large granular vesicles. Other nerves of unknown nature contain large opaque vesicles mixed with small agranular vesicles (Table 4).

The fact that varicosities contain several types of vesicles may mean that vesicles have a different appearance at different stages of filling. It could also mean that a single axon may synthesize several transmitters simultaneously. The idea of 'one-nerve, one-transmitter' has been abandoned.

Terminal nerve fibres wander among muscle bundles, approaching the muscle cells closely at points. The axons extend a long way among muscle bundles, releasing transmitters over their whole length. Transmitters are applied to the muscle cells as a whole tissue, and they affect a single muscle cell over its whole surface.

Neuronal Physiology of the Intramural Nerves of the Gut (Wood, 1987)

Introduction

There are, conceptually, three functional classes of intramural neurons: sensory neurons, internuncial neurons (that communicate among neurons within the plexuses), and motor neurons. All three classes are presumed to be present in both submucous and myenteric plexuses.

Two other functional classifications of intramural neurons exist based upon neurophysiological methods. Intramural enteric nerves are studied with intracellular microelectrodes inserted into ganglia exposed *in vitro*, and with extracellular electrodes. No correlations are yet possible either between these electrophysiological classifications, or between them and the morphological classification.

The Two Classes of Enteric Nerves Found with Intracellular Recordings

Electrophysiological studies reveal two classes of enteric neurons, called Type 1 and Type 2 neurons, distinguished on the basis of six electrophysiological features (Table 5). About one-third of myenteric plexus neurons in the intestine are Type 2, while only a very small fraction of submucous plexus neurons are Type 2.

The Classes of Enteric Nerves Found with Extracellular Electrodes

Another functional classification of enteric

Table 5. Electrophysical characteristics of myenteric plexus neurons. From Davison (1983), with permission.

Type 1	Type 2
Low resting membrane potential relative to Type 2	High resting membrane potential relative to Type 1
High input resistance relative to Type 2	Low input resistance relative to Type 1
Discharge spikes continuously in response to depolarization by intracellular injection of a current pulse—discharge frequency proportional to current intensity	Discharge 1 or 2 spikes only at the onset of injection of a depolarizing current pulse
Excitation at the termination of intracellular injection of a hyperpolarizing current pulse	No excitation at the termination of intracellular injection of a hyperpolarizing current pulse
No hyperpolarizing after-potential	Hyperpolarizing after-potential associated with action potential discharge
Tetrodotoxin-sensitive action potentials	Tetrodotoxin-resistant action potentials

neurons is based on their patterns of discharge in spontaneous and evoked activity. These patterns are *burst patterns, mechanically induced patterns* and *single-spike patterns*.

Burst pattern neurons discharge action potentials in bursts. Action potentials occur in short bursts with interspersed long periods of electrical silence. Some neurons, called '*steady burst neurons*', discharge this way constantly. Others, called '*erratic burst neurons*', do so intermittently, reverting at times to the continuous discharge of action potentials (Figure 17).

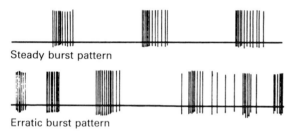

Figure 17. A diagram of the burst patterns of spike discharges from myenteric plexus neurons. From Davison (1983), with permission.

Mechanically induced pattern neurons are silent at rest but discharge action potentials in response to mechanical deformation of the intestinal wall. There are three kinds of patterns (Figure 18). In

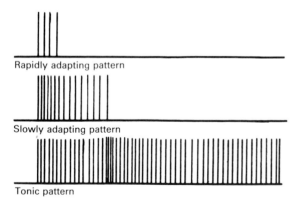

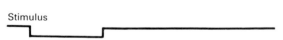

Figure 18. A diagram of the patterns of response of mechano-responsive neurons in the myenteric plexus. From Davison (1983), with permission.

the 'on' or '*on-off response*', the neuron discharges with a brief burst of spikes at the onset of the wall deformation and, occasionally, at the offset of the deformation. This is the pattern that would be expected from the excitation of a rapidly adapting mechanoreceptor. In the '*sustained response*', the discharge of action potentials begins at the onset of the wall deformation and continues to the end of the deformation. This is the pattern that would be expected from the excitation of a slowly adapting mechanoreceptor. In the '*tonic response*', the discharge of neuronal action potential begins at the onset of the wall deformation and continues for up to 40 seconds after the offset.

Single-spike pattern neurons discharge single spike action potentials continuously at a low frequency.

These patterns of discharge imply a further way to group enteric neurons into classes. '*Steady burst neurons*' are considered to be spontaneous pacemakers. The neurons showing an '*on*' or '*on-off response*' to mechanical stimulation are probably sensory neurons connected to rapidly adapting mechanoreceptors. Those with the '*sustained response*' are thought to be sensory neurons connected to slowly adapting mechanoreceptors. Those with the '*tonic response*' may be internuncial neurons, communicating between sensory and motor neurons.

Functional Specialization Within a Neuron

A neuron is not necessarily a single functional unit, always transmitting every stimulus that it receives from its dendrites to its axon. Instead, the membranes of the different parts of a neuron (dendrites, soma, axon hillock and axon) have different electrophysiological properties. A neuron may thus be able to isolate activity in one process, or preferentially to select or to direct the transmission of activity. This capacity would allow a single neuron to be a multifunctional unit.

Synaptic Transmission in Intramural Enteric Nerves

When one nerve cell transmits a signal to another, the membrane of the receiving cell (the postsynaptic cell) shows an immediate small change in membrane potential. This is a 'pre-potential' which may or may not lead to the discharge of an action potential by the receiving neuron. A fall in resting membrane potential is called an *excitatory postsynaptic potential* (EPSP), while an increase in resting membrane potential is called an *inhibitory postsynaptic potential* (IPSP). These are shown in Figure 19. EPSPs can be 'fast' (less than 50 msec long) or 'slow' (more than 50 msec long), while IPSPs are always 'slow'.

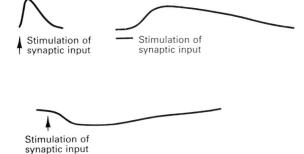

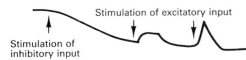

Figure 19. Diagrams of excitatory postsynaptic potentials (EPSPs) and inhibitory postsynaptic potentials (IPSPs). The top pair of tracings show fast (left) and slow (right) EPSPs. The middle tracing is an IPSP. The diagram at the bottom shows fast EPSPs superimposed on an IPSP. From Davison (1983), with permission.

Fast EPSPs occur in nerve cells of both submucous and myenteric plexuses, in both Type 1 and Type 2 cells. They are mediated by acetylcholine. Slow EPSPs occur only in Type 2 cells. IPSPs occur in Type 1 cells.

Transmitter Substances of Enteric Neurons

Many substances seem to be neurohumoral transmitters in the nerves of the gut. For a *candidate transmitter*, two criteria are required: its presence in nerve terminals, and its ability to act on muscle or nerve at low ('physiological') concentrations. For an *established transmitter*, other criteria are required. These include evidence of its

release on nerve stimulation, and a full description of mechanisms for its synthesis, release, degradation and reuptake into nerve terminals. These latter criteria are not easily satisfied. Nerve-to-nerve and nerve-to-muscle communication is very complicated. Many nerves contain several candidate transmitters. Some substances may act in usual or 'normal' circumstances, while others may be released only in special or 'abnormal' circumstances. Also, transmission could perhaps be electrotonic, mediated by local electrical current flow rather than by neurohumoral transmitters. The best established neurohumoral transmitters are acetylcholine, norepinephrine, serotonin, substance P, gamma-aminobutyric acid, and the adenine nucleotides. The candidate transmitters include the many recently studied peptides, especially vasoactive intestinal polypeptide (VIP).

The Physiology of Sympathetic Integration—the Prevertebral Ganglia (Wood, 1987)

Introduction

The prevertebral ganglia of the sympathetic system have several functions. They provide the means to suppress gastrointestinal motility during generalized sympathetic arousal. They are stations for the relay of afferent information from the gut to the central nervous system. And they integrate sensory information and relay it back to the gut over motor pathways to influence motility.

Functional Organization of the Prevertebral Ganglia

Each prevertebral ganglion cell receives synaptic inputs from all fibres that enter the ganglion. Thus, every such cell can integrate information both from the gut and from the central nervous system. The axons from these cells pass to the gut and to the other prevertebral ganglia. Thus, the three prevertebral ganglia provide for interactions among all parts of the gut, and between the gut and the central nervous system (Figures 20 and 21). Some entero-enteric reflex interactions take place only through the prevertebral ganglia, inde-

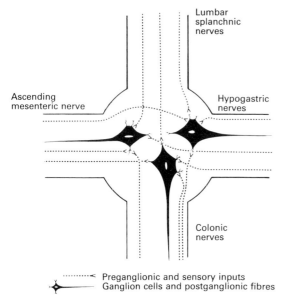

Figure 20. Pathways through the inferior mesenteric ganglion. Note that every ganglion cell receives inputs from all four groups of nerves, and that postganglionic axons pass to all except the lumbar splanchnic nerves. Some fibres pass through the ganglion without making synapse. From Davison (1983), with permission.

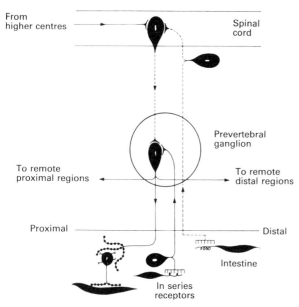

Figure 21. Pathways for peripheral sympathetic reflexes (solid lines). The dotted lines show the long reflex pathway through the spinal cord which reinforces the peripheral reflex pathway. The long pathway is shown as a monosynaptic path, but poly-synaptic pathways could be involved. From Davison (1983), with permission.

pendent of the central nervous system. Such 'local' pathways may be duplicated by longer pathways through the central nervous system.

Although the nerve cells in these ganglia are thought to be functionally homogeneous, they are not morphologically homogeneous. A small pro-portion of cells is found to be especially intensely stained by catecholamine fluorescence. These are called SIF (small intensely fluorescent) cells. Their special function is unknown.

Transmission in the Prevertebral Ganglia

The prevertebral ganglion cells seem to be phy-siologically homogeneous. Nerve stimulation evokes both 'fast' and 'slow' EPSPs, but no IPSPs. That is, all inputs to these nerve cells are excit-atory, both those from the preganglionic fibres of central nervous system origin, and those from the walls of the viscera. A postspike hyperpolarization, like that of the Type 2 cells of the myenteric plexus, is the means of termination of the evoked discharge in these cells.

The Efferent Projections of the Prevertebral Ganglion Cells

The ganglion cell axons pass to the other pre-vertebral ganglia and to the gut. Those to the gut terminate mainly in relation to enteric ganglion cells and blood vessels. The transmitters of these efferent fibres are catecholamines.

The Physiology of Parasympathetic Integration (Wood, 1987)

Introduction

The *long extrinsic pathways* of the craniosacral pathways have been examined almost entirely in the cranial system. The sacral outflow is relatively neglected.

Sensory Functions in the Vagi

Vagal sensory endings detect both mechanical and chemical stimulation of the gut. There are two types of sensory endings. The *mucosal ending* acts both as a sensitive rapidly adapting mechano-receptor and as a slowly adapting chemo-receptor, responsive to a variety of substances. The *intramuscular ending* acts as a slowly adapting mechanoreceptor, behaving as though arranged in series with the muscle bundles. It is therefore called an 'in-series tension receptor'. These receptors can follow gut volume as well as contractile force. For example, they probably monitor gastric volume in the regulation of gastric emptying.

Vagal sensory fibres are processes from the bipolar ganglion cells of the nodose ganglion. These cells have a somatotopic organization in that ganglion. That is, discrete regions of that ganglion receive separate inputs from the separate organs. This somatotopy probably projects into the central nervous system.

Motor Functions in the Vagi

The vagus contains both sensory fibres and motor fibres of several kinds. One set of these motor fibres is somatic, innervating the striated muscle of the proximal oesophagus. There are two types of autonomic motor fibres: *sympathetic* post-ganglionic fibres that enter the vagus from the superior cervical ganglion, and *parasympathetic* preganglionic fibres that arise in the vagal nuclei. The parasympathetic fibres serve the long reflex pathways that are important in motility.

Vago-vagal Reflexes

Vago-vagal reflexes are generally initiated by the stimulation of the intramuscular in-series tension receptors. The responding vagal motor fibres discharge continuously for a long time, well beyond the duration of the stimulus. The cells of the vagal nuclei have both excitatory and inhibitory inputs, so that vago-vagal reflexes may involve either or both excitation and inhibition of either or both excitatory and inhibitory motor fibres. Some of these reflex responses are reversed when the intensity of stimulation of the sensory limb of the reflex is increased. That is, a stimulus that *excites* activity at a low intensity may *inhibit* activity at a greater intensity. Also, as one group of nerve cells in the vagal nuclei is excited, another group is inhibited.

Thus, a high degree of plasticity is possible in the long parasympathetic reflexes within the vagal nuclei.

The Central Centres Involved in Gut Motility

Three general methods are used to identify the central nervous system structures that may influence gut motility. *First*, intracellular dyes can be used to trace extrinsic nerve trunks back into the central nervous system. *Second*, gut motility can be examined after stimulation or destruction of central structures. *Third*, the existence of 'centres' can be inferred from observations of motility.

Each method has limitations. Dye tracing methods identify only the immediate central projections of the peripheral nerves which are stained. The stimulation or destruction of specific central structures may stimulate or destroy not only the nerve cell bodies of that structure but also fibre tracts that pass through the structure without actually involving the function of the structure. And 'centres' are physiological abstractions, integrators whose existence must be postulated to explain the observed integration of the motor behaviour of the gut, but whose morphological correlates are not demonstrated.

Some generally accepted facts about some central nervous system structures in the control of motility are presented in Table 6.

Methods to Study the Morphology of the Nerves of the Gut (Costa et al, 1987)

Introduction

Nervous tissue is stained nonspecifically by many metachromatic stains, but the non-selectivity of such stains limits their usefulness. Some empirical stains, like silver impregnation, are more selective for nervous tissue. Other even more specific stains are based on the biochemical features of nerves and their associated structures. These include immunohistochemical stains, depending upon the binding of antibodies to proteins or polypeptides

Table 6.   Motility responses evoked by stimulating some CNS areas. From Davison (1983), with permission.

Area	Motility responses	Peripheral nerve pathways
Cortex	Excitatory and inhibitory responses from stomach, small intestine and colon, depending on precise area stimulated.	Excitatory effects are mediated through parasympathetic nerves, inhibitory effects through parasympathetic and sympathetic nerves. Vagal fibres project to somatosensory cortex and orbital gyrus.
Thalamaus	Excitatory gastric responses to stimulation of reticular nucleus, anterior nucleus ventralis, lateral pulvinar and endopeduncular nuclei. Inhibitory gastric responses to stimulation of ventral nucleus and antero-medial nucleus.	Excitatory and inhibitory pathways are parasympathetic.
Amygdaloid complex nuclei	Defecation, including postural responses.	Pelvic nerves and spinal motor neurons.
Hypothalamus	Excitatory and inhibitory responses affecting the entire gut.	Excitatory effects involve parasympathetic pathways. Inhibition involves excitation of nonadrenergic, noncholinergic inhibitory pathways, inhibition of cholinergic pathways (both parasympathetic) and excitation of sympathetic pathways.
Mesencephalon and pons	Stimulation of superior colliculi, fasciculus longitudinalis, and reticular substance of pons excites the stomach. Stimulation of dorsal tegmentum, medial lemniscus and reticular substance of pons inhibits the stomach.	Excitatory effects are parasympathetic. Inhibitory effects are sympathetic.
Cerebellum	Increased gastric, intestinal and colonic motility.	Sympathetic, probably due to suppression of sympathetic inhibitory tone.
Medulla	Excitatory and inhibitory effects on the entire gut.	Excitation and inhibition are mediated by parasympathetic pathways. A splanchnic motor area has also been identified.

that are concentrated in nerve cells. The immuno-histochemical methods apply especially to the localization of polypeptides that are candidate neurohumoral transmitters.

General Stains

Silver Impregnation

The affinity of silver for nerves is the basis for many methods still used. The many techniques differ only in details, but these details seem to be important, for the students of one or another structure use one or another of these techniques selectively. All modern methods are based on a two-stage silver impregnation. The formalin-fixed tissue is exposed to silver salts in two steps, the first a solution of silver nitrate and the second a solution of ammoniacal silver nitrate, with the ultimate reduction of the silver in a reducing solution. Some methods are capricious, with the quality of staining varying a great deal from tissue to tissue for no apparent reason. The technique of Richardson (1960) is reliable, controllable and predictable.

Supravital Methylene Blue

Most living cells take up methylene blue, but nerve cells show somewhat greater avidity for the dye than most other cells of the gut wall. The fresh tissue is exposed under standard conditions *in vivo* or *in vitro* to a low concentration of the dye. Different workers use slightly different conditions of exposure. Nerve cell bodies are stained well, but their processes are shown poorly. The stain reveals little structural detail of nerves.

The Osmic Acid-Zinc Iodide Stain (Maillet, 1959)

This simple method reveals a wealth of detail. Fresh tissue is immersed in a fresh mixture of osmic acid and zinc iodide for 20–24 hours, and then sectioned. Nerves are stained black while other tissues are stained grey, brown or yellow. The varicose nerve processes are stained black in fine detail, but the nerve cell bodies are stained rather poorly. This method is the best available way to examine neurites. The interstitial cells of Cajal are also stained with clarity. The method is somewhat capricious, so that the density of staining is not fully predictable. The staining reaction involves sulphydryl groups in membrane proteins.

Stains for Nerve Components That Are Not Transmitters

The Nissl Stain

Basic dyes like toluidine blue and thionin stain the acidic proteins of the endoplasmic reticulum, and the nucleic acids. Since these are relatively abundant in nerve cell bodies, the stain is selective for neuronal perikarya. Nerve processes are not well demonstrated.

The NADH Stain

The NADH stain is more specific than the Nissl stain for nerve cell bodies. The reaction depends on the relatively dense distribution of mitochondria, the source of NADH reductase, in nerve cell bodies. The tissue is quick-frozen and thawed, and then incubated in nitro-BT with NADH. The resulting dark blue stain is concentrated in nerve cell bodies. Processes are usually not stained well.

Quinacrine Fluorescence

Under suitable conditions of incubation, quinacrine is localized selectively in enteric neurons, and it can be visualized by fluorescence microscopy. The stain may be related to the binding of quinacrine to nucleic acids. Not all neurons are stained. Some but not all processes are stained.

Stains for the Enzymes Related to Established Neurohumoral Transmitters

Acetylcholinesterase Stains

The enzyme that degrades acetylcholine should be localized to regions where acetylcholine is produced. There are several stains for the localization of this enzyme, using various substrates and inhibitors (to inhibit nonspecific cholinesterases). The method stains many nerve cell bodies and processes. Unfortunately, it cannot be considered to be selective for cholinergic neurons.

Catecholamine Fluorescence

Catecholamines produce fluorescent compounds when reacted with aldehydes. This reaction allows the use of fluorescence microscopy to localize catecholamines in the enteric nerves. It shows the localization of catecholamine-containing (sympathetic) terminal nerves in the plexuses.

Immunohistochemical Demonstration of Peptides

The localization of peptides in enteric nerves can now be studied with the use of antibodies raised to these peptides. Several techniques have been developed, but all rely on the specific binding of labelled antibody to the peptide in fresh tissue. By these techniques, one can discover the localization of any peptide for which an antibody exists. In this way, nerves reactive to many peptides, candidate transmitters, have been discovered.

Acknowledgement

Work supported by Grants AM 11242, AM 34986 and DK 34392 from the National Institutes of Health.

References

Christensen, J., and Robison, B. A., (1982), Anatomy of the myenteric plexus of the opossum esophagus. *Gastroenterology*, **83:** 1033–42.

Christensen, J., Rick, G. A., Robison, B. A., Stiles, M. J., and Wix, M. A., (1983), The arrangement of the myenteric plexus throughout the gastrointestinal tract of the opossum. *Gastroenterology*, **85:** 890–9.

Christensen, J., Stiles, M. J., Rick, G. A., and Sutherland, J., (1984), Comparative anatomy of the myenteric plexus of the distal colon in eight mammals. *Gastroenterology*, **86:** 706–13.

Christensen, J., and Rick, G. A., (1985a), Shunt fascicles in the gastric myenteric plexus in five monogastric species. *Gastroenterology*, **88:** 1020–5.

Christensen, J., and Rick, G. A., (1985b), Nerve cell density in submucous plexus throughout the gut of cat and opossum. *Gastroenterology*, **89:** 1064–9.

Christensen, J., and Rick, G. A., (1987), The distribution of myelinated nerves in the ascending nerves and myenteric plexus of the cat colon. *Am. J. Anat.*, **178:** 250–8.

Christensen, J., Rick, G. A., and Soll, D. J., (1987), Intramural nerves and interstitial cells revealed by the Champy-Maillet stain in the opossum esophagus. *J. Auton. Nerv. Syst.*, **19:** 137–51.

Costa, M., Furness, J. B., and Llewellyn-Smith, I. J., (1987), Histochemistry of the enteric nervous system. In: *Physiology of the Gastrointestinal Tract* (Eds. Johnson, L. R., Christensen, J., Jackson, M. J., Jacobson, E. D. and Walsh, J. H.) 2nd Ed., Vol. 1, pp. 1–40, Raven Press, New York.

Daniel, E. E., and Posey-Daniel, V., (1984), Neuromuscular structures in opossum esophagus: role of interstitial cells of Cajal. *Am. J. Physiol.*, **246:** G305–15.

Davison, J. S., (1983), Innervation of the gastrointestinal tract. In: *A Guide to Gastrointestinal Motility* (Eds. Christensen, J., and Wingate, D. L.) Chapter 1, pp. 1–47, Wright-PSG, Bristol, London, Boston.

Dogiel, A. S., (1899), Ueber den bau der ganglien in den geflechten des darmes und der gallenblase des menschen und der säugetiere. *Arch. Anat. Physiol., Anat. Abt.*, 130–58.

Gabella, G., (1979), Innervation of the gastrointestinal tract. *Int. Rev. Cytol.*, **59:** 129–93.

Gabella, G., (1987), Structure of muscles and nerves in the gastrointestinal tract. In: *Physiology of the Gastrointestinal Tract* (Eds. Johnson, L. R., Christensen, J., Jackson, M. J., Jacobson, E. D., and Walsh, J. H.) 2nd Ed., Vol. 1, pp. 335–82, Raven Press, New York.

Maillet, M., (1959), Modifications de la technique de Champy au tetraoxyde d'osmium-iodure de potassium. Resultats de son application à l'étude des fibres nerveuses. *C. R. Soc. Biol.*, **153:** 939–41.

Richardson, K. C., (1960), Studies on the structure of autonomic nerves in the small intestine, correlating the silver-impregnated image in light microscopy with the permanganate-fixed ultrastructure in electron-microscopy. *J. Anat.*, **94:** 457–72.

Rodrigo, J., Hernandez, C. J., Vidal, M. A., and Pedrosa, J. A., (1975), Vegetative innervation of the esophagus. III. Intraepithelial endings. *Acta Anat.*, **92:** 242–58.

Rodrigo, J., de Filipe, J., Robles-Chillida, E. M., Perez Anton, J. A., Mayo, I., and Gomez, A., (1982), Sensory vagal nature and anatomical access paths to esophageal laminar nerve endings in myenteric ganglia. Determination by surgical degeneration methods. *Acta Anat.*, **112:** 47–57.

Rumessen, J. J., and Thuneberg, L., (1982), Plexus muscularis profundus and associated interstitial cells. I. Light microscopical studies of mouse small intestine. *Anat. Rec.*, **203:** 115–27.

Rumessen, J. J., Thuneberg, L., and Mikkelsen, H. B., (1982), Plexus muscularis profundus and associated interstitial cells. II. Ultrastructural studies of mouse small intestine. *Anat. Rec.*, **203:** 129–46.

Stach, W., (1972), Der plexus entericus extremus des Dickdarmes und seine Beziehungen zu den interstiellen Zellen (Cajal). *Z. mikrosk.-anat. Forsch.*, **85:** 245–72.

Stach, W., (1980), Zur neuronalen organisation des plexus myentericus (Auerbach) im schweine-dünndarm. I. Typ I-neurone. *Z. mikrosk.-anat. Forsch.*, **94:** 833–49.

Stach, W., (1981), Zur neuronalen organisation des plexus myentericus (Auerbach) im schweine-dünndarm. II. Typ II-neurone. *Z. mikrosk.-anat. Forsch.*, **95:** 161–82.

Stach, W., (1982a), Zur neuronalen organisation des plexus myentericus (Auerbach) im schweine-dünndarm. III. Typ III-neurone. *Z. mikrosk.-anat. Forsch.*, **96:** 497–516.

Stach, W., (1982b), Zur neuronalen organisation des plexus myentericus (Auerbach) im schweine-dünndarm. IV. Typ IV-neurone. *Z. mikrosk.-anat. Forsch.*, **96:** 972–94.

Stach, W., (1985), Zur neuronalen organisation des plexus myentericus (Auerbach) im schweine-dünndarm. V. Typ V-neurone. *Z. mikrosk.-anat. Forsch.*, **99:** 562–82.

Thuneberg, L., (1982), Interstitial cells of Cajal: intestinal pacemaker cells. *Adv. Anat. Embryol. Cell Biol.*, **71:** 1–130.

Wood, J. D., (1987), Physiology of the enteric nervous system. In: *Physiology of the Gastrointestinal Tract* (Eds. Johnson, L. R., Christensen, J., Jackson, M. J., Jacobson, E. D. and Walsh, J. H.) 2nd Ed., Vol. 1, pp. 67–110, Raven Press, New York.

3
STRUCTURE OF SMOOTH MUSCLE

Giorgio Gabella
University College London, London, UK

The chief muscular component of the wall of the stomach and intestine of vertebrates is the muscle coat or muscularis externa, which ranges in thickness from 50 μm or less in the mouse to 1 mm or more in man. The muscle coat is compact, has well-defined boundaries and has no perimysium.

It is crossed by laminae of connective tissue, the intramuscular septa. Additional musculature forms the muscularis mucosae and the media of intramural blood vessels.

The muscle coat is usually made of two layers of musculature, the longitudinal (outer) layer and

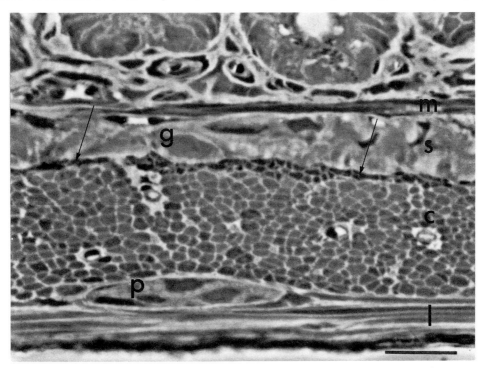

Figure 1. Transverse section of the rat ileum photographed unstained in phase contrast microscopy. The mucosa is at the top, the serosa at the bottom. c, circular muscle layer; l, longitudinal muscle layer; m, muscularis mucosae; s, submucosa. Between the two muscle layers is a ganglion of the myenteric plexus (p) and in the submucosa there is a ganglion of the submucosal plexus (g). At the innermost part of the circular muscle, note a thin layer of small and dark muscle cells (arrows). (Reproduced from Gabella, 1987.) Calibration bar: 30 μm.

the circular (inner) layer (Figure 1); it is not uncommon to find bundles of muscle cells that pass from one layer to the other. The muscle cells lie on planes that are parallel to the serosal surface, but they run orthogonal to one another in the two layers. Longitudinal and circular muscle layers are firmly anchored to each other; in the interstice between them, one also finds the myenteric plexus, connective tissue, blood vessels and lymphatic vessels. In the innermost part of the circular layer of the small intestine there are special muscle cells that are smaller and denser (s.a.d. cells) than those of the main circular layer (Figure 1) and can be distinguished without difficulty by their characteristic ultrastructure and by the features of the connective tissue surrounding them (Gabella, 1987). They usually form a layer that is one or two cells thick and extends over the entire small intestine but it is not found in the large intestine.

In the caecum (of mammals) and in parts of the colon the longitudinal musculature is condensed into cords, or taeniae. Between the taeniae the wall bulges outward forming numerous regular evaginations (haustrations) where the muscle coat is made almost exclusively of circular muscle: the lumen has a profile that ranges from an equilateral triangle (where the circular muscle is fully contracted and runs in straight segments between any two taeniae) to a clover leaf (where the circular muscle is relaxed and bulges out under the pressure of the luminal contents). The taeniae act as longitudinal pillars over which the transverse (circular) musculature hinges inward and outward. This architecture gives a certain rigidity to the organ, despite its bulk, and it allows great, although localized, variations in luminal size to take place.

The intestinal musculature is not just an assembly of muscle cells. Smooth muscle is a complex tissue; in addition to the principal cell type, smooth muscle cells (which are packed to a density of 190 000/mm³), there are nerve fibres, Schwann cells, interstitial cells, fibroblasts and cells of lymphatic and blood vessels, mainly endothelial cells (Figure 2). The extracellular space amounts to 20–30% of the tissue volume, and has a fluid component, the rest being occupied mainly by collagen fibrils and elastic fibres. The collagen fibrils form networks close to the surface of muscle cells and link the cells to one another and to larger arrays of collagen, such as the intramuscular septa or the submucosa or, in some cases, the serosa. The collagen concentration in intestinal muscles is generally higher than that of skeletal and cardiac muscles. The materials of the extracellular space, collagen included, are probably synthesized and secreted, for the most part, by the muscle cells themselves.

Smooth Muscle Cells

Muscle cells of the gastrointestinal tract are uninucleated and approximately spindle-shaped; they are 400–600 μm long and measure about 2000 to 4000 μm³ in volume. The maximum diameter of a muscle cell at rest does not exceed 4 or 5 μm, so that no part of the sarcoplasm is further away from the cell membrane than about 2.5 μm (Figure 3). The surface to volume ratio is relatively high, as there are usually about 1.5 μm² of cell surface for every cubic micron of cell volume. The surface of the cells at rest is smooth and regular, except for occasional cell processes. However, when the muscle is fully stretched the cell surface develops shallow longitudinal grooves, whereas in isotonically contracted muscle cells the membrane is thrown into many lamellar evaginations.

Caveolae

Caveolae, cell-to-cell junctions, cell-to-stroma junctions, and dense bands are the main structural specializations found at the cell membrane. Caveolae are stable flask-like invaginations of the cell membrane, about 120 nm long and 70 nm wide; they open into the extracellular space through a neck measuring about 35 nm across. Caveolae are often associated with flattened sacs or with tubules of sarcoplasmic reticulum, although there are no obvious structural links between the two components. Caveolae are mostly grouped into bands, one to four caveolae across, which run parallel to the cell length (Figure 4). There are between 20 and 35 caveolae per square micron of cell surface, and their number does not seem to be affected by

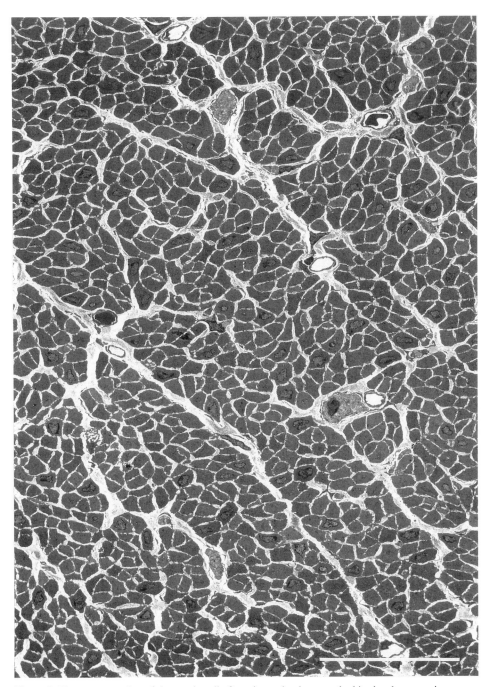

Figure 2. Transverse section of the taenia coli of a guinea-pig photographed in the electron microscope. In addition to smooth muscle cell profiles, one can recognize capillaries, small nerve bundles, interstitial cells, fibroblasts and intramuscular septa. Calibration bar: $2\,\mu$m.

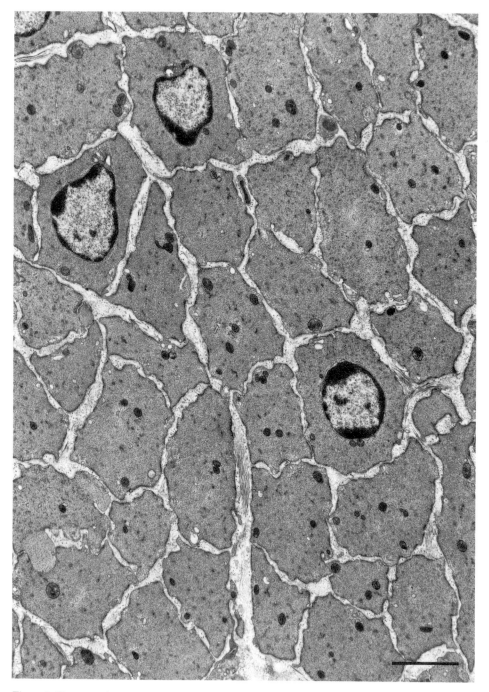

Figure 3. Electron micrograph of a guinea-pig taenia coli in transverse section. Some of the muscle cell profiles display the nucleus; the dark particles are mitochondria. The cells are surrounded by collagen fibrils (small dots in the extracellular space). Calibration bar: 2 μm.

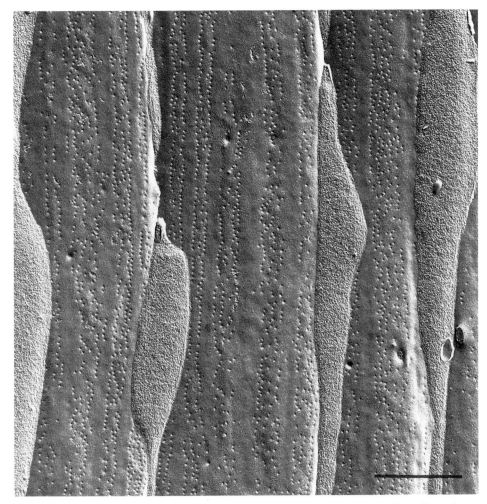

Figure 4. Freeze-fracture preparation of circular muscle of the guinea-pig ileum. The cell membrane shows rows of caveolae arranged longitudinally. Calibration bar: 2 μm.

stretch or contraction of the muscle. On the whole the caveolae increase the amount of cell membrane by about 70% over the area of the cell surface proper.

Dense Bands

Dense bands are patches of electron-dense material, measuring 0.2–0.4 μm in width and 1 or 2 micron long, bound to the cell membrane and located between rows of caveolae; the felt of electron-dense material measures 30 nm or more in thickness. Dense bands are spread over the entire surface of a muscle cell and they occupy between 30 and 50% of the cell profile; towards the tapering ends of the cell this percentage increases and in some small profiles the entire cell membrane is encrusted by dense bands.

A compact bundle of actin filaments penetrates into the felt of electron-dense material, and the contractile apparatus is thus linked to the cell membrane. The actin filaments approach the cell membrane at a very small angle, but the link with the membrane is probably a flexible one that can change during muscle contraction. Also some intermediate filaments reach the dense bands, independently of the actin filaments. Alpha-actinin (Bagby, 1980) and vinculin (Geiger et al, 1981), two proteins that have been localized at the dense bands by immunocytochemistry, are probably involved in linking actin filaments and cell membrane.

Intermediate Junctions

One type of cell-to-cell junction found in intestinal muscles involves the apposition of two dense bands in adjacent cells (Figure 5A). These junctions (intermediate junctions) are of the adherens type, they are elongated (fasciae) and provide mechanical coupling between the two cells. The intercellular gap measures up to 60 nm and is occupied by a layer of electron-dense material that is continuous with the basal laminae investing the two cells and often shows ill-defined periodic densities.

Other junctions, which may constitute a separate type of junction, are small and patch-like (maculae), have an intercellular gap of about 20 nm, and do not have a clear association with bundles of intracellular filaments (Figure 5B). This type of junction is also occasionally observed between a muscle cell and a Schwann cell or an interstitial cell; on rare occasions it is found between a muscle cell and a varicose axon.

Gap Junctions

In many intestinal muscles muscle cells are linked by gap junctions (nexuses). These are symmetrical patches (maculae) of the membrane of two cells, occupied by special channels that permit a private exchange of ions and small molecules between two cells and hence provide ionic and metabolic coupling. Their ultrastructure is identical to that analysed in detail in hepatocytes and other cell types (Figure 6). The structural units of the nexus (connexons) bridge the 3 nm gap between the

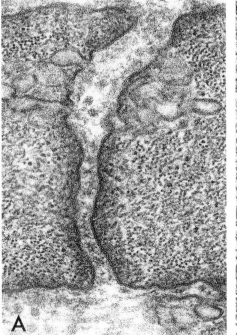 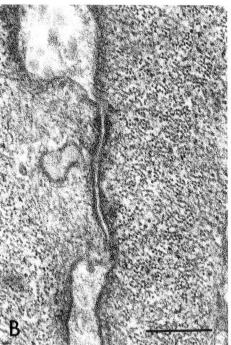

Figure 5. Transverse section of the taenia coli of a guinea-pig. A. Intermediate junction between two muscle cells. The intercellular gap measures about 50 nm and is occupied by electron-dense material with a faint periodic appearance. Actin filaments and intermediate filaments are associated with the dense bands on either side of the junction. B. Another type of junction with an intercellular gap of only about 15 nm. Calibration bar (for both micrographs): 0.2 μm.

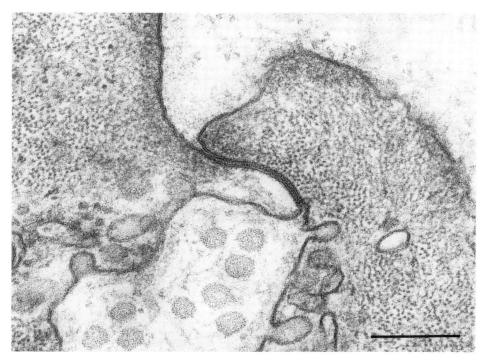

Figure 6. Transverse section of rabbit taenia coli. The two muscle cells are connected by a gap junction. Microfibrils and transversely sectioned collagen fibrils are present in the extracellular space. Calibration bar: 0.2 μm.

membranes; in freeze-fracture preparations the connexons appear as intramembrane particles of 8–10 nm diameter and they remain invariably attached to the cytoplasmic (P) leaflet of the membrane (Figure 7A). The packing density of connexons in a junction is about $7000/\mu m^2$. The area of the junction rarely exceeds 0.2 μm, and some junctions are made of only a few connexons (Figure 7B).

Gap junctions are not present uniformly in the various intestinal muscles. In the circular muscle of the small intestine they are abundant in all the species studied. In the circular muscle of the caecum gap junctions are less numerous than in the ileum, and in the colon there are very few (Figure 7B). In many animal species the longitudinal musculature of small and large intestine is virtually devoid of gap junctions. In species where gap junctions are also found in the longitudinal musculature, they are rare and exceedingly small. The great variability in the extent of gap junctions in different muscles and their absence in some muscles is difficult to reconcile with the electrophysiological evidence of electrical coupling.

Cell-to-Stroma Junctions

Except at the level of specialized junctions the cell membrane is lined by a basal lamina. This has a fuzzy appearance that in certain preparations can be resolved into a fine fibrillar texture. Microfibrils of 11 nm diameter and amorphous materials link the basal lamina, especially where it lies over a dense band, and collagen fibrils and elastic fibres. Junctions between the contractile apparatus of the cell and the stroma of the muscle are thus produced, and these provide a crucial mechanical link for force transference.

Sarcoplasmic Reticulum

The sarcoplasmic reticulum is well represented in intestinal muscle cells and constitutes about 2% of the cell volume. Flat and broad cisternae, tubules, networks of tubules and concave sacs are some of the most common forms of smooth sarcoplasmic reticulum. Some cisternae of sarcoplasmic reti-

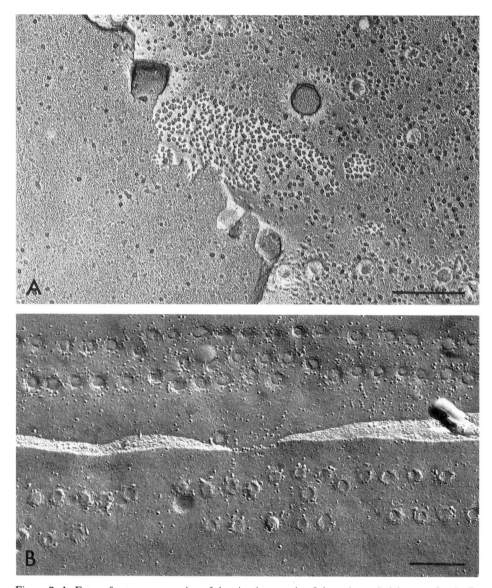

Figure 7. A. Freeze-fracture preparation of the circular muscle of the guinea-pig jejunum. On the P-face (cell on the right) are the opening of several caveolae, surrounded by a ring of intramembrane particles. In the centre a gap junction is recognizable as a loose aggregation of particles. The adjacent cell (on the left) shows its E-face. B. Freeze-fracture preparation of the guinea-pig distal colon. The two muscle cells are joined by a very small gap junction, made of only few connexons. Caveolae are seen on the P-face (cell on top) and on the E-face (cell at bottom). The light band across the micrograph is the extracellular space. Calibration bars: 0.2 μm.

culum lie parallel to the cell membrane, and the 10–20 nm gap between the two structures is bridged by dense periodic structures 20–25 nm apart, an arrangement similar to the peripheral coupling between cell membrane and sarcoplasmic

reticulum in cardiac muscle cells. The sarcoplasmic reticulum of smooth muscles can accumulate calcium ions and participates in the regulation of calcium concentration in the sarcoplasm (Bond et al, 1984). However, the muscles have only a very limited ability of contracting in the absence of extracellular calcium (Casteels and Raeymaekers, 1979).

Myosin Filaments

Up to 90% of the cell volume is occupied by filaments, of which there are three main classes: thick filaments of myosin, thin filaments of actin, and intermediate filaments (Bagby, 1983). Myosin filaments measure 15–17 nm in diameter and have a rather irregular profile. They are labile structures and are easily altered or disrupted by preparative procedures. Myosin molecules isolated from smooth muscles are identical in appearance to those obtained from striated muscles (Elliott et al, 1976), but they are chemically distinguishable (Small and Sobieszek, 1980). There are also major differences in the way the molecules are packed into filaments, although the exact packing is not yet known. According to one model, myosin molecules are assembled into side-polar filaments having cross-bridges with the same polarity along the entire length of one side of the filaments and the opposite polarity along the other side (Craig and Megerman, 1977). The concentration of myosin in smooth muscle (about 16 mg/kg) is about a quarter of that found in skeletal muscle (Murphy et al, 1977). Despite the relatively low myosin content, intestinal smooth muscle can generate an amount of force per unit sectional area that is comparable to that of skeletal muscle.

Actin Filaments

Actin filaments measure about 7 nm in diameter and are readily preserved in most preparations. They are often arranged in bundles or cables of 10–20 with a square lattice. The bundles split and merge with each other, rather than forming discrete entities, and because of this arrangement many actin filaments do not interact with a myosin filament, at least over part of their length. In a muscle cell in transverse section the apparent ratio of actin filaments to myosin filaments is approximately 12:1 (Bois, 1973). The weight ratio of actin to myosin ranges between two and four, and these values are six to 10 times higher than those found in skeletal muscles. Actin filaments penetrate into the dense bodies attached to the cell membrane and into dense bodies (Ashton et al, 1975). The latter are electron-dense structures scattered through the sarcoplasm, elongated and extremely variable in size and appearance: a bundle of actin filaments penetrates into each end of a dense body. The polarity of the actin filaments inserted into dense bodies or into dense bands is fixed: the arrowheads formed by decoration of the filaments with the fragment S-1 of myosin always point away from the point of insertion (Bond and Somlyo, 1982). The polarity of the actin filaments is therefore opposite at either side of a dense body, an arrangement similar to that found in actin filaments inserted into Z lines in skeletal muscles.

Intermediate Filaments

Intermediate filaments measure 10 nm in diameter and in intestinal muscle cells are made of a fibrous protein called desmin or skeletin. They are often closely associated with the amorphous material of dense bands and surround some of the dense bodies, and probably form a mechanical link with them.

Smooth Muscle Contraction

Intestinal smooth muscles are able to generate an amount of force that is comparable to that produced by skeletal muscles which have a much higher myosin content (hence a much larger number of potential cross-bridges) (Murphy et al, 1977); moreover, they maintain the contraction with little energy expenditure, probably through the formation of attached non-cycling cross-bridges (Siegman et al, 1976; Dillon et al, 1981), and can shorten, in certain conditions, to as little as one-fifth of their resting length. The shortening of a smooth muscle in an isotonic contraction is accompanied by lateral expansion of the muscle, such that the increase in sectional area of the muscle is about equal to the decrease in muscle

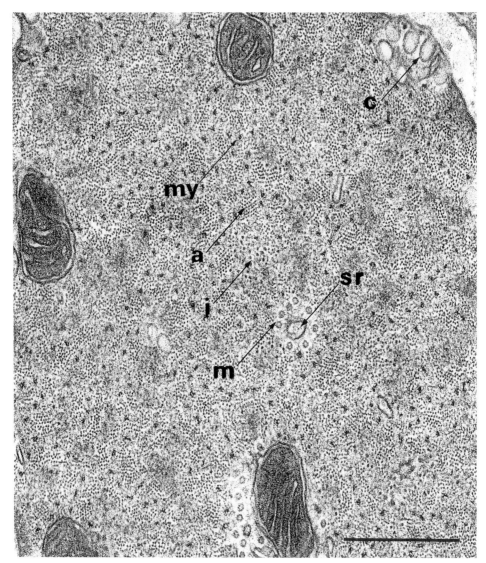

Figure 8. Cytoplasm of a muscle cell of the guinea-pig taenia coli showing mitochondria, microtubules (m), sacs of sarcoplasmic reticulum (sr) and caveolae (c). a, actin filaments; i, intermediate filaments; my, myosin filaments. Calibration bar: 0.5 μm.

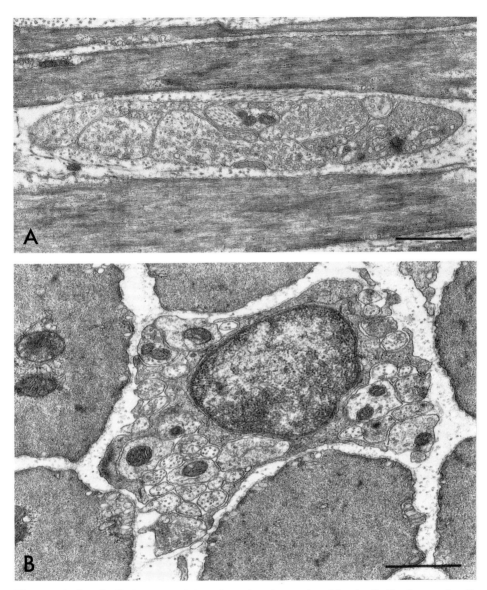

Figure 9. A. Longitudinal muscle of the guinea-pig colon sectioned longitudinally. A nerve bundle containing three axons (varicosities) packed with synaptic vesicles runs between the muscle cells. B. Taenia coli of a guinea-pig, in transverse section. A nerve bundle containing several axons runs between the muscle cells. The Schwann cell is sectioned at the level of its nucleus. Calibration bars: 1 μm.

length. The lateral expansion of the muscle during shortening affects both width and thickness of the muscle. There is no evidence of a substantial change in muscle volume or in muscle cell volume during contraction. The structural changes of the contracting muscle are mirrored by changes in the individual muscle cells. Cells from contracted muscles are shorter and fatter than those from resting muscles, and so is their nucleus. With extensive shortening the muscle cells also undergo some axial torsion and no longer lie exactly parallel to one another. Their surface is thrown into tall projections that are mainly laminar and run at an angle to the cell length, interdigitating with those from adjacent cells. While the membrane of these projections bears numerous caveolae, the deep grooves between projections almost invariably show dense bands. An extensive rearrangement of the pericellular collagen fibrils accompanies cell shortening. Whereas in the muscle at rest the collagen fibrils run longitudinally, either parallel to or forming a small angle with the axis of the muscle cells, in the shortened muscle the fibrils are wound around the cells and run obliquely or almost transversely to the cell length (Gabella, 1987).

Other Cell Types

Non-muscle cells found in intestinal muscles include fibroblasts and interstitial cells of Cajal. Most intestinal muscles are well vascularized, an exception being the taenia coli of the rabbit, an elastic smooth muscle in which blood vessels are rare. The intramuscular vessels are usually capillaries, most of which run along the muscle length. Large blood vessels traverse the muscle coat obliquely, running within large intramuscular septa. Large lymphatic vessels, which mainly drain lymph from the mucosa, are often seen traversing the circular muscle layer of the intestine; they then travel for considerable distances circumferentially within the interstice between the two muscle layers. The lymphatic vessels, easily recognized through their content, are very thin-walled, have no musculature but do have valves. Their extensive association with the muscle coat of the intestine probably assists lymph transport.

Nerve fibres and Schwann cells form nerve bundles that run between the muscle cells (Figure 7). Vesicle-containing varicosities are found within bundles of all sizes, but they are more frequent in the small ones (Figure 7A). Varicose axons running singly are less common than in other smooth muscles (e.g. vas deferens or iris), but they do occur in intestinal muscles too. Various configurations of intramuscular nerves can be observed, even within the same muscle: they range from isolated varicosities lying very close to, or partly embedded into, a muscle cell, to bundles containing varicosities, located at various distances from muscle cells and interstitial cells.

References

Ashton, F. T., Somlyo, A. V., and Somlyo, A. P., (1975), The contractile apparatus of vascular smooth muscle: Intermediate high voltage stereo electron microscopy. *J. Mol. Biol.*, **98:** 17–29.

Bagby, R. M., (1980), Double immunofluorescent staining of isolated smooth muscle cells. I. Preparation of anti-chicken gizzard alpha actinin and its use with anti-chicken gizzard myosin for co-localization of alpha actinin and myosin in chicken gizzard cells. *Histochemistry*, **69:** 113–30.

Bagby, R. M., (1983), Organization of contractile/cytoskeletal elements. In: *Biochemistry of Smooth Muscle* (Ed. Stephens, N. L.), pp. 1–84, CRC Press, Boca.

Bois, R. M., (1973), The organization of the contractile apparatus of vertebrate smooth muscle. *Anat. Rec.* **93:** 138–49.

Bond, M., Kitizawa, T., Somlyo, A. P., and Somlyo, A. V., (1984), Release and recycling of calcium by the sarcoplasmic reticulum in guinea-pig portal vein smooth muscle. *J. Physiol.* (*Lond.*), **355:** 677–95.

Bond, M., and Somlyo, A. V., (1982), Dense bodies and actin polarity in vertebrate smooth muscle. *J. Cell Biol.*, **95:** 403–13.

Casteels, R., and Raeymaekers, L., (1979), The action of acetylcholine and catecholamines on an intracellular calcium store in the smooth muscle cells of the guinea-pig taenia coli. *J. Physiol.* (*Lond.*) **294:** 51–68.

Craig, R., and Megerman, J., (1977), Assembly of smooth muscle myosin into side-polar filaments. *J. Cell Biol.*, **75(3):** 990–6.

Dillon, P. F., Adksoy, M. O., Driska, S. P., and Murphy, R. A., (1981), Myosin phosphorylation and the cross-bridge cycle in arterial smooth muscle. *Science*, **211:** 495–7.

Elliott, A., Offer, G., and Burridge, K., (1976), Electron

microscopy of myosin molecules from muscle and non-muscle sources. *Proc. Roy. Soc. Lond. Series B*, **193**: 45–53.

Gabella, G., (1987), Structure of muscles and nerves in the gastrointestinal tract. In: *Physiology of the Gastrointestinal Tract* (Ed. Johnson, L. R.), pp. 335–81. Raven Press, New York.

Geiger, B., Dutton, A. H., Tokuashi, K. T., and Singer, S. J., (1981), Immunoelectron microscope studies of membrane-microfilament interactions: distributions of a-actinin, tropomyosin, and vinculin in intestinal epithelial brush border and chicken gizzard smooth muscle cells. *J. Cell Biol.*, **91**: 614–28.

Murphy, R. A., Driska, S. P., and Cohen, D. M., (1977), Variations in actin to myosin ratios and cellular force generation in vertebrate smooth muscles. In: *Excitation–Contraction Coupling in Smooth Muscle* (Ed. Casteels, R.), pp. 417–24, Elsevier/North-Holland, Amsterdam.

Siegman, M. J., Butler, T. M., Mooers, S. U., and Davies, R. E., (1976), Calcium-dependent resistance to stretch and stress relaxation in resting smooth muscle. *Am. J. Physiol.*, **231**: 1501–8.

Small, V. J., and Sobieszek, A., (1980), The contractile apparatus of smooth muscle. *Int. Rev. Cytol.*, **64**: 241–306.

II
METHODOLOGY OF MOTILITY

4
RADIOLOGY

Enrico Corazziari, Aldo Torsoli
Università 'La Sapienza', Rome, Italy

Radiology offers qualitative or semiquantitative information on the motor behaviour of the alimentary canal. Following the administration of a carefully selected contrast material, X-rays can indirectly reveal wall contractions, as well as displacement of contents. The degree of luminal distension can provide some information on tonicity and/or capacitance of the viscus.

Radiological Techniques

Fluoroscopic observation is the most valuable radiological test for the investigation of motor activity of the gastrointestinal tract. Image intensifier systems (Wolf and Khilnani, 1966) offer a better resolution of the images, significantly reduce radiation, and make telefluorography, photofluorography, cinefluorography, and magnetic tape recording possible (Gebauer et al, 1967).

Cinefluorography enables the evaluation of rapid motor sequences by slow motion or still picture analysis (Cohen and Wolf, 1968).

Fluoroscopic images converted into video signals and recorded on magnetic tape or disk can be immediately displayed by playback. Adequate radiological evaluation of rapid motor sequences can thus be obtained by spot-camera imaging.

Limitations of Radiological Technique

Radiology carries the risk of radiation exposure and, therefore, only few and short-lasting motor events can be observed. With the exception of the colon, radiological description concerns motor events, elicited by intraluminal distension due to

contrast medium, which are not physically and chemically comparable to those induced by food.

Radiology detects wall movement caused by contraction of the circular muscle layer but it is inadequate in the investigation of motor events of the longitudinal layer. Finally, radiological observations are essentially qualitative in nature and, with a few exceptions, do not allow quantification of the data.

Radiological Evaluation of Deglutition and Defecation

Deglutition and defecation are functions controlled at a conscious level and performed by integrated actions of several striated muscles. These events are rapid and can only be evaluated by means of slow motion or frame-by-frame analysis of cinefluorographic or videotape recordings.

Deglutition

The mechanism of normal deglutition is described in Figure 1 (Mantesi et al, 1987).

Altered patterns of deglutition can often be identified by cineradiography in patients with oropharyngeal dysphagia. The most common abnormalities include partial or total paresis of pharyngeal constrictors (Figure 2), defective closure of the laryngeal vestibule followed by entrance of contrast medium into the upper airways, partial mobility or immobility of the epiglottis (Figure 3), cricopharyngeal dysfunction (Figure 4) identified as a permanent posterior indentation during the transit of barium. Any of

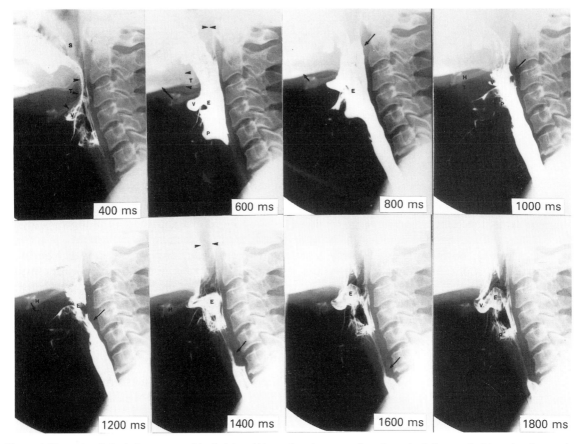

Figure 1. Normal radiological sequence of deglutition. 400 ms after the onset of swallow, the bolus, pushed into the pharynx by the tongue, is displaced posteriorly (arrows) and the valleculae (V) become evident. The tongue and the hyoid bone move slightly forward. After 600 ms the bolus is filling the pharynx, the base of the tongue moves forward, the valleculae and the piriform recesses (P) are distended; the palatopharyngeal isthmus (facing arrows) is closed; the hyoid bone moves upward and forward; the epiglottis (E) is in a horizontal position. After 800 ms, the bolus has reached the cervical oesophagus; concomitantly the crico-pharyngeal muscle relaxes and the peristaltic contraction of the superior pharyngeal constrictor occurs (long arrow); a small amount of barium can be detected in the subepiglottic space. After 1000 ms the bolus is pushed by the peristaltic contraction of the medial pharyngeal constrictor (long arrow), the hyoid bone (H) has reached its highest level close to the mandible and the thyroid cartilage; the epiglottis is almost completely inverted, the valleculae and the pyriform sinuses are no longer outpouching. After 1200 ms the bolus is pushed distally by the peristaltic contraction. After 1400 ms the palatopharyngeal isthmus opens, the hyoid bone and the larynx move downward, the epiglottis moves upright and air fills the larynx. After 1600–1800 ms the pharyngo-laryngeal structures are back to the resting position and the primary peristaltic contraction of the cervical oesophagus (arrow) pushes the bolus into the thoracic oesophagus. From Montesi et al, 1987 with permission.

these may present as the only abnormality but the concomitant presence of two or more abnormalities may frequently occur in the same patient (Ekberg and Nylander, 1982a, 1982b).

Defecation

Following the rectal injection of a contrast medium, carefully prepared to simulate physical characteristics of faeces, the dynamic events during straining and defecation can be visualized. The radiological examination is performed by taking the lateral pelvic view at rest, during straining and defecation with the patient sitting on a radiolucent commode (Mahieu et al, 1984a). At rest, the anorectal angle is about 90° and the anorectal junction which identifies the level of the pelvic floor is located less than 2 cm below the

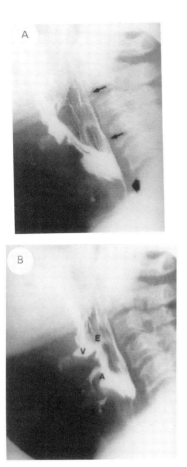

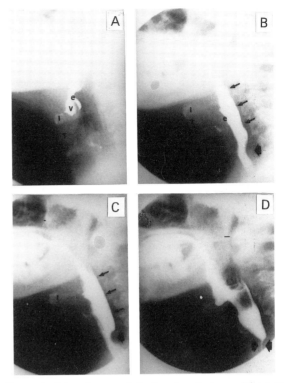

Figure 4. Crico-pharyngeal dysfunction. In image B and C lack of contraction of the pharyngeal constrictor (long arrows) and lack of relaxation of the crico-pharyngeal muscle (thick arrow); in image D retention of barium in the hypopharynx. e = epiglottis, v = ventricle, I = hyoid bone, T = thyroid cartilage. By courtesy of A. Montesi.

Figure 2. Paresis of the pharyngeal constrictors. Retention of the bolus in the oro- and hypopharynx due to lack of contraction of the pharyngeal constrictors. A. Failure of elevation of the hyoid bone and larynx. B. Aspiration of contrast into the larynx. A, arytenoid cartilage; V, ventricle; E, epiglottis. By courtesy of A. Montesi.

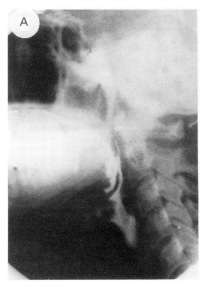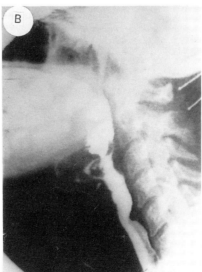

Figure 3. Immobile epiglottis. During the passage of the bolus through the (A) oro- and (B) hypopharynx the epiglottis remains still. By courtesy of A. Montesi.

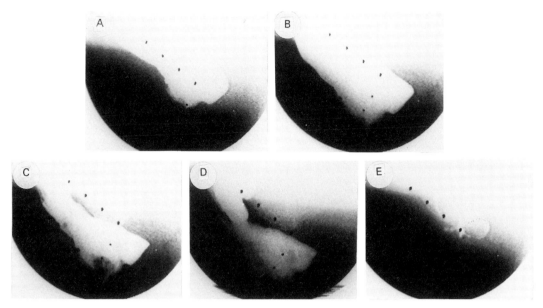

Figure 5. Normal radiological sequence of defecation. Defecography in latero-lateral view. Dotted line indicates the anorectal angle in resting conditions. A. Resting conditions; B, C. straining, progressive lowering of the pelvic floor, widening of the anorectal angle and opening of the distal rectum and anal canal; D. evacuation; E. post-evacuation image with pelvic floor and anorectal angle back to resting conditions. By courtesy of V. Piloni and A. Montesi.

pubococcygeal line. During straining, the pelvic floor descends by no more than 2 cm and as tone of the puborectalis decreases, the anorectal angle straightens out to about 137°.

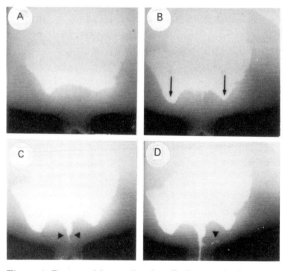

Figure 6. Rectoanal incoordination. Defecography in antero-posterior projection. A, B. Failure of rectoanal relaxation during attempts of defecation. C. Incomplete opening of the anal canal. A fistulous tract is evident in D. By courtesy of V. Piloni and A. Montesi.

During defecation, as the pelvic floor descends the distal rectum and the anal canal open up and are progressively filled by contrast medium. At the end of defecation the lumen of the anal canal and distal rectum close, the pelvic floor rises, and the anorectal angle is restored (Figure 5). Altered proctograms at rest include a recto-anal junction located more than 2 cm below the pubococcygeal line and a widened anorectal angle. Altered pattern of defecation includes a pelvic floor which does not descend or descends more than 2 cm; a puborectalis which either fails to relax or contracts (Figure 6); intrarectal or intra-anal intussusception; rectal prolapse (Figure 7); rectocele; retained contrast medium at the end of defecation (Mahieu et al, 1984b). By using a barium filled balloon (balloon proctography) instead of a semi-solid bolus, a simpler and better tolerated examination of the recto-anal tract can be performed. There is, however, loss of information concerning details of the rectal mucosa and overall emptying of the rectum (Preston et al, 1984).

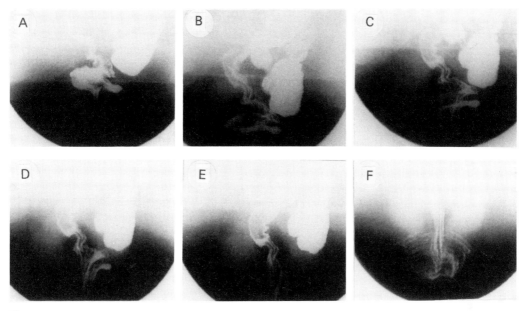

Figure 7. Rectal prolapse. Defecography in antero-posterior projection. A. Resting conditions; B, C. mucosal intussusception; D, E. perineal descent; F. external prolapse. By courtesy of V. Piloni and A. Montesi.

Wall Movements

Segmenting Stationary Contractions

Segmenting contractions appear radiologically as stationary nonpropagating ring-like indentations of the wall, which totally or partially occlude the lumen dividing the viscus into segments. These contractions may, however, give rise to pressure gradients determining displacement of contents in either direction.

In the oesophagus, local intermittent contractions (tertiary contractions) may appear isolated or simultaneously at different levels (Figure 8). Their infrequent occurrence is compatible with a normal oesophageal function. Their frequent and/or simultaneous occurrence at multiple levels, sometimes associated with curling of the oesophagus, is suggestive of an oesophageal motor abnormality (Figure 9).

In the stomach, stationary wall movements do not present the characteristic segmentary ring-like contractions, but rather appear as slow tonic variation. This type of motor activity, which takes place in the fundus and upper two-thirds of the corpus, can scarcely be investigated by radiology, as no critical or well-identifiable changes of the wall profile can be detected.

At the level of the small intestine, segmenting activity appears as 1–2 cm long annular contractions which occur at intervals of 3–4 cm. They are usually isolated (Figure 10) and sometimes simultaneous at different levels. Annular contractions may sometimes occur for short periods in adjacent intestinal tracts causing bidirectional displacement of contents ('to and fro' or 'pendular' movements) (Hertz, 1907).

At the level of the large intestine, segmenting activity is characterized by localized wall contractions which, partly or completely, involve the circumference of the colon (Ritchie, 1968). They represent more than 90% of the entire colonic motor activity (Figure 11) and originate, for the major part, at the level of the stable interhaustral folds (Torsoli et al, 1971b).

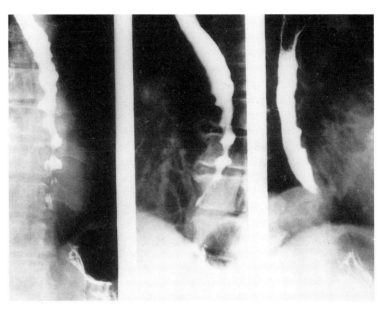

Figure 8. Segmenting contractions of the oesophagus. Three oesophagograms of the same patient showing segmenting contractions and their variability during a short observation period.

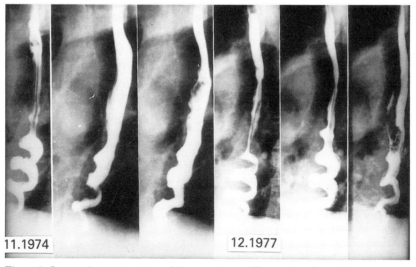

Figure 9. Segmenting contractions of the oesophagus. Two series of oesophagograms performed at three-year intervals in the same patient with diffuse oesophageal spasm. The two series are strikingly similar and show a corkscrew appearance of the oesophageal body despite the absence of any symptoms during the radiological examinations.

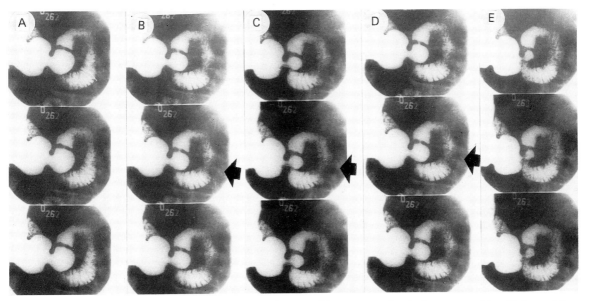

Figure 10. Segmenting contraction of the duodenum. Cinefluorographic sequence taken in the prone position. To be read from top to bottom. A. Duodenum filled with barium; B, C. ring-like constriction as indicated by arrows; D. duodenal wall starts relaxing without forward progression of either constriction or barium; E. duodenal wall fully relaxed and distribution of barium similar to that seen in A. From Torsoli et al, 1971, with kind permission.

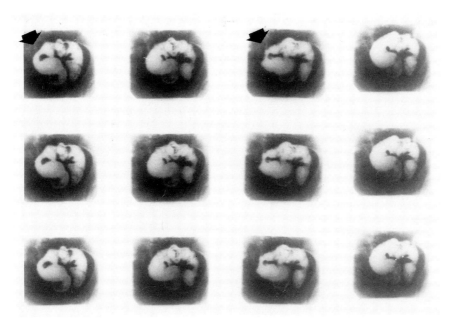

Figure 11. Segmenting contraction of the colon. Cinefluorographic sequence of the sigmoid colon contrasted with barium sulphate administered per os. To be read from top to bottom and from left to right. Annular segmenting contraction occurs twice in the sequence on the left side of the sigmoid (arrows).

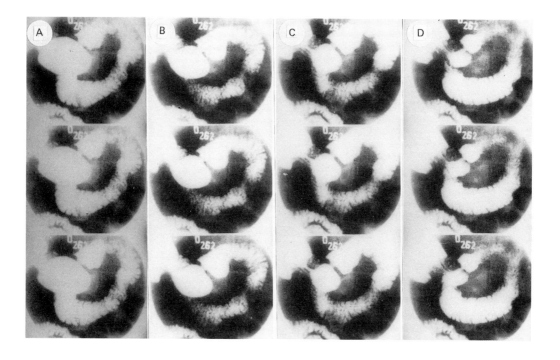

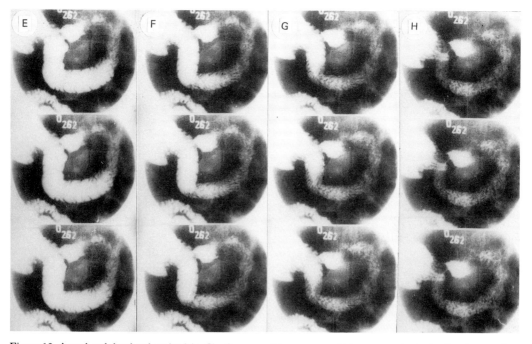

Figure 12. Antral and duodenal peristalsis. Cinefluorographic sequence of the antro-pyloric-duodenal tract taken in prone position. To be read from top to bottom. A. Annular contraction of the antrum moving distally (B, C and D) propelling barium into the duodenum, (B, C); D. constriction appearing just beyond the duodenal bulb and propelling barium into the ascending duodenum (E and F) and beyond the duodeno-jejunal flexure (G and H).

Peristalsis

The peristaltic motor event is visualized as an aborally directed ring-like contraction, which, at least in the oesophagus and small and large intestine, appears to follow a circumscribed dilatation of the walls.

In the oesophagus primary peristalsis follows an act of swallowing and it is seen to progress from the pharynx to the oesophagogastric junction. Secondary peristalsis is not preceded by the oropharyngeal phase of deglutition and usually originates in the middle–distal part of the oesophagus (Turano, 1957).

In the distal stomach, circular ring-like indentations which start in the corpus and move slowly towards the pylorus are visible on contrast examination (Smith et al, 1957). In some instances, the indentations are shallow and fade out at the antrum, do not reach the pylorus, or produce any substantial movement of the contents. In other instances, the indentations deepen as they move distally, occluding the lumen as they reach the incisura angularis; at 3–4 cm from the pylorus the antrum appears to contract simultaneously (antral systole). This type of contraction causes displacement of contents towards the pylorus and, as the terminal antral contraction takes place, barium may be either pushed forward into the duodenum if the pylorus is open (Figure 12), or propelled backwards into the stomach if the pylorus is closed (Smith et al, 1957; Carlson et al, 1966).

At the level of the small bowel, peristaltic movements displace contrast medium for short distances (4–5 cm). In the duodenum, however, movement of contents over longer distances (up to and beyond the ligament of Treitz) may be seen (Figure 12) (Torsoli et al, 1971a).

At the level of the colon, peristalsis begins with a progressive change in the spatial orientation of the colonic folds, which rapidly disappear. Then, a concentric contraction starts at the cranial end of the unsegmented tract and moves distally, preceded by dilatation of the lumen. Subsequently, haustrations first reappear in the segment proximal to the displaced contents and then at the level of the segment where contents have been displaced (Figure 13) (Torsoli et al, 1971b).

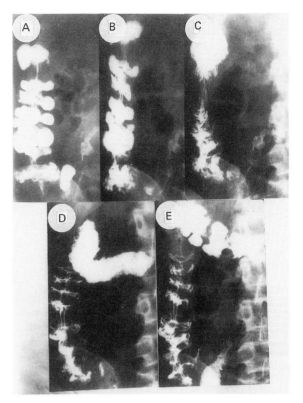

Figure 13. Lower gastrointestinal series showing a peristaltic movement (right colon). Haustra modify orientation (B) and then disappear (C) as contents are displaced distally (C and D). Haustra are present again in the segment proximal to the displaced contents (D) and then at the level of contents (E) after termination of the motor event. From Torsoli et al, 1966 with permission.

Retrograde motor activity

Retrograde displacement of contents for short distances can be detected occasionally in the small bowel, but a sequential wall contraction moving in oral direction has only been described in the duodenum (Figure 14) (Borgstrom and Arborelius, 1971; Torsoli et al, 1971a). Retrograde displacement of contents for medium and large distances, occurs in the colon, but the underlying motor mechanism is not clear.

Transit

Depending upon the anatomic structure, the specific motor pattern of each segment and the physi-

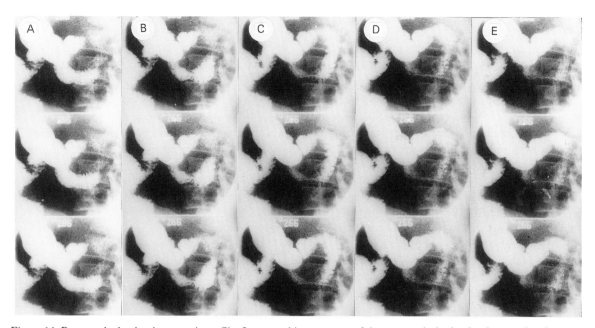

Figure 14. Retrograde duodenal contractions. Cinefluorographic sequences of the antro-pyloric-duodenal tract taken in prone position. A. Barium contrast in the stomach and the ascending part of the duodenum. B, A duodenal constriction appears just before the ascending duodenal loop and moving backward propels barium into the descending duodenal loop (C and D) and then into the duodenal bulb and the stomach (D and E).

cal characteristics of the contents, the transit rate varies in different parts of the gastrointestinal tract. Since its earliest clinical application radiology has been used to evaluate the progression of a radio-opaque bolus. This approach has the advantage of simplicity but only gives a semiquantitative evaluation as it detects the head and, less precisely, the body and tail of the radio-opaque bolus. Furthermore, the great variability in viscosity and stability of the barium sulphate suspension may affect the final interpretation, even when the technique is standardized (Miller, 1967).

Oesophageal transit depends on gravity, consistency of the bolus and oesophageal motor activity. In the erect position, nonviscous boluses reach the oesophagogastric junction with the aid of oropharyngeal pressure and gravity. Peristaltic contractions occur after the passage of the bolus and empty the oesophageal body of any residual contents. Conversely, in the supine position oesophageal transit of a viscous bolus depends entirely upon pressure gradients caused by propulsive motor activity. To detect subtle changes in oeso-

phageal transit, it is necessary to challenge the oesophagus with a solid radio-opaque bolus swallow in the supine position (Figure 15).

The radiological demonstration of the passage of barium from the stomach into the oesophagus in the supine position, and in the absence of physical efforts which may increase the abdominothoracic pressure gradient, is a definite diagnostic sign of gastro-oesophageal reflux.

The gastric emptying of a barium meal cannot be considered an accurate method to evaluate transit of food through the stomach: however the retention of barium contrast in the stomach of fasting patients for several hours suggests an abnormally prolonged gastric emptying time. In the evaluation of patients with slow gastric emptying it might be useful to perform a radiological investigation with solid food impregnated with barium or with corpuscolate radio-opaque markers to detect delayed gastric emptying of solid components (Bertrand et al, 1980), in the presence of normal liquid emptying.

Detection of contrast medium in the stomach

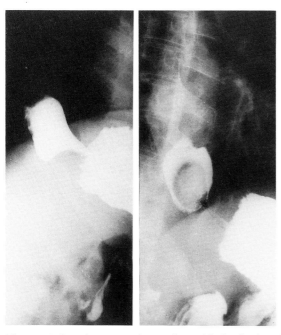

Figure 15. Oesophagograms in a patient with dysphagia and recurrent episodes of chest pain after a Nissen fundoplication for reflux oesophagitis. Liquid barium is emptied from the oesophagus into the stomach; conversely (on the right) a solid bolus (marshmallow) is retained above the fundoplication. By courtesy of F. I. Habib.

subsequent to its introduction directly into the duodenum via a fine catheter has been used to detect duodenogastric reflux. Evaluation of the small bowel transit by means of a barium meal is inaccurate (Thompson and Saunders, 1972).

Particulate radio-opaque markers (3×5 mm, polyethylene and 20% w/w barium sulphate) are more suitable for measuring transit of semisolid–solid contents through the large bowel. Following the ingestion of markers, X-ray films or fluoroscopic observation of the abdomen at regular time intervals (Hinton et al, 1969; Chaussade et al, 1986) can be used to detect their location within the large bowel. The distribution of markers in various segments of the colon and rectum can provide valuable information on transit in patients with constipation (Corazziari et al, 1975) (Figures 16–19).

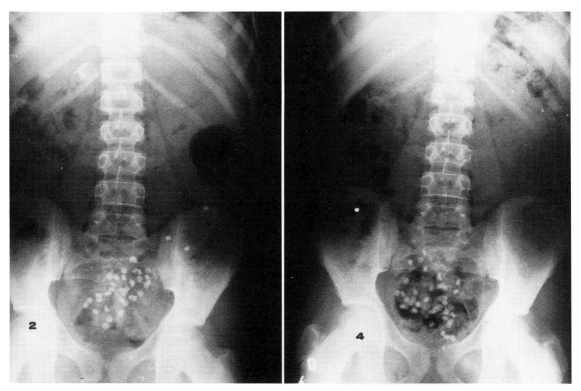

Figure 16. Large bowel segmental transit time. Chronic nonorganic constipation with rectal slowing of transit (dyschezia). On day 2 and 4 after ingestion, radio-opaque markers are retained in the rectal ampulla.

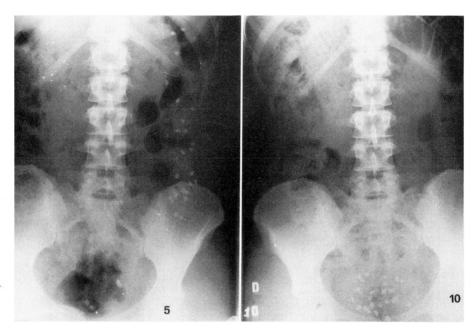

Figure 17. Large bowel segmental transit time. Chronic nonorganic constipation with colonic and rectal slowing of transit. On day 5 after ingestion, radio-opaque markers are retained in the left colon in the presence of an empty rectum; on day 10 markers are retained in the rectal ampulla.

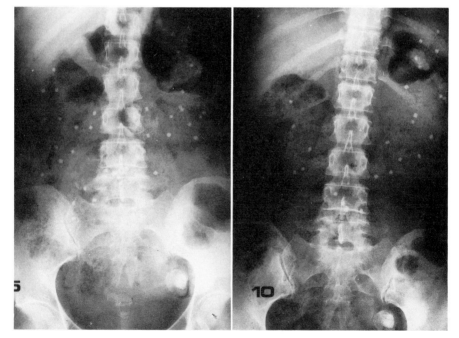

Figure 18. Large bowel segmental transit time. Chronic nonorganic constipation with colonic slowing of transit in a patient with colostomy performed at the level of the distal left colon after a stercoral perforation. On day 5 and 10 after ingestion, markers are retained in the colon proximal to the colostomy.

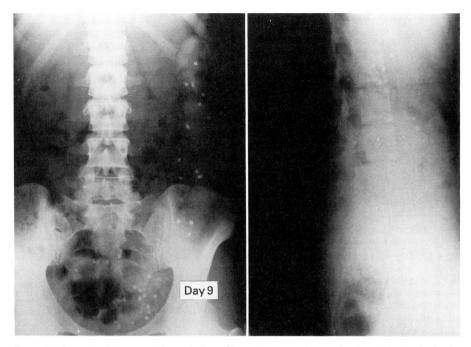

Figure 19. Large bowel segmental transit time. Chronic nonorganic constipation with colonic slowing of transit. X-ray discrimination between sigmoid and rectal location of the markers by means of a radiogram performed in lateral view. On day nine after ingestion, an anteroposterior view of the abdomen depicts markers scattered along the descending colon and within the pelvis (in the rectum?); a lateral view shows an empty rectum indicating that markers are retained in the descending colon and sigmoid only.

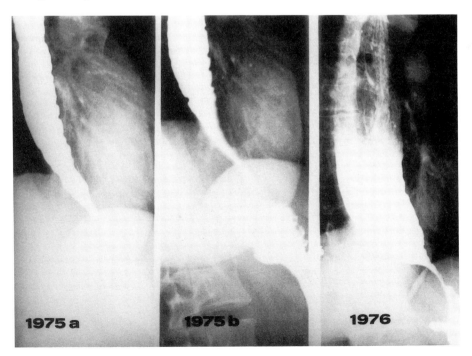

Figure 20. Mega-oesophagus. Oesophagograms of a patient with achalasia, performed at different times. Note progressive dilatation of the oesophageal body.

Dilatation of the Lumen

Capacitance and tone of the alimentary canal may vary widely and cannot be measured accurately. Nonetheless, abnormal dilatation of the lumen, indicated by the prefix 'mega', is easily detected radiologically and indicates the presence of either a functional or mechanical obstruction distally or loss of tone in the dilated viscus. Accordingly, mega-oesophagus (Figures 20–22), megastomach, megacolon and megarectum (Figures 23 and 24) are common findings in the presence of ineffective relaxation of the lower oesophageal sphincter, the pylorus and the anal canal, respectively. Less commonly, however, one or more segments of the alimentary tract appear dilated in the presence of wall hypotonicity secondary to either myopathies or neuropathies (Figure 25).

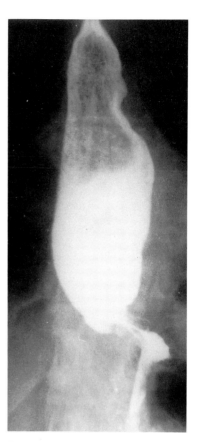

Figure 22. Mega-oesophagus. Oesophagogram showing dilated oesophageal body with retention of barium and air level in a patient with scleroderma.

In conclusion, radiology is still the most reliable method to evaluate motor function of the striated muscles at the level of the oropharynx and the anorectum and to measure transit through the large bowel. In other areas, it should be used to complement methods that offer quantitative measurements.

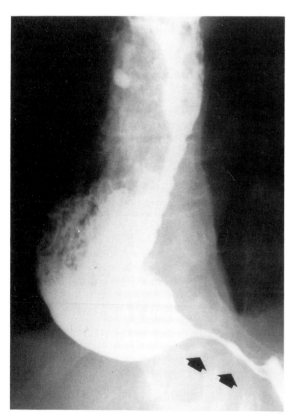

Figure 21. Mega-oesophagus. Oesophagogram showing dilated oesophageal body with retention of barium and ingesta secondary to leiomyoma (arrows) located at the oesophagogastric junction.

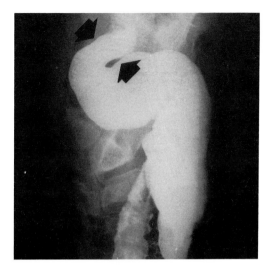
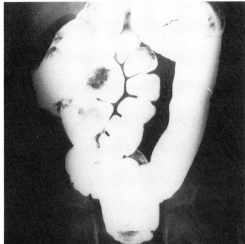
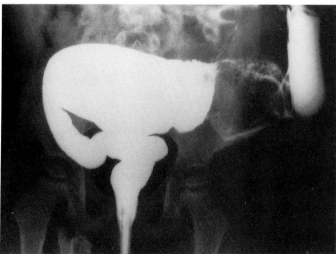

Figure 23. Megacolon in Hirschsprung's disease. Barium enema in three patients affected by Hirschsprung's disease. Note different length of the aganglionic segment and large bowel distension proximal to it. On the left involvement of the distal part of the rectum, in the middle involvement of the entire rectum, on the right involvement of the rectum and sigmoid. Transition zone is better appreciated in the lateral view (arrows) of a barium enema performed without previous large bowel preparation. Transition zone cannot be detected in patients with ultra-short Hirschsprung's disease.

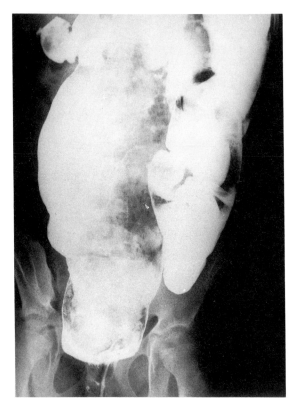

Figure 24. Megarectum and megacolon in chronic idiopathic constipation. Barium enema shows extremely distended rectum and colon in the absence of any transition zone.

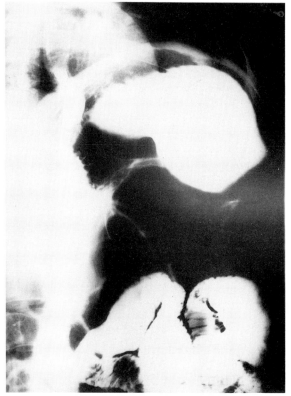

Figure 25. Megastomach and mega-small bowel in chronic idiopathic intestinal pseudo-obstruction. Upper gastro-intestinal series of a patient with recurrent episodes of intestinal obstruction who has been previously submitted to total colectomy and a negative laparotomy. Note gaseous distension of the stomach and the small bowel.

References

Bertrand, J., Metman, E. H., Dorval, E. D., Rouleau, P. H., D'Hueppe, A., and Philippe, L., (1980), Etude du temps d'evacuation gastrique de repas normaux au moyen de granules radio-opaque. Applications cliniques et validation. *Gastroenterol. Clin. Biol.*, **4**: 770–6.

Borgstrom, S., and Arborelius, M. Jr., (1971), A technique for studying propulsion and the displacement of contents in the duodenum and proximal jejunum. *Rendic. Gastroenterol*, **3**: 174–7.

Carlson, H. C., Code, C. F., and Nelson, R. A., (1966), Motor action of canine gastroduodenal junction: a cineradiographic, pressure and electric study. *Am. J. Dig. Dis.*, **11**: 155–72.

Chaussade, S., Roche, H., Khyara, A., Couterier, D., and Guerre, J., (1986), Measure du temps de transit colique (TTC): description et validation d'une nouvelle technique. *Gastroenterol. Clin. Biol.* **10**: 385–9.

Cohen, B. R., and Wolf, B. S., (1968), Cineradiographic and intraluminal pressure correlations in the pharynx and oesophagus. In: *Alimentary Canal.* (Ed. code, C. F.) American Physiological Society. Washington DC (*Handbook of Physiology*, vol. IV, sect. 6, pp. 1841–60).

Corazziari, E., Dani, S., Pozzessere, C., Anzini, F., and Torsoli, A., (1975), Colonic segmental transit times in chronic nonorganic constipation. *Rendic. Gastroenterol.*, **7**: 67–9.

Ekberg, O., and Nylander, G., (1982a), Cineradiography of the pharyngeal stage of deglutition in 150 individuals without dysphagia. *Brit. J. Rad.*, **55**: 253–7.

Ekberg, O., and Nylander, G., (1982b), Cineradiography of the pharyngeal stage of deglutition in 250 dysphagial patients. *Brit. J. Rad.*, **55**: 258–62.

Gebauer, A., Lissner, J., and Schott, O., (1967), *Roent-*

gen Television. Grune & Stratton, New York, London.

Hertz, A. F., (1907), The passage of food along the alimentary canal. *Guy. Hosp. Rep.*, **61**: 389–427.

Hinton, J. M., Lennard-Jones, J. E., and Young, A. C., (1969), A new method for studying gut transit times using radioopaque markers. *Gut*, **10**: 842–7.

Mahieu, P., Pringot, J., and Bodart, P., (1984a), Defecography: I. Description of a new procedure and results in normal patients. *Gastrointest. Radiol.*, **9**: 247–51.

Mahieu, P., Pringot, J., and Bodart, P., (1984b), Defecography: II. Contribution to the diagnosis of defecation disorders. *Gastrointest. Radiol.*, **9**: 253–61.

Miller, R. E., (1967), Barium sulphate as a contrast medium. In: *Alimentary Tract Roentgenology.* (Eds. Margulis, A. R., Burheune, H. J.) Mosby, Saint Louis, pp. 25–36.

Montesi, A., Piloni, V., Pesaresi, A., Antico, E., and Blasetti, R., (1987), Le tube digestif. Approche radiologicque fonctionelle. Radiology in mobile organs: the gastrointestinal tract. *Radiologie du Cepur*, **7**: 95–103.

Preston, D. M., Lennard-Jones, J. E., and Thomas, B. M., (1984), The balloon proctogram. *Brit. J. Surg.*, **71**: 29–32.

Ritchie, J. A., (1968), Colonic motor activity and bowel function. Part I. Normal movement of contents. *Gut*, **9**: 442–56.

Smith, A. W. M., Code, C. F., and Schlegel, J. F., (1957), Simultaneous cineradiographic and kimographic studies of human gastric antral motility. *J. Appl. Physiol.*, **11**: 12–16.

Thompson, J. R., and Sanders, I., (1972), Lactose barium small bowel study. Efficacy of a screening method. *Am. J. Roentgen.*, **116**: 276–8.

Torsoli, A., Corazzari, E., Waller, S. L., and Anzini, F., (1971a), Duodenal peristalsis in man. *Rendic. Gastroenterol.*, **3**: 168–73.

Torsoli, A., Ramorino, M. L., Ammaturo, M. V., Capurso, L., Arcangeli, G., and Paoluzi, P., (1971b), Mass movements and intracolonic pressures. *Am. J. Dig. Dis.*, **16**: 693–6.

Turano, L., (1957), Malattie non neoplastiche dell'esofago. In: *Atti Congr. Ital. Med. Intern.* (Ed. Pozzi, L.) Rome, pp. 1–72.

Wolf, B. S., and Khilnani, M. T., (1966), Progress in gastroenterological radiology. *Gastroenterology*, **51**: 542–59.

5
MANOMETRY

Sven Gustavsson and Richard Tucker
University Hospital, Uppsala, Sweden, and St. Mary's
Hospital, Rochester, USA

Introduction

Manometry is the technique for recording mechanical activity of the bowel by detecting and quantitating changes in intraluminal pressure caused by contractions of the gut wall. Manometry is an established routine procedure for the evaluation of oesophageal and anorectal motility, including diagnostic studies in disease. Research studies have generated a large body of information on manometric patterns from most other parts of the gastrointestinal tract (for a review see Malagelada et al, 1986) and, in the near future, information obtained by gastric, biliary and small intestinal manometry will be required for a thorough evaluation of some patients with symptoms of gut intestinal dysfunction. Even if manometry is relatively easy to perform, interpretation of tracings requires care and experience if overinterpretations are to be avoided.

Intraluminal pressure recordings can be obtained from all regions of the gastrointestinal tract using miniature intraluminal transducers or the low-compliance water-perfused manometry tube system, which nowadays should be considered to be the standard equipment. In this chapter we will review some basic principles of performing manometric investigations with a bias towards methods that are in routine use at the Gastroenterology Unit at the Mayo Clinic. Miniature transducers, though used extensively by some laboratories (Mathias et al, 1985), have not had the broad use of perfused systems. Sleeve manometry is also a special technique, designed particularly for the study of sphincters.

The Manometry Tube

There are commercially available multilumen manometry tubes of standard construction intended for oesophageal, intestinal, biliary and anorectal application (see Appendix for manufacturers). However, many studies, and especially those of a research character, require a specific configuration of the tube with respect to tube length, location of manometry ports, size of mercury and air balloon in the tip, etc.

Tubing best suited for construction of a manometry tube is polyvinyl chloride (PVC), because it can be bonded together easily and still be flexible enough for transport through the gastrointestinal tract. PVC tubing may be obtained in single, double or triple lumen. Single-lumen tubes from Dural Plastics (SV 50) have inner diameter of 0.75 mm and outer diameter of 1.45 mm. Triple-lumen tubings from the same manufacturer (TV 8) have an inner diameter of 0.78 mm and outer diameter of 2.0 mm. A radio-opaque single-lumen tube (paediatric opaque from Ferraris, inner diameter 0.039″ and outer 0.079″) is often incorporated into the assembly for checking the position of tubes fluoroscopically.

Perfusion through the small lumens of tubing such as these is very restricted, but for manometry distilled water at a slow infusion rate (0.5–1 ml/min or even up to 3 ml/min) works well. Perfusates with high viscosity cannot be perfused through these small lumens. Aspiration is not possible through small multi-lumen tubes, and one must use a larger single-lumen tube which will increase the diameter of the composite tube. It

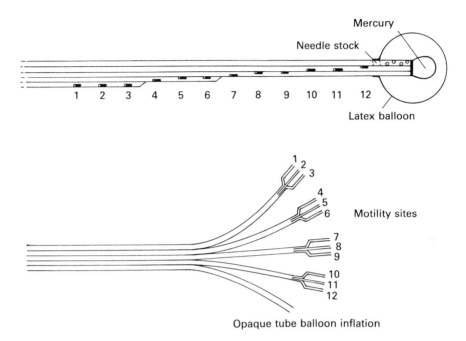

Figure 1. The 13-lumen tube (schematic).

is important not to enlarge an assembly beyond patient tolerance; this is more likely to occur if multiple aspiration sites are required. However, with the small triple-lumen PVC tubing, it has been possible to have up to 12 motility sites by putting together four of these tubes. The recording sites can be spaced closely (1 cm apart), or further, depending on the aims of the study (Figure 1).

Side-holes in the tube are cut by using needle stock of the same diameter as the inside of the tubing. The needle stock should be about 5 cm long and sharpened on the end for easier cutting. Because of the possibility of cutting the membrane inside a triple-lumen tubing, it is helpful to insert a fine wire into the lumen to the point where the hole is to be cut. When the holes are cut, the distal extent of the tube, beyond the site of the hole, must be plugged with stainless steel wire (about 1 cm will suffice), so that perfusates cannot go beyond this point. It is helpful to add a small radio-opaque tube to your assembly; it can be used to infuse air into the balloon at the tip of the assembly, this approach being helpful for rapid tube placement (see below).

After all tubes are cut to the proper length, the holes made and stainless steel wires inserted, the tube is ready to be assembled. A 13-lumen tube, featuring four triple-lumen PVC tubes, and one radio-opaque tube constitutes an assembly which is approximately 6 mm in diameter. The tubes are put together, two at a time, using tetrahydrofuran as a cement. It is best not to carry all tubes to the tip; this leaves the distal portion of the tube more flexible and more easily able to pass along the bowel.

Care of Manometic Tubes

Tubes must be checked for leaks by submerging the assembly in water and infusing air through all lumens. When each study is completed, tubes must be washed with warm water and soap, and air dried for at least one hour. After drying, tubes are coiled and wrapped in a large bath towel. Any balloons should be left inflated with about 10 ml of air. With proper care it is possible to use tubes for multiple studies.

Placement of the Tube

A firm but relaxed attitude helps to allay the patient's uncertainties and will facilitate passage of the assembly. If not contraindicated, local anaesthetic is sprayed in the hypopharynx and tubing is swallowed with the subject in a sitting position. The tube will be least uncomfortable when kept lateral to the teeth, and moved about as little as possible.

For small bowel intubation, tubes can be placed over a guide wire, which can be introduced either by a steerable radio-opaque catheter or through the working channel of an endoscope. The manometry assembly is then fed upon the guide wire into position. This approach will often be needed in patients with gastroparesis in whom assemblies are slow to leave the stomach. For intubation of bowel segments distal to the ligament of Treitz, a mercury weight is added to the tip and is used to pull the tube across the stomach to the pylorus. When the tube has advanced to the second or third portion of the duodenum, air is infused into a balloon at the tip (see above). This speeds transit of the tube through the jejunum and ileum and even into the colon. Once in position, the balloon must be deflated to avoid further advancement of the assembly (Kerlin et al, 1983).

Recording Equipment

The hydraulic capillary infusion system achieves high fidelity recording of intraluminal pressure at a desirably low infusion rate. Reservoir water is maintained at a high constant pressure (1000 mmHg) and is reduced to atmospheric pressure by capillary tubing which has high resistance to flow (Figure 2). Pressure events in the gastrointestinal tract will always have little effect on flow rate because manometry tube lumen pressure always remains low in comparison with the pressure of the reservoir. With the compliance of the infusion system minimized, the manometric catheter itself becomes the major source of compliance in the recording system. The most common capillaries are made of stainless steel. Instead of a tank, perfusion fluids can be fed through capillaries

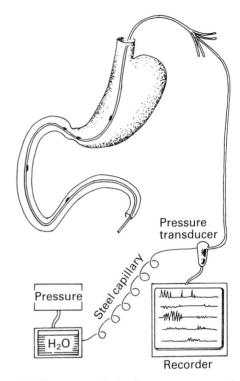

Figure 2. The pneumo-hydraulic system connected to a multi-lumen tube assembly.

from a plastic bag compressed in the same way as blood is for rapid transfusion. Both systems are available commercially, see Appendix.

The Sleeve Manometry Tube

The simple side-hole perfusion tube could be considered a standard tool for routine manometry. However, in manometry of sphincters, displacement of the side-hole from the region of maximal pressure occurs to a variable degree in different individuals and can be caused by even minor movements. This inherent limitation in the continuous perfused side-hole tube has prompted the development of sleeve tubes.

The Dent sleeve (Dent, 1976) is a 6 cm long pressure sensor developed to measure lower oesophageal sphincter pressure continuously in spite of movement of the sphincter relative to the sensor. Simultaneous recording from conventional side-holes and a sleeve showed a consistent pattern with

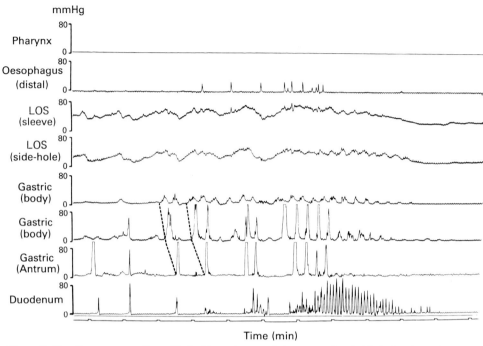

Figure 3. Simultaneous recording with the Dent sleeve and the conventional side-hole tube. LOS, Lower oesophageal sphincter. Reproduced with permission from Dent et al, 1983.

lower pressures being recorded by the side-hole tube (Figure 3). The observation that the lower oesophageal sphincter moves relative to the recording catheter with oesophageal peristalsis has led to doubt as to the significance of the side-hole recorded drop in sphincter pressure seen with swallowing. But also when recorded with the sleeve, the lower oesophageal sphincter pressure drops to zero with swallowing and, thus, this drop cannot be due to side-hole displacement. For different sphincters sleeves with different physical characteristics can be prepared (Quigley et al, 1987).

The Kraglund tube (manufactured by Cook Europe, see Appendix) is constructed by gluing a 6 cm long PVC cuff over a side-hole opening of a multi-lumen tube (Figure 4). While the conventional Dent sleeve only measures pressure in one direction, the Kraglund cuff tube permits reliable circumferential recordings. It is arguable, however, how much asymmetry should be expected in a sphincteric segment (see also Chapter 20). Both the Dent sleeve and the Krag-

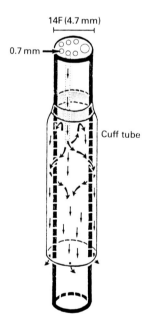

Figure 4. The Kraglund cuff tube (schematic). The tube is made of PVC. The cuff is glued to the multi-lumen tube. Courtesy Dr Karsten Kraglund, Department of Surgical Gastroenterology, Aarhus Kommunehospital, Denmark.

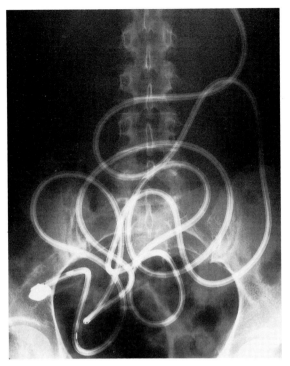

Figure 5. The long multi-lumen assembly placed with the Kraglund tube in the ileo-colonic sphincter area of a healthy volunteer. The proximal and distal end of the cuff is marked by radio-opaque steel rods.

lund cuff can pick up tonic elevations of pressure in the lower oesophageal sphincter. One problem with sleeve manometry is that when it is applied to the lower oesophageal sphincter some part of the sleeve is located in the stomach and will thus pick up gastric contractions.

The Kraglund cuff tube has also been adapted to a long multi-channel assembly for measurement of ileocaecal sphincter pressure. In unpublished experiments on healthy volunteers (Gustavsson et al, 1987), the Kraglund cuff was placed across the ileocolic junction (Figure 5) but there was no tonic elevation of base-line pressure, either during basal conditions or after stimulation of contractions with morphine sulphate (Figure 6). Thus recordings with the Kraglund cuff tube in this area seem to support earlier side-hole manometric findings (Quigley et al, 1985) that there is no high pressure zone in the ileocaecal sphincter in man. Our experiments also indicate that the ileocolonic junction might be less suitable for sleeve manometry because in some individuals the sleeve area will be subjected to a longitudinal bend which might create an artificial tonic elevation of pressure (Figures 7 and 8).

Morphine sulphate i.v. 1 mg/10 kg body weight

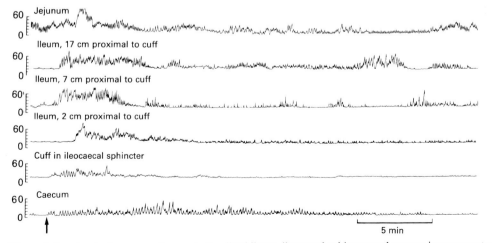

Figure 6. Intraluminal pressure changes in the distal ileum, ileocaecal sphincter and caecum in response to intravenous morphine. No tonic elevations of pressure could be recorded in the ileocaecal area with the cuff tube.

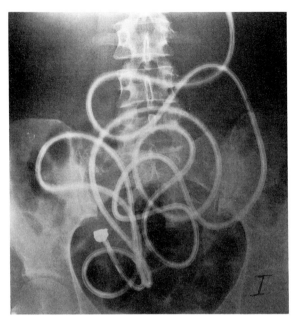

Figure 7. The long multilumen assembly with the tip placed near but not across the ileocaecal valve. Note the sharp bend of the tube at the location of the cuff as outlined by the steel rods.

Miniature Electronic Transducers

As an alternative to the low-compliance open-tip perfused-tube system, manometry can also be performed through tube-mounted strain gauges.

Miniature pressure transducers are available for use as motility probes (see Appendix for manufacturers).

In theory, small changes in intraluminal pressure might be recorded even more accurately, since distortion of only part of the circuit within the strain gauge is necessary to generate a signal. In an elegant experimental study in dogs, Valori et al (1986) compared the motor activities recorded from the antrum and duodenum by two simultaneously applied intraluminal techniques, the tube-mounted strain gauge and the perfused tube system (Figure 9), with those obtained from serosal mounted strain gauges. The results showed that the tube-mounted strain gauge recorded fewer phasic contractions than the perfused tube (Figure 10) but the tube-mounted strain gauge was less sensitive to regional and anatomical variation and recorded tonic contractions as well or better than the perfused tube. For most studies the tube-mounted strain gauge will provide essentially the same information as the pneumo-hydraulic systems.

The electronic transducers are attractive because they can be used in portable systems, one of which is illustrated in Figure 11. Registrations on freely moving individuals outside the laboratory environment will be possible (Figure 12). Together with expansion of portable data-storing

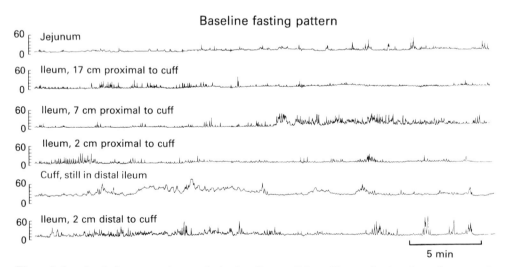

Figure 8. Intraluminal pressure changes during baseline conditions. Note tonic elevations of pressure in cuff recording probably secondary to longitudinal bend of the cuff.

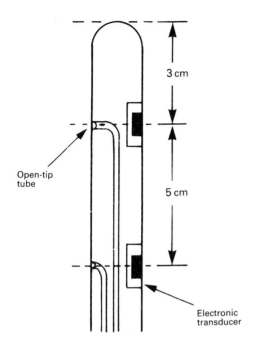

Figure 9. Tube for simultaneous recording of pressure with electronic transducer and conventional open-tip tube. Reproduced with permission from Valori et al, 1986.

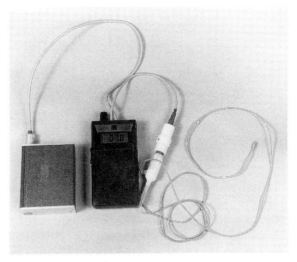

Figure 11. Portable manometry system from Gaeltec in use at the Gastroenterology Unit, The London Hospital. By courtesy of Dr D. Kumar.

equipment, registrations of motility patterns in outpatients will be possible during periods of 24 hours or even longer.

The problems with the electronic transducers are the high cost and relative fragility. It is also difficult to mount the transducers closely spaced and there is a limit to the number of transducers that can be used at the same time.

Limitations of Manometry

It has been suggested that the manometry tube optimally records pressure changes within a sealed cavity and its ability to detect more subtle changes in pressure, not associated with lumen obliterating contractions, has been questioned. There are also well-known difficulties in getting good signals from the gastric fundus and parts of the colon and recordings in small bowel segments affected by heavy dilatation. Manometry in the upper digestive tract in the postprandial state is disturbed by solid food components, not to speak about manometry in the unprepared colon.

Another area of concern regarding the very long manometry tubes intended for investigation of the entire small bowel is the distortion of the normal anatomy induced by the tube. Probably small bowel loops will telescope onto the tube with unknown effects on motility patterns.

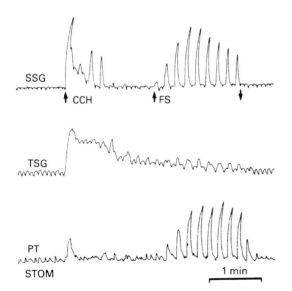

Figure 10. Comparison of serosal strain gauge (SSG), electronic transducer (TSG) and open-tip tube (PT) recording in the stomach (STOM) in response to intra-arterial carbachol (CCH) and local field stimulation (FS). Reproduced with permission from Valori et al, 1986.

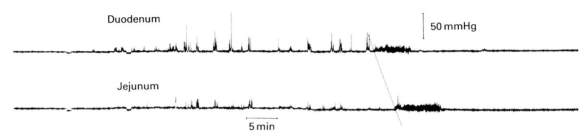

Figure 12. Manometry tracing from a freely moving volunteer recorded by miniaturized transducers. By courtesy of Dr D. Kumar.

Acknowledgements

We are grateful to Dr Karsten Kraglund and Dr Devinder Kumar for providing illustration material and to Dr Sidney F. Phillips for valuable comments upon the manuscript.

References

Arndorfer R. C., Stef, J. J., Dodds, W. J., Linehan, J. H., and Hogan, W. J., (1977), Improved infusion system for intraluminal esophageal manometry. *Gastroenterology*, **73**: 23–27.

Dent, J., (1976), A new technique for continuous sphincter pressure measurement. *Gastroenterology*, **71**: 263–7.

Dent J., Dodds, W. J., Schiguchi, T., Hogan, W. J., and Arndorfer, R. C., (1983), Interdigestive phasic contractions of the human lower esophageal sphincter. *Gastroenterology*, **84**: 453–60.

Gustavsson, S., Kraglund, K., and Phillips, S. F., (1987), Experiments with the Kraglund cuff tube for measurement of ileocecal sphincter pressure. To be published.

Kerlin, P., Tucker, R., and Phillips, S. F., (1983), Rapid intubation of the ileo-colonic region of man. *Aust. NZ. J. Med.*, **13**: 591–3.

Malagelada, J.-R., Camilleri, M., and Stanghellini, V., (1986), *Manometric Diagnosis of Gastrointestinal Motility Disorders*. Thieme Inc., New York.

Mathias, J. R., Sninsky, C. A., Millar, H. D., Clench, M. H., and Davis, R. H., (1985), Development of an improved multi-pressure-sensor probe for recording muscle contraction in human intestine. *Dig. Dis. Sci.*, **30**: 119–23.

Quigley, E. M. M., Borody, T. J., Phillips, S. F., Wienbeck, M., Tucker, R. L., and Haddad, A., (1985), Motility of the terminal ileum and ileocecal sphincter in healthy humans. *Gastroenterology*, **87**: 857–66.

Quigley, E. M. M., Dent, J., and Phillips, S. F., (1987), Manometry of canine ileocolonic sphincter: comparison of sleeve method to point sensors. *Am. J. Physiol.*, **252**: G585–91.

Valori, R. M., Collins, S. M., Daniel, E. E., Reddy, S. N., Shannon, S., and Jury, J., (1986), Comparison of methodologies for the measurement of antroduodenal motor activity in the dog. *Gastroenterology*, **91**: 546–53.

Appendix

Manufacturer of triple- and single-lumen tubings:
Dural Plastics & Eng Pty Ltd
Dural, NSW 2158
Australia

Manufacturer of opaque tubings:
Ferraris Development & Eng Co Ltd
26 Lea Valley Trading Estate, Angel Road
Edmonton, London N18
UK

Manufacturer of manometry tubes and pneumohydraulic systems:
Arndorfer Medical Specialities Inc
5656 Grove Terrace
Greendale, Wisconsin 53129
USA

Manufacturer of manometry tubes, including cuff tubes and steel capillaries:
William Cook Europe A/S
Sandet 8, Bjaeverskov
DK 4632, Denmark

Manufacturer of electronic transducers:
    Gaeltec Ltd
    Dunvegan
    Isle of Skye
    IV55 8GU
    UK

Millar Instruments Inc
USA

Synectics AB
Renstiernas g12
Stockholm, Sweden

6
RADIOTELEMETRY

Roland Valori
Selly Oak Hospital, Birmingham, UK

Introduction

The first reports of radiotelemetry used to measure gastrointestinal motility emerged in the late 1950s. After some initial enthusiasm, its popularity declined until 20 years later when it became an accepted method of monitoring motility (Thompson et al, 1982). Three factors were important in this renaissance. First, tethering of the radiotelemetric capsules or radio-pills allowed measurement of motility in a single position. Second, it became possible to use more than one sensor to examine migrating activity (Figure 1) and finally, miniaturization of recording equipment and the new 24-hour ECG cassette recorders allowed more prolonged studies on fully ambulant patients.

Description

Radio-pills are small capsules (28×8 mm) made up of three compartments: a pressure-sensing device, usually housed in the nose-cone of the capsule; some micro-electronics and a radio-transmitter in the centre; and a battery compartment in the rear. One or two radio-pills are tied to a long thread covered with a radio-opaque tubing (Figure 2) and then swallowed by the subject. When in the correct position (determined

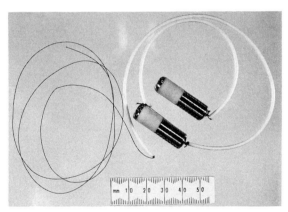

Figure 2. Two radio-pills attached, 15 cm apart, to silk thread. The thread is covered with radio-opaque tubing proximal to and between the radio-pills.

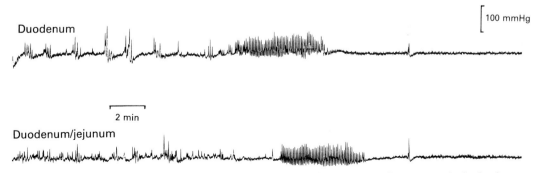

Figure 1. Recordings of fasting motor activity obtained from two radio-pills tethered 15 cm apart in the duodenum. The recording shows phases II, III and I sequentially. The migratory nature of phase III is clearly visible.

fluoroscopically), the thread is tethered to the subject's cheek. The radio-pills are retrieved orally by gentle traction, or the thread can be cut and the capsules recovered later from the stools.

Radio-pills can use either the AM or FM radio wavebands for transmission. The signal is usually fairly weak and directional and it is received by three aerials placed around the subject's trunk in three planes at right angles (Figure 3). The radio signal is processed and amplified by a radio receiver and then recorded onto a chart recorder or onto a slow-moving 24-hour cassette tape. The 24-hour tape is analysed after a study at high speed (24-hour tape in 24 minutes).

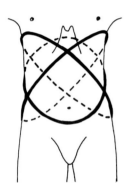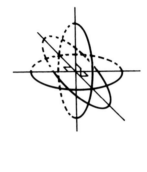

Figure 3. Schematic diagram of aerial arrangement. Three aerials in planes at 90° to each other optimize radio-reception.

Comparison with Other Systems

Like a new drug, a new manometric system must be compared to the best available systems (Table 1). Currently, low-compliance perfused catheters and miniature sensors mounted on the end of cables offer the best alternatives to radio-telemetry.

Low-compliance perfused catheters are much more popular than pressure sensors on cables. They have good pressure-response characteristics, unlike balloons and water-filled catheters, and replacement catheters are easy to make and cheap to buy. Unfortunately, the perfusion apparatus is cumbersome and too heavy to be carried around, restricting its use to the recumbent subject. Like pH profiles, prolonged motility recordings in patients suspected of having motility disorders

Table 1. Comparison of high fidelity manometric systems used to measure gastrointestinal motility.

	Perfused tube	Cable-mounted sensor	Radio-pills
Fidelity	+ + +	+ + +	+ + +
Reliability	+ + +	+ +	+ +
Ambulant studies	0	+ +	+ + +
Flexibility of sensor arrangement	+	0	+ + +
Patient comfort	+ +	+ +	+ + +
Durability	+ + +	+ +	+ + +
Availability	+ + +	+ +	+ +
Current popularity	+ + +	+	+ +
Maximum number of sensors	12	6	2

+ + +   Excellent
+ +   Good
+   Acceptable
0   Poor/not suitable

will almost certainly need to be in ambulant patients. While much helpful information about motility has been obtained in stationary subjects, the perfused catheter obviously has limitations in its future role as a diagnostic tool.

Both radio-pills and cable-mounted sensors are ideally suited to ambulant recordings of motility. In this mode, they have been used successfully to investigate healthy volunteers and patients (Thompson et al, 1980; Valori et al, 1986). How will the future investigator of gastrointestinal motility decide which system to use? Each system works well for extended periods (24 hours or more) with minimal supervision and the cost per sensor is very similar. Currently, radio-pills are restricted to two sensors while the thickness of the cable and the number of available recording channels determines the maximum number of sensors used in the cable-mounted system. In the future, there is no reason why radio-pill systems could not accommodate more sensors and without any need to increase the diameter of the tethering thread.

The position of radio-pills on the tethering thread within the gut can be varied for each individual subject. Once cable-mounted sensors are

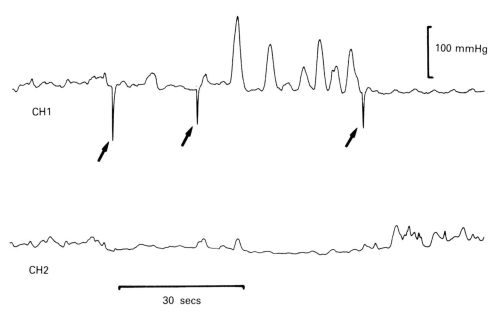

Figure 4. Dual radio-pill recordings demonstrating three episodes of signal loss (marked with arrows).

constructed, changing the position of the sensors is very costly. The cable itself is vulnerable to damage: sharp teeth cutting through thread tethering radio-pills may prematurely abort an experiment, but they will not delay the next one by very long. The main disadvantage of radio-pills is signal loss. Current receiving equipment has minimized this problem and decoding circuits can make sure signal loss is easily recognized as a sharp negative deflection from the baseline (Figure 4). Most published data suggest that signal loss occurs less than 5% of the time. Finally, there is a theoretical problem with dual radio-pills which has not been examined. It is possible that the bowel may sleeve over the distal radio-pill leading to an underestimation of propagation velocity because the

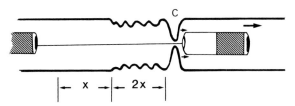

Figure 5. Illustrations of the theoretical appearance of sleeving. As the contraction (C) propels the distal radio-pill forward, bowel 'gathers' up behind it and the length of bowel between the radio-pills increases.

actual length of gut between the sensors has increased (Figure 5). This is less likely to occur in the other systems.

In conclusion, for those clinicians wanting good recording fidelity in ambulant subjects the choice is between radio-pills and 'transducers-*in-situ*'. The former are certainly more versatile but they may be less reliable. There is little to choose between cost, patient acceptability and the durability of the sensors themselves.

Availability

Two radio-pill systems (Rigel and Gaeltec) have been used regularly during the past 10 years. The Rigel radio-pill uses the same principle of pressure-sensing and radio transmission (FM) as when it was first used in the early 1960s. Two radio-pills need two receiving systems but provided the radio-pills transmit at well-separated frequencies there is no radio interference. The radio-pills can be purchased from Remote Control Systems, 12 Leconfield Rd, London NW1, UK and the receiver from Warwick Instruments, Nottingham Science Park, University Boulevard, Nottingham, UK.

The Gaeltec radio-pill is much newer: it uses a pressure-sensitive strain-gauge transducer with pulsed modulation of the pressure signal and it transmits in the MW band. It is available from Gaeltec Ltd, Dunvegan, isle of Skye, IV55 8GU, UK. Details of a dual receiving and playback system have been published (Browning et al, 1983) but the system is not available commercially. The Gaeltec radio-pill is probably superior to the Rigel radiopill but currently the interested investigator would have to construct the receiving and replay system.

References

Browning, C., Valori, R. M., and Wingate, D. L., (1983), Receiving, decoding and noise limiting systems for a new pressure-sensitive ingestible radio-telemetric capsule. *J. Biomed. Eng.*, **5**: 262–6.

Thompson, D. G., Wingate, D. L., Archer, L., Benson, M. J., Green, W. J., and Hardy, R. J., (1980), Normal patterns of human upper small bowel motor activity recorded by prolonged radiotelemetry. *Gut*, **21**: 500–6.

Thompson, D. G., Valori, R. M., and Wingate, D. L., (1982), Radiotelemetry of human jejunal pressure activity: retrospect and prospect. In: *Motility of the Digestive Tract* (Ed. Wienbeck, M.), pp. 255–8, Proceedings of the 8th International Symposium on GI Motility, Raven Press, New York.

Valori, R. M., Kumar, D., and Wingate, D. L., (1986), Effects of different types of stress and of 'prokinetic' drugs on the control of the fasting motor complex in humans, *Gastroenterology*, **90**: 1890–1900.

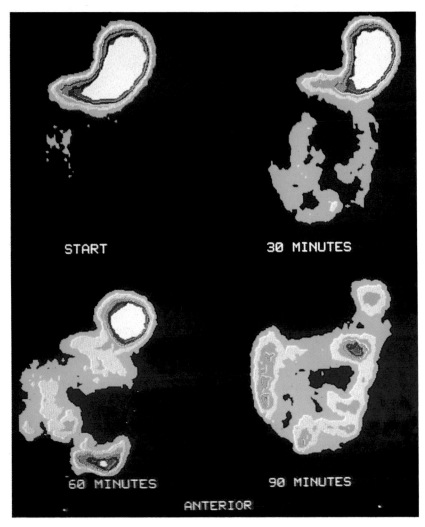

Figure 1. Gamma camera images of orally ingested ^{99m}Tc-DTPA reaching the stomach, small intestine and colon. Courtesy of the Gastroenterology Unit, Mayo Clinic, Director Dr S. F. Phillips.

7
SCINTIGRAPHY

Sven Gustavsson
University Hospital, Uppsala, Sweden

Introduction

Scintigraphy is a rapidly developing area of modern motility research and practice. This chapter reviews the use of gamma cameras for detection of radionuclide tracers in gastrointestinal transit studies. As is evident from Figure 1 an orally ingested radiopharmaceutical agent such as ^{99m}Tc-DTPA will successively reach the stomach, duodenum, small and large intestine and produce an image of each part of the entire gastrointestinal tract. Also the liver parenchyma, the bile ducts, the gall-bladder and the intestine, respectively, can be visualized scintigraphically by intravenous injection of the bile-excreted ^{99m}Tc-HIDA (Figure 2). As is evident from these figures the scintigraphic pictures cannot compete with ordinary contrast X-ray pictures with respect to image resolution. However, the strength of scintigraphy lies in the possibilities of varying the physical characteristics of the radioactive test meal and the avoidance of unphysiological contrast media. Furthermore, the computer-assisted modern scintigraphic technique allows easy quantification of the movement of luminal contents.

Choice of Isotope and Radiopharmaceutical Preparation

The isotope of choice should be a gamma-emitting radionuclide with no associated beta emissions and short half-life. [99m]Technetium, which has been the standard isotope since the 1960s for detection by the gamma camera, comes very near this ideal since it has optimum photon energy for gamma camera detection, as well as widespread availability and affordable price and, finally, gives a low radiation dose due to a suitable half-life (6.0 h). ^{99m}Tc-tagged sulphur colloid or diethylenetriaminepentaaceticacid (DTPA) are the most universally employed radiopharmaceutical agents in motility studies since neither is absorbed from the gastrointestinal tract. Often there is a need for having two different labels in the same study, for

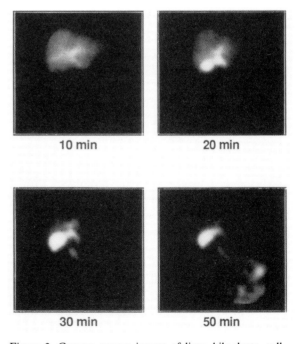

10 min   20 min

30 min   50 min

Figure 2. Gamma camera images of liver, bile ducts, gall-bladder and intestine after intravenous injection of ^{99m}Tc-HIDA. At 10 min the biliary ducts become visualized against the dense liver parenchyma. At 20 min activity is accumulating in the gall-bladder. At 30 min the radioactivity appears in the duodenum and later (50 min) also in the small bowel.

example when studying both liquid and solid gastric emptying. In such double isotope systems the photon energy of ^{99m}Tc (140 keV) can be combined for example with that of ^{111}In (247 keV). With suitable detection equipment overhearing between channels should be minimal.

In gastric emptying studies, the major advantage of isotope methods compared to older intubation techniques using recoverable markers or the use of non-physiologic contrast media, is the ability to assess non-invasively emptying of normal meals. For this purpose the radiolabel must behave, under *in vivo* conditions, like the food it is supposed to represent. This means that it must have a chemical or physical affinity for the food many times that of the surrounding gastric mucosa or unlabelled gastric contents. Also the food itself must be uniformly labelled. The test substance should be incorporated in a meal with normal palatability. The choice of test substance will also depend on whether nutrient or non-nutrient food is going to be studied.

A variety of methods for incorporating radiolabels into test substances has been developed and have correctly identified the behaviour of the test food under simulated or *in vivo* conditions. The emptying of both solid and liquid food components can be studied. To incorporate isotopes into solid meals, the most sophisticated method employs *in vivo* labelling of chicken liver (Meyer et al, 1976). The rapid phagocytosis of circulating colloidal nuclides (^{99m}Tc or ^{113m}In) by the Kupffer cells of the liver of living donor animals has produced test meals with the radiolabel firmly trapped inside cells. However, it has been shown that *in vitro* labelling of liver or egg is a practical alternative with relatively little loss of accuracy (McCallum et al, 1980). So the practical test substance that has emerged for liquid phase gastric emptying is ^{113m}In-DTPA (Heading et al, 1971) and ^{99m}Tc labelling of egg for solids. ^{57}Co and ^{59}Fe could also be used to label hepatocytes. Further, starch has a high affinity for iodine and the cyclotrone-produced ^{123}I has appropriate photon energy for gamma camera detection and is a favourable test substance. Obviously there are many alternatives in creating test substances that mimic ordinary food and there are ample oppor-

tunities to create a test substance that is adequate for the study the researcher has in mind.

Also in studies of oesophageal transit the physical characteristics of the test meal will be of crucial importance for the reproducibility of the test. The strength of oesophageal scintigraphy lies in the possibilities of varying the bolus composition.

An alternative way to get access to the gastrointestinal tract is by means of *in vivo* labelling of bile. ^{99m}Tc-HIDA has a rapid blood clearance after intravenous injection, early concentration in the liver and rapid transit through the liver cells to reach a high concentration in bile. Gall-bladder filling could be studied as well as gall-bladder emptying with or without stimulation of gall-bladder smooth muscles with cholecystokinin. The fate of the radioactivity in the duodenum and small bowel can be monitored to obtain information on small bowel transit and duodenogastric reflux (Wilén et al, 1982, Gustavsson et al, 1982).

Administration of the Radiopharmaceutical Agent

In gastric emptying studies the isotope is generally administered with a normal meal. However, the administration of the tracer by normal eating has inherent problems. In liquid emptying studies the stomach starts the emptying process momentarily and in some instances, e.g. after vagotomy, before all the liquid meal is taken. There are indications that this early emptying of food could quantitatively be of greater importance than the slower emptying during the ensuing hour(s) especially after vagotomy (Gustavsson et al, 1978). Thus it is important not only to consider variables like emptying half-time but also the degree of early emptying. As proposed by Elashoff et al (1982) time 0 is defined as the point at which meal ingestion begins.

Scintigraphic oesophageal transit studies and demonstration of gastro-oesophageal reflux are performed by administration of ^{99m}Tc-tagged sulphur colloid perorally and subsequent scanning of the oesophagus with the gamma camera. Normally the oesophagus is rapidly cleared already by the first swallow (Tolin et al, 1979). These very rapid events pose great demands on the fidelity of the recording equipment. Provocation tests like Valsalva manoeuvre or straight leg raising are used in the reflux part of the study. Also an inflatable abdominal belt could be used to apply a standardized pressure over the abdomen.

Administration of the radioactive, bile-excreted, label is easy since after simple intravenous injection ^{99m}Tc-HIDA is rapidly excreted in the bile. The fate of the radioactivity can be easily followed with the gamma camera (Figure 2).

In small bowel transit studies Read et al (1980) and Caride et al (1984) administered the radioactive tracers perorally, thus measuring also the gastric emptying. However, input of the meal into the small bowel is variable and dependent on gastric emptying. For quantitative studies of small bowel transit isolated from the gastric emptying rate the test substance has to be administered through a naso-jejunal catheter (Read et al, 1983). Another way of administering the isotope to the small bowel is through *in vivo* labelling of bile that eventually reaches the small bowel. Of course this method is dependent on the rate of hepatic clearance, and gall-bladder filling and emptying which limits its usefulness in man. In animals and especially in rats, that lack a gall-bladder, the method has been used extensively for quantitative studies of small intestinal transit (Wilén et al, 1980).

Colonic transit scintigraphy requires intubation of the caecum with a tube that is passed orally and avoids administering isotope in the small bowel, which otherwise would overlap the caecum to some extent. ^{111}In-DTPA or ^{99m}Tc-DTPA is infused with a few millilitres of ileal electrolyte solution and sequential images are recorded (Krevsky et al, 1986). This method also allows estimation of colo-ileal reflux.

Detection Techniques

The rectilinear scanner was used for gastric emptying studies in the early days of gastrointestinal scintigraphy (Griffith et al, 1966). Also in small intestinal transit studies Read et al (1980) scanned the right iliac fossa with a scintillation probe to monitor the appearance of a radio-

labelled marker that had been added to the meal. However, the development of the gamma camera has greatly facilitated detection of radioactivity in motility studies, one advantage being the possibility of separate analysis of different areas of interest in the gamma camera image. At present the computer-assisted gamma camera with a large field of view is the standard equipment for motility studies.

Geometry has to be taken into consideration since the distance between the isotope and the detection camera is of great importance in the measurement of the density of the image and, hence, for quantification of radioactivity in a region of interest. Preferably a geometric mean should be calculated based on anterior and posterior detection cameras. Anterior imaging alone will overestimate radioactivity moving forwards, and radioactivity moving backwards (away from the gamma camera) will be underestimated in the quantitative calculation of radioactivity in an area of interest. Whether the extra trouble and expense of two camera heads and more complicated data handling really pay off in improving data quality in all types of scintigraphic studies is uncertain.

Gamma camera images are stored on magnetic disks and data are processed in a computer. A light pen system on the computer is ideal for selecting regions of interest corresponding to areas under study like the distal oesophagus in gastro-oesophageal reflux studies, the proximal or distal stomach in gastric emptying studies, or the gastric remnant in duodenogastric reflux studies and the right part of the colon in small bowel transit studies (Figure 3). An external ^{99m}Tc point source is used for purposes of body alignment and allows for adequate repositioning of the subject between the images.

Calculation of volumes from gamma camera images can be made, for example, in studies of colonic transit. This requires anterior and lateral gamma camera heads and a computer.

Presentation of the Results

The computer-generated time–activity curves for different regions of interest often need to be nor-

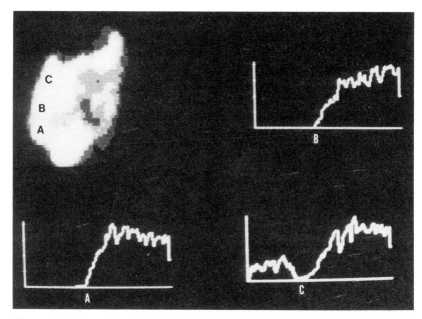

Figure 3. Selection of regions of interest in studies of small intestinal transit. The images consist of separate frames of information concerning activity in the caecum (A), ascending colon (B) and hepatic flexure (C). Time–activity curves are generated from each region. Reproduced with permission from Caride et al, 1984.

malized to 100% at time zero. In gastric emptying studies curves are constructed for liquids and solids versus time expressed as a percentage of the total meal remaining in the stomach versus time. An index for very early emptying as well as the lag period before the commencement of emptying should be given. Alternative ways of presenting emptying data have been discussed by Dugas et al (1982). Due to a significant inter- and intra-individual variation both in liquid and solid emptying and the sensitivity of the test, also for small variations in the test procedure, each laboratory must use its own reference ranges, derived from a large number of normal as well as patient studies. Standardization issues for reporting gastric emptying data have been reviewed by Elashoff et al (1982).

Computer-assisted methods for calculation of intestinal transit of solid and liquid markers have been described (Malagelada et al, 1984).

Clinical Applications

Oesophageal Transit and Gastro-oesophageal Reflux

Beginning with the studies of Kazem (1972) interest in oesophageal radionuclide scintigraphy has increased (Tolin et al, 1979; Ebel and Treves, 1985). The potential advantages of the scintigraphic techniques are that they are rapid, non-invasive, quantitative and associated with a small radiation burden (Figure 4). Scintigraphy gives an oesophageal transit time and an estimation of the efficacy of the oesophageal clearance mechanisms as well as the occurrence of gastro-oesophageal reflux. Further, scintigraphy can be used to assess the effect of position, pharmacological agents, and bolus composition on oesophageal motor function. Theoretically, test substances that adhere to inflamed mucosa can be used as a marker for oesophagitis.

However, the information obtained by scintigraphy can also be obtained by alternative methods and the use of oesophageal scintigraphy

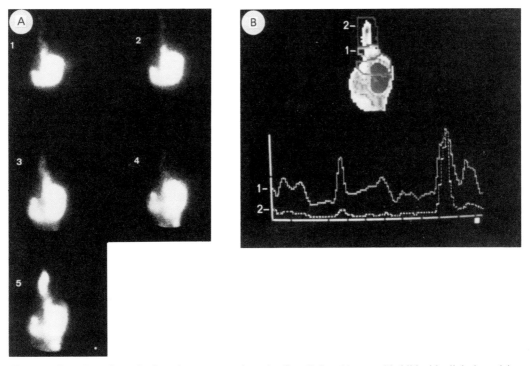

Figure 4. Oesophageal transit, A. and gastro-oesophageal reflux, B. in a 14-year-old child with clinical suspicion of gastro-oesophageal reflux but with normal conventional X-ray studies. Reproduced with permission from Ebel and Treves, 1985.

in clinical practice is limited to centres with special interest (Fisher and Malmud, 1981).

Gastric Emptying of Liquid and Solids

Scintigraphic tests for the emptying of one or two isotopes incorporated into a test meal are increasingly available in hospitals. Emptying of both liquids and solids can be evaluated (Figure 5). It is likely that eventually such tests will be the standard clinical method for assessing gastric emptying. However, using scintigraphic tests to evaluate patients, the physician should always remember that clinical correlation is sketchy at present and that the clinical significance of minor or even moderate abnormalities in gastric emptying is uncertain.

Gall-bladder Motility and Duodenogastric Reflux

Visualization of the gall-bladder (Figure 2) in patients with acute abdomen speaks against the presence of acute cholecystitis. The usefulness of cholescintigraphy for diagnosis of jaundice has declined with the development of ultrasonography, computed tomography, percutaneous trans-hepatic cholangiography and ERCP. Demonstration of biliary reflux to the stomach either in patients with intact gastrointestinal tract or in postgastrectomy states is a widely applied technique (Figure 6). However, the clinician has to remember that scintigraphy cannot differentiate between symptomatic and asymptomatic reflux and the clinical significance of duodenogastric reflux has probably been overemphasized previously. Thus the clinical usefulness of reflux tests is limited.

Small Intestinal Transit

In healthy volunteers the small intestinal transit time after peroral ingestion of ^{99m}Tc-DTPA and lactulose ranged from 31 to 139 min and correlated well with the results of simultaneously applied

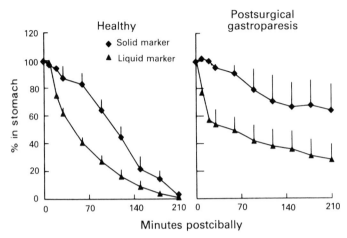

Figure 5. Gastric emptying of liquids and solids in health and in patients with postsurgical gastroparesis. Reproduced with permission from Azpiroz and Malagelada, 1987.

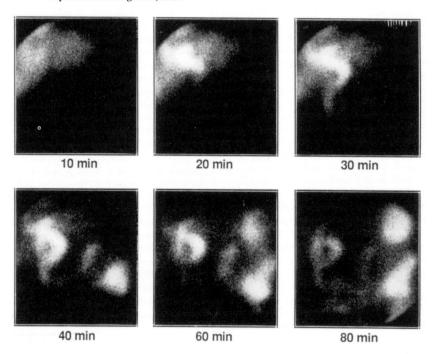

Figure 6. Duodenogastric reflux as demonstrated by cholescintigraphy in a patient with previous subtotal gastrectomy according to Billroth II.

hydrogen breath test (Caride et al, 1984). Using both solid (^{131}I-labelled fibre) and liquid (^{99m}Tc-DTPA) markers, Malagelada et al (1984) showed that both markers progressed along the small bowel separately but at similar speeds. Small bowel scintigraphy is an interesting research tool that has generated new information on small bowel physiology.

Colonic Transit

Colonic transit scintigraphy is a method to monitor, quantitatively, the progression of a marker from caecal instillation to defecation. The caecum and ascending colon was found to empty rapidly with an initial logarithmic progression of

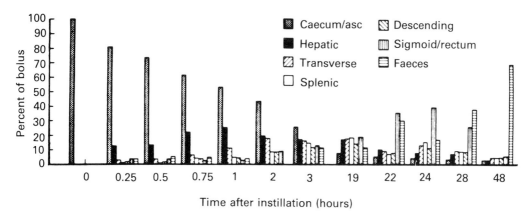

Figure 7. Progression of radionuclide through different parts of the colon as measured by colonic scintigraphy. At 48 hours most of the activity has been excreted. Reproduced with permission from Krevsky et al, 1986.

activity (half emptying time 87.6 ±27 min) (Krevsky et al, 1986). The progression through the remaining colon was slower and linear with time (Figure 7). Scintigraphic studies of colonic transit suggest that the transverse colon, not the caecum and ascending colon, as the primary site of faecal storage. This method provides a tool for further evaluation of normal and abnormal large intestinal physiology.

Limitations of Scintigraphy

The most common problem with the scintigraphic technique is poor image resolution, which makes it difficult or impossible definitely to ascribe radio-activity in the gamma camera image to a specific organ, especially in cases where overlap between organs is present. The problem is particularly pro-nounced in studies of duodenogastric reflux where small bowel loops could be superimposed on the stomach, in small bowel transit studies where ileal loops could be superimposed on the caecum and ascending colon and in colonic transit studies where reflux into the ileum could be superimposed on the sigmoid colon. Special care has to be used in analysing the temporal pattern and differential counting in carefully outlined regions of interest.

Variability of gastric emptying measurement with the standardized radiolabelled meals is rela-

tively large. In a recent study, the mean solid half-emptying time was 58 ± 17 min (range 29–92) while the mean liquid half-emptying time was 24 ± 8 min (range 12–37) (Brophy et al, 1986). When the same individuals were investigated on four different occasions there was a moderate intrasubject variability for solid emptying and high intrasubject variability for liquid emptying. Thus the day-to-day variations in gastric emptying must be considered in the interpretation of individual study results.

It has been established that meals of larger weight and caloric content are associated with longer emptying times for both solids and liquids (Moore et al, 1981). Thus a strict standardization of volume, temperature, palatability, and caloric content of the test meal is of utmost importance to reduce variability. Also the body size will affect the results of gastric emptying tests (Lavigne et al, 1978).

In scintigraphic studies the radioactive test meal comes in close contact with the mucosa and radi-ation exposure has to be considered. The radiation exposure is calculated on the assumption that all activity in the colon will remain there indefinitely, which means that the female gonads will be at risk. At the end of all studies the colon should be checked for remaining activity and evacuation by enemas should be undertaken to diminish exposure.

References

Azpiroz, F., and Malagelada, J.-R., (1987), Gastric tone measured by an electronic barostat in health and postsurgical gastroparesis. *Gastroenterology*, **92**:934–43.

Brophy, C. M., Moore, J. G., Christian, P. E., Egger, M. J., and Taylor, A. T., (1986), Variability of gastric emptying measurement in man employing standardized radiolabeled meals. *Dig. Dis. Sci.*, **31**:799–806.

Caride, V. J., Prokop, E. K., Troncale, F. J., Buddoura, W., Winchenbach, K., and McCallum, R. W., (1984), Scintigraphic determination of small intestinal transit time: Comparison with the hydrogen breath technique. *Gastroenterology*, **86**:714–20.

Dugas, M. C., Schade, R. R., Lhotsky, D., and van Thiel, D., (1982), Comparison of methods for analysing gastric isotopic emptying. *Am. J. Physiol.*, **243**:G237–42.

Ebel, K.-D., and Treves, S., (1985), Pädiatrische nuklearmedizin. In: *Handbuch der Medizinischen Radiologie*, (Ed. Hundeshagen, H.) Band XV/3, pp 465–86. Springer Verlag, Berlin, Heidelberg, New York, Tokyo.

Elashoff, J. D., Reedy, T. J., and Meyer, J. H., (1982), Analysis of gastric emptying data. *Gastroenterology*, **83**:1306–12.

Fisher, R. S., and Malmud, L. S., (1981), Esophageal scintigraphy: are there advantages? *Gastroenterology*, **80**:1066–7.

Griffith, G. H., Owen, G. M., Kirkman, S., and Shields, R., (1966), Measurement of the rate of gastric emptying using chromium-51. *Lancet*, **i**:1244–5.

Gustavsson, S., Hemmingsson, A., Jung, B., Nilsson, F., and Wadin, K., (1978), Gastric emptying in duodenal ulcer patients before and after truncal vagotomy with pyloroplasty and parietal cell vagotomy. *Acta Chir. Scand.*, **144**:379–85.

Gustavsson, S., Enander, L.-K., Jung, B., and Krog, M., (1982), Scintigraphic assessment of biliary reflux into the residual stomach after subtotal gastrectomy and gastrojejunostomy. *Acta Radiologica Diagnosis*, **21**:639–43.

Heading, R. C., Tothill, P., Laidlaw, A. J., and Shearman, J. C., (1971), An evaluation of [113m]indium DTPA chelate in the measurement of gastric emptying by scintiscanning. *Gut*, **12**:611–15.

Kazem, I., (1972), A new scintigraphic technique for the study of the esophagus. *Am. J. Roentgenol. Rad. Ther. Nucl. Med.*, **115**:681–8.

Krevsky, B., Malmud, L. S., D'Ercole, F., Maurer, A. H., and Fisher, R. S., (1986), Colonic transit scintigraphy. A physiologic approach to the quantitative measurement of colonic transit in humans. *Gastroenterology*, **91**:1102–12.

Lavigne, M. E., Wiley, Z. D., Meyer, J. H., Martin, P., and MacGregor, I. L., (1978), Gastric emptying rates of solid food in relation to body size. *Gastroenterology*, **74**:1258–60.

McCallum, R. W., Saladino, T., and Lange, R., (1980), Comparison of gastric emptying rates of intracellular and surface labelled chicken liver in normal subjects. *J. Nucl. Med.*, **21**:67.

Malagelada, J.-R., Robertson, J. S., Brown, M. L., Remington, M., Duenes, J. A., Thomforde, G. M., and Carryer, P. W., (1984), Intestinal transit of solid and liquid components of a meal in health. *Gastroenterology*, **87**:1255–63.

Malmud, I. S., Fisher, R. S., Knight, I. C., and Rock, E., (1982), Scintigraphic evaluation of gastric emptying. *Sem. Nucl. Med.*, **12**:116–24.

Meyer, J. H., MacGregor, I. L., Guellar, R., Martin, P., and Cavalieri, R., (1976), ^{99m}Tc-tagged chicken liver as a marker of solid food in the human stomach. *Am. J. Dig. Dis.*, **21**:296–304.

Moore, J. G., Christian, P. E., and Coleman, R. E., (1981), Gastric emptying of varying meal weight and composition in man. *Dig. Dis. Sci.*, **26**:16–22.

Read, N. W., Miles, C. A., Fisher, D., Holgate, A. M., Kime, N. D., Mitchell, M. A., Reeve, A. M., Roche, T. B., and Walter, M., (1980), Transit of a meal through the stomach, small intestine, and colon in normal subjects and its role in the pathogenesis of diarrhoea. *Gastroenterology*, **79**:1276–82.

Read, N. W., Aljanabi, M. N., Bates, T. E., and Barber, D. C., (1983), Effect of gastrointestinal intubation on the passage of a solid meal through the stomach and small intestine in humans. *Gastroenterology*, **84**:1568–72.

Tolin, R. D., Malmud, L. S., Reilly, J., and Fisher, R. S., (1979), Esophageal scintigraphy to quantitate esophageal transit (quantitation of esophageal transit). *Gastroenterology*, **76**:1402–8.

Tothill, P., McLaughlin, G. P., and Heading, R. C., (1978), Techniques and errors in scintigraphic measurements of gastric emptying. *J. Nucl. Med.* **19**:256–61.

Wilén, T., Gustavsson, S., and Jung, B., (1980), Study of small bowel transport pattern in fasted, conscious rats with an intact gastrointestinal tract. *Eur. Surg. Res.*, **12**: 283–93.

8

ULTRASONOGRAPHY

Peter M. King, R. C. Heading

Edinburgh Royal Infirmary, Edinburgh, UK

Ultrasonic imaging has been employed increasingly as a method for visualizing internal body structures since the early 1970s. Initially widely used as a technique to allow the prenatal examination and diagnosis of fetal abnormalities *in utero*, it has subsequently become a routine diagnostic tool available in most X-ray departments. Ultrasonic imaging is non-invasive and, although in experiments ultrasound has been associated with adverse biological effects produced both by thermal damage to tissues and by cavitation (Liebeskind et al, 1979; Stratmeyer, 1980), human diagnostic ultrasonic imaging is considered to be safe (Kinnear Wilson and Waterhouse, 1984; Cartwright et al, 1984).

The creation of an ultrasonic image is based on the fact that when a beam of very high frequency sound impulses (1.5–10 MHz) is sent into a subject they are reflected back to a varying degree depending on the density of the medium through which they are passing (Donald et al, 1958). As in radar and sonar, the detection of the returning echoes can be used to generate information about the position and nature of the object being scanned. Each returning echo produces a single dot on the screen, the position of which reflects the distance between the transducer and the point of reflection, and the brightness of the dot depends on the density of the reflecting substance (Kikuchi et al, 1957). Strong echoes appear white on the screen whereas low level echoes are dark grey and those of intermediate strength lie at an appropriate point on a grey scale range between white and black. Fluid-filled areas, such as the lumen of the gall-bladder or distended urinary bladder, which do not reflect the ultrasound beam appear black, whereas organ boundaries, which are strongly echogenic, appear white. The parenchyma of tissues such as the liver or kidney appear on the screen as mid-grey. Although differences in the density of most tissue substances are not great, those of bone and particularly air differ markedly from the others and very strong reflections occur at bone–soft tissue or air–soft tissue interfaces. Reflections from these substances are so great that they significantly attenuate the ultrasonic beam and, for all practical purposes, it can be considered impossible to visualize structures lying behind bone or to scan through air-filled bowel. The ultrasonic image is continuously updated at a speed which produces a dynamic picture of the motion of the internal body structures. This type of imaging is termed 'real-time'.

Ultrasonic scanning of the stomach was first performed in attempts to detect and examine disease of the gastric walls (Lutz et al, 1973 and 1976; Walls, 1976). Adequate assessment of the stomach was, however, frequently found to be hampered by the presence of intragastric gas (Warren et al, 1978). However, filling the stomach with liquid to displace the intragastric gas and distend the gastric walls results in an echo-free fluid-filled lumen (Holm, 1971), allowing the stomach wall to be more easily identified and also providing a sonic window to deeper structures such as the tail of the pancreas (Holmes et al, 1973; Sample et al, 1975). During the course of ultrasonic examinations with the stomach filled with fluid, contractions of the antral walls were often noted, but because the rapid emptying of the fluid from the stomach made the technique somewhat transient and unreliable (Weighall et al, 1979), the subjects were often given an injection of hyoscin-N-butylbromide (Buscopan) or glucagon to inhibit gastric peristalsis and, by delaying gastric emptying, prolong gastric distension.

Real-time ultrasonic imaging has subsequently been used in attempts to measure directly the rate of emptying of liquid (Bateman and Whittingham, 1982) and mixed solid–liquid test meals (Bolondi et al, 1985) from the human stomach. In the former technique a real-time linear array scanner consisting of 60 or more transducers was used to produce a series of parallel two-dimensional cross-sectional images of the liquid-filled stomach. From the multiple two-dimensional cross-sections a three-dimensional representation of the stomach was constructed and the intragastric volume calculated. By repeating each multiple scan at regular intervals after ingestion of a liquid test meal, its rate of emptying from the stomach could be calculated. In the latter technique a high-resolution real-time scanner linked to a 3.5 MHz linear array transducer was used to measure the changes in cross-sectional area of the gastric antrum at 30-minute intervals after the ingestion of the solid–liquid test meal. Calculation of gastric emptying rates using ultrasound has recently been shown to correlate well with more conventional methods such as scintigraphy (Holt et al, 1986).

Ultrasonic imaging has also been used specifically in attempts to assess gastric contractile activity. Bateman and co-workers (1977) recorded gastric antral contraction rates using a B-scan plus time-motion (T-P mode) scan technique. However T-P mode does not produce an easily recognizable image of the area of the stomach under examination and thus provides only limited information about contractions. Holt and co-workers (1980) then suggested that real-time ultrasound would provide a dynamic image of the intragastric events and thus might permit an assessment to be made of the spatial relationships between movement of the stomach walls and the luminal contents. Adam and co-workers (1982) subsequently reported the results of a small pilot study in which, using real-time imaging, they

attempted to examine the relationship between gastric motility and the movement of echogenic particles of ground-up biscuit ingested along with a liquid test meal.

Since then we have developed a reliable technique for studying the motility of the gastro-duodenal region using real-time ultrasound imaging and have reported the results of some of our investigations both in normal subjects and patients (King et al, 1984, 1985, 1987). In this chapter we will discuss our method in some detail and the accompanying illustrations will be used to highlight certain points. We make no excuses for the nature of the discussion, as we feel strongly that the illustrations, which are single frames from a continuous recording of events visualized as they occur, cannot really impart to the reader the dynamic nature of the technique. We rather hope that the description of our method will stimulate others to use and subsequently further develop real-time ultrasonic imaging as a method for studying gastrointestinal pathophysiology.

The image produced by real-time ultrasonic imaging can be considered two-dimensional

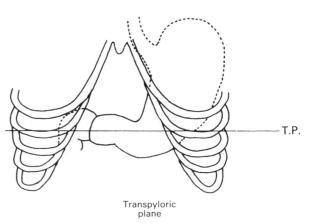

Transpyloric
plane

Ultrasound probe positioned to
obtain a transverse section

Figure 1. Line drawing of transpyloric plane. Ultrasonic examinations are begun by positioning the handheld probe on the anterior abdominal wall of the subject at the midpoint of the transpyloric plane (T.P.). The pylorus lies deep to this point. Adjustments are then made to the orientation of the probe to allow visualization of the gastroduodenal region.

representing a cross-section through the under-lying structures being examined. In order to obtain simultaneous visualization of a number of intra-abdominal structures, it must be possible to orientate the probe so that the imaging plane transects them all. Variations in subject anatomy may sometimes make it difficult to determine the precise location and orientation of the more mobile intra-abdominal organs such as the fundus and proximal antrum of the stomach. However, the retroperitoneal structures are relatively fixed in position, and their relationships to other struc-tures can be used as a reference to facilitate orien-tation of the ultrasonic image. In most subjects the first part of the human duodenum and pylorus lie retroperitoneally (Oliva et al, 1981), and in any individual the pylorus is said to lie deep to the midpoint of a transverse plane (Figure 1) situated half-way between the xiphisternum and the umbilicus (transpyloric plane). Consequently we begin the examination of any subject by posi-tioning the ultrasonic probe at the midpoint of the transpyloric plane and scanning transversely. Thereafter small adjustments are made to the orientation of the probe to bring the stomach and/or duodenum into view.

The fluid-filled lumen of the stomach appears as a black sonolucent area when examined using ultrasound. Although this echo-free area enhances visualization of the gastric walls, the lack of echoes makes it impossible to determine whether there is any movement of the intraluminal fluid. It is therefore necessary to incorporate in the test meal a particle of a suitable size which, when suspended in the luminal contents, would be detectable by the ultrasound technique. The visible movement of the particles will then reflect the movement of the liquid. The particles should be large enough to render them sufficiently echogenic to be visible ultrasonically, but not so large that their behaviour would represent that of intraluminal solids rather than liquids; and since the emptying charac-teristics of solids less than 2 mm in diameter have been shown to be indistinguishable from liquids (Meyer et al, 1981), a particle size of up to 2 mm should be permissible. In order to maintain the individual particle size once ingested along with a test meal, they should neither be susceptible to

breakdown by the digestive processes nor exhibit any tendency to aggregate into larger clumps. Ingestion of the particles should not expose the subject to any risk and, in addition, their com-position should not influence the physical charac-teristics of the test meal (e.g. negligible calorific value).

Natural bran flakes, which are actually the outer layers (husks) of wheat grain removed during the milling process, are readily available from health food shops and are inexpensive. These bran flakes vary in size from powder to around 0.5 cm. By a process of alternately sieving the flakes through wire mesh of two different sizes, discarding the material less than 1 mm, chopping up that greater than 2 mm in a blender and then repeating the whole process, it is possible to manufacture a large quantity of uniformly sized small bran particles. Multiple random sampling of the particles once they have been immersed in the test meals shows the majority to have a wet particle size of 1.5 mm. *In vitro* exposure of the bran to gastric juice revealed it to be indigestible, and the particles themselves exhibit no tendency to aggregate into larger clumps. The particles do tend after a while to settle out of suspension, but when ingested remain suspended in the liquid phase long enough to reflect its movement for the duration of each study. We have found that adding 0.5 g of the chopped and sieved bran particles to each 500 ml test meal (Figure 2) results in a sufficient density of echogenic particles suspended in the stomach to allow the detection of intraluminal fluid move-ment.

In order to confirm that the movement of the bran particles did in fact reflect that of the liquid we compared their gastric emptying charac-teristics using scintigraphic techniques. The radionuclides utilized were [113m]In to label the bran particles, and ^{99m}Tc as the liquid-phase marker. Each subject, who was standing, consumed a labelled 500 ml liquid test meal containing 0.5 g of labelled bran particles. Then, using a dual isotope gamma camera, the abdomen of each subject was scintiscanned at regular intervals during the fol-lowing 60 minutes. The amount of each isotope remaining in the stomach after successive intervals was measured and from these results the emptying

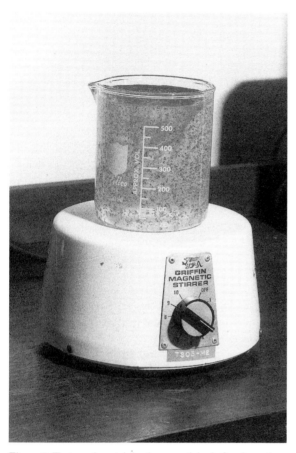

Figure 2. Test meal containing bran particles before ingestion. All test meals contain 0.5 g of fine bran particles which, when suspended in the gastric contents, produce recognizable ultrasonic echoes. The movements of these particles reflects that of the test meal in which they are suspended.

an anechoic periphery representing the ultrasonic appearance of the muscle in the gastric wall, and an echogenic centre composed of gastric mucosa, mucus, and the difference in acoustic impedance between the gastric wall and lumen (Fakhry and Berk, 1981). This olive-shaped area lies anterior to the aorta, inferior vena cava and lumbar spine (Figure 4). The easily recognizable sonolucent area of the gall-bladder, which often lies close to the duodenum, also provides a useful landmark. Respiratory and other movements by the patient rendered it necessary for the orientation of the probe on the anterior abdominal wall to be maintained by hand so that minor adjustments could be made continuously to compensate for these movements. The subjects are examined seated upright because in this position any intragastric gas which if present in the area under examination would scatter and attenuate the ultrasonic beam, collects high in the fundus well away from the distal stomach (Warren et al, 1978). In addition, in the upright position overlying gas containing bowel such as the transverse colon tends to hang down below the level of the pylorus. Posture, however, is said to have little effect on gastric emptying of nutrient liquids in normal individuals (Hunt et al, 1965; Burn-Murdoch et al, 1980; Muller-Lissner et al, 1983), thus we feel it is not unreasonable to compare the results of the ultrasonic studies performed in seated subjects with

characteristics of the ^{113m}In and ^{99m}Tc could be calculated. During the first 10 to 20 minutes after ingestion of the test meal there was no significant difference between the emptying of the ^{113m}In and ^{99m}Tc. Thereafter, however, their emptying characteristics were significantly different. This was presumed to be due to ^{113m}In-labelled bran particles settling out of the liquid and being left behind in the stomach as the liquid emptied.

The ultrasonic examinations are performed after an overnight fast in subjects who are seated upright (Figure 3). In fasted subjects the proximal antrum and fundus of the stomach are usually not readily identifiable. The pylorus, however, can often be visualized as an olive-shaped area with

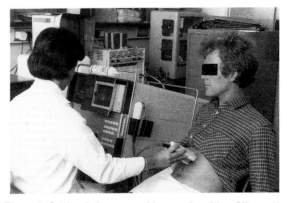

Figure 3. Subject being scanned in seated position. Ultrasonic scanning of the upper abdomen is performed with the subject seated upright. Any intragastric gas, which tends to reflect and scatter the ultrasonic beam and distort the image, collects in the gastric fundus well away from the areas under observation.

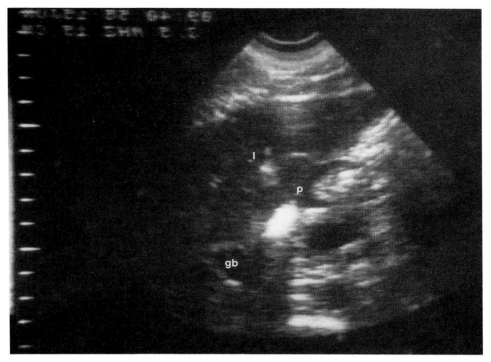

Figure 4. Ultrasonic image of the gastroduodenal region before ingestion of liquid. Transverse B-scan, using a 3.5 MHz probe, of the upper abdomen at the level of the transpyloric plane. The anterior abdominal wall is at the top of the image. The pylorus (p) can be seen as an olive shaped area just to the right of centre of the image, lying below the liver (1). The sonolucent area of the gall-bladder (gb) is situated to the left of centre towards the bottom of the image.

those of the many other investigators who have performed their studies on gastroduodenal function in recumbent subjects.

We use a test meal of 500 ml as this volume has been found by several investigators who have previously examined the stomach with ultrasonic imaging (Warren et al, 1978; Weighall et al, 1979) to induce moderate gastric distension and the anechoic fluid-filled lumen renders visualization of the walls of the gastric antrum, pylorus and proximal duodenum much easier. Subsequently test meals of this volume were also used in studies where ultrasonic imaging was specifically applied to the investigation of gastric function (Bateman et al, 1977; Holt et al, 1980; Bateman and Whittingham, 1982). Ingestion of a volume of 500 ml is known to interrupt the interdigestive cycle of fasting individuals (Rees et al, 1979) and results in a pattern of gastroduodenal motor activity which resembles that of the postprandial period.

The test meals are warmed to a temperature of 37°C. Variations in the temperature of ingested material may influence its rate of emptying from the stomach and, in addition, lower temperatures are associated with inhibition of gastric contractions (Bateman et al, 1977). At present the test meals used in our investigations have all been at 37°C so that temperature-induced variations in gastric emptying and gastroduodenal motility between different subjects would be eliminated. However, we did assess the effect of altering other physical characteristics of the test meals such as pH, osmolality and calorific value according to the criteria of the particular study in which the effect of their variation was being assessed.

Our subjects ingest the 500 ml test meals over one to two minutes, and during this time the passage of the liquid into the stomach was monitored with the ultrasonic techniques. The actual ingestion of the test meal is accomplished by the subject drinking it through a straw, which reduces the amount of air swallowed while drinking and helps to minimize the artefacts produced by air bubbles in the liquid (Crade et al, 1978). Subsequently, when the observations were reviewed and then analysed, the time at which ingestion of the test meal was completed was deemed time zero (the actual start of the observations). Calculation of the interval between time zero and the start of the subsection of the observations in which the relationships between the gastroduodenal contractions and intraluminal fluid movements were analysed in detail was necessary to ensure that the results from each subject came from a comparable portion of the postprandial period.

The ultrasonic imaging technique is used to allow simultaneous visualization of the motor activity of the distal stomach, pyloric canal and proximal duodenum and also the associated movements of the intraluminal contents. To do this, the video recordings of the ultrasonic observations made following the ingestion of any test meal are reviewed to identify those periods when a clear image of the above structures has been maintained without interruption and is coupled with a sufficient density of bran particles suspended in the luminal contents to identify movement across the pylorus. Figure 5 is taken from such a period of recording. In the context of studies where the primary objective is the investigation of transpyloric flow, we take the view that even momentary loss of the plane of imaging through the pyloric channel is not permissible, and so the sections of the recordings that are considered suitable for detailed analysis are often of short duration. We feel, however, that a section to be analysed should last at least two minutes.

Identification of the sections of the recordings suitable for analysis is usually more rapidly accomplished by viewing a fast replay of the obser-

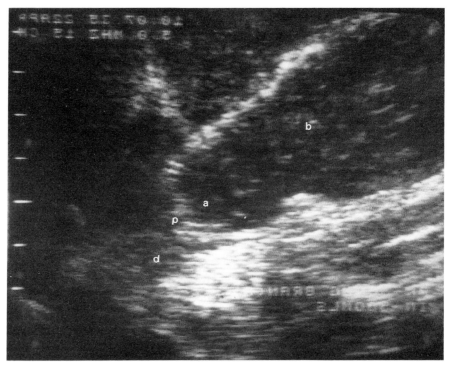

Figure 5. Ultrasonic image of the gastroduodenal region illustrating the criteria for analysis. Transverse B-scan using a 5 MHz probe. The recorded image is considered suitable for analysis when the gastric antrum (a), pylorus (p) and first part of the duodenum (bulb) (d) are visualized simultaneously, in conjunction with a sufficient concentration of echogenic bran particles (b) suspended in the luminal contents to allow the detection of transpyloric movement.

vations, since the resultant time-scale compression markedly enhances the appreciation of movement. The selected sections are subsequently analysed at normal speed.

Our detailed observations on intraluminal fluid movement have been confined to the pyloric channel. It must be appreciated that particle movement in and out of the imaging plane can lead to a false impression of movement, particularly in the relatively voluminous gastric antrum and duodenal bulb. However, because the pyloric channel is comparatively narrow and transpyloric fluid movement tends to be linear in a gastroduodenal direction (forward flow [FF]) or a duodenogastric direction (retrograde flow [RF]) we feel that by maintaining the imaging plane through this region, any observed particle movement should be a true representation of the events.

In an effort to minimize errors due to observer variability the section of the recorded observations undergoing detailed analysis is reviewed on several occasions, so that each event (i.e. TAC, DC, FF, RF) is studied by two independent observers on at least six occasions. The transfer of the timing and duration of the intra-abdominal events visualized on the ultrasound screen on to 'hard copy' is accomplished by using a simple push-button event-marking system and a continuous four-channel chart recorder (Figure 6). One observer

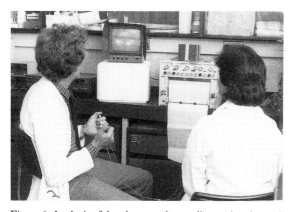

Figure 6. Analysis of the ultrasound recordings using the push-button event-marking system. Analysis is performed by two independent observers who use a push-button event-marking system to transfer the observed events (i.e. terminal antral and proximal duodenal contractions and gastroduodenal and duodenogastric particle movement across the pylorus) onto a four-channel chart recorder.

with a separate push-button in each hand watches the video recording for the occurrence of terminal antral and proximal duodenal contractions and presses the appropriate button whenever these events occur. The observer also has two push-buttons and uses them to denote the occurrence and direction of particle movement through the pylorus. After the third review of each section undergoing analysis, the observers swap over.

An example of repeated analysis of a section from a video record with the event-marking system is illustrated in Figure 7. An event is judged to have occurred if two or more closely grouped observations by separate observers are marked on the chart paper. However, in order to provide a 'best estimate' of the timing and duration of each event judged to have occurred, an average is made of the individual observations on that event. Some observer variation can be seen in Figure 7, particularly in regard to duodenogastric flow (RF). An indication of this variation can be seen from the number of individual observations on the chart which cannot be included in any group of observations. Each time a subject is scanned by the ultrasonic technique and satisfactory visualization of the events at the gastroduodenal junction achieved, a chart plot is constructed from the analysed section of the video recording. The chart plots allow not only calculation of the temporal relationships between the contractile activity of the terminal antrum and proximal duodenum and transpyloric fluid movement in individual studies, but also the comparison of results from several studies.

Figures 8–11 are taken from a section of the video recording from one subject and illustrate the result of the analysis of the ultrasound observations and the subsequent transfer of the timing and duration of the events on to a completed chart plot. An ultrasound scan is shown in the top half of each figure and, below, plotted on a time-scale calibrated in seconds, are the timing and duration of the terminal antral (TAC) and proximal duodenal (DC) contractions and episodes of gastroduodenal (FF) and duodenogastric (RF) flow through the pylorus. Three consecutive gastric cycles have been plotted, with the ultrasound pictures corresponding to the events of the middle

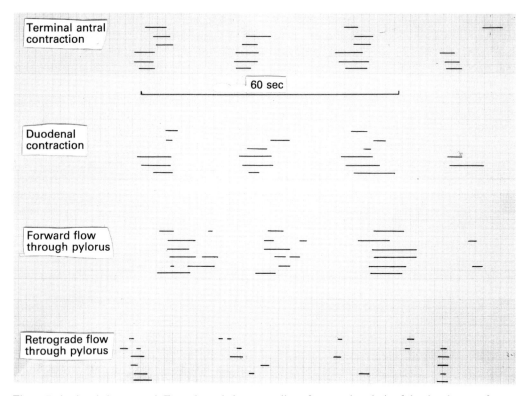

Figure 7. Analysed chart record. Four-channel chart recording of repeated analysis of the timed events from a single subject. Individual observations represented by a single line, on each event are subsequently compared and averaged to provide a 'best estimate' of the timing and duration of terminal antral and proximal duodenal contractions and particle movement through the pylorus.

cycle. The black arrow at the top of the plot shows the time in the cycle at which the picture was taken. In Figure 8 the events are in mid-cycle. There is no antral wave visible in the distal stomach (letter a on figure) and the pyloric (p) and proximal duodenal (d) lumina are widely patent. Ten seconds later (Figure 9), an antral wave (w) has migrated distally and is just about to end in the terminal antral contraction. The pylorus (p) and proximal duodenum (d) are still wide open. Although not apparent from these still pictures, the accompanying plot shows that a short episode of duodenogastric (RF) flow through the pylorus occurred as this antral wave approached the pylorus. A further five seconds later (Figure 10), the terminal and antral contraction (a), pyloric closure (p) and proximal duodenal (d) contraction have occurred and the ultrasound scan shows their lumina to be obliterated. In the final figure of this

series (Figure 11), the terminal antrum (a), pylorus (p) and proximal duodenum (d) have relaxed and their lumina are once again widely patent. Just after this, a short episode of gastroduodenal flow (FF) can be seen to have occurred. The cycle of events was then repeated.

Using the ultrasonic technique we have examined a large number of volunteer subjects and several groups of patients. In the normal subjects we have examined the effects of alterations in the nature of the liquid test meals on gastroduodenal motility and the associated patterns of liquid movement across this region. Our observations demonstrated that although the rhythmic contractile activity was largely unaltered by changes in the composition of the liquid test meals, there were subtle alterations in the patterns of fluid movement (King et al, 1984). In patients with proven gastro-oesophageal reflux we observed that

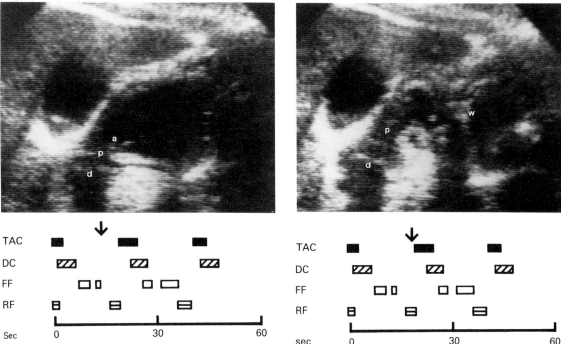

Figure 8. Ultrasonic image of the gastroduodenal region: events are in mid-cycle. Figures 8–11 are a consecutive series of images from a single analysed section of an ultrasound recording and illustrate the transfer of the timing and duration of the observed intra-abdominal events onto a chart plot illustrated in the lower half of each figure. The black arrow at the top of each plot indicates the point in the recording when the picture was taken. There is no antral wave visible in the distal stomach (a) and the pyloric (p) and proximal duodenal (d) lumina are widely patent. TAC, Terminal antral contraction; DC, proximal duodenal contraction; FF, gastroduodenal movement; RF, duodenogastric movement.

Figure 9. Ultrasonic image of the gastroduodenal region: distal migration of antral contraction. Five seconds later in the recording, an antral wave (w) is migrating distally and is about to end in a terminal antral contraction. The pylorus (p) and proximal duodenum (d) are still patent. For abbreviations see Figure 8.

although the pattern of their gastroduodenal contractions was similar to normal they exhibited a significant alteration in the pattern of transpyloric fluid movement (King et al, 1987). We have also examined patients after highly selective vagotomy or truncal vagotomy and pyloroplasty (King et al, 1986). After both types of vagotomy we found a significant increase in the number of episodes of gastroduodenal flow occurring in each gastric cycle compared to normal controls. In addition, we found that, although gastroduodenal motility was normal in patients who had undergone highly selective vagotomy, after truncal vagotomy and pyloroplasty we observed a significant reduction in the degree of antroduodenal co-ordination.

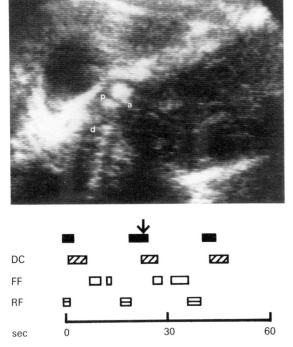

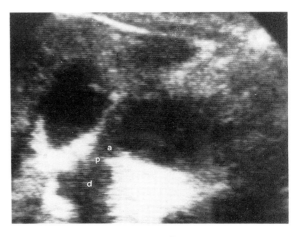

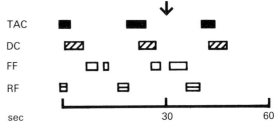

Figure 10. Ultrasonic image of the gastroduodenal region: terminal antral and pyloric contraction. After a further 5 seconds the terminal antrum (a) and proximal duodenum (d) have contracted and the pylorus (p) is closed. For abbreviations see Figure 8.

Figure 11. Ultrasonic image of the gastroduodenal region: relaxation has occurred and the lumina are widely patent. Ten seconds after the events in Figure 10, the terminal antrum (a), pylorus (p) and proximal duodenum (d) have relaxed. For abbreviations see Figure 8.

References

Adam, R. D., Heading, R. C., Anderson, T., and McDicken, W. N., (1982), Application of real-time ultrasonic imaging to the study of gastric motility. In: *Motility of the Digestive Tract* (Ed Wienbeck, M.) Raven Press, New York.

Bateman, D. N., Leeman, S., Metreweli, C., and Willson, K., (1977), A non-invasive technique for gastric motility measurement. *Br. J. Radiol.*, 50:526–7.

Bateman, D. N., and Whittingham, T. A., (1982), Measurement of gastric emptying by real-time ultrasound. *Gut*, 23:524–7.

Bolondi, L., Bortolotti, M., Santi, V., Calletti, T., Gaiani, S., and Labo, G., (1985), Measurement of gastric emptying time by real-time ultrasonography. *Gastroenterology*, 89:752–9.

Burn-Murdoch, R., Fisher, M. A., and Hunt, J. N., (1980), Does lying on the right side increase the rate of gastric emptying? *J. Physiol.*, 302:395–8.

Cartwright, R. A., McKinney, P. A., Hopton, P. A.,

Birch, J. M., Hartley, A. L., Mann, J. R., Waterhouse, J. A. H., Johnston, H. E., Draper, G. J., and Stiller, C., (1984), Ultrasound examinations in pregnancy and childhood cancer. *Lancet*, ii:999–1000.

Crade, M., Taylor, K. J. W., and Rosenfield, A. T., (1978), Water distension of the gut in the evaluation of the pancreas by ultrasound. *Am. J. Roentgenol.*, 131:348.

Donald, I., MacVicar, J., and Brown, T. G., (1958), Investigation of abdominal masses by pulsed ultrasound. *Lancet*, i:1188–95.

Fakhry, J. R., and Berk, R. N., (1981), The 'Target' Pattern: Characteristic sonographic feature of stomach and bowel abnormalities. *Am. J. Radiol.*, 137:969–72.

Holm, H. H., (1971), Ultrasonic scanning in the diagnosis of space-occupying lesions of the upper abdomen. *Br. J. Radiol.*, 44:24.

Holmes, J. H., Findley, L., and Frank, B., (1973), Diagnosis of pancreatic pathology using ultrasound. *Trans. Am. Clin. Climatol. Assoc.*, 85:224.

Holt, S., McDicken, W. N., Anderson, T., Stewart, I. C., and Heading, R. C., (1980), Dynamic imaging of the stomach by real-time ultrasound—a method for the study of gastric motility. *Gut*, **21**:597–601.

Holt, S., Cervantes, J., Wilkinson, A. A., and Wallace, J. H. K., (1986), Measurement of gastric emptying rate in humans by real-time ultrasound. *Gastroenterology*, **90**:918–23.

Hunt, J. N., Knox, M. T., and Oginski, A., (1965), The effect of gravity on gastric emptying with various test meals. *J. Physiol.*, **178**:92–7.

Kikuchi, Y., Tanaka, K., Wagai, T., and Uchida, R., (1957), Early cancer diagnosis through ultrasonics. *J. Acc. Soc. Am.*, **29**:824–33.

King, P. M., Adam, R. D., Pryde, A., McDicken, W. N., and Heading, R. C., (1983), Relationships of human antroduodenal motility and transpyloric fluid movement: non-invasive observations with real-time ultrasound. *Gut*, **25**:1384–91.

King, P. M., Pryde, A., and Heading, R. C., (1984), Human transpyloric fluid movement and related gastroduodenal motor activity. The effects of four different test meals. Presented at the 2nd European Symposium on Gastrointestinal Motility, Oxford. September, 1984.

King, P. M., Heading, R. C., and Pryde, A., (1985), The co-ordinated motor activity of the human gastroduodenal region. *Dig. Dis. Sci.*, **30**:219–24.

King, P. M., Pryde, A., and Heading, R. C., (1986), Effects of truncal vagotomy and pyloroplasty and highly selective vagotomy on antroduodenal motility and transpyloric fluid movement. *Gut*, **27**:1256.

King, P. M., Pryde, A., and Heading, R. C., (1987), Transpyloric fluid movement and antroduodenal motility in patients with gastro-oesophageal reflux. *Gut*, **28**:545–8.

Kinnear Wilson, L. M., and Waterhouse, J. A. H., (1984), Obstetric ultrasound and childhood malignancies. *Lancet*, **ii**:997–9.

Liebeskind, D., Bases, R., Elequin, F., Neubort, S., Leifer, R., Goldberg, E. E., and Koenigsberg, M., (1979), Diagnostic ultrasound: effects on the DNA and growth patterns of animal cells. *Radiology*, **131**:177–84.

Lutz, H., and Rettenmaier, G., (1973), Sonographic pattern of tumors of the stomach and the intestine. *Exc. Med. Int. Cong. Ser.*, **277**:67 (Abst).

Lutz, H., and Petzoldt, R., (1976), Ultrasonic patterns of space occupying lesions of the stomach and the intestine. *Ultr. Med. Biol.*, **2**:129.

Meyer, J. H., Ohashi, H., Jehn, D., and Thomson, J. B., (1981), Size of liver particles emptied from the human stomach. *Gastroenterology*, **80**:1489–96.

Muller-Lissner, S. A., Fimmel, C. J., Sonnenberg, A., Will, N., Muller-Duysing, W., Heinzel, F., Muller, R., and Blum, A. L., (1983), Novel approach to quantify duodenogastric reflux in healthy volunteers and in patients with type I gastric ulcer. *Gut*, **24**:510–18.

Oliva, L., Biggi, E., Derchi, L. E., and Cicio, G. R., (1981), Ultrasonic anatomy of the fluid-filled duodenum. *J. Clin. Ultras.*, **9**:245–8.

Rees, W. D. W., Go, V. L. W., and Malagelada, J. R., (1979), Antroduodenal motor response to solid-liquid and homogenised meals. *Gastroenterology*, **76**:1438–42.

Sample, W. F., Po, J. B., Gray, R. K., (1975), Greyscale ultrasonography, techniques in pancreatic scanning. *Appl. Radiol.*, **4**:63.

Stratmeyer, M. E., (1980), Research in ultrasound bioeffects: A public health view. *Birth Fam. J.*, **7**:92–100.

Walls, W., (1976), The evaluation of malignant neoplasms by ultrasonic B-scanning. *Radiology*, **118**:159.

Warren, P. S., Garrett, W. J., and Kossoff, G., (1978), The liquid filled stomach: An ultrasonic window to the upper abdomen. *J. Clin. Ultras.*, **6**:315.

Weighall, S. L., Wolfman, N. T., and Watson, N., (1979), The fluid-filled stomach: A new sonic window. *J. Clin. Ultras.*, **7**:353–6.

9
ELECTROMYOGRAPHY

Nathaniel J. Soper, Michael G. Sarr
Mayo Medical School, Rochester, Minnesota, USA

Gastrointestinal electromyography represents the extracellular recording of changes in electrical potential generated by the smooth muscle in the wall of the gut. Similar to electrocardiography and electroencephalography, electromyography is the myoelectric correlate of events occurring in the individual array of smooth muscle cells in a given region of interest. Alvarez and Mahoney (1922) were the first to record myoelectric activity from the serosal surface of the feline stomach. They used calomel electrodes implanted on the stomach *in vitro* to send electrical signals to a string galvanometer. Since then, improvements in the fidelity of electronic recording techniques have led to increased interest in electromyography and to the expansion of its indications for use in research and, recently, in clinical practice.

Physiology of Electromyography

The smooth muscle in the wall of the stomach and the intestine generates cyclic changes in electrical potential that can be recorded extracellularly. This cyclic change in electrical potential forms the basis of electromyography. From a cellular standpoint, as measured by intracellular microelectrodes, the smooth muscle cells of the gut undergo a cyclic change in cellular potential related to membrane depolarization/repolarization. When measured by an extracellular electrode, the electrical potential represents the integration of the changes in membrane potential of all the smooth muscle cells in that region and takes the form of slow, rhythmic changes in electrical potential called the 'slow waves' (Szurszewski, 1987). These slow waves are

omnipresent whether the smooth muscle is at rest or contracting (Figure 1). Superimposed on the slow wave may be bursts of rapid changes in electrical potential termed 'spike potentials' (Figure 1). Again, from a cellular standpoint, smooth muscle contraction is associated with a sudden depolarization in membrane potential called the action potential. Action potentials (and thus muscular contraction) can occur only during the depolarization phase of the cyclic change in membrane potential (Bass et al, 1961). The spike potentials measured by the extracellular electrode are the summation of action potentials occurring in individual smooth muscle cells in the region of the electrode. Thus, spike potentials represent the

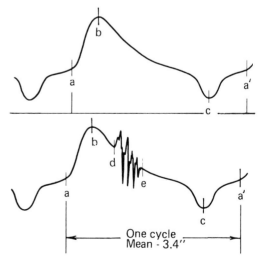

Figure 1. Two cycles of the duodenal slow wave, with and without spike potentials. Reprinted with permission from Bass et al, 1961.

myoelectric correlates of contractile activity
(Figure 2). Because electromyography can distinguish the frequency, amplitude, and morphology of slow waves in the absence or presence
of spikes, it gives information about resting as well
as contracting gastrointestinal smooth muscle,
respectively.

The smooth muscle cells in the wall of the
stomach and in the wall of the small bowel form
an electrically coupled syncytium such that
changes in membrane potential are conducted
rapidly from cell to cell. Although the spontaneous
oscillations of slow waves were originally thought
to be of myogenic origin, recent studies suggest
that a specialized group of closely aligned and
electrically coupled myoneural cells called the
'interstitial cells of Cajal' serve as the 'pacemaker
cells' to induce these cyclic changes in membrane
potential (Thuneberg, 1982). Both the stomach
and small intestine have 'pacemaker' regions in
which these cyclic changes in membrane potential
are generated at a frequency more rapid than the
surrounding areas. The pacemaker in the stomach
is located in the mid-corpus (Hinder and Kelly,
1977), while the pacemaker of the small intestine is
located about 1 cm distal to the pylorus (Herman-
Taylor and Code, 1971). No dominant pacemaker
region is evident in the large intestine. The cyclic
changes in electrical potential, the slow waves,
emanate from their respective pacemaker regions
to pass down the stomach and aborally along the

small intestine by spreading along the smooth
muscle syncytium. Because contractions (spike
potentials) occur only during a specific phase of
the slow wave, the pacemaker regions serve to co-
ordinate the frequency of contractions of the gut.
Whether or not an individual slow wave is
accompanied by spike activity (and thus contraction) is not determined by the slow wave, but
likely by superimposed excitatory or inhibitory
input from neurohormonal stimuli (Weisbrodt,
1987). Thus, while the slow wave co-ordinates the
maximum frequency and direction of propagation
of contractions, other mechanisms control the
excitability of the muscle and the actual pattern of
contractions between different regions.

The frequency of the slow waves, and therefore
the maximum frequency of contractions, varies in
different regions of the gastrointestinal tract. The
normal frequency of the slow wave in the human
stomach is 3 cycles per minute, while in the canine
stomach it is 5 cpm. In most mammals there is a
gradient in the frequency of slow waves in the
small intestine that decreases aborally. In man,
the frequency of the slow wave is greater in the
duodenum than in the ileum (12 versus 8 cpm
respectively); in the dog, these frequencies are 19
and 14 cpm, respectively. The reported frequency
of the slow waves in the human colon is highly
variable, ranging from 2 to 10 cpm in the different
anatomic regions (Szurszewski, 1987).

Gastrointestinal myoelectric activity in man and

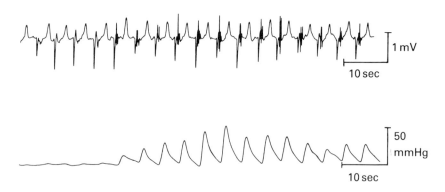

Figure 2. Simultaneous myoelectric activity (top panel) and motor activity (perfused intraluminal catheter; bottom panel) of canine jejunum. Spike potentials are recorded concurrently
with muscular contractions.

in most other nonruminant mammals exhibits characteristic patterns during fasting and after feeding. In the fasted or 'interdigestive state', the migrating myoelectric (or motor) complex (MMC) occurs cyclically throughout the stomach and small intestine. Each cycle of the MMC is composed of four phases (Code and Marlett, 1975). Phase I has little or no electrical spike activity and thus no measurable contractions; Phase II has intermittent spike activity; Phase III, the activity front, has numerous spikes of large amplitude superimposed on virtually every slow wave and is therefore associated with strong contractile activity (Figure 3); and Phase IV is a brief period of intermittent spike potentials leading back to the quiescence of Phase I. In man, the duration of each complete cycle (the period of the MMC) is approximately 90–120 min. The MMC appears first in the lower oesophageal sphincter and stomach and then in the duodenum from where it migrates aborally in an orderly fashion to the terminal ileum, at which time a new cycle begins again in the lower oesophageal sphincter and stomach. The contractions associated with Phase III of the MMC are truly peristaltic and sweep over 30–50-cm lengths of bowel (Dusdieker and

Summers, 1980). These high amplitude contractions are believed to sweep debris from the upper gastrointestinal tract and may thereby function as the 'interdigestive housekeeper' (Code and Schlegel, 1974). Eating abolishes the MMC and induces a pattern of intermittent spike activity which appears similar to Phase II (Figure 3); the duration of this postprandial 'fed' pattern is determined both by the caloric content and the type of nutrient in the meal (DeWever et al, 1978).

Applications of Electromyography

Electromyography has been used extensively *in vivo* to characterize the myoelectric activity from most regions of the gastrointestinal tract in many species of animals. These studies have provided the foundation for much of the current understanding of normal patterns of gastrointestinal smooth muscle activity, and of alterations in contractile activity induced by drugs, by hormones and after various operations (Szurszewski, 1987; Weisbrodt, 1987). Temporary serosal electrodes have been applied to the human gut, but the indications for, and ethics of such investigations are

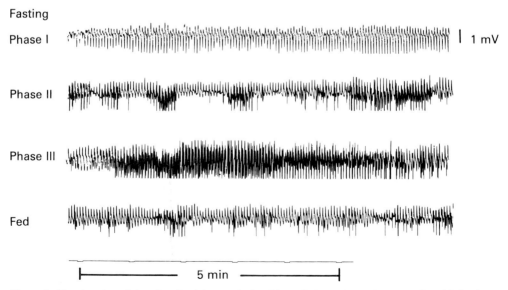

Figure 3. Myoelectric activity of canine jejunum during Phases I, II, and III of the MMC and following a meal. Phase IV is not shown.

Table 1. Advantages of electromyography for the assessment of gastrointestinal motility

Advantages	Disadvantages
Serosal electrodes	
1) Information gained dynamically about non-contracting as well as contracting muscle 2) Avoid stimulation of mucosal receptors 3) Recording sites stationary and precisely localized 4) May study many sites simultaneously 5) Chronic studies possible 6) Electrodes small and inexpensive	1) Require coeliotomy for placement and replacement 2) Intraperitoneal wires may cause adhesive small bowel obstruction 3) Potential risk of erosion into intestinal lumen or adjacent structures 4) Role in human studies not well defined 5) Indirect relationship between electrical and mechanical activity
Mucosal electrodes	
1) Information gained dynamically about non-contracting as well as contracting muscle 2) Relatively easy to position in proximal and distal GI tract 3) Human studies well established 4) May be combined with strain gauges on probes 5) May study many sites simultaneously (multiple electrodes) on a single probe	1) Loss of mucosal contact and thus loss of the signal may occur during study 2) Hazardous if used for long periods; only applicable for acute studies 3) Less precise localization; electrode placement may change with contractions 4) Need for luminal intubation and possibility of motility disorder secondary to intraluminal probe 5) Indirect relationship between electrical and mechanical activity

unclear. In recent years, investigators have used various types of electrodes attached to intubation systems to measure human electromyographic signals in a transmucosal fashion (Fleckenstein, 1978; Frexinos et al, 1985) (see below). When compared to other objective techniques of measuring gastrointestinal motility such as perfused intraluminal catheters and strain gauges, electromyography has distinct advantages and drawbacks, which are displayed in Table 1.

Electrode Systems

Myoelectric activity of the gut is detected by electrodes which monitor a small area of muscle. Many different metals can be used for construction of electrodes, including platinum (Bass, 1968), silver-silver chloride (Code and Marlett, 1975), copper (Fleckenstein, 1978), stainless steel (Richter and Kelly, 1986), and nickel–chrome alloy (Frexinos et al, 1985). Recording electrodes may be either monopolar or bipolar. When a monopolar electrode is placed in contact with the gut wall, an indifferent reference electrode must be placed in an area of minimal electrical potential activity distant from the intestine. The electrodes are connected to an amplifying-recording device. The recorder then measures the dynamic differences in electrical potential between the intestinal and reference electrodes. Bipolar recordings measure electropotential differences between two electrodes closely spaced within the same tissue. Any one of a number of amplifier-recorders may be used. We are most familiar with Grass Model D polygraphs and Gould Brush recorders. When recording electroenterograms, it is necessary to have a frequency response from d-c to approximately 50 Hz to reproduce accurately the slow waves as well as the rapid oscillations of spike potentials. In general, alternating current amplifiers and a time constant of 1 sec yield satisfactory recordings. Using different band pass filtering systems, it is possible to record only slow waves or only spike activity if so desired.

Serosal Electrodes

Either bipolar or monopolar electrodes may be used for chronic recordings. In general, bipolar electrodes give a better signal-to-noise ratio from the stomach, while monopolar electrodes are adequate for the small intestine. We have used the following technique for recording gastric and intestinal myoelectric activity in the Gastroenterology Unit at the Mayo Clinic for over 15 years (Akwari et al, 1975). The electrodes, made of silver wire (1mm diameter), project 1 mm from where they are embedded in an acrylic disk. The electrode shafts are insulated with vinyl paint, but their tips are exposed and coated electrolytically with silver-silver chloride. The shafts of bipolar electrodes are spaced 5 mm apart in a similar acrylic disk. The electrodes are soldered to an insulated copper wire, the junction of which is also embedded (and thus protected) within the acrylic disk. The copper wires are attached to a multi-pinned socket mounted within a flanged stainless steel cannula. The electrodes are implanted on the serosal surface of the bowel by sewing the acrylic disk to the bowel wall. The flanged stainless steel cannula carrying the leads to the surface is positioned within the abdominal wall and fixed to the posterior abdominal fascia with wire sutures. In subsequent recording sessions, this metal cannula is used as the indifferent electrode for monopolar recordings. The components used in our chronic studies are shown in Figure 4.

We have placed temporary serosal electrodes on the duodenum and on the jejunum to monitor myoelectric activity in 16 human subjects after coeliotomy (Richter and Kelly, 1986). Stainless-steel epicardial pacemaker wire electrodes (Ethicon, Inc., Somerville, NJ), 1 mm in diameter, were passed obliquely through the tunica muscularis, such that 6–8 mm of the bare wire was in contact with the muscle. Two wires comprising each bipolar pair were placed 5 mm apart along the longitudinal axis of the gut at each site of insertion. The electrodes were anchored in place with 4-0 absorbable chromic sutures tied around the electrode at its points of entry into, and exit from, the muscularis (Figure 5). The leads were exteriorized through puncture sites in the anterior

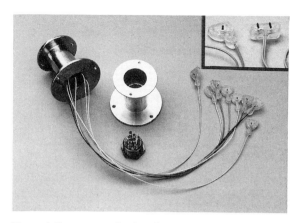

Figure 4. Components for chronic recording of gastrointestinal myoelectric activity in the laboratory animal. Recording unit consists of several electrodes, a flanged stainless steel cannula for implantation within the abdominal wall, and an electrical connector. A bipolar and a monopolar electrode are shown in insert; each consists of silver wire embedded in dental acrylic.

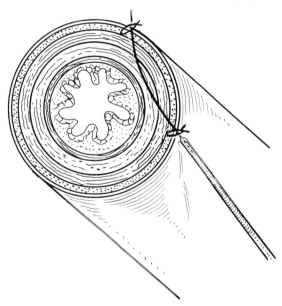

Figure 5. Placement of temporary seromuscular electrode on the human gut. The electrode is orientated obliquely to assure a broad area of contact between the bare wire and intestinal muscularis. Absorbable sutures (4-0 chromic) anchor the electrode in place.

abdominal wall. When recording sessions were completed, the electrodes were removed easily by slow, steady traction. We experienced no complications related to the electrodes.

Mucosal Electrodes

Many different types of electrodes have been attached to probes and used to record trans- mucosal electromyograms in the upper and lower gastrointestinal tract. Recently, investigators in Copenhagen (Fleckenstein, 1978) and Toulouse (Frexinos et al, 1985) have used bipolar ring elec- trodes to monitor human small intestinal and colonic electrical activity, respectively. The ring electrodes are made from two strands of copper or nickel-chrome wire wound around the probe; a 4– 5 mm distance was left between electrode pairs for bipolar recordings. Multiple electrodes at known intervals may be incorporated on a single probe. The tracings published by these groups appear to be reproducible with minimal artefacts (Figure 6). Suction, wick, and clip electrodes have been used in the past, but concerns about their safety and reliability have minimized their use in recent years.

Interpretation of Electromyograms

Electromyography has been performed success-

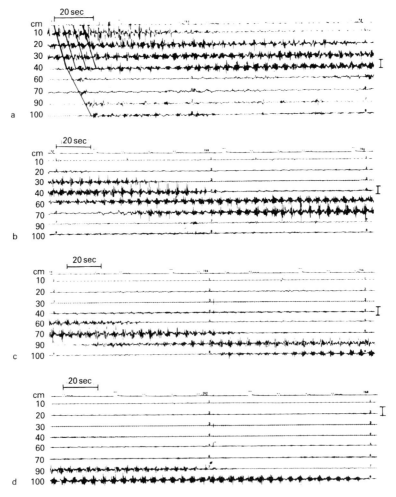

Figure 6. Transmucosal electromyogram from the small intestine in man. Record- ings from bipolar electrodes at various distances from pylorus (vertical axis). Panels a–d represent consecutive recordings of Phase III. Vertical bars = 150 μV. Reprinted with permission from Fleckenstein, 1978.

fully in the stomach, duodenum, jejunum, ileum and colon. In each location, the configuration of the slow waves and the spike potentials differs. An extensive literature has been developed on the electromyographic patterns in the dog, pig, rat, sheep and, more recently, in man. Normal patterns are well described, but the interpretation of changes in myoelectric patterns secondary to

disease states is still in its infancy. Normal gastric slow waves and spike activity are shown in Figure 7A, while Figure 7B portrays tachygastria of the canine gastric antrum. Normal gastric slow wave frequency is 3 cpm in humans and 5–6 cpm in dogs (Kim and Malagelada, 1986). Gastric dysrhythmias, including bradygastria, tachygastria, and gastric arrhythmia, have been described in both

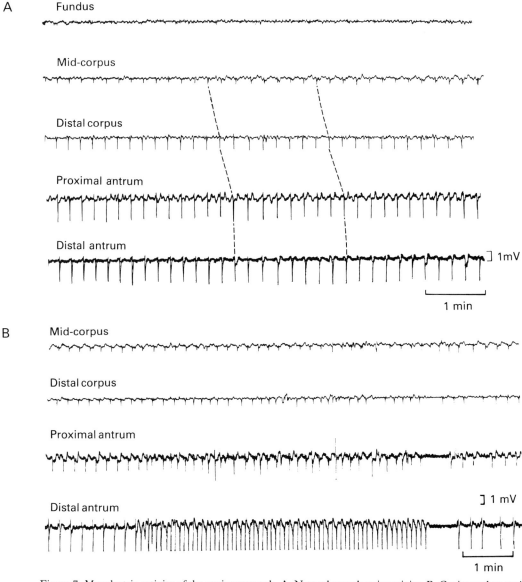

Figure 7. Myoelectric activity of the canine stomach. A. Normal myoelectric activity. B. Canine tachygastria (induced by close arterial infusion of prostaglandin E_2). Reprinted with permission from Kim and Malagelada, 1986.

dogs and humans (Kim and Malagelada 1986), although the clinical importance of these findings has not been established precisely.

Human duodenal electromyographic activity, as recorded by two temporary bipolar serosal electrodes, is shown in Figure 8. This recording was obtained 48 hours following cholecystectomy. The frequency of the slow wave (approximately 12 per minute) is normal. Ten minutes following intramuscular administration of morphine sulphate, spike activity is apparent in both leads, beginning first at the aborad duodenal electrode.

Figure 9 contrasts slow wave and spike morphology of canine jejunum and ileum. Fast paper speeds highlight the configuration of brief individual electropotential events (Figures 1, 2, 7 and

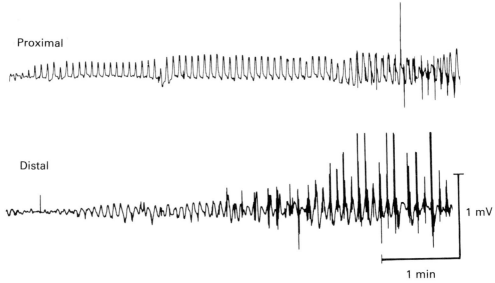

Figure 8. Human duodenal myoelectric activity. Top panel: Bipolar electrodes located 2 cm distal to pylorus. Bottom panel: Electrodes located 8 cm distal to pylorus. Normal slow wave appearance and frequency with superimposed spike potentials following intramuscular administration of morphine sulphate.

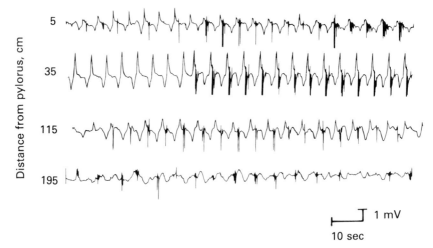

Figure 9. Myoelectric activity of the canine jejunum and ileum measured by multiple serosal electrodes implanted at various distances from pylorus. The configuration and frequency of the slow wave are different in the proximal and distal small intestine.

13). Conversely, Figure 10 displays a multiple-electrode recording with a much slower paper speed which is useful for observing patterns of myoelectric activity, such as the MMC, which occur over a period of hours.

Gastrointestinal electromyographic recordings

are associated with various artefacts which must be recognized as such. The characteristic 'waxing and waning' amplitude of intestinal myoelectric potentials is evident in Figures 3, 8, 10 and 14. This phenomenon is thought to be due to variable synchrony of adjacent populations of smooth

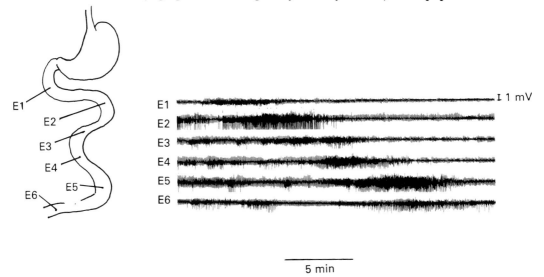

Figure 10. Interdigestive migrating myoelectric complex of the canine jejunum as measured by multiple monopolar electrodes. Phase III spike activity migrates from proximal to distal jejunum.

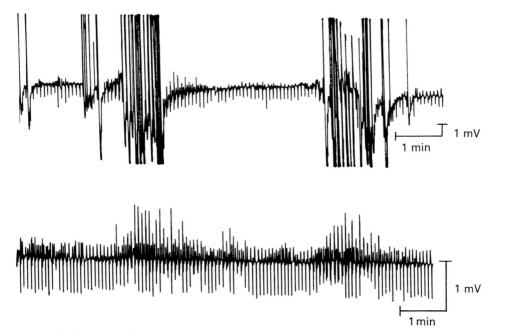

Figure 11. Recording of canine jejunal myoelectric activity using two closely spaced monopolar electrodes. Top panel: degenerating electrode, manifested by intermittent high-amplitude interference occurring only in one electrode. Bottom panel: normal slow wave and spike activity.

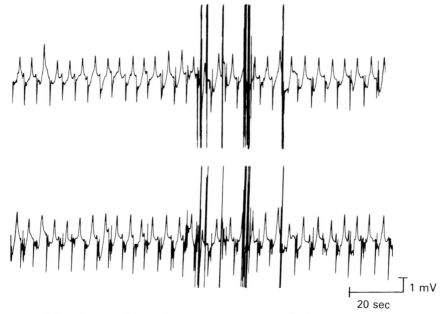

Figure 12. Myoelectric activity of the canine jejunum measured using two closely spaced monopolar electrodes; extrinsic 60 Hz electrical interference occurs simultaneously in both electrodes.

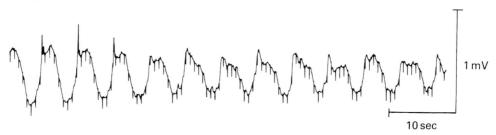

Figure 13. Myoelectric activity of the human duodenum; normal slow waves with superimposed cardiac electrical potentials.

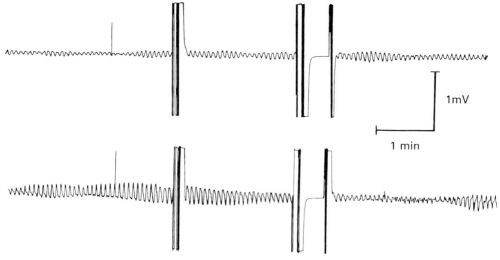

Figure 14. Myoelectric activity of the human duodenum; motion artefact recorded simultaneously from bipolar electrodes placed 2 cm (top panel) and 8 cm (bottom panel) distal to pylorus.

muscle cells in close proximity to an electrode, leading to a diminution or to an amplification of the summed potentials detected by the surface electrode (Szurszewski, 1987). Some other frequently occurring artefacts are depicted in Figures 11–14. These include the degenerating electrode (thought to be due to connective tissue ingrowth or leaching of the metal at the electrode/tissue interface), 60 Hz electrical interference, transmitted cardiac electrical potentials, and motion artefact. In general, extrinsic electrical artefacts occur simultaneously in all channels, while intrinsic events are seen only in individual electrodes.

Future Applications

As is apparent from the foregoing discussion, great strides have been made in the implementation and interpretation of electromyography. In recent years, a number of computer software programs have been developed to assist with electromyographic interpretation. Further refinements of these systems and more familiarity with their use should simplify the analysis of electromyographic data. Continued improvements in probe-directed mucosal electrode systems may lead to wider clinical applications of electromyography and to a greater understanding of intestinal dysmotility syndromes. More widespread use of recording systems employing serosal electrodes in humans awaits the clarification of indications for this diagnostic technique and further refinements in technology, which may include the application of wireless radiotelemetry transmitting electrodes.

References

Akwari, O. E., Kelly, K. A., Steinbach, J. H., and Code, C. F., (1975), Electric pacing of intact and transected canine small intestine and its computer model. *Am. J. Physiol.*, 229:1188–97.

Alvarez, W. C., and Mahoney, L. J., (1922), Action current in the stomach and intestine. *Am. J. Physiol.*, 58:476–93.

Bass, P., Code, C. F., and Lambert, E. H., (1961), Motor and electric activity of the duodenum. *Am. J. Physiol.*, 201:287–91.

Bass, P., (1968), In vivo electrical activity of the small bowel. In: *Handbook of Physiology*, Section 6, Vol. 4: Motility (Ed. Code, C. F.), pp. 2051–75, Williams and Wilkins, Baltimore.

Code, C. F., and Schlegel, J. F., (1974), The gastrointestinal housekeeper. In: *Gastrointestinal Motility* (Ed. Daniel, E. E.), pp. 631–3, Mitchell Press, Vancouver.

Code, C. F., and Marlett, J. A., (1975), 'The interdigestive myoelectric complex of the stomach and small bowel of dogs. *J. Physiol.* (*London*) 246:289–309.

DeWever, I., Eeckhout, C., Vantrappen, G., and Hellemans, J., (1978), Disruptive effect of test meals on interdigestive motor complex in dogs. *Am. J. Physiol.*, 235:E661–5.

Dusdieker, N. S., and Summers, R. W., (1980), Longitudinal and circumferential spread of spike bursts in canine jejunum *in vivo*. *Am. J. Physiol.*, 239:G311–18.

Fleckenstein, P., (1978), Migrating electrical spike activity in the fasting human small intestine. *Am. J. Dig. Dis.*, 23:769–75.

Frexinos, J., Bueno, L., and Fioramonti, J., (1985), Diurnal changes in myoelectric spiking activity of the human colon. *Gastroenterology*, 88:1104–10.

Herman-Taylor, J., and Code, C. F., (1971), Localization of the duodenal pacemaker and its role in the organization of duodenal myoelectric activity. *Gut*, 12:40–7.

Hinder, R. A., and Kelly, K. A., (1977), Human gastric pacesetter potential: site of origin, spread, and response to gastric transection and proximal gastric vagotomy. *Am. J. Surg.*, 133:29–33.

Kim, C. H., and Malagelada, J-R., (1986), Electrical activity of the stomach: clinical implications. *Mayo Clin. Proc.*, 61:205–10.

Richter, H. M., and Kelly, K. A., (1986), Effect of transection and pacing on human jejunal pacesetter potentials. *Gastroenterology*, 91:1380–5.

Szurszewski, J. H., (1987), Electrical basis for gastrointestinal motility. In: *Physiology of the Gastrointestinal Tract*, 2nd Edition (Ed. Johnson, L. R.), pp. 383–422, Raven Press, New York.

Thuneberg, L., (1982), Interstitial cells of Cajal: intestinal pacemaker cells? In: *Advances in Anatomy, Embryology and Cell Biology*, Vol. 71 (Eds. Beck, F., Hild, W., van Kimbrorgh, J., Ortmann, R., Pauley, J. E., and Schiebler, T. H.), pp. 1–130, Springer-Verlag, Berlin.

Weisbrodt, N. W., (1987), Motility of the small intestine. In: *Physiology of the Gastrointestinal Tract*, 2nd Edition (Ed. Johnson, L. R.), pp. 631–3, Raven Press, New York.

10
IMPEDANCE

J. A. Sutton
Roussel Laboratories Limited, Swindon, UK

Impedance methods have long been established as non-invasive and accurate for monitoring the volume of various organs. Non-invasiveness is due to low current densities several orders of magnitude below those which would depolarize cell membranes including the sensitive neuronal synapse (Brown, 1983). Also, current frequencies do not invoke significant displacement-current effects such as heating.

Impedance methods also offer high sensitivity. Darby et al (1982) demonstrated its superior accuracy to manometry in monitoring intestinal contractions. Murray (1981) calculated that the neonatal skull monitor of Reigel et al (1977) would detect a haemorrhage as little as 10 ml.

Previous attempts to harness the impedance principle have foundered on the complexity of tissues beneath the skin and their variation between individuals which precluded accurate calibration. Current cardiac methods circumvent the problem by nomograms (Bomed Ltd., Irvine, Ca, USA). For filling or emptying rates there is no need for referral to absolute volumes when the rate of change provides the information required. Electrode–skin interface problems have been eased by silver-silver chloride electrodes which make good, stable contact with skin.

Overall impedance is directly proportional to volume when specific impedance remains constant (Pethig 1979; Brown 1983). In diagnostic equipment this simplifies data handling and avoids the need for highly trained personnel. It provides a continuous output signal which is more accurate than periodic sampling methods. Equipment is relatively simple and it is portable to the patient and relatively inexpensive. The result appears immediately and in an easily interpretable form.

Sutton and McClelland (1983) reported that a simple four-electrode device detected faster gastric emptying after an intravenous dose of metoclopramide in healthy volunteers. Subsequently it was compared with three different methods measuring gastric emptying: scintigraphy (Sutton et al, 1985), dye dilution (McClelland and Sutton, 1985) and paracetamol absorption (Sutton, 1988) with significant correlations between methods in each case. It detected slower emptying of glucose solutions compared with water and faster gastric emptying after oral metoclopramide (McClelland and Sutton, 1985). Rainbird and colleagues (1987) found that it detected faster emptying of a liquid meal of healthy volunteers who sat upright compared with supine.

When a suitable liquid is drunk the device detects an increase in overall impedance across the epigastric zone during gastric filling (Figure 1). Typically an increase of 1–2 ohms occurs after 500 ml of water or orange flavoured drinks which contain no conductive ionized particles. Natural orange juice contains free ions and is conductive and may not produce the impedance increase. Sutton (1988) showed that this increase is directly proportional to volume of meal. It is followed by a gradual decline, the slope of which indicates the gastric emptying rate.

Subjects are best prepared by an overnight or 6-hour fast. A comfortable posture is essential since the torso must not move throughout the test. Most practical is a 45° semi-supine position shown

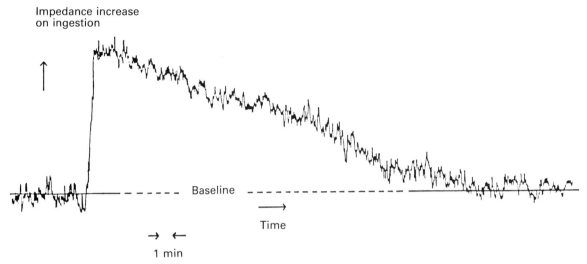

Figure 1. An example of an epigastric impedance trace during gastric filling with 500 ml dilute orange squash (Quosh^(R) 80 ml, tap water 420 ml) and subsequent emptying. The increase typically is 1–2 ohms.

in Figure 2 because it is comfortable and the liquid test 'meal' can be drunk easily. Variations in upright posture can influence the result (Rainbird et al, 1987) but not enough to cause misdiagnosis of pathologically delayed gastric emptying.

Electrodes are positioned such that the stomach lies between anterior and posterior input electrodes (Figure 3). However, the position of the stomach may vary such that in 20 of 77 normal volunteers Sutton (1988) found no deflection on ingestion of a test meal. These were reduced from 20 to 8 by applying the adjustment described in Figure 3. These eight subjects tended to be overweight and Pickworth (1984) showed that the stomach in the obese was displaced cranially, suggesting that higher positions of the electrodes may be necessary.

Further electrode sites are being explored by a multi-electrode device (London Medical Electronics, Northampton, UK). This machine monitors a larger zone and thereby increases the detection rate. Also Brown and colleagues (1985) have developed a 16-electrode device to produce images of the entire stomach. This may improve data on gastric location and the optimal electrode position.

Over 200 measurements suggest that normal volunteers fall in one of three groups: fast emptiers ($T_{\frac{1}{2}}$ below 8 min approx), moderate ($T_{\frac{1}{2}}$ below 16 min approx) and slow emptiers ($T_{\frac{1}{2}}$ 16–30 min). These figures apply to a dilute orange squash liquid test 'meal' and compare favourably with scintigraphic studies using similar meals (Dooley et al, 1984). The method of calculation of half emptying time is shown in Figure 4.

Gastric secretions increase conductivity of gastric contents; increased conductivity would reduce overall impedance and produce unduly rapid emptying rates. However, compared with dye-dilution, impedance emptying times were, if anything, slower (Sutton, 1988). Moreover, reduction of acid secretion by H2 blockers did not change gastric emptying rates. Possibly, the current pathway is the peritoneal surface of the stomach until the conductivity of gastric contents exceeds a threshold value. Once the threshold is exceeded the pathway becomes intragastric. This would explain the effect of highly ionized liquid meals which produce a zone of reduced overall impedance in the gastric imaging techniques used by Brown et al (1985).

Figure 5 illustrates delayed gastric emptying in diabetic autonomic neuropathy. Both patients with gastric symptoms exceeded the normal limit

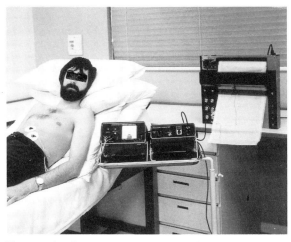

Figure 2. A volunteer on test. Note the 45° semi-upright position and the trace emerging from the chart recorder. In this case the generator of the 4 mA peak-to-peak, 100 kHz current is connected to the electrodes. The return signal is amplified by a separate amplifier to reduce induction current interference.

of 30 min for gastric $T_{\frac{1}{2}}$ (Gilbey and Watkins, 1987). Similarly, Sutton (1988) has demonstrated delayed gastric emptying in migraine and a significant correlation between the severity of pain and delayed gastric emptying. This demonstrates the suitability of the method for unwell and frail patients.

The epigastric impedance method is in its infancy but appears to provide accurate and simple measurements of emptying. Also, it appears to detect gastric contractility (McClelland and Sutton, 1985); Van der Schee, personal communication) which may be quantifiable by Fourier analysis. If it could be validated by further experiments it will be the first method capable of measuring both gastric functions simultaneously.

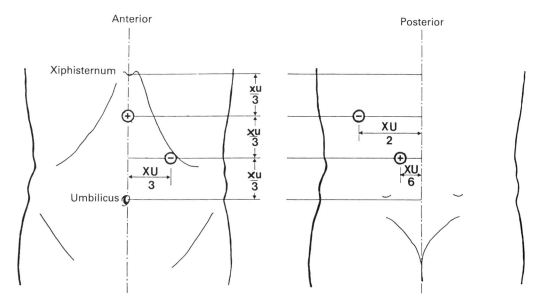

Figure 3. Electrode positions using the xiphisternum and umbilicus as reference points. In this case where the distance X–U is 18 cm the anterior input electrode ⊕ is 6 cm inferior to the xiphisternum in the mid-line. The detector electrode ⊖ is the same distance further inferior and to the left. Posterior electrodes are 9 and 3 cm to the left at the same levels. A second position, used when the first detects no gastric filling, places the anterior electrodes at: input ⊕ XU/6 in mid-line and detector ⊖ to XU/2 inferior and XU/2 to the left of the xiphisternum. The posterior pair positions are unchanged.

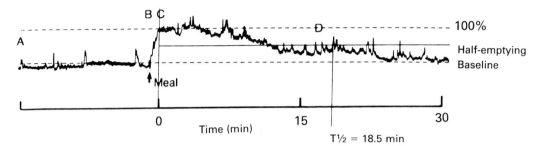

Figure 4. Calculation of the half emptying time. This is the time when the descending trace finally recrosses the 50% level of the initial deflection. It compares closely with computer curve fitted values (Sutton, 1988). The time is calculated from the filling peak and excludes the drinking time.

Diabetic patient with autonomic neuropathy plus gastric symptoms T½ > 30 min

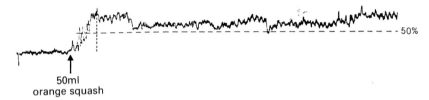

Diabetic patient with autonomic neuropathy plus gastric symptoms T½ > 30 min

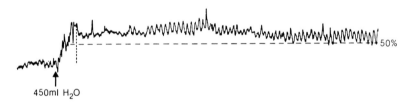

Diabetic patient – no gastric symptoms T½ = 16 min

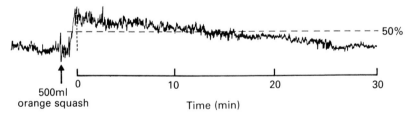

Figure 5. Two retarded ($T_\frac{1}{2} > 30$ min) and one normal gastric emptying trace in patients with diabetic autonomic neuropathy. Only the two slow emptiers had gastric symptoms (e.g. bloating, nausea and regurgitation).

REFERENCES

Brown, B. W., (1983), Tissue impedance methods. In: *Imaging with Non-ionising Radiations*. (Ed: Jackson, D. F.) pp 85–110. Surrey University Press.

Brown, B. H., Barber, D. C., and Seager, A. D., (1985), Applied potential tomography; possible clinical applications. *Clin. Phys. Physiol. Meas.*, 6, 2:109–21.

Darby, C. F., Hammond, P., Taylor, I., and Morris, I. R., (1982), A method for the simultaneous detection of motility and myoelectrical activity in smooth muscle. *Clin. Phys. Physiol. Meas.*, **3**:283–91.

Dooley, C. P., Reznik, J. B., and Valenzuela, J. E., (1984), Variations in gastric and duodenal motility during gastric emptying of liquid meals in humans. *Gastroenterology*, **87**:1114–9.

Gilbey, S., and Watkins, P., (1987), Delayed gastric emptying in diabetic autonomic neuropathy demonstrated by the epigastric impedance method. *Diabetic Medicine.* In press.

McClelland, G. R., and Sutton, J. A., (1985), Epigastric impedance: a non-invasive method for the assessment of gastric emptying and motility. *Gut*, 26, **6**:607–14.

Murray, P. W., (1981), Field calculations in the head of a newborn infant and their application to the interpretation of transcephalic impedance measurements. *Med. Biol. Eng. Comput.*, **19**:538–46.

Pethig, R., (1979), *Dielectric and Electronic Properties of Biological Materials.* John Wiley and Sons, Chichester, UK.

Pickworth, M. J. W., (1984), *Impedance Measurements for Gastric Emptying.* MSc Thesis, Surrey University.

Rainbird, A. L., Pickworth, M. J. W., Lightowler, C., Mitchell, M., and Wingate, D. L. (1987), Effect of posture and cold stress on gastric emptying measured by the method of epigastric impedance. *Pharmaceutical Medicine.* In press.

Reigel, D. H., Dallman, D. E., Scarff, T. B., and Woodford, J., (1977), Transcephalic impedance measurement during infancy. *Develop. Med. Child. Neurol.*, **19**:295–304.

Sutton, J. A., and McClelland, G. R., (1983), Epigastric impedance: a pharmacological test of a new non-invasive method of measuring gastric emptying. *Br. J. Anaesth.*, **55**:913.

Sutton, J. A., Thompson, S., and Sobnack, R., (1985), Measurement of gastric emptying rates by radioactive isotope scanning and epigastric impedance. *Lancet*, April 20th. 898–900.

Sutton, J. A. (1988), *Epigastric Impedance Measurements of Gastric Emptying.* MD Thesis, University of London.

11
ELECTROGASTROGRAPHY

Chung H. Kim
Mayo Clinic, Rochester, USA

Introduction

Evaluation of patients who present with symptoms of chronic nausea, vomiting and abdominal bloating without an anatomical lesion demonstrable on radiological or endoscopic examination can be a frustrating experience for the clinicians. Recent evidence suggests that up to 75% of patients with such functional gastrointestinal symptoms can have abnormalities in gut motility (Malagelada and Stanghellini, 1985). Because gastrointestinal motility is controlled by its electrical activity, increasing efforts are being made to characterize the underlying electrical disturbances in various disorders of gut motility. In this chapter, the electrical activity of the stomach, both in health and disease, is briefly reviewed and the application of electrogastrography in the detection of gastric dysrhythmia is discussed.

Gastric Electrical Activity: Normal Pattern

The stomach can be divided into two regions based on its electrical properties. The proximal portion which includes the fundus and the oral third of the body, exhibits a constant nonfluctuating electrical activity whereas the remainder of the stomach (the distal portion) is characterized by oscillating electrical potentials which occur at regular time intervals (Hinder and Kelly, 1977). These oscillating potentials have been labelled as slow waves, pacesetter potentials, basic electrical rhythm, or control potentials and they all refer to the same phenomenon.

Gastric slow waves are generated by spontaneous depolarization and subsequent repolarization of the smooth muscle cell membrane. When the smooth muscle cell membrane is depolarized beyond a criticial threshold, contraction is elicited (Morgan and Szurszewski, 1980). In an intact stomach, an area in the mid-body along the greater curve behaves as a gastric pacemaker because it has the highest intrinsic rate of slow wave production and, therefore, sets pace for the entire stomach. From the pacemaker site, the slow waves propagate circumferentially and aborally towards the pylorus at a rate of three cycles per minute (Hinder and Kelly, 1977). Recent *in vitro* experiments have shown that the slow waves propagate at a faster speed along the parallel axis of the circular smooth muscle than along its perpendicular axis (Bauer et al, 1985). The end result is a co-ordinated motor response whereby waves of concentric contractions sweep across the distal stomach in a peristaltic fashion. An example of the normal postprandial electromechanical pattern of the stomach is shown in Figure 1.

Gastric Electrical Activity: Abnormal Patterns

Three types of abnormal gastric electrical rhythms have been recognized; unusually fast rhythm (tachygastria), slow rhythm (bradygastria), and irregular rhythm (arrhythmia). A mixture of tachygastria and arrhythmia is sometimes referred to as tachyarrhythmia and is illustrated in Figure 2. Tachygastria and bradygastria have distinct electrical characteristics on electromyography. Tachy-

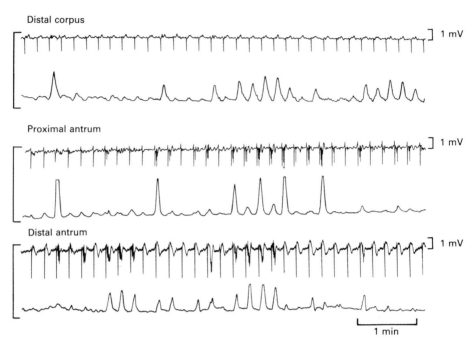

Figure 1. Electromyogram showing a normal electromechanical pattern of the canine stomach following a meal. For each region of the stomach the top line represents electrical activity and the bottom line contractile activity.

gastria usually originates from an ectopic focus in the distal antrum and its slow waves propagate orally. Furthermore, tachygastria is predominantly confined to the antrum and seldom affects the body of the stomach (Code and Marlett, 1974; Kim et al, 1986a). Bradygastria, on the other hand, usually appears in both the body and the antrum simultaneously and its slow waves propagate aborally (Kim et al, 1986a).

The aetiological mechanism of gastric dysrhythmia remains unclear at the present time. However, gastric dysrhythmia can be experimentally induced, both in humans and animals, using pharmacological agents such as glucagon, epinephrine, prostaglandin E_2, and enkephalins (Stoddard et al, 1981; Abell and Malagelada, 1985;

Kim et al, 1986a). Recent experiments in dogs have shown that some of these drugs induce gastric dysrhythmia by stimulating the synthesis of endogenous prostaglandins (Kim et al, 1987a). Whether or not spontaneously occurring dysrhythmias in the human stomach are mediated by a similar mechanism remains to be seen.

Gastric Dysrhythmia and its Clinical Consequences

Gastric dysrhythmias have been described in a variety of conditions including diabetic gastroparesis (Abell et al, 1985a; Hamilton et al, 1986), anorexia nervosa (Abell et al, 1985b), and idio-

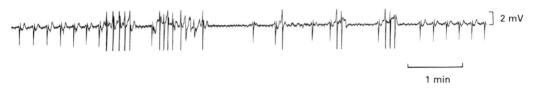

Figure 2. An example of canine gastric dysrhythmia detected by electromyography. Both tachygastria and arrhythmia are shown in this example.

pathic gastroparesis (Telander et al, 1978; You et al, 1980; Geldof et al, 1986). However, gastric dysrhythmias are not observed exclusively in diseases that are characterized by gastric stasis. They also have been described in healthy volunteers (Stoddard et al, 1981; Abell et al, 1985a), during the immediate postoperative period (Sarna et al, 1973; Bertrand et al, 1984), and in a variety of unrelated clinical conditions (Hinder and Kelly, 1977; Geldof et al, 1983; Koch et al, 1987). Although the role of gastric dysrhythmia in human disease is yet to be established, evidence suggests that gastric motility can be significantly impaired in the presence of dysrhythmia. Recently, two groups of investigators working separately, each reported a patient with severe gastric retention who underwent a subtotal gastrectomy for relief of intractable nausea and vomiting. When the surgically resected antrum was examined *in vitro* with electromechanical probes, it demonstrated persistent tachygastria and a concomitant lack of contractions (Telander et al, 1978; Sanders et al, 1979). We recently examined, in conscious dogs, the mechanical consequences of gastric dysrhythmia and found that antral motility was significantly lower during episodes of dysrhythmia than during episodes of normal electrical rhythm (Kim et al, 1987b). This evidence suggests that gastric motility is adversely affected in the presence of dysrhythmia; however, it is still controversial whether gastric dysrhythmia is a direct cause of gastroparesis or an epiphenomenon.

Electrogastrography: Technical Considerations

Surgical implantation of electrodes as used in electromyography provides a reliable and excellent recording of gastric electrical activity with minimal background noise. This is possible because the tip of the electrode is securely positioned in the gastric musculature where the slow waves are generated. Electromyographic recordings typically show distinct and easily recognizable triphasic gastric potentials separated by a stable baseline potential (Figures 1 and 2). Furthermore, interfering signals such as respiration or move-

ment artefacts and cardiac potentials are easily identified. In spite of its superior quality, however, electromyography is seldom used in clinical practice because of its invasive nature.

Electrogastrography measures gastric electrical activity with the aid of electrodes placed either in the gastric mucosa (mucosal electrode) and/or epigastric skin surface (cutaneous electrode). Because of its noninvasive nature, electrogastrography is an attractive alternative to electromyography, but it is associated with several technical problems. First, the mucosal or cutaneous electrode does not come in direct contact with the gastric smooth muscle. This increases the probability that electrical potentials from non-gastric sources may be picked up by the mucosal or cutaneous electrode and interfere with the detection of gastric slow waves. Such interfering signals or the background noise can be reduced with the use of appropriate filters (Hamilton et al, 1986); however, the background noise can be excessive and some investigators have used a computer in their data analysis to sort out various electrical frequencies represented in the electrogastrographic recording (Geldof et al, 1986).

Another technical problem associated with electrogastrography has been its inconsistent success rate in obtaining prolonged recordings of good quality. In our experience, gastric electrical activity can be satisfactorily recorded with cutaneous electrodes if the patient has a thin abdominal wall and a stomach which lies well below the costal margin. Similarly, the mucosal electrode can provide an excellent tracing of gastric electrical activity if it remains securely attached to the gastric mucosa (Figure 3). However, our own experience and that of others suggests that many patients do not have a suitable body habitus for cutaneous electrogastrography and that the mucosal electrode (suction electrode, in particular) often becomes detached for such reasons as gastric contractions and build-up of secretions around the electrode.

To overcome the aforementioned problems which limited the use of electrogastrography in the past, a technique which utilizes a magnetic force was recently introduced (Abell and Malagelada, 1985). In brief, the mucosal electrode is

a. Normal

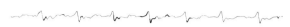

b. Tachyarrhythmia

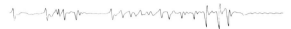

c. Tachygastria

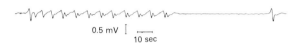

0.5 mV $\vert$ $\longmapsto$
                      10 sec

Figure 3. Examples of human gastric dysrhythmia detected by electrogastrography using a suction mucosal electrode. Note that both tachyarrhythmia and tachygastria are followed by an electrically silent period. Reproduced with kind permission from You et al, 1983.

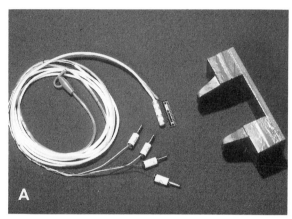

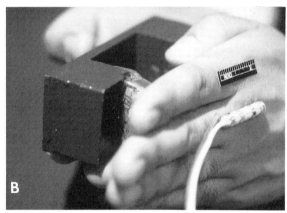

Figure 4. Improved electrogastrographic technique using magnetic force. The mucosal electrode (A) has a pair of bipolar silver-silver chloride circular electrodes mounted around a small 'Alnico' magnet covered with a polyvinyl tube. The mucosal electrode is brought in apposition with gastric mucosa, represented in (B) by the dorsum of the hand, by placing a larger 'rare earth' magnet over the epigastric skin surface (represented here by the palm of the hand). The magnetic field created by the two magnets on each side of the gastric wall allows the mucosal electrode to be securely attached to the gastric mucosa.

constructed so that a pair of bipolar silver-silver chloride circular electrodes is mounted around a small core of 'Alnico' magnet covered with a polyvinyl tube (Figure 4A). The mucosal electrode which is introduced orally is held in apposition with gastric mucosa by a larger 'rare earth' magnet placed over the epigastric skin surface (Figure 4B). Using this technique, we recently recorded gastric electrical activity in 44 healthy subjects for a minimum of three hours in each subject. The overall quality of the electrogastrographic recording was excellent and the gastric slow waves were easily recognizable on visual inspection in about 80% of the individual recordings (Kim et al, 1986b). The correlation between simultaneously recorded mucosal and cutaneous recordings was excellent and the background noise was minimal (Figure 5). We also had an opportunity to perform a 24-hour electrogastrography using the same technique in a patient suspected of having gastric dysrhythmia. The patient tolerated the procedure well and the quality of the 24-hour tracing was excellent with approximately 80% of the tracing demonstrating distinct gastric slow waves with minimal background noise (Kim, unpublished data).

In summary, there has been a slow but steady progress in electrogastrography since it was first put to use in 1922 (Alvarez, 1922). Technological advances in recent years made it possible to change electrogastrography from a primitive research tool into a modern diagnostic tool. The role of electrogastrography in the investigation of patients with functional gastrointestinal symptoms is just beginning to be explored.

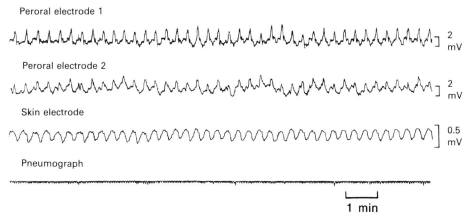

Figure 5. An example of a normal human electrogastrogram using the improved electrogastrographic technique. Note the gastric slow waves are easily recognizable on visual inspection and the correlation between the mucosal recordings (peroral electrodes 1 and 2) and the cutaneous recordings (skin electrode) is excellent.

References

Abell, T. L., and Malagelada, J.-R., (1985), Glucagon-evoked gastric dysrhythmias in humans shown by an improved electrogastrographic technique. *Gastroenterology*, **88**:1932–40.

Abell, T. L., Camilleri, M., and Malagelada, J.-R., (1985a), High prevalence of gastric electrical dysrhythmias in diabetic gastroparesis (abstract). *Gastroenterology*, **88**:1299.

Abell, T. L., Lucas, A. R., Brown, M. L., and Malagelada, J.-R., (1985b), Gastric electrical dysrhythmias in anorexia nervosa (AN) (abstract). *Gastroenterology*, **88**:1300

Alvarez, W. C., (1922), The electrogastrogram and what it shows. *JAMA*, **78**:1116–19.

Bauer, A. J., Publicover, N. G., and Sanders, K. M., (1985), Origin and spread of slow waves in canine gastric antral circular muscle. *Am. J. Physiol.*, **12**:G800–6

Bertrand, J., Dorval, E. D., Metman, E. H., de Calan, L., and Ozoux, J. P., (1984), Electrogastrography and serosal electrical recording of the antrum after proximal vagotomy in man (abstract). *Gastroenterology*, **86**:1026.

Code, C. F., and Marlett, J. A., (1974), Canine tachygastria. *Mayo Clinic Proceedings*, **49**:325–32

Geldof, H., van der Schee, E. J., van Blankenstein, M., and Grashuis, J. L., (1983), Gastric dysrhythmia: an electrogastrographic study (abstract). *Gastroenterology*, **84**:1163.

Geldof, H., van der Schee, E. J., van Blankenstein, M., and Grashuis, J. L., (1986), Electrogastrographic study of gastric myoelectrical activity in patients with unexplained nausea and vomiting. *Gut*, **27**:799–808.

Hamilton, J. W., Bellahsene, B. E., Reichelderfer, M.,

Webster, J. G., and Bass, P., (1986), Human electrogastrograms: comparison of surface and mucosal recordings. *Dig. Dis. Sci.*, **31**:33–9.

Hinder, R. A., and Kelly, K. A., (1977), Human gastric pacesetter potential: site of origin, spread, and response to gastric transection and proximal gastric vagotomy. *Am. J. Surg.*, **133**:29–33.

Kim, C. H., Azpiroz, F., and Malagelada, J.-R., (1986a), Characteristics of spontaneous and drug-induced gastric dysrhythmias in a chronic canine model. *Gastroenterology*, **90**:421–7.

Kim, C. H., Hanson, R., Abell, T., and Malagelada, J. (1986b), The role of prostaglandins in the regulation of human gastric electromechanical activity (abstract). *Gastroenterology*, **91**:1058.

Kim, C. H., Zinsmeister, A. R., and Malagelada, J.-R., (1987a). Mechanisms of canine gastric dysrhythmia. *Gastroenterology*, **92**:993–9.

Kim, C. H., Zinsmeister, A. R., and Malagelada, J.-R., (1987b), Effect of gastric dysrhythmias on postcibal motor activity of the stomach. *Dig. Dis. Sci.* (in press).

Koch, K. L., Stern, R. M., Dwyer, A., and Vasey, M., (1987), Temporal relationships between tachygastria and symptoms of motion sickness (abstract). *Gastroenterology*, **92**:1473.

Malagelada, J.-R., and Stanghellini, V., (1985), Manometric evaluation of functional upper gut syndrome. *Gastroenterology*, **88**:1223–31.

Morgan, K. G., and Szurszewski, J. H., (1980), Mechanisms of phasic and tonic actions of pentagastrin on canine gastric smooth muscle. *J. Physiol. (Lond).*, **301**:229–42.

Sanders, K., Menguy, R., Chey, W., You, C., Lee, K., Morgan, K., Kreulen, D., Schmalz, P., Muir, T., and Szurszewski, J., (1979), One explanation for human antral tachygastria (abstract). *Gastroenterology*, **76**:1234.

Sarna, S. K., Bowes, K. L., and Daniel, E. E., (1973), Postoperative gastric electrical control activity (ECA) in man. In: *Proceedings of the Fourth International Symposium on Gastrointestinal Motility*. (Ed Daniel, E. E.) pp 73–83. Mitchell Press, Vancouver.

Stoddard, C. J., Smallwood, R. H., and Duthie, H. C., (1981), Electrical arrhythmias in the human stomach. *Gut*, **22**:705–12.

Telander, R. L., Morgan, K. G., Kreulen, D. L., Schmalz, P. F., Kelly, K. A., and Szurszewski, J. H., (1978), Human gastric atony with tachygastria and gastric retention. *Gastroenterology*, **75**:497–501.

You, C. H., Lee, K. Y., Chey, W. H., and Menguy, R., (1980), Electrogastrographic study of patients with unexplained nausea, bloating, and vomiting. *Gastroenterology*, **79**:311–14.

You, C. H., Lee, K. Y., and Chey, W. Y. (1983), Gastric electromyography in normal and abnormal states in humans. In: *Functional Disorders of the Digestive Tract*. (Ed Chey, W. Y.) pp 167–173. Raven Press, New York.

12
HYDROGEN BREATH TEST

Hasse Abrahamsson

Sahlgren's Hospital, Gothenberg, Sweden

The relative inaccessibility of the small intestine has stimulated research for simple indirect methods, not requiring intubation, to assess transit along the intestine. Transit through a particular part of the gut can be estimated by an ingested substance that is not absorbed in that part but is rapidly absorbed distal to the organ. For example, gastric emptying can be indirectly estimated if a solution of paracetamol is ingested and

blood levels of the drug followed, since this drug is poorly absorbed in the stomach but rapidly absorbed in the small intestine. A similar principle has been used to assess orocaecal transit time: the pulmonary excretion of hydrogen is measured after ingestion of carbohydrates which are poorly absorbed in the small intestine but rapidly fermented in the colon (Figure 1).

Some disaccharides, e.g. lactulose and raffinose, as well as dietary fibre polysaccharides, pass undigested through the small intestine. In the colon hydrogen is formed from the carbohydrates by the colonic bacteria. Hydrogen is rapidly diffused to the blood and exhaled from the lungs.

Sometimes this principle cannot be used for measurement of the orocaecal transit time, e.g. in subjects with bacterial overgrowth of the stomach and small intestine, and in individuals without H_2-generating bacteria in the colon.

In basic studies Bond and Levitt (1975) established the hydrogen breath test to determine the orocaecal transit time. After ingestion of lactulose and unabsorbable polyethylene glycol (PEG) the rise in breath hydrogen correlated well with the appearance of PEG in the distal ileum (Figure 2).

In these early studies hydrogen was sampled by a complicated closed-circuit rebreathing method and hydrogen concentrations were measured by gas chromatography. However, simplified methods to sample hydrogen and to determine hydrogen concentrations have led to widespread use of H_2 breath tests. Also, application of the H_2 breath test to solid test meals has prompted physiological and clinical transit studies. Today, the H_2 breath test is used not only in motility studies primarily aimed to calculate orocaecal

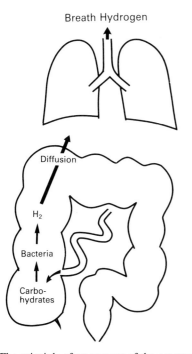

Figure 1. The principle of assessment of the orocaecal transit time by breath hydrogen analysis. When the nonabsorbable carbohydrates of a test meal are emptied into the caecum, breath hydrogen concentrations increase within a few minutes.

125

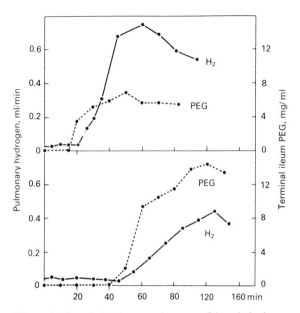

Figure 2. Correlation between increase of breath hydrogen and increase of polyethylene glycol (PEG) concentration in terminal ileum in two subjects following ingestion of a lactulose-PEG mixture. (Modified from Bond and Levitt, 1975.)

transit time, but also in studies of carbohydrate malabsorption and in the diagnosis of bacterial overgrowth.

Principle of Measurement

Various sampling techniques have been applied to sample *end expiratory air*, for analysis of breath hydrogen:

(1) The subject expires through a Haldane-Priestley tube and at the end of the expiration, air is aspirated into a syringe at the proximal end of the tube. The sample is then injected into the H_2 monitor.

(2) The subject expires through a Y-piece to which a syringe is connected. During the last phase of expiration the Y-piece's exit to the atmosphere is covered and the syringe filled.

(3) The subject expires through a Y-piece with one exit to atmosphere and the other to the H_2 monitor. During the last phase of expiration

the exit to atmosphere is covered so that end expiratory air flows directly into the monitor.

With these three sampling techniques the lowest H_2 concentrations are obtained with the Haldane-Priestley tube and the highest values with expiration directly into the H_2 monitor (Brummer et al, 1985). The Y-piece syringe method gives intermediate values. All three methods seem to be satisfactory for clinical and scientific purposes. Breath sampling in a gas-tight syringe has the advantage that the sample can be stored until analysis. Sample volumes vary from 20 to 50 ml in published studies.

Hydrogen Analysis

Hydrogen concentration of air samples can now be measured by a relatively inexpensive device using an electrochemical cell (Corbett et al, 1981). Modern monitors immediately yield the hydrogen concentration of a sample in ppm (parts per million).

Test Meal Procedure

Subjects are usually examined after an overnight fast. On the day before the examination, fibre-rich food containing nonabsorbable carbohydrates should be avoided while rice and meat are allowed. Antibiotics are not allowed during the week before the study.

Two types of test meal are common in clinical studies of orocaecal transit time. A solution of a nonabsorbable carbohydrate, usually lactulose 10–30 g, has often been used. However, a solid meal is more representative of the physiological situation and is usually preferred, as discussed in more detail below.

Hydrogen Profile and Orocaecal Transit Time

After a test meal expiratory air is sampled, usually with intervals of 10–15 min, and the orocaecal

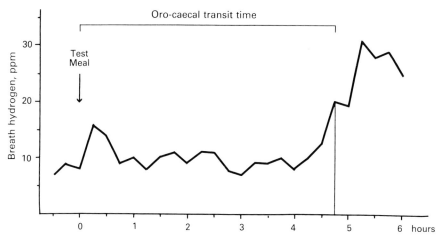

Figure 3. Calculation of the orocaecal transit time from the breath hydrogen curve obtained after a test meal containing oatmeal porridge.

transit time calculated from the hydrogen values obtained. Figure 3 shows a representative hydrogen profile curve in one subject after a standard test meal. End expiratory air was exhaled directly into the H_2 monitor with 15 minutes interval. After the test meal two H_2 peaks appear. The initial H_2 peak may have a duration of half an hour or more, and is the result of fermentation of ingested carbohydrates by oropharyngeal bacteria. This peak can be largely abolished by washing the mouth with chlorhexidine (Thompson et al, 1986). It has also

been advocated that emptying of ileal contents (from a previous meal) into the colon may contribute to the initial H_2 peak after a test meal.

The second rise in breath hydrogen represents the arrival of the test meal in the caecum. There is no generally accepted rule as to how the transit time should be calculated from the hydrogen curve. Some investigators use the time when a certain increase of H_2 in ppm above the level after the initial peak is obtained. Increases of 4–10 ppm have been used in published studies. Other

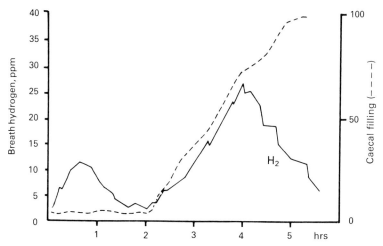

Figure 4. Breath hydrogen profile and caecal radioactivity after ingestion of a radiolabelled meal containing baked beans by a normal subject. Note the simultaneous rise of caecal radioactivity and breath hydrogen after about two hours, and the time difference between maximum values of caecal radioactivity and the second hydrogen peak. (Modified from Read et al, 1985).

workers define orocaecal transit from a *relative* increase in H_2, e.g. 50% above the mean values observed 1–2 hours after a test meal (Armbrecht et al, 1986).

Simultaneous measurements of breath hydrogen and caecal filling after ingestion of an isotope test meal have confirmed that the beginning of the second H_2 peak closely correlates with the arrival of the front of the test meal to the caecum (Figure 4). The time when all of the meal has entered the colon cannot be calculated from the hydrogen excretion curve.

Aspects of Test Meals

Considerable intra- and inter-individual differences in orocaecal transit time are obtained with solid test meals and with lactulose meals (Read et al, 1980; Korth et al, 1984). The reproducibility of the lactulose test to determine orocaecal transit can be improved by the combination of lactulose with a liquid meal containing fat, protein and carbohydrates (La Brooy et al, 1983). The transit time of lactulose solutions is much shorter than that of solid meals. This difference may partly be explained by the rapid gastric emptying of liquids. However, other factors may also be of relevance since the orocaecal transit time after a standard meal decreases when increasing amounts of lactulose are added to the test meal (Figure 5). The discrepancies between results from studies with lactulose and with standard test meals indicate that the lactulose test does not reflect the physiological situation. Also, there is no significant correlation between transit times obtained with a lactulose meal and a solid meal in the same subject (Read et al, 1980). Therefore, results from lactulose tests should be interpreted with caution.

Some Factors Influencing Breath Hydrogen

The use of the H_2 breath test to study orocaecal transit times presupposes that the bulk of H_2-generating bacteria is confined to the colon. An altered bacterial flora may markedly affect the hydrogen test. In patients with abnormal flora proximal to the colon, e.g. achlorhydric and gastrectomy patients, the test cannot be used for motility studies of orocaecal transit (Figure 6). Likewise, the test may not be reliable in patients recently treated with antibiotics. Furthermore, a number of extra-intestinal influences may affect hydrogen excretion. Physical exercise and hyperventilation are followed by a reduction of breath hydrogen concentration. In contrast, breath

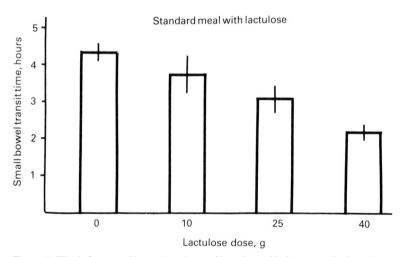

Figure 5. The influence of increasing doses of lactulose added to a standard meal on small intestinal transit time in six normal subjects. (Based on data presented by Read et al, 1980.)

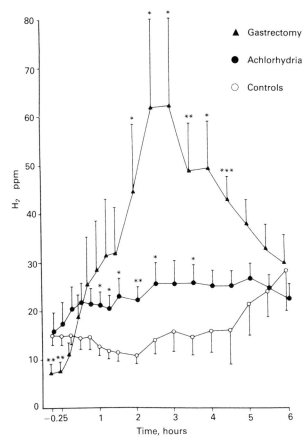

Figure 6. Breath hydrogen profiles after a standard meal in 10 normal subjects, 16 patients with achlorhydria, and 12 Billroth II patients. (From Armbrecht et al, 1985.)

expensive and laborious methods, e.g. scintigraphy, are not available or feasible.

References

Armbrecht, U., Bosaeus, I., Gillberg, R., Seeberg, S., and Stockbrügger, R., (1985), Hydrogen (H_2) breath test and gastric bacteria in acid-secreting subjects and in achlorhydric and postgastrectomy patients before and after antimicrobial treatment. *Scand. J. Gastroenterol.*, **20**:805–13.

Armbrecht, U., Jensen, J., Edén, S., and Stockbrügger, R., (1986), Assessment of orocaecal transit time by means of a hydrogen (H_2) breath test as compared with a radiological control method. *Scand. J. Gastroenterol.*, **21**:669–77.

Bond, J. H., and Levitt, M. D., (1975), Investigation of small bowel transit time in man utilizing pulmonary hydrogen (H_2) measurements. *J. Lab. Clin. Med.*, **85**:546–55.

Brummer, R.-J. M., Armbrecht, U., Bosaeus, I., Dotevall, G., and Stockbrügger, R. W., (1985), The hydrogen (H_2) breath test. Sampling methods and the influence of dietary fibre on fasting level. *Scand. J. Gastroenterol.*, **20**:1007–13.

Cann, P. A., Read, N. W., Brown, C., Hobson, N., and Holdsworth, C. D., (1983), Irritable bowel syndrome: relationship of disorders in the transit of a single solid meal to symptom patterns. *Gut*, **24**:405–11.

Corbett, C. L., Thomas, S., Read, N. W., Hobson, N., Bergman, I., and Holdsworth, C. D., (1981), Electrochemical detector for breath hydrogen determination: measurement of small bowel transit time in normal subjects and patients with the irritable bowel syndrome. *Gut*, **22**:836–40.

Korth, H., Müller, I., Erckenbrecht, J. F., and Wienbeck, M., (1984), Breath hydrogen as a test for gastrointestinal transit. *Hepatogastroenterol.*, **31**:282–4.

La Brooy, S. J., Male, P.-J., Beavis, A. K., and Misiewicz, J. J., (1983), Assessment of the reproducibility of the lactulose H_2 breath test as a measure of mouth to caecum transit time. *Gut*, **24**: 893–6.

Read, N. W., Miles, C. A., Fisher, D., Holgate, A. M., Kime, N. D., Mitchell, M. A., Reeve, A. M., Roche, T. B., and Walker, M., (1980), Transit time of a meal through the stomach, small intestine, and colon in normal subjects and its role in the pathogenesis of diarrhoea. *Gastroenterology*, **79**:1276–82.

Read, N. W., Al-Jamabi, M. N., Bates, T. E., Holgate, A. M., Cann, P. A., Kinsman, R. I., McFarlane, A., and Brown, C., (1985), Interpretation of the breath

hydrogen is markedly increased during cigarette smoking (Thompson et al, 1985).

Application of the Hydrogen Breath Test

With the hydrogen method the effect of various factors such as drugs and stress on intestinal transit has been studied. In clinical investigations the hydrogen breath test has revealed interesting correlations between symptoms and transit time in patients with functional gut disorders (Cann et al, 1983). It seems that the hydrogen breath test is a good alternative for physiological and clinical studies of orocaecal transit time when more hydrogen profile obtained after ingestion of a solid meal containing unabsorbable carbohydrate. *Gut*, **26:** 834–42.

Thompson, D. G., Binfield, P., DeBelder, A., O'Brien, J., and Warren, S., (1985), Extra intestinal influences on exhaled breath hydrogen measurements during the investigation of gastrointestinal disease. *Gut*, **26:**1349–52.

Thompson, D. G., O'Brien, J. D., and Hardie, J. M., (1986), Influence of the oropharyngeal microflora on the measurement of exhaled breath hydrogen. *Gastroenterology*, **91:**853–60.

13

THE ROLE OF COMPUTERS IN THE ANALYSIS OF GUT MOTILITY

Robert W. Summers

Veterans Administration Medical Center and University of Iowa Hospitals and Clinics, Iowa, USA

Introduction

Information about gastrointestinal motility comes from a variety of sources. The most direct qualitative and quantitative data are obtained through the study of mechanical and myoelectric properties of the hollow organs. Radiological, scintigraphic and metabolic techniques (e.g. postprandial breath hydrogen analysis) also yield important data regarding swallowing, gastro-oesophageal reflux, gastric emptying and intestinal or colonic transit. These applications are indirect measures which reflect smooth muscle activity. Although a great deal of information can be obtained by observation, quantitation of the data from any of these techniques is also necessary. Hand measurement of the many characteristics exhibited by the waveforms generated from the pharynx to the anus is a difficult if not impossible task. This is increasingly true as the number of sensors and recording times increases. Analysis by hand is a time-consuming and tedious task, subject to error and interpretation. Computer analysis of data is feasible and desirable because of its efficiency, objectivity and relatively low cost. Its main application has been to analyse the more well-defined waveforms such as the slow waves (electrical control activity), spike bursts (electrical response activity) and contraction waves (mechanical activity). Analytical computer programs have been applied to the study of hydrogen ion

concentration in the oesophagus (and stomach) and gastric emptying. Many of the more indirect methods of studying motility are descriptive and are analysed by observation. Monitoring of oesophageal (or gastric) pH and gastric emptying are two methods where computer analysis has been useful.

Oesophageal pH Monitoring

Although not a direct measure of motility, pH monitoring of the lower oesophagus is an indirect measure of lower oesophageal sphincter function. Initially monitoring of pH was performed for short periods under conditions designed to provoke reflux, such as the reverse Trendelenberg position, leg lifts or acid loading of the stomach. Extended ambulatory recordings for 24 hours under ordinary daily conditions has become the preferred technique to evaluate indeterminant symptoms, especially non-cardiac chest pain, to determine the severity of reflux or to assess the effectiveness of treatment strategies. After positioning appropriate electrodes at one or more sites in the oesophagus (and/or stomach), repetitive pH measurements are recorded at regular time increments using an analogue portable tape or digital solid state recorder. At the end of the recording period, playback to an analyser or computer is performed. The data are summarized and compared with values obtained from recordings of normal subjects (Stanciu et al, 1977; DeMeester et al, 1980; Schindbeck et al, 1987). Values such as the total number of reflux episodes (pH < 4.0) per time period, fraction of total time below pH 4.0 or duration of reflux episodes can readily be computed or the data can be expressed in terms of timing in relation to symptoms, meals, posture (upright or supine) or medication. Fortunately, a number of these analytical programs are commercially available (Figure 1).

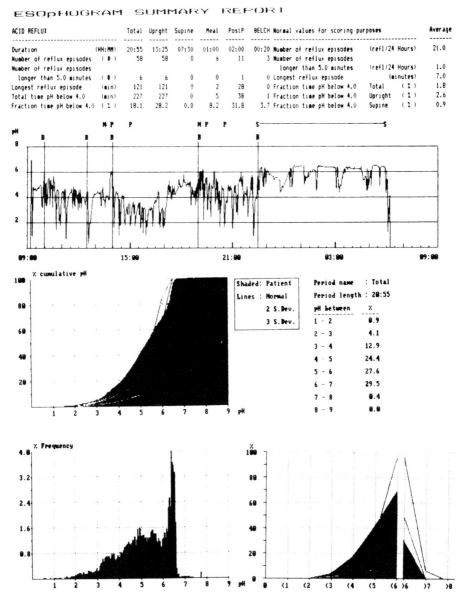

Figure 1. Example of a computer printout, displaying data from a 24-hour pH-monitoring device.

Gastric Emptying

The evaluation of gastric emptying is an indirect measure of gastric motor activity, although the forward propulsion of stomach contents can also be influenced by anatomical and mechanical factors outside of the stomach walls. Computer analysis has been applied in a variety of methods used to study gastric emptying. In order to account for absorption and secretion in addition to exit of liquid contents from the stomach, the dye dilution method of George (1968) has been modified by Dubois et al (1977). This sophisticated approach is facilitated through the use of the computer. Radioscintigraphy is more commonly utilized and the computer is convenient to analyse counts from defined regions of interest, to correct for isotope decay, to calculate a geometric mean count from anterior and posterior detectors, etc. It may also be used to describe the emptying curve mathematically by using the power exponential or other equations (Meyer et al, 1976; Tothill et al, 1978, 1980; Elashoff et al, 1982; Heading, 1982; Sheiner, 1984).

The newest application of the computer to monitor gastric emptying is the technique called applied potential tomography (Barber and Brown, 1984; Avill et al, 1987). In this method, a high-frequency, high-voltage current is applied to one of an array of electrodes mounted circumferentially on the lower chest. The change in tissue resistivity recorded from each of the other electrodes is serially compared with baseline after ingestion of food or a beverage. An emptying curve can then be calculated using tomographic images generated from the impedance data after identifying regions of interest from the gastric profile. This method has the great advantage of being non-invasive and of eliminating radiation exposure. Measurements of gastric emptying can be performed repetitively and at relatively low cost.

Electrical and Mechanical Signals

The origin of the signal is an important determinant of the analytical result and its interpretation. Electrical signals are derived from electrodes usually placed surgically on the serosa or intraluminally in small catheters. There are two major kinds of electrical signals: a recurring slow pacemaker potential called the slow wave or electrical control activity, and an intermittent series of fast action potentials, intermittently superimposed on the slow wave, called a spike burst or electrical response activity.

Electrical signals from the stomach can also be detected percutaneously. Signals occurring as a result of mechanical activity are derived from serosal strain gauges which measure changes in wall tension or intraluminal catheters which detect intraluminal pressure. The characteristics of the electrical and mechanical signals vary from organ to organ and from species to species so that a program must be able to recognize the event in each region and experimental subject.

The analytical approaches to computer analysis of motor events have been extremely varied. The remainder of this review will be organized according to the major waveforms recorded from the gastrointestinal tract.

Slow Waves (Electrical Control Activity)

In order to describe these pacemaker or pacesetter potentials, some comment about terminology is in order. The term slow wave frequency is often used, but frequency has two connotations which are often confused or used inappropriately. Regular repetitive electrical events occur with an intervening period or interval and 'rate of occurrence' would be a better term than frequency. Unfortunately, the term slow wave frequency is often applied in this context rather than slow wave rate. The frequency of a wave is related to the 'rise and fall' times or changes in voltage with respect to time, dV/dt. The units are in cycles per second or Hertz (Hz).

Several techniques have been widely utilized to analyse slow waves from the stomach, small bowel and colon and these have recently been reviewed (Kingma, 1987). When signals are clearly defined, have uniform morphology and are devoid of excessive extraneous frequencies, the time between the crossing of a fixed reference can readily be analysed by the computer. This approach is often called the zero-crossing method.

When signals are contaminated by noise or when frequencies are variable, it is often useful to incorporate signal filtering to facilitate the analysis. It is imperative to know which frequencies to enhance and which to suppress in order to avoid rejecting important but unanticipated frequencies. Filtering may be accomplished by active or passive analogue devices or digitally using the computer. A self-optimizing filtering routine called adaptive filtration is a special program approximating a band reject filter (van der Schee et al, 1982). Filtering may transform an unrecognizable frequency into one which can be analysed by the zero-crossing method.

When signals are composites of a variety of frequencies and waveforms are obscure, analysis may be facilitated by computing frequency power spectra. Methods used include the fast Fourier transform method and the Walsh transform method. Fourier transforms have been most used to analyse periodic components of the electrical signal (slow waves) which were not always apparent on visual inspection (Nelsen and Becker, 1968; Diamant et al, 1970; Sarna et al, 1971; Brown et al, 1975; Linkens and Connell, 1974; Linkens and Mhone, 1979). These efforts have been particularly useful in the colon where waveforms are more complex and constantly changing (Postaire et al, 1978; Stoddard et al, 1979). Because both methods analyse a signal for only a brief time increment, a running spectral analysis may be useful by creating consecutive frequency spectra and plotting frequency versus power versus time.

Electrogastrography (EGG)

Electrogastrography, a technique to record gastric periodic electrical activity, requires special analytic approaches. Alvarez (1922) was the first to record 3 cpm sinusoidal waves percutaneously over the stomach of a thin elderly woman. Although there were subsequent investigations of this phenomenon, significant advances in recording techniques and waveform analysis did not

occur until 1980. A group of Rotterdam investigators advanced the physiological understanding and meaning of this waveform and facilitated its analysis and interpretation in a series of articles (Smout et al, 1979, 1980a, 1980b; van der Schee et al, 1981). The computer was used to calculate the fast Fourier transform, but instead of applying this method to long recording periods of the EGG, the power spectra of short, overlapping segments were displayed as a function of time (van der Schee et al, 1982). A pseudo three-dimensional or grey-scale plot can be used to display the data; this technique is called running spectrum analysis. It has greatly facilitated the clinical application of this technique.

Spike Bursts (Electrical Response Activity)

In order to achieve data reduction for more efficient data processing, several investigators have utilized hardware devices prior to signal analysis by the computer. Wingate and his co-workers recorded the unamplified signal on a low recording speed cassette tape recorder for subsequent replay and analysis at 60 times the recording speed (Wingate et al, 1976, 1977; Wingate and Barnett, 1978). The electrical signal was divided between an active low-pass and a high-pass filter for analysis of slow waves and spike bursts, respectively. Schmitt triggers (comparators) with variable thresholds were then utilized to convert the data into brief square wave pulses. The signal was then analysed to obtain pulse-density histograms. The system integrated spike activity over time, resulting in a summation of all of the electrical spike activity. The detection and quantification of spike activity by similar methods have been utilized in the small intestine by other investigators (Latour, 1973; Hiesinger et al, 1978; Sinar and Charles, 1983). A similar approach has been used in the colon (Latour et al, 1983; Cherbut and Ruckebusch, 1984; Hacket et al, 1985).

As pointed out by Groh et al (1984), these methods do not give a one-to-one profile of electrical and mechanical activity because each contraction is heralded by a burst composed of several

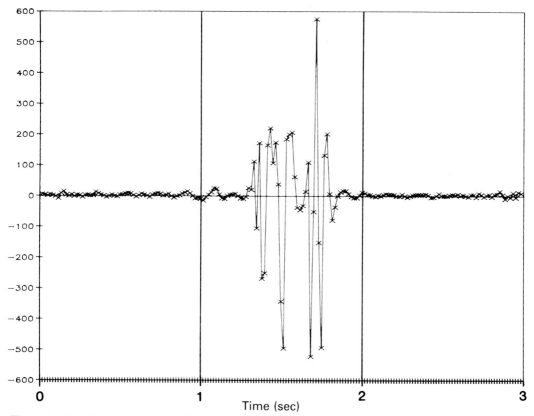

Figure 2. Most signals are recorded in an analogue scale and must be transformed to numerical form (A to D conversion) for computer analysis. This waveform is an actual spike burst, recorded at a rapid chart speed and sampled at short, regular intervals (60 Hz).

spikes rather than a single event. For this reason, the preferable method of estimating intestinal contractile activity is to count each spike burst as a single event. This method has been adopted by Summers et al (1982), Groh et al (1984) and Flatt and Summers (1987) (Figures 2 and 3).

Bandpass filtration of the signal can be accomplished through computerized digital filtration methods (Summers et al, 1982), but the computer time and memory requirements are excessive. The use of external analogue filters eliminates the need for computer filtering and improves efficiency considerably (Wingate et al, 1976; Groh et al, 1984; Flatt and Summers, 1987).

After the spike bursts or contractions have been detected, the computer can be utilized to construct frequency histograms of contraction intervals (Hiesinger et al, 1978; Christensen et al, 1971; Engstrom et al, 1979; Pousse et al, 1979). This

application has limited usefulness but was an important indirect method to establish the slow wave interval from recordings of mechanical activity.

Contraction Waves (Mechanical Activity)

The first applications of the computer to intestinal motor activity were directed towards the mathematical analysis of intestinal contraction waves (Farrar, 1960). Analogue-to-digital conversion itself was a major task but the efforts of Farrar and co-workers pointed the way to improvements in automated analysis, making it more efficient, more accurate and more comprehensive in scope than was possible with visual analysis. Early computers were primitive, slow, and had limited memory. A

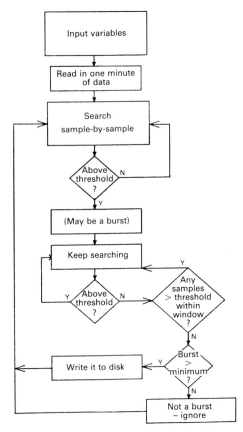

Figure 3. Flow diagram of the logic for a spike detection program.

tractions is technically difficult and attempts to analyse them using the computer are very limited (Hacket et al, 1986). But the intestinal contraction has been studied since the early 1960s (Christensen et al, 1971; Farrar, 1960; Misiewicz et al, 1968). Misiewicz et al (1968) designed a system to analyse five variables describing intraluminal intestinal pressures. These included the number of contractions, their amplitudes and durations, the percentage of recorded time during which contractions occurred and the area under the curve. Similar approaches have been adopted by others (Schemann et al, 1985; Flatt and Summers, 1987) (Figure 4).

significant amount of hand labour was still required to prepare the signal for analysis. Improvements in hardware have made most of the early analytical techniques obsolete; however, many of the principles of analysis remain the same.

Only a few attempts to develop programs to analyse oesophageal motor activity have been published, although a number of other programs are in use (Castell et al, 1984; Castell and Castell, 1986). The parameters analysed in body contractions usually include the wave amplitude, duration and velocity of peristalsis as well as the maximum dP/dt and area under the contraction curve. Those in the sphincter region include the baseline gastric and sphincter pressures and the degree and duration of relaxation.

The recording of gastric and colonic con-

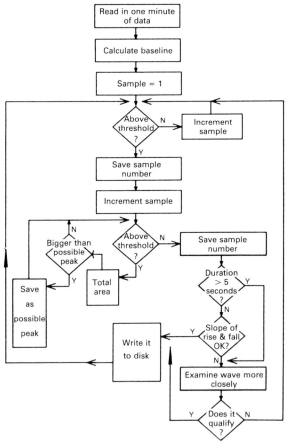

Figure 4. Flow diagram for analysis of contraction waves.

Spread or Migration of Spike Bursts or Contractile Waves

In addition to the recognition and quantification of motor events, it is essential to analyse their temporal and spatial relationships. Most methods quantitate motor events at a single site and provide a summation of activity over a regular time increment. It has been our contention that integration over time cannot provide an adequate understanding of propulsion or transit of a bolus (Dusdieker and Summers, 1980; Summers and Dusdieker, 1981). Consideration of space and time

are inherent in an understanding of propagation or migration of contractile events. Therefore the analysis must consider patterns of motor events and it must describe what is happening at two or more points.

A great deal of information has been obtained from computer analysis of contractile events from just two points. Engstrom et al (1979) have analysed wave intervals between two serosal transducers placed 2.5 cm apart on the dog intestine. A preponderance of contractions are propagated in an aborad direction. Similarly Reddy et al (1981) characterized directions of propagation as aborad,

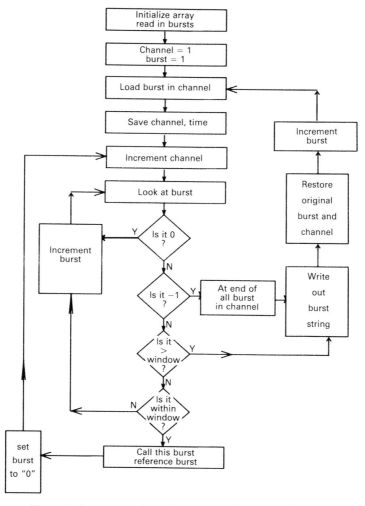

Figure 5. Flow diagram for analysis of spike burst migration.

local or orad. A statistical pattern recognition technique was utilized to classify contractile activity. Feature vectors were employed in algorithms according to Baye's classification technique. This approach was able to differentiate between patterns recorded during meals of different compositions; however, it did not describe the patterns in any way, and is not helpful in conceptualizing or describing propulsion.

The introduction of the concept of myoelectric timing has facilitated description of some of the complex events in the antroduodenal region. The term 'antroduodenal co-ordination' has been introduced and the computer-aided study of the phenomenon has aided our understanding of gastric emptying (Ehrlein and Hiesinger, 1982; Engstrom et al, 1979; Roelofs et al, 1987).

Through the use of closely spaced electrical or mechanical sensors, contractile events in the small bowel can be characterized as non-migrating or migrating ('segmental' or 'propulsive'). The principles of analysis include consideration of both temporal and spatial relationships of motor activity from multiple sensors. Our early attempts to do this were laboriously done by hand (Dusdieker and Summers, 1980; Summers and Dusdieker, 1981), but now the computer is capable of performing the analysis much more rapidly, objectively, thoroughly and accurately than thought possible a decade ago (Summers et al, 1982; Schemann et al, 1985). Our programs analysed spread of myoelectric activity (Summers et al, 1982) while Schemann et al (1985) adopted the same principle to quantitate the same propulsive patterns from recordings of mechanical activity. We have modified our initial programs considerably, but the theoretical considerations remain essentially the same (Flatt and Summers, 1987) (Figure 5).

Several investigators have utilized the computer to identify the various phases of the MMC and determine their length and periodicity (Sarna et al, 1971; Wingate et al, 1976). However, automated analysis of more complex motility patterns has developed more slowly. This is partly because the logic is more difficult, but also because definitions are somewhat arbitrary and generate more controversy.

Other Computer Applications

The computer has been utilized to analyse a number of other variables related to small intestinal motility. The purpose of intestinal motor activity is to produce movement of intestinal contents. The analysis of transit has been approached using the computer although further developments in this area of interest are needed (Lundquist et al, 1974). The ability of the intestine to perform work is the topic of studies by Weems et al using *in vitro* techniques (Weems and Seygal, 1981; Weems and Weisbrodt, 1984; Weems et al, 1985). The program developed by this group could be adapted to *in vivo* studies and either approach constitutes a powerful technique applicable to physiological and pharmacological studies. The computer has even been utilized to study bowel sounds (Dalle and Devroede, 1975).

Future Developments

When investigating repetitive and nearly identical events, the computer may not ultimately be the analytical technique of choice. The previously noted use of the tape recorder to avoid on-line processing of data and the use of hard-wired filters to reduce memory requirements are examples of devices replacing the computer. Many of the analyses already described as performed by the computer can be accomplished by instruments using analogue circuits (Crenner et al, 1982). Future developments may incorporate more of such devices rather than computer software. Hardware circuits, though somewhat more difficult to modify than software, cost nothing in terms of computer time or storage space once constructed. If a device can carefully define important characteristics (e.g filtering frequencies), there is nothing to be gained by doing that task in software. Eventually combinations of analogue devices and digital computers will likely be utilized to achieve maximum efficiency and accuracy with minimum cost and time commitment.

Future efforts should be directed towards the analysis of motor events in the stomach, biliary tree and colon because of the dearth of applications in those organs. In addition much effort should be directed towards analysis of motility patterns because of the importance of both spatial and temporal orientation of contractions in determining propulsion of intraluminal contents.

Acknowledgement

This study was supported in part by Veterans Administration Research funds and NIH Digestive Disease Core Center Grant AM34986.

References

Alvarez, W. C., (1922), The electrogastogram and what it shows. *JAMA*, **78**:1116–19.

Avill, R., Manguall, Y. F., Bird, N. C., Brown, B. H., Barber, D. C., Seagar, A. D., Johnson, A. G., and Read, N. W., (1987), Applied potential tomography: a new noninvasive technique for measuring gastric emptying. *Gastroenterology*, **92**:1019–26.

Barber, D. C., and Brown, B. H., (1984), Applied potential tomography. *J. Phys. E. Sci. Inst.*, **17**:723–33.

Brown, B. H., Duthie, H. L., Horn, A. R., and Smallwood, R. H., (1975), A linked oscillator model of electrical activity of human small intestine. *Am. J. Physiol.*, **229**:384–8.

Castell, J. A., and Castell, D. O., (1986), Computer analysis of human esophageal peristalsis and lower esophageal sphincter pressure. II An interactive system for on-line data collection and analysis. *Dig. Dis. Sci.*, **31**:1211–16.

Castell, D. O., Dubois, A., Davis, C. R., Cordova, C. M., and Norman, D. O., (1984), Computer-aided analysis of human esophageal peristalsis. I. Technical description and comparison with manual analysis. *Dig. Dis. Sci.*, **29**:65–72.

Cherbut, C., and Ruckebusch, Y., (1984), Modifications de l'électromyogramme du côlon liées à l'ingestion de particules non digestibles chez le chien. *Gastroenterol. Clin. Biol.*, **8**:955–9.

Christensen, J., Glover, J. R., Macagno, E. O., Singerman, R. B., and Weisbrodt, N. W., (1971), Statistics of contractions at a point in the human duodenum. *Am. J. Physiol.*, **221**:1818–23.

Crenner, F., Lambert, A., Angel, F., Schang, J. C., and Grenier, J. F., (1982), Analogue automated analysis of small intestinal electromyogram. *Med. Biol. Eng. Comput.*, **20**:151–8.

Dalle, D., and Devroede, G., (1975), Computer analysis of bowel sounds. *Comput. Biol. Med.*, **4**:247–56.

DeMeester, T. R., Wang, Ch.-I., Wernly, J. A., Pellegrini, C. A., Little, A. G., Klementschitsch, P., Bèrmudez, G., Johnson, L. F., and Skinner, D. B., (1980), Techniques, indications, and clinical use of 24 hour esophageal pH monitoring. *J. Thoracic. Cardiovas. Surg.*, **79**: 656–70.

Diamant, N. E., Rose, P. K., and Davison, E. J., (1970), Computer simulation of intestinal slow-wave frequency gradient. *Am. J. Physiol.*, **219**:1684–90.

Dubois, A., Van Eerdewegh, P., and Gardner, J. D., (1977), Gastric emptying and secretion in the Zollinger-Ellison syndrome. *J. Clin. Invest.*, **59**:255–63.

Dusdieker, N. S., and Summers, R. W., (1980), Longitudinal and circumferential spread of spike bursts in canine jejunum in vivo. *Am. J. Physiol.*, **239**:G311–18.

Ehrlein, H.-J., and Hiesinger, E., (1982), Computer analysis of mechanical activity of gastroduodenal junction in unanesthetized dogs. *Quart J. Exp. Physiol.*, **67**:17–29.

Elashoff, S. D., Reedy, T. J., and Meyer, J. H., (1982), Analysis of gastric emptying data. *Gastroenterol.*, **83**:1306–12.

Engstrom, E., Webster, J., and Bass, P., (1979), Analysis of duodenal contractility in the unanaesthetized dog. *IEEE Trans. Biomed. Eng. BME*, **26**:517–23.

Farrar, S. T., (1960), Use of a digital computer in the analysis of intestinal motility records. *IRE Trans. Med. Electron. ME*, **7**:259–63.

Flatt, A. J., and Summers, R. W., (1987), Computer analysis of intestinal motor activity. *Automedica*, **7**:221–36.

George, J. D., (1968), New clinical method for measuring the rate of gastric emptying: the double sampling test meal. *Gut*, **9**:237–42.

Groh, W. J., Takahashi, I., Sarna, S., Dodds, W. J., and Hogan, W. J., (1984), Computerized analysis of spike-burst activity of the upper gastrointestinal tract. *Dig. Dis. Sci.*, **29**:442–6.

Hacket, T., Bueno, L., Fioramonti, J., and Rode, C., (1986), The use of a compact portable microcomputer system (Epson HX20) to measure on-line the contractile activity of the digestive tract from light channels. *J. Pharm. Meth.*, **16**:171–80.

Hacket, T., Bueno, L., Fioramonti, J., and Frexinos, J., (1985), 'Off-line four channel measurement of colonic myoelectrical activity in humans using a compact portable microcomputer (Epson HX20). *Int. J. Bio-Med. Comput.*, **17**:115–21.

Heading, R. C., (1982), Gastric emptying: a clinical perspective. *Clin. Sci.*, **63**:231–5.

Hiesinger, E., Hoernicke, H., and Ehrlein, H.-J., (1978), Computer analysis of electrical and mechanical activity of stomach, duodenum and cecum over long periods. In: *Gastrointestinal Motility in Health and Disease* (Ed Duthie, H. L.), pp 275–84, MTP Press, Lancaster.

Kingma, Y. J., (1987), Spectral analysis of gastro-intestinal electrical signals. *Automedica*, 7:237–48.

Latour, A., (1973), Un dispositif simple d'analyse quantitative de l'electro-myogramme intestinal chronique. *Ann. Rech. Vet.*, 4:347–53.

Latour, A., Bueno, L., and Fioramonti, J., (1983), Quantitative measurement of human colonic electrical activity by a micro-computerized system. *Int. J. Bio-Med. Comput.*, 14:7–16.

Linkens, D. A., and Connell, A. E., (1974), Interactive graphics analysis of gastrointestinal electrical signals. *IEEE Trans. Biomed. Eng. BME*, 21:335–9.

Linkens, D. A., and Mhone, P. G., (1979), Frequency transients in a coupled oscillator model of intestinal myoelectric activity. *Comput. Biol. Med.*, 9:131–44.

Lundquist, H., Jung, B., and Nilsson, F., (1974), A theoretical analysis of some measures used in studies of small bowel propulsion and their dependence on gastric evacuation pattern. *Acta. Chir. Scand.*, 140:410–15.

Meyer, J. H., MacGregor, I. L., Gueller, R., et al (1976), ^{99m}Tc-tagged chicken liver as a marker of solid food in the human stomach *Am. J. Dig. Dis.*, 21:296–304.

Misiewicz, J. J., Waller, S. L., Healy, M. J. R., and Piper, E. A., (1968), Computer analysis of intra-luminal pressure records. *Gut*, 9:232–6.

Nelsen, T. S., and Becker, J. L., (1968), Simulation of the electrical and mechanical gradient of the small intestine. *Am. J. Physiol.*, 214:749–57.

Postaire, J. G., Van Houtte, N., and DeVroede, G., (1978), A computer for quantitative analysis of gastrointestinal signals. *Comput. Biol. Med.*, 9:295–303.

Pousse, A., Mendel, C., Kashelhoffer, J., and Grenier, J. F., (1979), Computer program for intestinal spike bursts recognition. *Pflugers Archiv.*, 381:15–18.

Reddy, S. N., Dumpala, S. R., Sarna, S. K., and Northcott, P. G., (1981), Pattern recognition of canine duodenal contractile activity. *IEEE Trans. Biomed. Eng. BME*, 28:696–701.

Roelofs, J. M. M., Akkermans, L. M. A., and Schuurkes, J. A. J., (1987), Computer-aided analysis and mechanical activity of stomach and duodenum. *Z. Gastroenterologie*, 25:107–11.

Sarna, S. K., Daniel, E. E., and Kingma, Y. J., (1971), Simulation of slow-wave electrical activity of small intestine. *Am. J. Physiol.*, 221:166–75.

Schemann, M., Ehrlein, H.-J., and Sahyoun, H., (1985), Computerised method for pattern recognition of intestinal motility: functional significance of the spread of contractions. *Med. Biol. Eng. Comput.*, 23:143–9.

Schindbeck, N. E., Heinrich, C., König, A., et al (1987), Optimal thresholds, sensitivity and specificity of long-term pH-metry for the detection of gastro-esophageal reflux disease. *Gastroenterol.*, 93:85–90.

Sheiner, H. J., (1984), Isotope methods in measuring gastric emptying. In: *Gastric and Duodenal Motility* (Eds Akkermans, L. M. A., Johnson, A. G., and Read, N. W.), pp 148–157, Praeger, Eastbourne.

Sinar, D. R., and Charles, L. G., (1983), Glucose is the major component controlling irregular spike activity after feeding in primates. *Gastroenterol.*, 85:1319–25.

Smout, A. J. P. M., van der Schee, E. J., and Grashuis, J. L., (1980a), What is measured in electro-gastrography? *Dig. Dis. Sci.*, 25:179–87.

Smout, A. J. P. M., van der Schee, E. J., and Grashuis, J. L., (1980b), Postprandial and interdigestive gastric electrical activity in the dog recorded by means of cutaneous electrodes. In: *Gastrointestinal Motility* (Ed Christensen, J.), pp 187–94, Raven Press, New York.

Smout, A. J. P. M., van der Schee, E. J., and Grashuis, J. L., (1979), Gastric pacemaker activity in conscious dogs. *Am. J. Physiol.*, 237:E279–83.

Stanciu, C., Hoare, R. C., and Bennett, S. R., (1977), Correlation between manometric and pH tests for gastroesophageal reflux disease. *Gut*, 18:536–40.

Stoddard, C. J., Duthie, H. L., Smallwood, R. H., and Linkens, A., (1979), Colonic myoelectric activity in man; comparison of recording techniques and methods of analysis. *Gut*, 20:476–83.

Summers, R. W., Cramer, J., and Flatt, A. J., (1982), Computerized analysis of spike burst activity in the small intestine. *IEEE Trans. Biomed. Eng.*, 29:309–14.

Summers, R. W., and Dusdieker, N. S., (1981), Patterns of spike burst spread in the canine small intestine. *Gastroenterol.*, 81:742–50.

Tothill, P., McLoughlin, G. P., and Heading, R. C., (1978), Techniques and errors in scintigraphic measurements of gastric emptying. *J. N. M.*, 19:256–61.

Tothill, P., McLoughlin, G. P., Holt, et al (1980), The effect of posture on errors in gastric emptying measurements. *Phys. Med. Biol.*, 25:1071–7.

van der Schee, E. J., Kentie, M. A., Grashuis, J. L., and Smout, A. J. P. M., (1981), Adaptive filtering of canine electrogastrography signals, Part 2: filter performance. *Med. Biol. Eng. Comput.*, 19:765–9.

van der Schee, E. J., Smout, A. J. P. M., and Grashuis, J. L., (1982), Application of running spectrum analysis to electrogastrographic signals recorded from dog and man. In: *Motility of the Digestive Tract* (Ed. Wienbech, M.), pp 241–50, Raven Press, New York.

Weems, W. A., Seidel, E. R., and Johnson, L. R., (1985), Induction in vitro of a specific pattern of jejunal propulsive behaviour by cholecystokinin. *Am. J. Physiol.*, 248:G470–9.

Weems, W. A., and Seygal, G. E., (1981), Fluid propulsion by cat intestine segments under conditions requiring hydrostatic work. *Am. J. Physiol.*, 240:G147–57.

Weems, W. A., and Weisbrodt, N. W., (1984), Comparison of colonic and ileal propulsive capabilities under conditions requiring hydrostatic work. *Am. J. Physiol.*, **246**:G587–93.

Wingate, D. L., and Barnett, T., (1978), The logical analysis of the electroenterogram. *Am. J. Dig. Dis.*, **23**:553–8.

Wingate, D. L., Barnett, T., Green, R., and Armstrong, J. M., (1977), Automated high-speed analysis of gastrointestinal myoelectric activity. *Am. J. Dig. Dis.*, **22**:243–51.

Wingate, D. L., Barnett, T. G., and Green, W. E. R., (1976), The analysis of gastrointestinal myoelectric activity. *Post. Grad. Med. J. (Suppl. 7)*, **52**:157.

III
NORMAL GASTROINTESTINAL MOTILITY

14
OESOPHAGUS

J. Janssens and G. Vantrappen
University Hospital Leuven, Leuven, Belgium

The Normal Oesophagus

The main function of the oesophagus is the transport of food and drink from the pharynx into the stomach. Swallowing induces a contraction wave which starts high up in the pharynx and progresses down the oesophagus until it reaches the cardia. This primary peristaltic contraction pushes a solid bolus down the oesophagus into the stomach. Fluids taken in the upright position reach the cardia prior to the arrival of the primary peristaltic contraction due to gravitational forces, but in the head-down position fluids are also propelled by the deglutitive contractions. In the resting state, in between deglutitions, the oesophagus is closed at both ends by sphincter mechanisms. The upper oesophageal (pharyngo-oesophageal) sphincter prevents air from entering the oesophagus during inspiration. The lower oesophageal (gastro-oesophageal) sphincter is of primary importance in the prevention of gastro-oesophageal reflux. Both sphincters relax temporarily after deglutition to allow the passage of the swallowed bolus. If reflux occurs, it gives rise to a secondary peristaltic contraction which propels the refluxed material back into the stomach (Hellemans and Vantrappen, 1974; Christensen, 1987).

Examination Techniques

The motor function of the oesophagus can be studied in several ways.

Radiology with Contrast Material

Using contrast material that coats the mucosa, high-speed cine- or videorecording and radiographic methods will show, apart from morphological abnormalities, flow of intraluminal material and motion of the wall. This technique is at present essential in the study of normal and disordered motor function of pharynx and pharyngo-oesophageal region, and may yield important information on the motility of the oesophageal body and lower oesophageal sphincter (LOS) as well.

Manometry

Manometric techniques have been widely used to examine the motor function of the oesophagus and its sphincters. For clinical purposes a bundle of tubes having distal lateral openings at different levels is used in connection with externally placed strain gauges and a continuous low compliance perfusion technique (Arndorfer et al, 1977). Details of the manometric methods have been published in many recent publications and are discussed in Section II. Intraluminal pressure measurements yield information on tension developed in circular muscles, but not on changes in longitudinal muscle tension. This technique is particularly useful in studying motor events in the LOS and the oesophageal body; its frequency response, however, is at the very limit for an adequate recording of the fast motor events occurring in pharynx and upper oesophageal sphincter. Intraluminal solid state transducers have a much

higher frequency response and prevent the need
for perfusion, but they are more expensive and
vulnerable. Solid state transducers are used in ambulatory recording systems that monitor oesophageal pressures (and pH) for prolonged periods of
time in patients with angina-like chest pain of
noncardiac origin (Figure 1) (Vantrappen et al,
1982; Janssens et al, 1986).

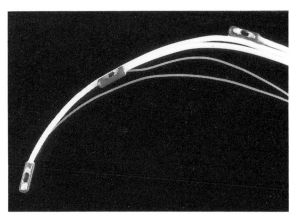

Figure 2. Assembly of small bipolar suction electrodes suitable
for electromyographic recording in the human oesophagus.

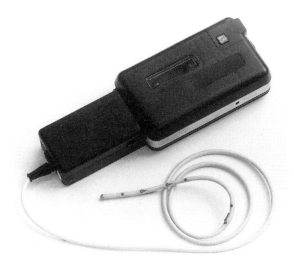

Figure 1. Ambulatory 24-hour pH and pressure recording
system.

Electromyography

Electromyographic techniques are the only way to
distinguish contractile activity of striated muscles
in the upper part of the oesophagus from that
of smooth muscles in the lower gullet. The best
recordings in man are currently obtained with
small bipolar suction electrodes. This technique,
however, is still in the experimental stage (Figure
2) (Hellemans et al, 1974).

Scintiscanning

Oesophageal scintiscanning during the passage of
a radiolabelled bolus has proved to be a reliable
technique in quantitative measurements of oesophageal transit.

Gastro-oesophageal reflux is best evaluated by
intra-oesophageal pH measurements or by scinti-

scanning. Several systems using small intraluminal glass electrodes with a combined intraluminal reference electrode and capable of
recording intra-oesophageal pH over a 24-hour
period in ambulatory patients are now commercially available. Oesophageal scintiscanning
following the administration of a radiolabelled
meal is another way to detect reflux especially in
children because it prevents the use of an intra-
oesophageal tube. The limited duration of the
recording period, however, is a major disadvantage of this technique.

Pharyngeal and Oesophageal Motility 'at rest'

Pharynx

Striated muscles of pharynx and parapharyngeal
structures exhibit some activity during the respiratory cycle giving rise to intrapharyngeal
pressure variations in between $+1.4\,\mathrm{mmHg}$
(expiration) and $-0.2\,\mathrm{mmHg}$ (inspiration) (Goyal
et al, 1970). This activity is best demonstrated by
electromyography.

Upper Oesophageal Sphincter

The upper oesophageal sphincter zone begins
immediately below the hypopharyngeal air
column and is 2–4 cm in length. It exhibits marked

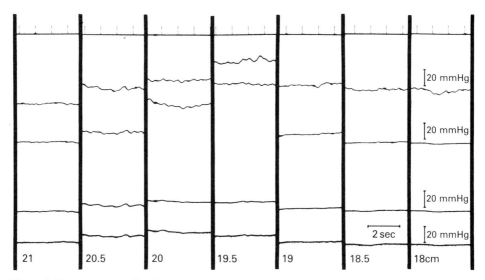

Figure 3. Manometric profile of upper oesophageal sphincter in a control subject, using four radially orientated continuously perfused catheters and a stepwise pull-through technique (steps indicated cm from incisors). Line 1: dorsally, 2: anteriorly, 3: left laterally, 4: right laterally.

radial and axial asymmetry, pressures being higher anteriorly and posteriorly than laterally (Figures 3 and 4) (Welch et al, 1979; Hellemans et al, 1981). Its normal maximal value during the resting state is fairly high, up to 100–130 mmHg above atmospheric pressure. The striated musculature of the sphincter generates continuous spiking activity which varies somewhat with respiration. The number of spike potentials is directly proportional to the resting pressure (Figures 5 and 6).

Oesophageal Body

The oesophageal body exhibits no rhythmic or tonic contractions at rest. All pressures are passively transmitted by respiratory variations (the intra-oesophageal pressure reflecting closely the intrapleural pressure), from −5 to −15 mmHg at inspiration to −2 to +5 mmHg at expiration, and by cardiovascular pulsations from aorta, left atrium and ventricle (Code and Schlegel, 1968). Electromyographically the oesophageal body is quiescent at rest.

Lower Oesophageal Sphincter

The high pressure zone of the LOS shows a bell-shaped configuration and is 2–4 cm in length. The sphincter has radial asymmetry with maximal pressures left laterally, primarily due to the crus sinistra of the diaphragm and the angled aspect of the lower oesophagus (Figure 7) (Welch and Drake, 1980). Some asymmetry, however, persists even in hiatal hernia patients and may be related to the spiral nature of the circular muscle fibres of the LOS. Because of this asymmetry LOS resting pressures should be evaluated manometrically using three or four tubes, with the lateral openings facing in different directions 120° or 90° apart. In most instances the LOS is situated around the pressure inversion point (PIP), at which the respiratory pressure swings with respiration change from inspiratory positive (intra-abdominal) to inspiratory negative (intrathoracic), and which usually corresponds to the level of the diaphragm (Figure 8). In case of hiatal hernia a double PIP may exist (Figure 9) (Harris and Pope, 1966).

In addition to the respiration related pressure changes, the LOS pressure may also vary with the different phases of the migrating motor complex, pressures being highest during phase 3 and lowest during phase 1 (Figure 10) (Dent et al, 1983; Smout et al, 1985).

The LOS pressure can also be evaluated by means of a rapid pull-through, which usually measures a slightly higher LOS pressure than the

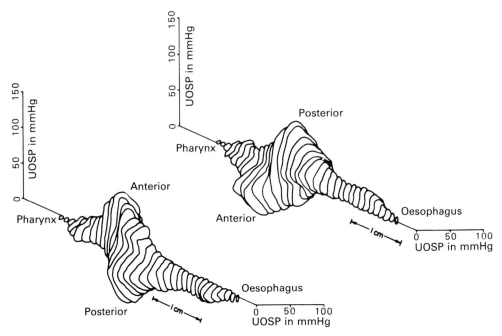

Figure 4. Three-dimensional pressure profiles of the upper oesophageal sphincter. Pressures are higher in antero-posterior position than laterally. (Welch et al, 1979.)

slow step-wise pull-through (Welch and Drake, 1980) (Figure 11). The best way to monitor continuously maximal LOS pressure over a prolonged period of time is performed with the Dent sleeve (Dent, 1976).

In addition to intra-subject variations (i.e. due to the MMC cycle) the normal LOS pressure also shows marked inter-subject variations. Normal values are accepted to vary from $+10$ to $+40$ mmHg (as compared to the intrafundic zero level).

Human electromyographic data are scarce. Whether or not the human LOS generates spontaneous electrical signals at rest, still remains con-

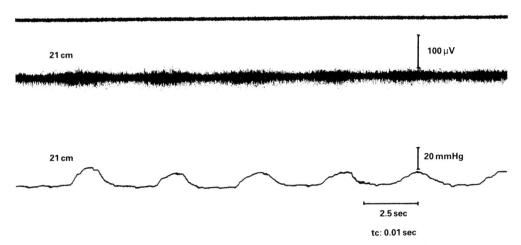

Figure 5. Simultaneous recording of electromyographic and intraluminal pressure in the human upper oesophageal sphincter at rest (21 cm from the incisors). The continuous spiking activity fluctuates with respiration.

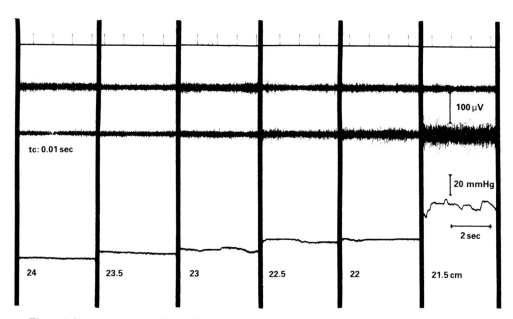

Figure 6. Simultaneous recording of electromyographic and intraluminal pressure in the human upper oesophageal sphincter at rest; stepwise pull-through from 24–21.5 cm from incisors. Line 1: EMG of the suprahyoid muscle showing the absence of deglutition. Line 2: EMG of the upper oesophageal sphincter showing an increase in number and amplitude of spike potentials together with an increase in sphincter pressure (line 3).

troversial (Hellemans et al, 1974; Asoh and Goyal, 1978). The competence of the LOS in the prevention of gastro-oesophageal reflux is best evaluated by 24 hour intraoesophageal pH measurements. A few reflux episodes (less than 50 peaks/24 h, or pH < 4 < 42% of time/24 h) especially during the postprandial period represent the so-called physiological reflux (Figure 12) (De Meester et al, 1974; Galmiche et al, 1980; Johnson and De Meester, 1986).

Pharyngeal and Oesophageal Motility after Swallowing

Pharynx

The swallowing movement starts with the onset of activity in the myelohyoid muscle. The sequence of pharyngeal and extrapharyngeal muscle contractions that occurs after swallowing gives rise to a wave of pharyngeal peristalsis that travels down the oropharynx and hypopharynx at a speed of about 15 cm/sec to reach the upper

oesophageal sphincter after about 0.7 sec. The hypopharyngeal peristaltic wave has a peak amplitude of about 200 ± 150 mmHg and a mean duration of 0.3–0.5 sec (Figure 13) (Dodds et al, 1975).

Upper Oesophageal Sphincter

The upper oesophageal sphincter relaxes after deglutition to allow easy passage of the swallowed bolus. The relaxation may even reach subatmospheric pressures. It starts upon swallowing, lasts for about 0.5–1.0 sec and is followed by a contraction which is the start of a primary peristaltic contraction in the oesophageal body. Occasionally a short increase in pressure, related to the inspiratory contraction of the sphincter, may precede the onset of relaxation. Electromyographically the relaxation is accompanied by the cessation of all spiking activity; during the post-deglutitive contraction there is an increase in spiking activity which lasts as long as the contraction itself (Figure 14) (Fyke and Code, 1955; Pelemans, 1983).

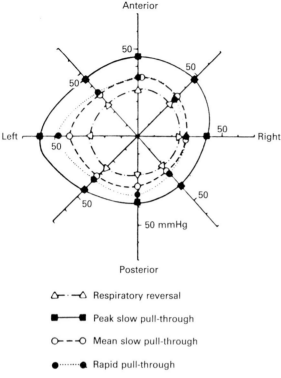

△—·—△ Respiratory reversal

■——■ Peak slow pull-through

○— —○ Mean slow pull-through

●······● Rapid pull-through

Figure 7. Radial asymmetry of the lower oesophageal sphincter in 18 normal subjects. With all methods pressures leftwards were significantly greater than rightwards (from Welch and Drake, 1980).

Oesophageal Body

The manometrically recorded deglutitive contraction of the oesophageal body may comprise of several components (Figure 15) (Vantrappen and Hellemans, 1967; Goyal and Cobb, 1981). The initial pressure change (A-wave) is a negative deflection which starts about 0.2 sec after the onset of swallowing and lasts for about 0.3–0.5 sec. It is probably due to a short inspiration just prior to the swallowing movement ('Schluckatmung') (Figure 16). In about 87% of the swallows this initial negative deflection is followed by a positive pressure change (B-wave), probably caused by the transmission of pharyngeal pressure through the swallowed bolus (Butin et al, 1953). A second positive wave (C-wave) is recorded in the distal part of the oesophagus after about one-third of the swallows and is probably caused by the increased pressure between the advancing bolus and the LOS (Figure 17) (Vantrappen and Hellemans, 1967; Hellemans, 1970). A, B and C-waves are passively transmitted pressure phenomena, not related to the peristaltic contraction itself. If present, they start simultaneously in different segments of the oesophageal body.

The main pressure component of the normal

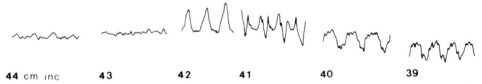

44 cm inc   **43**   **42**   **41**   **40**   **39**

Figure 8. Stepwise pull-through of the lower oesophageal sphincter showing the pressure inversion point (PIP) at the level of 41 cm from incisors.

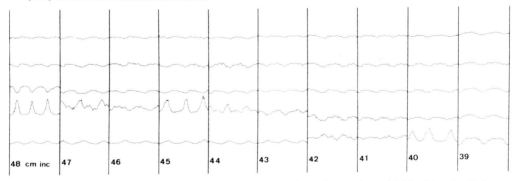

Figure 9. Stepwise pull-through of the lower oesophageal sphincter in a patient with hiatal hernia. Catheter assembly with 5 perfused catheters with side openings 5 cm apart. Centimetres from incisors indicated for the most distally located side opening. A double pressure inversion point (double PIP) is observed at 42 and 39 cm from incisors at line 5 and at 41 and 38 cm (46 – 5 cm and 43 – 5 cm) at line 4.

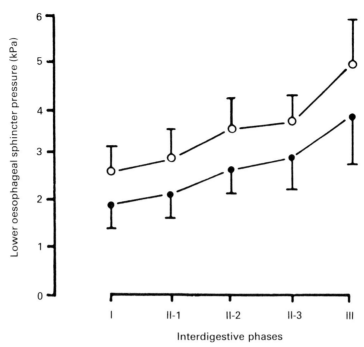

Figure 10. Mean lower oesophageal sphincter pressure (± SEM) in six healthy patients during various phases of the migrating motor complex after placebo (●) and cisapride (○) (0.5 mg/h i.v.) (from Smout et al, 1985).

deglutition complex is a large positive pressure wave which represents the peristaltic contraction. In most instances it is a single-peaked wave (E-wave) but double-peaked waves (M-waves) are seen in healthy volunteers after about 11% of wet swallows (Figure 18) (Richter et al, 1987). The amplitude of the peristaltic contraction varies considerably from one individual to another and, in the same individual, from one segment of the oesophageal body to another. Measured with intra-

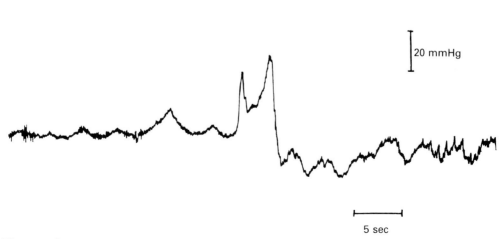

Figure 11. Lower oesophageal sphincter pressure evaluated by rapid pull-through from stomach (left) to oesophageal body (right).

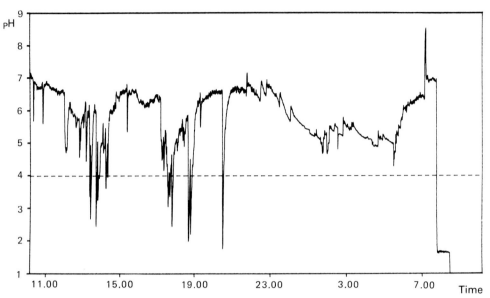

Figure 12. 24-hour pH plot showing intra-oesophageal pH (measured at 5 cm above the lower oesophageal sphincter) versus time in a patient with minimal complaints of heartburn during the postprandial period.

luminal solid state transducers the amplitude was found to be 69.5 ± 12.1 mmHg in the lower oesophagus, 53.4 ± 9.0 mmHg in the upper gullet and 35.0 ± 6.4 mmHg in the mid-oesophageal segment which corresponds to the transition zone between striated and smooth oesophageal muscle (Humphries and Castell, 1977). The speed of progression of the peristaltic wave increases from 3 cm/sec in the upper segment to 5 cm/sec in the lower oesophagus, but slows down again to 2.5 cm/sec just above the LOS. The peristaltic contraction reaches the LOS 5–6 sec after swal-

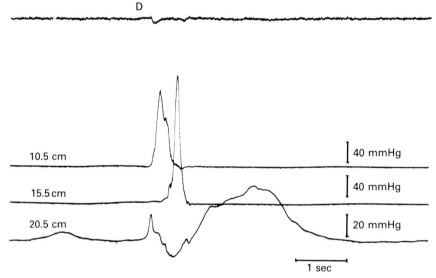

Figure 13. Pressure measurement in the pharyngo-oesophageal region. Catheter assembly with three solid state intraluminal microtransducers at 10.5, 15.5 and 20.5 cm from incisors. The most distal catheter is located in the upper oesophageal sphincter.

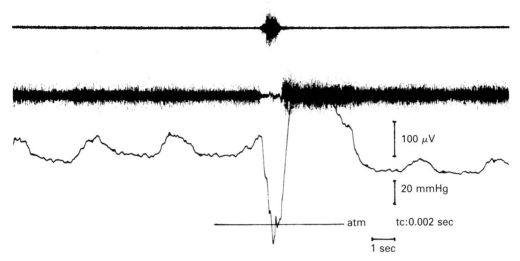

Figure 14. Simultaneous electromyographic (line 2) and intraluminal pressure (line 3) recording in the human upper oesophageal sphincter. Line 1 is the deglutitive signal (EMG of the suprahyoideal muscle).

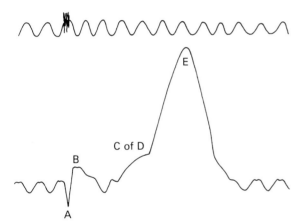

Figure 15. Schematic representation of the various components of the deglutitive contractions in the oesophageal body.

lowing. The duration of a single peaked peristaltic wave varies from 2 to 4 sec but never exceeds 6.5 sec (Vantrappen and Hellemans, 1967).

Some parameters of the normal deglutition complex may change with age. The most consistent finding is an increase in the number of non-peristaltic contractions (up to 30% of the deglutitive contractions being simultaneous) and in the number of repetitive (triple or more) waves, up to 7%. The manometric tracing may even look like diffuse oesophageal spasm. The amplitude of contractions may decrease somewhat with age but this

is certainly not a consistent finding (Hellemans, 1970; Richter et al, 1987).

Electromyographic studies with intraluminal suction electrodes have shown that contraction in the upper oesophagus is accompanied by a burst of striated muscle spikes, the intensity of which is directly proportional to the amplitude of the contraction; the spike burst lasts as long as the contraction. In the lower oesophageal segment the spike burst that accompanies the contraction wave is of the smooth muscle type: smooth muscle spikes have a greater amplitude and a markedly longer duration and their rhythm is much slower than that of striated muscle spikes. In contrast to the response in the striated muscle oesophagus, smooth muscle action potentials never occur after the peak pressure of the deglutitive pressure wave has been reached (Figure 19). At the level of the transition zone between striated and smooth muscles both types of spikes are seen intermingled; the trace usually begins with spikes of the striated muscle type (Figure 20) (Hellemans et al, 1974).

If swallows are taken in rapid succession, no peristaltic wave appears until after the last swallow because a new deglutition inhibits the activity of the previous swallow (Figure 21). In the zone where the spike burst consists entirely of striated muscle spikes, a second deglutition results in

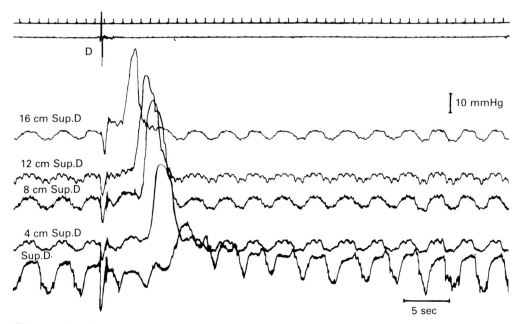

Figure 16. Intraluminal pressure measurement with a catheter assembly consisting of five perfused catheters with side openings at different levels above the diaphragm (Sup. D). The post-deglutitive (D) contraction shows an example of an A-wave ('Schluckatmung').

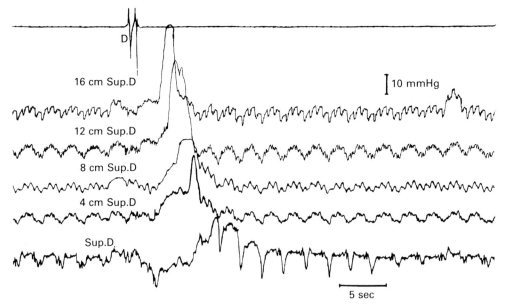

Figure 17. Intraluminal pressure measurement with a catheter assembly consisting of five perfused catheters with side openings at different levels above the diaphragm (Sup. D). The post-deglutitive (D) contraction shows an example of a C-wave at the level of 12, 8 and 4 cm above the diaphragm.

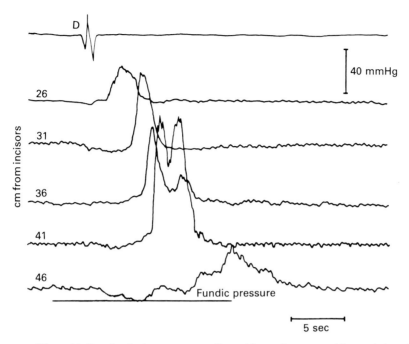

Figure 18. Intraluminal pressure recording with a catheter assembly consisting of five perfused catheters with side openings 5 cm apart. The post-deglutitive (D) peristaltic contraction shows an M-shaped pressure wave at the level of 41 cm from the incisors.

immediate disappearance of all spiking activity of the previous swallow and is accompanied by a decrease in intraluminal pressure. Swallowing also inhibits the spiking activity in the transitional zone where striated and smooth muscles are intermingled. In the distal segment, consisting of smooth muscles, the pattern is different. If the second deglutition occurs immediately before or during the initial phase of a spike burst, it does not interrupt the spiking activity in this oesophageal segment; yet the distal progression of the spike burst is halted and the deglutitive wave does not proceed further distally (Figure 22) (Hellemans et al, 1974; Janssens, 1978).

Lower Oesophageal Sphincter

The lower oesophageal sphincter relaxes upon deglutition to allow easy passage of the swallowed bolus. The relaxation may start with the onset of deglutition but in many instances it is delayed for 2–3 seconds after the initiation of swallowing. In normal individuals the relaxation is complete (or almost complete) with a mean reduction of $85\% \pm 5\%$ of the resting LOS pressure. The relaxation lasts 5–10 seconds and is followed in the upper part of the sphincter by an after-contraction which lasts 7–10 seconds. In the lower part of the sphincter the pressure returns to baseline level after the relaxation without the presence of an after-contraction (Figure 23) (Goyal and Cobb, 1981; Christensen, 1987; Jian et al, 1987).

Electromyographic studies in the human oesophagus were unable to demonstrate a clear electromyographic correlate for the sphincter relaxation, although in the opossum a cessation of the continuous spiking activity was described. The after-contraction is accompanied by a spike burst of the smooth muscle type, as in the oesophageal body (Figure 24) (Hellemans et al, 1968, 1974; Asoh and Goyal, 1978).

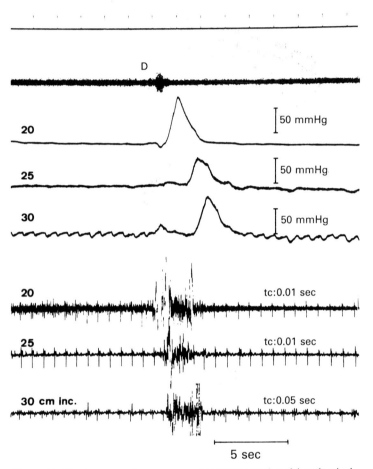

Figure 19. Simultaneous electromyographic (lower part) and intraluminal pressure (upper part) measurements at three different levels in the human oesophagus.

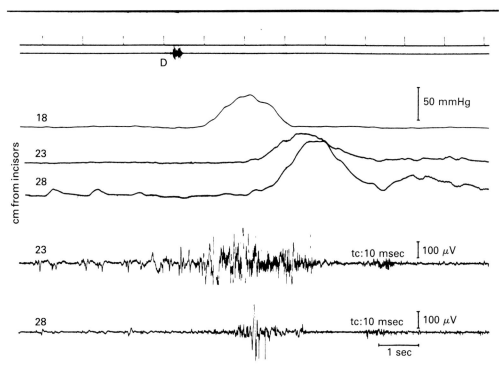

Figure 20. Simultaneous electromyographic (lower part) and intraluminal pressure (upper part) recording in the human oesophagus. The electrical tracing at 23 cm from incisors was recorded in the transitional zone where striated and smooth muscle spikes occur intermingled.

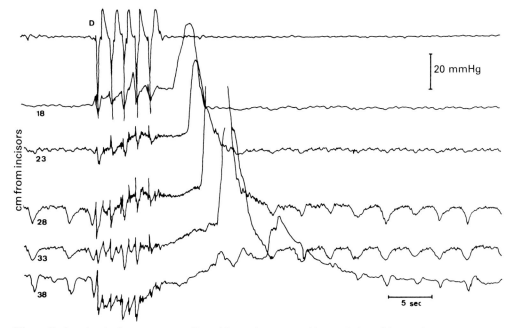

Figure 21. Intraluminal pressure recording with a catheter assembly consisting of five perfused catheters with side openings 5 cm apart. When a series of deglutitions is taken in rapid succession, only one oesophageal contraction is elicited starting after the last swallow.

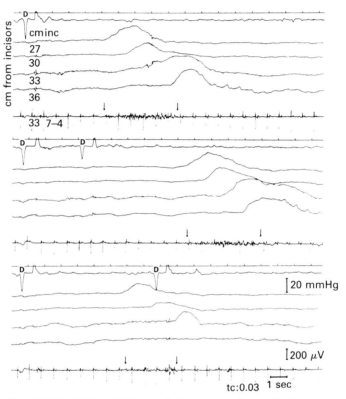

Figure 22. Deglutitive inhibition in the human oesophagus. Simultaneous intraluminal pressure measurements at 27, 30, 33 and 36 cm from incisors and EMG at 33 cm. Upper part: normal deglutitive response. Middle part: a deglutition 3.5 cm after a previous swallow eliminates the deglutitive response to the first deglutition. Lower part: if the second deglutition occurs during the spike burst of a previous swallow, it does not inhibit the spiking activity in this oesophageal segment but the distal progression is halted. (From Hellemans et al, 1974.)

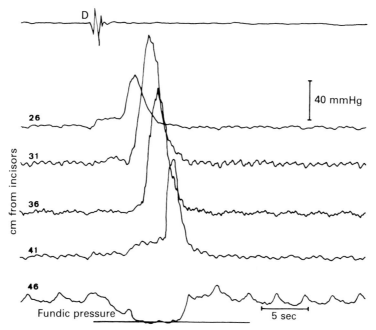

Figure 23. Intraluminal pressure recording with a catheter assembly consisting of five perfused catheters with side openings 5 cm apart. The distal opening is located in the lower part of the lower oesophageal sphincter. The pressure returns to baseline level after the relaxation without the presence of an after-contraction.

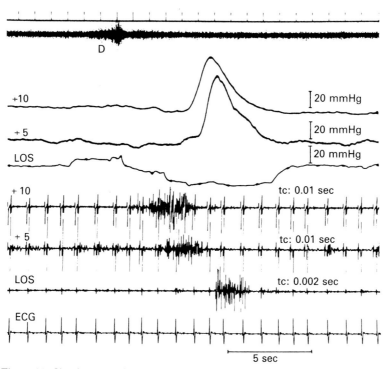

Figure 24. Simultaneous electromyographic (lower part) and intraluminal pressure (upper part) recording at two different levels in the oesophagus (5 and 10 cm above the lower oesophageal sphincter) and in the lower oesophageal sphincter in a normal subject. There is no clear correlate for the sphincter relaxation. ECG, electrocardiogram; LOS, lower oesophageal sphincter; D, deglutitive signal.

References

Arndorfer, R. C., Stef, J. J., Dodds, W. J., Linehan, J. H., and Hogan, W. J., (1977), Improved infusion system for intraluminal oesophageal manometry. *Gastroenterology*, **73**:23–7.

Asoh, R., and Goyal, R. K., 1978), Electrical activity of the opossum lower oesophageal sphincter in vivo. *Gastroenterology*, **74**:835–40.

Butin, J. W., Olsen, A. M., Moersh, H. J., and Code, C. F., (1953), A study of oesophageal pressures in normal persons and patients with cardiospasm. *Gastroenterology*, **23**:278–93.

Christensen, J., (1987), Motor functions of the pharynx and oesophagus. In: *Physiology of the Gastrointestinal Tract* (Ed. Johnson, L. R.), pp. 595–612, Raven Press, New Work.

Code, C. F., and Schlegel, J. F., (1968), Motor actions of the oesophagus and its sphincters. In: *Handbook of Physiology, Section 6, Alimentary Canal, Vol. IV Motility*, pp. 1821–39, American Physiological Society, Washington DC.

De Meester, T. R., Johnson, L. F., and Kent, A. H., (1974), Evaluation of current operations for the prevention of gastroesophageal reflux. *Ann. Surg.*, **180**:511–25.

Dent, J., (1976), A new technique for continuous sphincter pressure measurement. *Gastroenterology*, **71**:263–7.

Dent, J., Dodds, W. J., Sekiguchi, T., Hogan, W. J., and Arndorfer, R. C., (1983), Interdigestive phasic contractions of the human lower esophageal sphincter. *Gastroenterology*, **84**:453–60.

Dodds, W. J., Hogan, W. J., Lyden, S. B., Stewart, E. T., Steff, J. J., and Arndorfer, R. C., (1975), Quantitation of pharyngeal motor function in normal human subjects. *J. Appl. Physiol.*, **39**:692–6.

Fyke, F. E., and Code, C. F., (1955), Resting and deglutition pressures in the pharyngoesophageal region. *Gastroenterology*, **29**:24–34.

Galmiche, J. P., Guillard, J. F., Denis, P., Boussakr, K., Lefrançois, R., and Colon, R., (1980), Etude du pH oesophagien en période post-prandiale chez le sujet normal et au cours de syndrome de reflux gastro-oesophagien. Intérêt diagnostique d'un score de reflux acide. *Gastroenterol. Clin. Biol.*, **4**:531–9.

Goyal, R. K., and Cobb, B. W., (1981), Motility of the pharynx, esophagus and esophageal sphincters. In: *Physiology of the Gastrointestinal Tract* (Ed. Johnson, L. R.), pp. 359–91, Raven Press, New York.

Goyal, R. K., Sangree, M. H., and Hersh, T., (1970), Pressure inversion point at the upper high pressure zone and its genesis. *Gastroenterology*, **59**:754–9.

Harris, L. D., and Pope, C. E. II, (1966), The pressure inversion point: its genesis and reliability. *Gastroenterology*, **51**:641–8.

Hellemans, J., (1970), *Invloed van de leeftijd op de*

motorische Functie van de Slokdarm. Thesis, Lannoo pvba., Tielt.

Hellemans, J., Pelemans, W., and Vantrappen, G., (1981), Pharyngoesophageal swallowing disorders and the pharyngoesophageal sphincter. *Med. Clin. North Am.*, **65**:1149–71.

Hellemans, J., and Vantrappen, G., (1974), Physiology. In: *Handbuch der Inneren Medizin, Diseases of the Esophagus* (Eds. Vantrappen, G., and Hellemans, J.), pp. 40–102, Springer-Verlag, Berlin, Heidelberg, New York.

Hellemans, J., Vantrappen, G., and Janssens, J., (1974), Electromyography of the esophagus. In: *Handbuch der Inneren Medizin, Diseases of the Esophagus* (Eds. Vantrappen, G., and Hellemans, J.), pp. 270–85, Springer-Verlag, Berlin, Heidelberg, New York.

Hellemans, J., Vantrappen, G., Valembois, P., Janssens, J., and Vandenbroucke, J., (1968), Electrical activity of striated and smooth muscle of the esophagus. *Am. J. Dig. Dis.*, **13**:320–34.

Humphries, T. J., and Castell, D. O., (1977), Pressure profile of esophageal peristalsis in normal humans as measured by direct intraesophageal transducers. *Am. J. Dig. Dis.*, **22**:641–5.

Janssens, J., (1978), *The Peristaltic Mechanism of the Esophagus*. Thesis, Acco, Leuven.

Janssens, J., Vantrappen, G., and Ghillebert, G., (1986), 24-Hour recording of esophageal pressure and pH in patients with noncardiac chest pain. *Gastroenterology*, **90**:1978–84.

Jian, R., Janssens, J., Vantrappen, G., and Ceccatelli, P., (1987), Influence of metenkephalin analogue on motor activity of the gastrointestinal tract. *Gastroenterology*, **93**:114–20.

Johnson, L. F., and De Meester, T. R., (1986), Development of the 24-hour intraesophageal pH monitoring composite scoring system. *J. Clin. Gastroenterol.*, **8** (suppl. 1):52–8.

Pelemans, W., (1983), *Functie van de faryngo-esofageale Overgangszone en Dysfunctie bij Bejaarden*. Thesis, Acco, Leuven.

Richter, J. E., Wu, W. C., Johns, D. N., Blackwell, J. N., Nelson, J. L., Castell, J. A., and Castell, D. O., (1987), Esophageal manometry in 95 healthy adult volunteers: variability of pressures with age and frequency of 'abnormal' contractions. *Dig. Dis. Sci.*, **32**:583–92.

Smout, A. J. P. M., Bogaard, J. W., Grade, A. C., Ten Thye, O. J., Akkermans, L. M. A., and Wittebol, P., (1985), Effects of Cisapride, a new gastrointestinal prokinetic substance, on interdigestive and post-prandial motor activity of the distal oesophagus in man. *Gut*, **26**:246–51.

Vantrappen, G., and Hellemans, J., (1967), Studies on the normal deglutition complex. *Am. J. Dig. Dis.*, **12**:255–6.

Vantrappen, G., Servaes, J., Janssens, J., and Peeters,

T., (1982), Twenty-four-hour esophageal pH- and pressure recording in outpatients. In: *Motility of the Digestive Tract* (Ed. Wienbeck, M.), pp. 293–7, Raven Press, New York.

Welch, R. W., and Drake, S. T., (1980), Normal lower esophageal sphincter: a comparison of rapid vs slow pull through techniques. *Gastroenterology*, **78**:1446–51.

Welch, R. W., Luckmann, K., Ricks, P. M., Drake, S. T., and Gates, G. A., (1979), Manometry of the normal esophageal sphincter and its alteration in laryngectomy. *J. Clin. Invest.*, **63**:1036–41.

15
STOMACH AND DUODENUM

Harry M. Richter

University of Illinois College of Medicine and Cook County Hospital, Chicago, Illinois, USA

Gastroduodenal motor activity accomplishes three interrelated digestive functions. First, the stomach is an expansile reservoir, enabling man to eat a complete meal without experiencing an uncomfortable sense of fullness. Of more fundamental importance, hunting animals eat intermittently according to the availability of prey, and eat rapidly to thwart scavenging competitors; thus, the gastric reservoir function is an asset for survival. Second, the stomach grinds solids into a fine particulate suspension, liquefying and mixing its content with saliva, pepsin, and hydrochloric acid. This action prepares nutrients for further digestion and absorption from the small bowel. Finally, the stomach and duodenum regulate the entry of nutrients into the small bowel, promoting complete processing and absorption. This chapter describes gastroduodenal motor patterns identified in man and experimental animals (chiefly dog and cat). More detailed discussions of the physiological control of gastric motility and emptying will be found in the reviews of Malagelada and Azpiroz (in press) and Meyer (1987).

Gastric Motor Regions

Walter B. Cannon's seminal fluoroscopic study of feline gastric motility identified specialization into two regions with distinct motor activity (Cannon, 1898). The proximal stomach subserved a reservoir function, storing ingesta and slowly compressing its content aborally via tonic contraction. The distal stomach featured peristaltic contractions sweeping from the mid-stomach aborally

to the pylorus. This regional specialization is confirmed by myoelectrical and manometric techniques as well. Because solid food must be reduced to fine particles before it will pass the pylorus, the peristaltic contractions of the distal stomach assume prime importance in regulation of solid emptying. Liquid emptying does not require antral contractions, but depends upon the presence of a gastroduodenal pressure gradient. Thus the pattern of tonic proximal gastric contraction is likely important in controlling liquid phase emptying.

Gastric Myoelectrical Activity

Contraction of gastrointestinal smooth muscle is triggered by a depolarization of the resting transmembrane electrical potential maintained by each individual cell (Szurszewski, 1987). Intracellular recordings from smooth muscle cells of the proximal gastric region demonstrate no spontaneous depolarization (action potential), but contraction can be brought about by stimuli which raise transmembrane potential, such as acetylcholine. Cells from the distal gastric region exhibit spontaneous action potentials, accompanied by contractions. Stimuli augment the action potential and strengthen the muscular contraction. The frequency of spontaneous cellular action potentials is greatest in the most orad extremity of the distal gastric region.

Subserosal electrodes implanted in the tunica muscularis of the gut will record a fluctuating electrical potential difference with respect to an

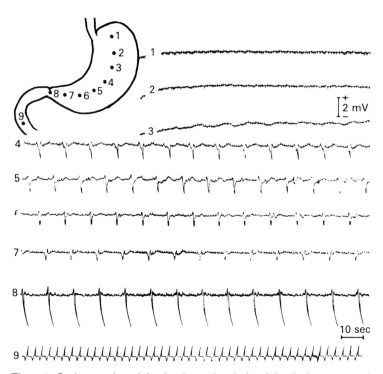

Figure 1. Canine gastric and duodenal myoelectrical activity during motor quiescence. Fundus and orad corpus are electrically silent, whereas a regular, distally propagating depolarization (pacesetter potential) is present in the distal stomach. Pacesetter potential frequency is approximately five per minute. (From Kelly et al, 1969 with permission.)

indifferent electrode placed elsewhere in the body. This potential represents a summation of electrical activity of the syncytium of smooth muscle cells in the immediate vicinity of the electrode. Prolonged simultaneous recordings of such myoelectric activity from a series of electrodes chronically implanted on the viscus under study demonstrates the regular pattern of electrical activity of that organ (see Chapter $\bar{9}$). Gastric myoelectrical recordings from the proximal region, including fundus and orad one-third of corpus, are silent (Figure 1). In contrast, the distal region, comprising antrum and distal two-thirds of corpus, displays omnipresent regular rhythmic depolarizations (representing underlying cellular action potentials) known as slow waves, pacesetter potentials, or electrical control activity (Figure 1). Although individual cells contract with each action potential, in the absence of excitatory stimuli (such as occurs after the ingestion of a

meal) these contractions are not sufficiently strong to generate a readily detected contraction of the gastric wall.

Slow waves propagate via the electrical syncytium of the tunica muscularis. An area of greater frequency of spontaneous depolarization will entrain an adjacent region of slower frequency to the higher rate. Since a decreasing cellular frequency gradient exists from the orad to the aboral extremity of the distal region, the frequency of slow waves is uniform throughout the stomach, determined by the rate of the proximal end. Furthermore, the direction of propagation of the slow waves is aboral. The controlling region known as the gastric pacemaker has been further localized to the vicinity of the junction of the orad and middle thirds of the corpus, along the greater curvature (Kelly and Code, 1971). Slow waves propagate much faster in the transverse than the longitudinal direction, so that a circumferential

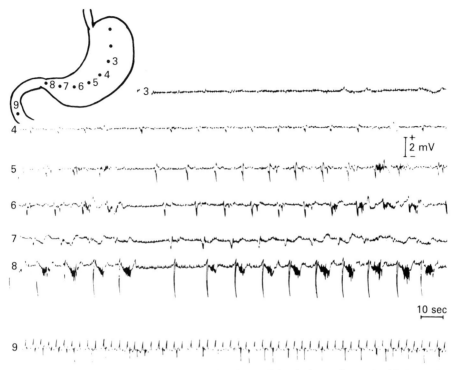

Figure 2. Canine gastric and duodenal myoelectrical activity during active peristalsis. Note that pacesetter potentials are followed by additional bursts of electrical activity (action potentials), seen most clearly in channel 8. Occurrence of a 'dropped beat' in this record facilitates clear identification of the aboral propagation of pacesetter potentials. (From Kelly et al, 1969, with permission.)

wave of gastric depolarization propagates repetitively from the corpus to the pylorus. Propagation is somewhat faster along the greater curvature than along the lesser, to make up for the greater distance travelled. Velocity of propagation increases distally. The frequency of gastric slow waves is approximately three per minute in man, and five per minute in the dog. At any given time, two or three waves of pacesetter potentials are present concurrently.

While distal gastric contractions do not accompany each slow wave, they clearly can occur only during the period of depolarization represented by the slow wave. When stimuli for contraction are present (e.g. vagal activity), slow waves are followed by further electrical activity, known as action potentials (but to be differentiated from the omnipresent cellular action potential), spike potentials, fast activity or electrical response activity (Figure 2). Under these circumstances,

contractions follow the pattern of propagation of the slow waves; that is, a circumferential wave of contraction arising near mid-corpus and propagating aborally (slightly faster along the greater curvature), and accelerating as it nears the pylorus. The local depth or strength of contraction depends upon the status of neurohumoral stimulation of that gastric region, so that some contractions may begin proximally but fade in mid-antrum, while others may be initially weak but gain strength as they approach the pylorus.

Gastric Motility—Response to Feeding

Proximal Stomach

Proximal gastric motor activity may be divided temporally into two phases. The first occurs during and perhaps shortly after the ingestion of

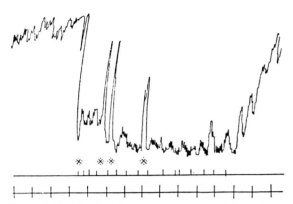

Figure 3. Gastric relaxation in response to repetitive swallows (✳)in the cat. Tracing reflects gastric volume, which increases abruptly with the first swallow, and remains constant during repetitive swallows. (From Cannon and Lieb, 1911, with permission.)

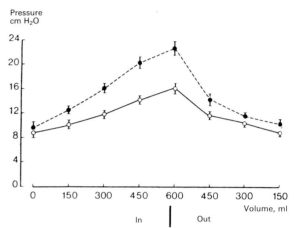

Figure 4. Intragastric pressure–volume relationship in patients with duodenal ulcer, before and after proximal gastric vagotomy. Note small increase in pressure during gastric inflation to 600 ml before vagotomy (open circles), and steeper increase in pressure during gastric inflation after vagotomy (closed circles). (From Stadaas, 1975, with permission.)

a meal, and consists of two relaxatory reflexes suitable to the reservoir function of that region. The second is a prolonged period of increasing tonic contraction thought to be responsible for maintaining a gastroduodenal pressure gradient, and for compressing solids into the distal stomach for processing.

Cannon and Lieb (1911) described the vagally mediated reflex relaxation of the proximal stomach in response to swallowing, and termed this reflex 'receptive relaxation', as it prepared the stomach to receive a swallowed bolus from the oesophagus. Wet swallows (of negligible volume) and sham feeding elicit the reflex, as does oesophageal distension. Repetitive swallows will maintain the relaxation of the fundus (Figure 3).

The second relaxatory response is the phenomenon of gastric accommodation. Again through a vagus-dependent mechanism, the proximal stomach progressively relaxes to accommodate increasing volume without undue increase in pressure, which could otherwise cause discomfort, cessation of eating, and perhaps precipitous gastric emptying (at least of liquids). Figure 4 illustrates the intragastric pressure–volume relationship in ulcer patients with intact stomachs, demonstrating the small rise in intragastric pressure as intragastric volume increases. After vagotomy of the

proximal stomach, accommodation is lost, leading to a steeper rise in pressure at similar volumes (Stadaas, 1975). Gastrin and cholecystokinin also cause fundic relaxation, augmenting gastric accommodation (Meyer, 1987).

The second phase of postcibal proximal gastric motility, consisting of a continuous tonic squeezing gastric content, was evident in Cannon's original fluoroscopic study. However, since tonic contraction occurs while producing virtually no acute change in luminal pressure, standard manometric techniques are incapable of recording this event. Its quantitation thus awaited the development of a novel technique, namely the gastric barostat. This apparatus consists of a flaccid bag introduced into the stomach and inflated with air to fill the proximal stomach. The bag is connected via a double-lumen tube to an injection/withdrawal pump system which maintains a constant intrabag pressure of 2 mmHg. Gastric tonic contraction causes the barostat to withdraw air to maintain the pressure, while relaxation triggers air injection to maintain pressure. Thus, intrabag volume is an inverse measure of proximal gastric tone.

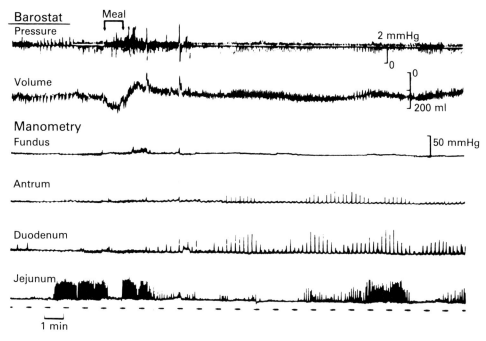

Figure 5. Canine gastric motor response to feeding measured by gastric barostat and manometry. Volume of barostat (second tracing) inversely measures proximal gastric tone. Thus, meal induces increase in volume (receptive relaxation) of proximal stomach, followed by increase in tone. Changes in fundic tone are not detected by manometry. Meal stimulates phasic antral and small bowel contractions. (From Azpiroz and Malagelada, 1985a, with permission.)

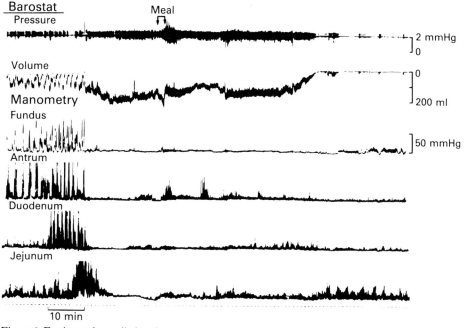

Figure 6. Fasting and postcibal canine gastrointestinal motility measured by barostat and manometry. Phase III of gastric MMC coincides with duodenal phase III. Proximal gastric tone is intermediate prior to ingestion of meal. Eating causes receptive relaxation followed by a steady increase in proximal gastric tone. (From Azpiroz and Malagelada, 1985a, with permission.)

Using the gastric barostat, Azpiroz and Malagelada (1985a) confirmed both the early postcibal relaxation of the proximal stomach and its subsequent tonic contraction (Figure 5 and 6). During the quiescent phase of fasting motility (see below), the proximal stomach is not totally relaxed, but instead maintains an intermediate level of tonic contraction (Figure 6). Eating causes gastric receptive relaxation, followed by relatively constant tone for a period of minutes, after which tone progressively increases. Nutrients perfused into the proximal small bowel (particularly lipid) and into the distal small bowel (particularly carbohydrate and protein) also relax the proximal stomach (Azpiroz and Malagelada, 1985b), providing a mechanism for feedback inhibition of gastric emptying. These enterogastric reflexes are mediated by a vagal non-cholinergic, non-adrenergic mechanism (Azpiroz and Malagelada, 1986). Maintenance of increased tone is also at least partly a vagal, cholinergic effect (Azpiroz and Malagelada, 1986).

Distal Stomach

In contrast to the tonic contractile activity of the proximal stomach, the motor pattern of the distal stomach consists of propagating phasic contractions conventionally called peristaltic contractions, or waves. As reviewed above, these contractions coincide with the rhythm and propagation of the gastric pacesetter potential when stimuli enhance contractility above the basal level. At least three prandial responses excite distal gastric contraction. These include vagal stimulation (Kelly and Code, 1971), gastrin release (Meyer, 1987), and gastric distension (Andrews et al, 1980). Negative feedback from nutrients in the bowel modulates this motility, and the physical consistency of gastric chyme also affects the depth of peristaltic contractions (Prove and Ehrlein, 1982).

Distal gastric peristalsis has been studied in several species, under a variety of experimental conditions, using diverse techniques, including fluoroscopy, manometry (Figures 7 and 8), endo-

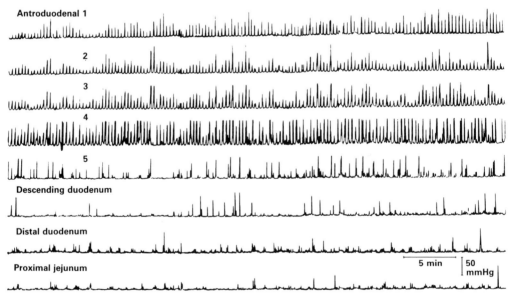

Figure 7. Human postcibal gastroduodenal motility—manometric study. Channels 1–4 are each separated by 1 cm registering antral peristaltic (phasic) contractions. Note that the most distal antral port (channel 4) reflects the powerful terminal antral contraction. (From Malagelada et al, 1986, with permission.)

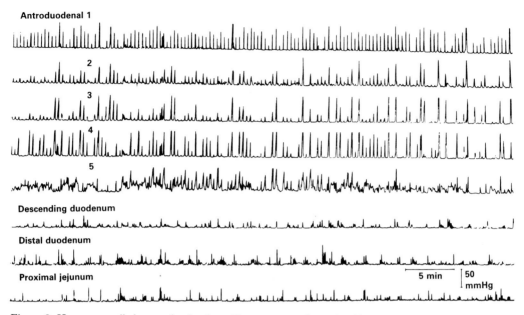

Figure 8. Human postcibal gastroduodenal motility—manometric study. Channels 1–5 are each separated by 1 cm. Channel 5 represents pyloric canal pressures: note tonic contraction evidenced by elevated baseline pressures (compare antral and duodenal ports), and alternating antral-type and duodenal-type contractile pattern, caused by manometry port migrating back and forth across the pyloric channel. From Malagelada et al, 1986, with permission.)

scopy, real-time ultrasonography and computed tomography. A description of the peristaltic cycle is thus of necessity merely schematic. The pattern illustrated in Figure 9 highlights specific features of canine postprandial motility (Carlson et al, 1966). Each peristaltic wave originates in mid-corpus as a shallow indentation. As the wave proceeds aborally to the antrum–corpus junction, it deepens, but does not completely occlude the antral lumen. The wave travels with increasing velocity until the distal 3–4 cm of antrum are reached, at which time the terminal antrum and pylorus appear to contract simultaneously. This final, powerful contraction, termed the terminal antral contraction or antral systole, most likely is the consequence of increasingly swift propagation of slow waves over the distal antrum. Although fluoroscopically the pylorus contracts in concert with the terminal antrum, transpyloric fluid flow ceases approximately two seconds before the terminal antral contraction (King et al, 1984). Pyloric closure probably precedes the terminal contraction by several seconds (Kumar et al, 1987),

even though maximal contraction of the pylorus does not (Prove and Ehrlein, 1982). The antecedent pyloric closure is explained by Szurszewski's hypothesis based upon the unique electromechanical properties of pyloric muscle (Szurszewski, 1987).

Relaxation of the terminal antrum is followed by pyloric opening, and emptying of liquid and suspended particles. At this point, the subsequent peristaltic wave is at the proximal antrum. It is natural to assume that the advancing wave accelerates liquid emptying (hence the 'antral pump' theory) but proof is lacking. Indeed, under certain conditions, fluid and suspended particles stream distally through the advancing wave, suggesting a greater pressure generated by the proximal stomach (Richter and Kelly, 1986).

The consequences of the gastric peristaltic cycle are striking. Liquids and solids within the distal antrum are compressed as the antral wave advances and deepens. Since the aperture of the wave is still greater than the pyloric lumen, liquid and suspended particles are retropelled through

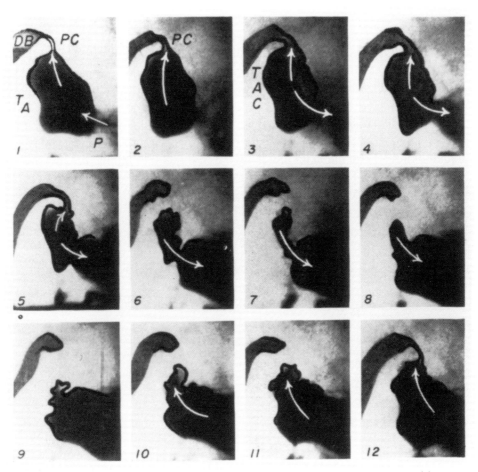

Figure 9. Cineradiographic study of canine antral peristaltic cycle. Frames are separated by one second. Arrows represent flow of barium. PC, pyloric canal; DB, duodenal bulb; TAC, terminal antral contraction. See text for detailed description. (From Code and Carlson, 1968.)

the wave. Larger or denser solids remain trapped ahead of the constriction. The pylorus closes, and the terminal antral contraction which follows forcefully grinds and then retropels the solids back into the proximal antrum (Figure 10). The grinding, combined with the sheer forces generated by retropulsion, break apart digestible solids and mix them thoroughly with gastric juice.

In health, digestible solids empty from the stomach only after they have been reduced to small particles; the vast majority of particles emptied are smaller than 1 mm (Meyer et al, 1979, 1981). While logically this 'sieving' may be ascribed to the narrow pyloric diameter, neither pyloroplasty nor pylorectomy alters the size distribution of solids leaving the stomach (Meyer et al, 1979; Hinder and San-Garde, 1982). Moreover, pylorus-sparing antrectomy preserves sieving, but antropyloric resection does not (Hinder and San-Garde, 1982). Therefore, the antrum alone can selectively retain solids in the absence of the pylorus, and the corpus can reduce solids provided that the pylorus retains them. After a meal, liquid emptying begins promptly, but solids are retained for a variable period before emptying commences. This 'lag period' represents the time required for solid particles to be reduced to the requisite small diameter. Once so reduced, the particles are suspended and dispersed in the liquid phase and emptied at a constant rate.

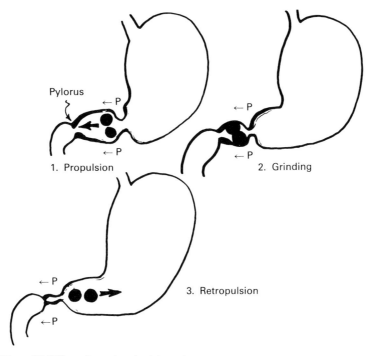

Figure 10. Effect of antral peristaltic cycle on solids. Advancing contraction carries solids distally, where they are retained by narrow pylorus. Terminal antral contraction grinds solids and finally retropels them into the proximal antrum. (From Kelly, 1981.)

Gastric Motility—Fasting Pattern

The gastrointestinal tract does not rest during fasting. Rather, the interdigestive period is characterized by a cyclic pattern of activity involving gut motility and secretion.

The cyclic pattern was first identified as a migrating band of intense phasic contractions, originating in the duodenum, and migrating slowly over the length of the small bowel. As one such activity front arrived at the terminal ileum, another was beginning in the duodenum; the cycle continued until interrupted by feeding. This pattern, called the migrating motor complex (MMC), is characterized at a given small bowel locus as follows: phase I quiescence; phase II irregular or random contractions; phase III high amplitude phasic contractions at the maximal frequency for the locus; phase IV decreasing con-

tractions, merging into phase I. Phase III of the complex is propulsive, and as it migrates the length of the bowel, it sweeps with it cellular debris, bacteria and indigestible residue into the colon (see Chapter 3). Code and Marlett (1975) demonstrated gastric involvement in the MMC, finding antral activity fronts coinciding with those in the duodenum.

Both proximal and distal gastric regions are involved in interdigestive cyclic motility (Figures 6 and 11), phases I and III of the MMC are clearly apparent. While phase II has been detected by serosal strain gauges in dogs (Gill et al, 1985), it is less distinct than its small bowel counterpart; phase IV does not occur in the stomach. Phase I features an absence of phasic contractions, but the proximal stomach maintains an intermediate tone, rather than complete relaxation (Azpiroz and Malagelada, 1985a). Phase III is characterized by powerful, co-ordinated contractions of proximal

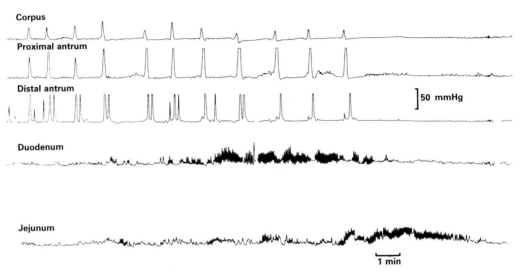

Figure 11. Canine interdigestive gastrointestinal motility. Phase III of the gastric MMC coincides with phases II and III of duodenal MMC. Antral phasic contractions during phase III are linked to proximal gastric contractions. Duodenal contractions are suppressed during gastric contractions.

and distal stomach, lasting about 20 minutes. The proximal contractions occur with a period of about 1.8 minutes and a duration of about 18 seconds (Azpiroz and Malagelada, 1984). During these fundic contractions, high amplitude peristaltic waves of the antrum occur; the antral waves coincide with slow waves accompanied by action potentials (Gill et al, 1985). In the intervals between fundic contractions the distal stomach is quiescent and slow waves lack action potentials. The gastric activity front (phase III) coincides with duodenal late phase II and phase III. During gastric contractions, duodenal contractions are inhibited.

Control of gastric cyclic motor activity is at least partly hormonal, as evidenced by cyclic activity in autotransplanted stomach pouches which remain co-ordinated with the small bowel MMC (Thomas and Kelly, 1979). The indigestible solid residue of a meal retained in the stomach is emptied during the first subsequent interdigestive phase III (Mroz and Kelly, 1977). Gastric bezoar formation in diabetic or post-vagotomy gastroparesis is associated with (or may be caused by) failure of the stomach to generate interdigestive activity fronts (Malagelada et al, 1980).

Duodenal Motility

The duodenum is the most orad portion of the small bowel, and as such its motility bears resemblance to the rest of the intestine. Myoelectrical control of duodenal motility parallels the gastric model; slow waves are omnipresent and propagate aborally. They phase the onset of action potentials, the myoelectric counterpart of contractions. The frequency of duodenal slow waves is greater, however, being about 12 per minute in man (and 18 per minute in dogs), and the potentials are not linked to antral electrical activity. The region of greatest frequency of spontaneous depolarization, the duodenal pacemaker, has been localized in dogs to the most proximal few centimetres of duodenum (Herman-Taylor and Code, 1971).

The duodenum is in the position of the receptacle of chyme emptied from the stomach. By offering greater or less resistance to gastric outflow, the duodenum may participate in the regulation of gastric emptying. Cinefluoroscopic evidence indicates that duodenal contractions are related to the antral peristaltic cycle so that gastric emptying is facilitated, while duodenogastric reflex is minimized. When the pylorus is open and chyme empties, the orad duodenum is relaxed; after pyloric closure and the terminal antral contraction, the duodenum contracts, sweeping its content distally. The bulb then again relaxes to accommodate the subsequent bolus of gastric content.

Antroduodenal myoelectrical recordings confirm this property of antroduodenal co-ordination. Thus, action potentials accompany duodenal slow waves only just after an antral action potential. This co-ordination depends upon connections of the antrum and duodenum via the intrinsic nervous system. When the duodenum is transected but only the mucosa rejoined, preventing intrinsic neutral continuity, antroduodenal co-ordination is lost (Bedi and Code, 1972).

Acknowledgement

Supported in part by a grant from the Hektoen Institute for Medical Research.

References

Andrews, P. L. R., Grundy, D., and Scratcherd, T., (1980), Reflex excitation of antral motility induced by gastric distension in the ferret. *J. Physiol.*, **298**:79–84.

Azpiroz, F., and Malagelada, J. R., (1984), Pressure activity patterns in the canine proximal stomach: response to distension. *Am. J. Physiol.*, **247**:G265–72.

Azpiroz, F., and Malagelada, J.-R., (1985a), Physiological variations in canine gastric tone measured by an electronic barostat. *Am. J. Physiol.*, **248**:G229–37.

Azpiroz, F., and Malagelada, J.-R., (1985b), Intestinal control of gastric tone. *Am. J. Physiol.* **249**:G501–9.

Azpiroz, F., and Malagelada, J.-R., (1986), Vagally mediated gastric relaxation induced by intestinal nutrients in the dog. *Am. J. Physiol.*, **251**:G727–35.

Bedi, B. S., and Code, C. F., (1972), Pathway of coordination of postprandial, antral and duodenal action potentials. *Am. J. Physiol.*, **222**:1295–8.

Cannon, W. B., (1898), The movements of the stomach studied by means of the rontgen rays. *Am. J. Physiol.*,

Cannon, W. B., and Lieb, C. W., (1911), The receptive relaxation of the stomach. *Am. J. Physiol.*, **29**:267–73.

Carlson, H. C., Code, C. F., and Nelson, R. A., (1966), Motor action of the canine gastroduodenal junction: a cineradiographic, pressure and electrical study. *Am. J. Digestive Dis.*, **11**:155–72.

Code, C. F., and Carlson, H. C., (1968), Motor activity of the stomach. In: *Handbook of Physiology, Section 6, Alimentary Canal, Volume IV. Motility* (Ed. Code, C. F.) pp. 1903–16, American Physiological Society, Washington DC.

Code, C. F., and Marlett, J. A., (1975), The interdigestive myo-electric complex of the stomach and small bowel of dogs. *J. Physiol.*, **246**:289–309.

Gill, R. C., Pilot, M.-A., Thomas, P. A., and Wingate, D. L., (1985), Organization of fasting and postprandial myoelectric activity in stomach and duodenum of conscious dogs. *Am. J. Physiol.*, **249**:G655–61.

Herman-Taylor, J., and Code, C. F., (1971), Localization of the duodenal pacemaker and its role in the organization of duodenal myoelectric activity. *Gut*, **12**:40–7.

Hinder, R. A., and San-Garde, B. A., (1982), Individual and combined roles of the pylorus and the antrum in the canine gastric emptying of a liquid and a digestible solid. *Gastroenterology*, **84**: 281–6.

Kelly, K. A., (1981), Motility of the stomach and gastroduodenal junction. In: *Physiology of the Gastrointestinal Tract*, 1st Edition (Ed. Johnson, L. R.) pp. 393–410, Raven Press, New York.

Kelly, K. A., and Code, C. F., (1971), Canine gastric pacemaker. *Am. J. Physiol.*, **220**:112–18.

Kelly, K. A., Code, C. F., and Elveback, L. R., (1969), Patterns of canine gastric electrical activity. *Am. J. Physiol.*, **217**:461–70.

King, P. M., Adam, R. D., Pryde, A., McDicken, W. N., and Heading, R. C., (1984), Relationships of human antroduodenal motility and transpyloric fluid movement: non-invasive observations with real-time ultrasound. *Gut*, **25**:1384–91.

Kumar, D., Ritman, E. L., and Malagelada, J.-R., (1987), Three-dimensional imaging of the stomach: role of pylorus in the emptying of liquids. *Am. J. Physiol.*, **253**:G79–85.

Malagelada, J.-R., Rees, W. W. D., Mazzotta, L. J., and Go, V. L. W., (1980), Gastric motor abnormalities in diabetic and postvagotomy gastroparesis: effect of metoclopramide and bethanecol. *Gastroenterology*, **78**:286–93.

Malagelada, J.-R., and Azpiroz, F., (In press), Determinant of gastric emptying and transit in the small intestine. In: *Handbook of Physiology Vol. IV: Motility and Circulation* (Ed. Wood, J. D.) American Physiological Society, Washington DC.

Malagelada, J.-R., Camilleri, M., and Stanghellini, V., (1986), *Manometric Diagnosis of Gastrointestinal Motility Disorders.* p. 48, Thieme Inc., New York.

Meyer, J., Thornson, J., Choen, M. B., Schadchehr,

A., and Mandiola, S. A., (1979), Sieving of solid food by canine stomach and sieving after gastric surgery. *Gastroenterology*, **76**:804–13.

Meyer, J., Ohaslis, H., Joh, D., and Thornson, J., (1981), Size of liver particles emptied from the human stomach. *Gastroenterology*, **80**:1489–96.

Meyer, J., (1987), Motility of the stomach and gastroduodenal junction. In: *Physiology of the Gastrointestinal Tract*, 2nd ed (Ed. Johnson, L. R.) pp. 613–29, Raven Press, New York.

Mroz, C. T., and Kelly, K. A., (1977), The role of the extrinsic antral nerves in the regulation of gastric emptying. *Surg., Gynec. Obstet.*, **145**:369–77.

Prove, J., and Ehrlein, H. J., (1982), Motor function of gastric antrum and pylorus for evacuation of low and high viscosity meals in dogs. *Gut*, **23**:150–6.

Richter, H. M., and Kelly, K. A., (1986), Intragastric movement of liquids and solids in the dog: Endoscopic observations. (Abstract) *Gastroenterology*, **90**:1603.

Stadaas, J. O., (1975), Intragastric pressure/volume relationships before and after proximal gastric vagotomy. *Scand. J. Gastroent.*, **10**:129–34.

Szurszewski, J. H., (1987), Electrical basis for gastrointestinal motility. In: *Physiology of the Gastrointestinal Tract*, 2nd ed. (Ed. Johnson, L. R.) pp. 383–422, Raven Press, New York.

Thomas, P. A., and Kelly, K. A., (1979), Hormonal control of interdigestive motor cycles of canine proximal stomach. *Am. J. Physiol.*, **237**:E192–7.

16
BILIARY TRACT

Aldo Torsoli, Enrico Corazziari
Università 'La Sapienza', Rome, Italy

Bile is continuously secreted from the liver into the biliary tree; it is then diverted into the gall-bladder or the duodenum depending upon the relative resistance to flow as determined by the contractile state of the gall-bladder and the choledochoduodenal junction.

Gall-bladder

The motor function of the gall-bladder consists of collection, storage and delivery of bile (Ivy, 1934; Banfield, 1975; Ryan, 1981).

Gall-bladder Filling

Bile enters the gall-bladder in the interdigestive period when the resistance of the choledochal sphincter to bile flow causes an increase in intra-choledochal pressure and therefore a favourable gradient between the common bile duct and the gall-bladder (Torsoli, 1961). There is, however, some evidence that filling of the gall-bladder may also take place after total sphincterotomy (personal unpublished data) and in the experimental animal in the absence of the sphincteric area (Castrini and Zicari, 1962). Intra-gall-bladder pressure is maintained low by its capacity actively to relax (Torsoli, 1964) and to reabsorb large amounts of fluid. In addition, flow of bile from the common duct into the gall-bladder is facilitated by the anatomical structure of the cholecystocystic junction which may act as a valve-like mechanism (Caroli et al, 1945a, 1945b).

In the interdigestive state, the human intra-gall-bladder pressure varies between 0 and 16 cm H_2O; spontaneous intragall-bladder pressure variations (Figure 1), sometimes with a rhythmic pattern, can be detected (Torsoli, 1961).

The presence of vasoactive intestinal polypeptide (VIP) in the nerve fibres contained in the human gall-bladder (Sundler et al, 1977) would support the possibility that VIP acts as a neurotransmitter and locally modulates the gall-bladder tone. Pancreatic polypeptide (PP), somatostatin and glucagon have been reported to inhibit the gall-bladder but their physiological role, if any, is still to be determined (Chernish et al, 1972; Creutzfeldt et al, 1975; Greenberg et al, 1978). It would appear that the tone of the gall-bladder may be affected by vagal fibres since gall-bladder dilatation follows vagotomy (Johnson and Boyden, 1952).

Gall-bladder Emptying

Emptying of the gall-bladder follows an active process of contraction of the viscus. It is generally held that gall-bladder emptying takes place after a meal, but a reduced rate of bile flow also occurs in the interdigestive state.

Tonic active contraction of the gall-bladder causes an increase of the intraluminal pressure followed shortly by volume reduction of the viscus and the outflow of bile (Figure 2). Gall-bladder emptying begins when the intragall-bladder pressure overcomes the resistance at the level of the cholecystocystic junction; the resistance opposing bile flow through the cholecystocystic junction is greater from the gall-bladder to the cystic duct

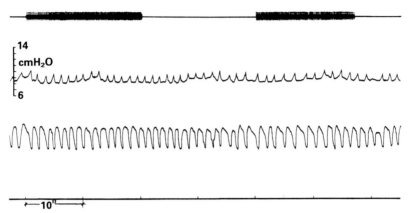

Figure 1. Intracholecystic recording performed during intra-operative cholangiography in a patient with a cholecystotomy. From top to bottom: synchronization signals between cinefluorography and manometric recordings; intracholecystic pressure variations; pneumograph. Besides respiratory induced variations, slow pressure variations of low amplitude are recorded from the gall-bladder. From Torsoli, 1961, with permission.

than in the opposite direction (Caroli et al, 1945a; Caroli et al, 1945b) and increases during rapid distension of the gall-bladder and morphine administration while it decreases after amyl nitrate administration (Figures 3 and 4; Torsoli 1964). The cholecystocystic junction, therefore, appears to be provided with a sphincter-like mechanism which is the most likely explanation of cystic duct occlusion in the absence of organic obstruction. The intraluminal pressure profile of the gall-bladder during contraction caused by, for example, a standard fatty meal is characterized by an initial rapid increase followed by a slow decline towards basal values (Torsoli, 1964). Duration and

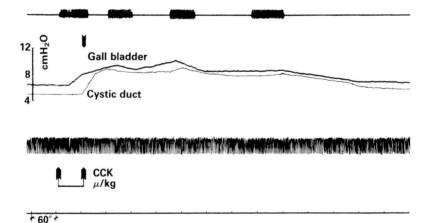

Figure 2. Intracholecystic and intracystic recording performed during postoperative cholangiography in dog. From top to bottom: synchronization signals between cinefluorography and manometric recordings; intracholecystic pressure variations, intracystic pressure variations; pneumograph. After CCK i.v. administration (1.0 IDU/kg) there is a rapid intracholecystic pressure rise followed by intracystic pressure increase and then a parallel decrease in pressure towards basal values. Flow of bile from the gall-bladder through the cystic duct is indicated by the upper arrow. From Torsoli, 1964, with permission.

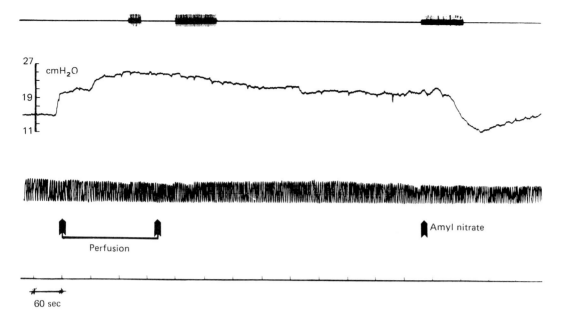

Figure 3. Effect of gall-bladder distension and of amyl nitrate on the cholecysto-cystic junction. Intracholecystic recording performed during operative cholangiography in man. From top to bottom: synchronization signals between cinefluorography and manometric recordings; intracholecystic pressure variations, pneumograph. Saline perfusion into the gall-bladder causes a persistent pressure increase which subsides following amyl nitrate administration; at the same time cinefluorographic images detect bile flow through the cholecystocystic junction. From Torsoli 1964, with permission.

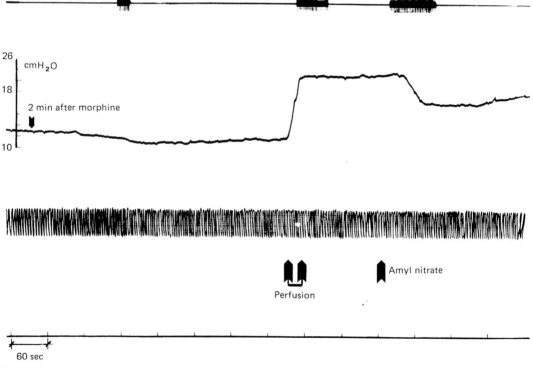

Figure 4. Intracholecystic recording performed during postoperative cholangiography in dog. From top to bottom: synchronization signals between cinefluorography and manometric recordings; intracholecystic pressure variations, pneumograph. Following morphine administration, a 20 sec saline perfusion into the gall-bladder causes a rapid and persistent pressure increase which partially subsides following amyl nitrate administration; at the same time cinefluorographic images detected bile flow through the cholecystocystic junction. From Torsoli, 1964, with permission.

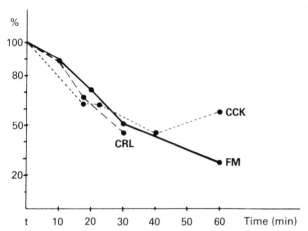

Figure 5. Gall-bladder emptying profiles after a standard fatty meal (FM, line); caerulein CRL (0.25 ng/kg/min) and cholecystokinin (CCK) (1.0 IDU/kg/min) i.v. infusion for 30 min.

strength of the contraction vary according to the stimulus; the standard fatty meal used to perform cholecystographic examination would generally cause a 40–70% gall-bladder emptying (Figure 5).

Limited amounts of bile are delivered in the fasting state and during phase II of the inter-digestive gastrointestinal migratory motor complex (Peeters et al, 1980; Itoh, 1980; Kraglund et al, 1984).

Gall-bladder contraction in response to a meal appears to be primarily mediated by the release of (cholecystokinins) CCK8 and CCK33. Although it has been shown that bombesin infusion causes gall-bladder contraction (Corazziari et al, 1974), and serum motilin increase is time-related with partial gall-bladder emptying in the interdigestive period (Mitznegg et al, 1976), a possible physio-logical role of gastrointestinal peptides besides CCK remains to be clarified.

Common Bile Duct

The human common bile duct does not exhibit phasic and peristaltic motor activity (Nebesar et al, 1966; Cassano et al, 1959). However, tone vari-ation has been reported to affect intracholedochal bile flow and pressure in the dog (Tansy et al, 1971). The tone variations may in part be due to passive elongation and recoil of the elastic fibres in response to the duodenal and/or sphincter of Oddi contractions respectively; in part it is due to active contractions of the longitudinal smooth muscle cells since *in vitro* preparations of the common bile duct show spontaneous rhythmical activity (Ludwick, 1966; Toouli and Watts, 1971).

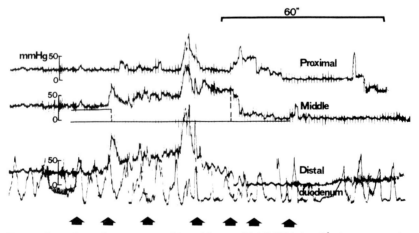

Figure 6. Perendoscopic manometry of the sphincter of Oddi. Withdrawing the manometric catheter from the common duct to the duodenum reveals a zone of elevated pressure at the three recording sites (proximal, middle, distal). The bottom tracing is from the duodenum. Arrow indicates a 0.5 cm catheter withdrawal. Solid line in the second tracing indicates duodenal pressure which is used as zero reference to measure intracholedochal and intrasphincteric resting pressure.

Sphincter of Oddi

At the terminal end of the common bile duct the sphincter of Oddi (SO) displays tonic and phasic motor activity which can be directly evaluated by means of perendoscopic (Csendes et al, 1979; Geenen et al, 1980; Carr-Locke and Gregg, 1981; Toouli et al, 1982), intra-operative (Funch-Jensen et al, 1984) and postoperative (T-tube) manometry (Torsoli et al, 1985).

Tonic activity can be detected in manometric recordings as a high pressure zone (Figure 6). Phasic inhibition of the SO does not occur, but the sphincter tone shows slow spontaneous variations (Torsoli et al, 1986) and it can be increased by morphine (Torsoli, 1964) and decreased by nitroglycerine (Staritz et al, 1984). SO phasic motor activity occurs as contractions which appear on manometric tracings as monophasic waves (Figure 7) measuring on average 114.3 ± 10.9 mmHg ($M \pm SE$) in amplitude and 6.9 ± 0.5 sec ($M \pm SE$) in duration (Torsoli et al, 1986). In the interdigestive period frequency of phasic contractions varies in accordance with the duodenal cyclical motor pattern (Honda et al, 1982; Torsoli et al, 1986). A phase of motor quiescence (phase I) is followed by a phase of intermediate (phase II) and maximal frequency (phase III) (Figure 8). Postprandial patterns of phasic contractions have not been sufficiently investigated in man, but there is some preliminary evidence that a prolonged inhibition of SO phasic motor activity ensues after a normocaloric meal (personal unpublished observations) (Figure 9). In the opossum, intraduodenal fat administration and mixed food increases SO contractions (Dubois and Hunt, 1932; Coelho et al, 1986).

Simultaneous long-lasting manometric recordings of the duodenal and SO motor activity have shown that all phasic contractions of the duodenal segment adjacent to the papilla are accompanied by SO phasic variations, while the opposite does not hold true. SO and duodenal contractions are closely associated during phase III and variably associated during phases I and II of the interdigestive migrating motor complex. Maximal frequency of sphincter and duodenal phasic activity coincides and is 11–12 c/min. This close associ-

ation raises the question whether the SO has its own pacemaker at the same frequency as the duodenum or its movements are paced by the duodenal pacemaker. Animal experiments have provided some evidence of independent pacemakers in the SO and the duodenum (Sarles et al, 1976; Honda et al, 1982), but in man this is not known.

Recordings performed by means of multiple manometric sensors closely spaced within the sphincter have also shown that the majority of phasic contractions occur simultaneously; alternatively an antegrade and, less frequently, a retrograde and bidirectional pattern of phasic contractions may be observed (Figure 10). The length of the sphincter high pressure zone coincides with the sphincter zone where phasic activity is recorded and, on average, it extends for 9.5 mm (Habib et al, in press).

The alternating manometric pattern of sphincteric contraction and relaxation corresponds to closing and opening movements of the choledochoduodenal junction seen on cinefluorography (Torsoli et al, 1961; Torsoli et al, 1970). The closing movement appears as a ring-like contraction which takes place about half-way down the sphincter and then extends upwards obstructing the ducts. At the same time, the lower end of the channel empties into the duodenum (Figures 11, 12 and 13). The opening movement appears as a progressive filling from the proximal to the distal part of the sphincter segment followed by flow of bile into the duodenum (Figures 14 and 15). Thus both contraction and relaxation of the sphincter are accompanied by entry of bile into the duodenum, but the relative bile flow rate differs markedly. The former actively squirts into the duodenum the tiny amount of bile retained in the ampulla, the latter is followed by flow of choledochal bile which varies according to the duct/duodenal pressure gradient.

There is general agreement that the release of CCK is the most important factor in enhancing flow through the SO (Sandblom et al, 1935). The effect of CCK on SO appears to be accomplished by different mechanisms in different animal species investigated. In man and dog CCK or caerulein administration is followed by a prompt

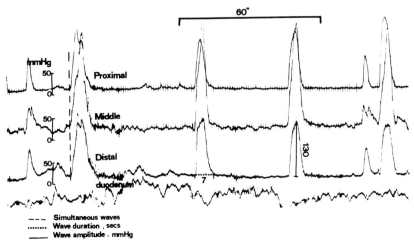

Figure 7. Perendoscopic manometry of the sphincter of Oddi. Three recording sites are located within the sphincter high pressure zone (proximal, middle, distal). Phasic contractions are superimposed on the sphincter resting pressure. The contractions appear simultaneously at the three levels. Dotted and solid lines indicate measurements of duration (7 sec) and amplitude (130 mmHg) of two phasic contractions.

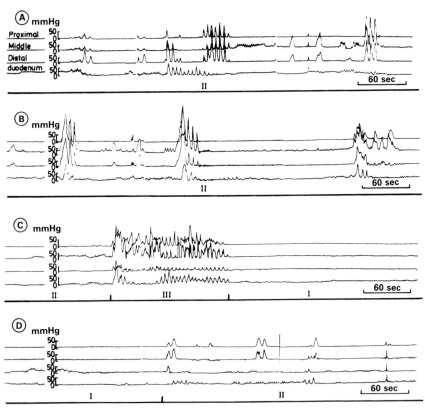

Figure 8. Postoperative transductal (T-tube) manometry. Sphincter of Oddi and duodenal phases of the interdigestive migrating motor complex in a prolonged manometric session. Three recordings (proximal, middle, distal) from the sphincter area by means of transductal (T-tube) manometry. Fourth tracing is recording from the duodenum by means of a naso-duodenal manometric catheter. The 35 min continuous recording shows phase II in A, B, and D; phase III in C; phase I in C and D. From Torsoli et al, 1986, with permission.

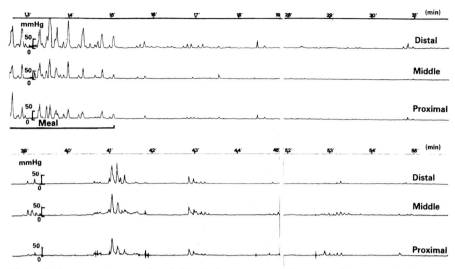

Figure 9. Postoperative transductal (T-tube) manometry. Three recordings (proximal, middle, distal) from the sphincteric area in a continuous tracing. Evidence of the inhibitory effect of a standard hospital meal on the sphincter of Oddi phasic activity. Minutes are indicated on the top of the two parts of the tracings. From Torsoli et al, 1985, with permission.

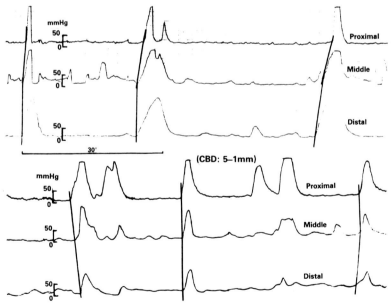

Figure 10. Perendoscopic manometry with three recordings (proximal, middle, distal) from the sphincteric area. During the same recording session retrograde (three events in the top tracings), antegrade (bottom left tracings), simultaneous (middle bottom tracings), and bidirectional (bottom right tracings) events are detected.

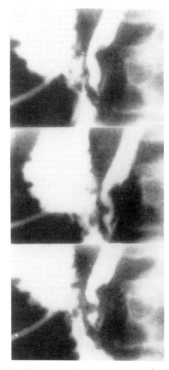

Figure 11. Cinefluorographic sequence performed in post-operative cholangiography in man. To be read from top to bottom. Frames show progression of the closing movement affecting the choledochal sphincter of Oddi.

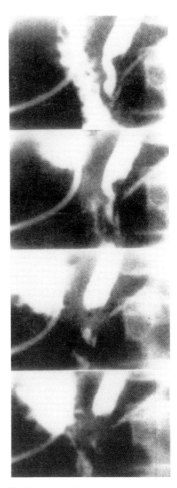

Figure 12. Cinefluorographic sequence performed in post-operative cholangiography in man. To be read from top to bottom. Frames show progression of the closing movement affecting both the choledochal and the pancreatic sphincter of Oddi.

inhibition of the phasic motor activity (Figure 16) and therefore a reduction in the sphincter resistance to flow (Lin, 1975; Corazziari et al, 1982). In the rabbit (Sarles et al, 1976) and in the opossum (Becker et al, 1982; Honda et al, 1983) CCK increases sphincter phasic activity and therefore enhances the flow of bile by means of a pump mechanism. The action, if any, on SO motor activity of secretin and other peptides which are released postprandially remains to be determined. The effect of adrenergic stimulation on SO is controversial; the exogenous administration of parasympathetic drugs increases the resistance to bile flow through the sphincter, while the effect of vagotomy on sphincter motor activity is still controversial. In summary, neuro-hormonal regulation of the SO motor activity is still poorly understood except for the physiological role of CCK.

The biliary tract is a link between the liver and intestine and appears to be a crucial factor in the regulation of the enterohepatic circulation of bile acids, since the rate of bile acid recycling, composition of bile and size of the bile acid pool is mainly determined by the integrated motor activity of the gall-bladder and the sphincter of Oddi.

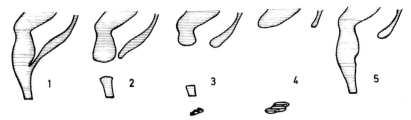

Figure 13. Diagrammatic representation of the sphincter of Oddi closing movement. In 1 the sphincter is open; in 2 a middle sphincteric contraction occludes the lumen of both the choledochal and pancreatic ducts and then (3 and 4) progresses distally, expelling a tiny amount of bile into the duodenum and proximally; in 5 an incomplete sphincter closing movement affecting only the pancreatic SO is depicted.

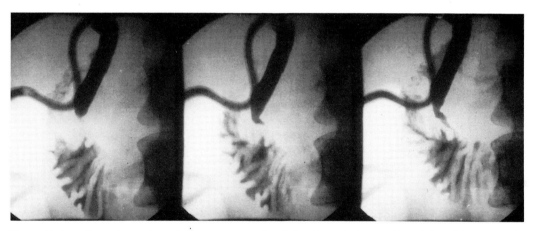

Figure 14. Spot-film series performed during postoperative cholangiography in man. From left to right, progression of the opening movement of the sphincter of Oddi can be seen.

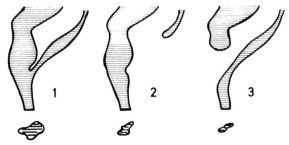

Figure 15. Diagrammatic representation of the sphincter of Oddi opening movement. In 1 complete opening of both chole-dochal and pancreatic sphincter of Oddi; in 2 and 3 incomplete opening affecting choledochal and pancreative sphincter of Oddi respectively.

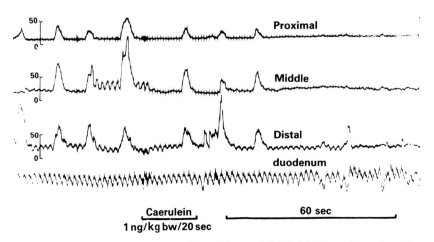

Figure 16. Perendoscopic manometry of the sphincter of Oddi. Inhibitory effect of caerulein (Ing/kg/20 sec) i.v. administration on phasic contractions of the sphincter. Three recordings (proximal, middle, distal) from the sphincteric area; the bottom tracing is recorded from the duodenum. From Corazziari et al, 1982, with kind permission of the authors and publisher.

References

Banfield, W. J., (1975), Physiology of the gallbladder. *Gastroenterology*, **69**:770–7.

Becker, J. M., Moody, F. G., and Zinsmeister, A. R., (1982), Effect of gastrointestinal hormones on the biliary sphincter of the opossum. *Gastroenterology*, **82**:1300–7.

Caroli, J., Varay, A., and Gilles, E., (1945a), Le fonctionnement du sphyncter vesiculaire chez l'homme, observation d'une double intubation, epreuve de la morphine et du repas gras. *Arch. Mal. App. Dig.*, **30**:352.

Caroli, J., Varay, A., and Gilles, E., (1945b), Le fonctionnement du sphyncter vesiculaire chez l'homme, observation d'une double intubation. *Arch. Mal.`App. Dig.*, **34**:350.

Carr-Locke, D. L., and Gregg, J. A., (1981), Endoscopic manometry of pancreatic and biliary sphincter zones in man: basal results in healthy volunteers. *Dig. Dis. Sci.*, **26**:7–15.

Cassano, C., Torsoli A., and Alessandrini, A., (1959), *Aspetti Dinamici di Fisiologia e Di Fisiopatologia Biliare*. XIII Congr. Soc. It. Gastro-enterol., Bologna.

Castrini, G., and Zicari, N., (1962), Studio della funzione della colecisti dopo abolizione dell'apparato sfinterico di Oddi. *La Chirurgia Generale*, **XI**:379–99.

Chernish, S. M., Miller, R. E., and Rsoenak, B. D., (1972), Hypotonic duodenography with the use of glucagon. *Gastroenterology*, **63**:392–8.

Coelho, J. C. U., Gouma, D. J., Moody, F. G., and Schlegel, J. F., (1986), Effect of feeding on myoelectric activity of the sphincter of Oddi and the gastrointestinal tract of the opossum. *Dig. Dis. Sci.*, **31**:202–7.

Corazziari, E., Torsoli, A., Melchiorri, P., and Delle Fave, G. F., (1974), Effect of bombesin on human gallbladder emptying. *Rendic. Gastroenterol.*, **6**:52–4.

Corazziari, E., De Masi, E., Gatti, V., Habib, F. I., De Simoni, A., Primerano, L., Torsoli, A., and Fegiz, G., (1982), Caerulein and sphincter of Oddi pressure activity. *Ital. J. Gastroenterol.*, **14**:238–41.

Creutzfeldt, W., Lankisch, P. G., and Folsch, U. R., (1975), Hemmung der sekretin- und cholezystokinin-pancreozymin-induzierten Saft-und Enzym-sekretion der Pankreas und der Gallenblasen-kontraktion deim Menschen durch Somatostatin. *Dtsch. Med. Wochenschr.*, **100**:1135–8.

Csendes, A., Kruse, A., Funch-Jensen, P., Oster, M. J., Ornsholt, J., and Amdrup, E., (1979), Pressure measurements in the biliary and pancreatic duct systems in controls and in patients with gallstones, previous cholecystectomy or common bile duct stones. *Gastroenterology*, **77**:1203–10.

Dubois, F. S., and Hunt, E. A., (1932), Peristalsis of the common bile duct in the opossum. *Anat. Rec.*, **53**:387–97.

Funch-Jensen, P., Diederich, P., and Kraglund, K., (1984), Intraoperative sphincter of Oddi manometry in patients with gallstones. *Scand. J. Gastroenterol.*, **19**:931–6.

Geenen, J. E., Hogan, W. J., Dodds, W. J., Stewart, E. T., and Arndorfer, R. C., (1980), Intraluminal pressure recordings from the human sphincter of Oddi. *Gastroenterology*, **78**:317–24.

Greenberg, G. R., Adrian, T. E., Baron, J. H., McCloy, R. F., Chadwick, V. S., and Bloom, S. R., (1978), Inhibition of pancreas and gallbladder by pancreatic polypeptide. *Lancet*, **ii**:1280.

Habib, F. I., Corazziari, E., Biliotti, D., Primerano, L., Viscardi, A., Torsoli, A., Speranza, V., and De Masi, E., (in press). Manometric measurement of human sphincter of Oddi length. *Gut*.

Honda, R., Toouli, J., Dodds, W. J., Sarna, S., Hogan, W. J., and Itoh, Z. (1982), Relationship of sphincter of Oddi spike bursts to gastrointestinal myoelectric activity in conscious opossum. *J. Clin. Invest.*, **69**:770–8.

Honda, R., Toouli, J., Dodds, W. J., Geenen, J. E., Hogan, W. J., and Itoh, Z., (1983), Effect of enteric hormones on sphincter of Oddi and gastrointestinal myoelectric activity in fasted conscious opossums. *Gastroenterology*, **84**:1–9.

Itoh, Z., (1980), Intradigestive cyclic activity—Signal in the gut. *Gastroenterology*, **79**:1337–9.

Ivy, A. C., (1934), The physiology of the gallbladder. *Physiol. Rev.*, **14**:1–102.

Johnson, F. E., and Boyden, E. A., (1952), The effect of double vagotomy on the motor activity of the human gallbladder. *Surgery*, **32**:591–601.

Kraglund, K., Hjermind, J., Jensen, F. T., Stoodkilde-Jorgensen, H., Oster-Jorgensen, E., and Pedersen, S. A., (1984), Gallbladder emptying and gastrointestinal cyclic motor activity in humans. *Scand. J. Gastroenterol.*, **19**:990–4.

Lin, T. M., (1975), Actions of gastrointestinal hormones and related peptides on the motor function of the biliary tract. *Gastroenterology*, **69**:1006–22.

Ludwick, J. R., (1966), Observations on the smooth muscle and contractile activity of the common bile duct. *Ann. Surg.*, **164**:1041–50.

Mitznegg, P., Bloom, S. R., Domschke, W., Domschke, S., Wuensch, E., and Demling, L., (1976), Release of motilin after duodenal acidification. *Lancet*, **ii**:888–9.

Nebesar, R. A., Pollard, J. J., and Potsaid, M. S., (1966), Cinefluorography, some physiological observations. *Radiology*, **86**:475–9.

Peeters, T. L., Vantrappen, G., and Janssens, J., (1980), Bile acid output and intraoperative migrating motor complex in normals and in cholecystectomy patients. *Gastroenterology*, **79**:678–81.

Ryan, J. P., (1981), Motility of the gallbladder and biliary tree. In: *Physiology of the Gastrointestinal Tract* (Ed. Johnson, L. R.) pp 473–94. Raven Press, New York.

Sandblom, P., Voegtlen, W. L., and Ivy, I. C., (1935), The effect of CCK on the choledochoduodenal mechanism (Sphincter of Oddi). *Am. J. Physiol.*, **93**:175–80.

Sarles, J. C., Bidart, J. M., Devaux, M. A., Echinard, C., and Castagnini, A., (1976), Actions of cholecystokinin and caerulein on the rabbit sphincter of Oddi. *Digestion*, **14**:415–23.

Staritz, M., Poralla, T., and Meyer zum Buschenfelds, K. H., (1984), Effects of nitroglycerin on the SO motility and baseline pressure. *Gut*, **25**:A1312.

Sundler, F., Alumets, J., Hakanson, R., Ingemansson, S., Fahrenkrug, J., and Schaffalitzky, O. B., (1977), VIP innervation of the gallbladder. *Gastroenterology*, **72**:1375–7.

Tansy, M. F., Mackowisk, R. C., and Chaffer, R. B., (1971), A vagosympathetic pathway capable of influencing common bile duct motility in the dog. *Surg. Gynecol. Obstet.*, **133**:225–36.

Toouli, J., and Watts, J. M., (1971), In vitro motility studies on canine and human extrahepatic biliary tracts. *Aus. N.Z.J. Surg.*, **40**:380–7.

Toouli, J., Geenen, J. E., Hogan, W. J., Dodds, W. J., and Arndorfer, R. C., (1982), Sphincter of Oddi motor activity: a comparison between patients with common bile duct stones and controls. *Gastroenterology*, **82**:111–17.

Torsoli, A., (1961), Sul meccanismo fisiologico di svuotamento della cistifellea. *Radiol. Med.*, **45**:57.

Torsoli, A., (1964), Studi sull'attivitá motoria biliare. *Il. Fegato*, **10**:133–221.

Torsoli, A., Ramorino, M. L., Palagi, L., Colagrande, C., Baschieri, I., and Ribotta, G., (1961), Observations roentgencinematographiques et electromanometriques sur la motilité des voies biliares. *Sem. Hop.*, **37**:790–802.

Torsoli, A., Ramorino, M. L., and Alessandrini, A. (1970), Motility of the biliary tract. *Rend. Gastroenterol.*, **2**:67–80.

Torsoli, A., Corazziari, E., Habib, F. I., Primerano, L., Giubilei, D., Mazzarella, R., De Masi, E., and Fegiz, G., (1985), Prolonged transductal manometry of the sphincter of Oddi. *Ital. J. Gastroenterol.*, **17**:35–7.

Torsoli, A., Corazziari, E., Habib, F. I., De Masi, E., Biliotti, D., Mazzarella, R., Giubilei, D., and Fegiz, G., (1986), Frequencies and cyclical pattern of the human sphincter of Oddi phasic activity. *Gut*, **27**:363–9.

17
SMALL BOWEL

Sidney F. Phillips

Mayo Clinic and Mayo Medical School, Rochester, Minnesota, USA

Introduction

Motility is a rubric applied to the functions of gastrointestinal smooth muscle. It covers a full spectrum; cellular properties, contractile activity, neuro-humoral control, and net effects of muscular activity on transit of contents. Also important are the mechanisms whereby muscular contractions are co-ordinated. This sequence is of particular importance in the small intestine, for finely co-ordinated contractions are the means whereby the muscular layers achieve their key teleological effects—the transit of chyme in a way which optimizes digestion and absorption.

The thrust of this text is towards the more applied aspects of motility, those which pertain to function of the *small intestine as an organ*. Thus, no attention will be directed towards the intrinsic, cellular properties of intestinal smooth muscle, to its intramural innervation by the enteric nervous system, and rather little to extrinsic innervation through the autonomic nervous system. Instead, the focus will be on the myoelectrical signals whereby the mechanical events, contractions of the tunica muscularis, are regulated. Attention will also be accorded to transit, this being the important end-result of contractions of individual cells as expressed by their groupings into tissues (e.g. segments of the longitudinal or circular muscle coats). Less can be said about the consequences of motility in the small intestine, the relationships that are presumed to exist between muscle contractions, transit and absorption. Unfortunately, data on these vital associations are sparse and incomplete.

The Small Intestine: Background Properties

Appreciation of the motor properties of the small bowel requires an understanding of several basic physiological phenomena. These include: (1) the electrical 'slow wave'; (2) action potentials, which are 'paced' by slow waves and which are the electrical equivalents of contractions; (3) co-ordination or propagation of contractile activity; (4) the interdigestive complex; and (5) postprandial motility. The story is not yet complete in man, extrapolations are needed from one species to another, and it is known that differences among species are not trivial. However, a credible overview can be fashioned, with primary attention to man. For those wishing more detailed analyses of certain aspects, the following reviews are recommended; Sarna (1985), Szurszewski (1987), Weisbrodt (1987), Wingate (1981).

Slow Waves in the Small Intestine

Designated variously (basal electrical rhythm, pacesetter potential, electrical control activity—ECA), 'slow waves' are rhythmic oscillations of the membrane potential of smooth muscle cells. The signals can be recorded by several techniques, intracellular micro-electrodes within individual cells *in vitro*, or from a group of cells, by extracellular electrodes *in vitro* or *in vivo* (Figure 1). Recordings *in vivo* are usually from needle electrodes placed within the tunica muscularis; for most experimental studies, electrodes are sewn onto the serosal surface of the bowel. Such

Canine jejunal motility

Action potentials trigger contractions

Electrical activity

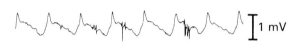

Intraluminal pressure

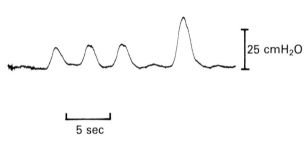

5 sec

Figure 1. Electrical and mechanical signals from the small intestine. Electrical activity was recorded by an extracellular electrode; it shows a slow wave (approximately 14 per minute) with action potential on the plateaus of several slow waves. When an action potential is recorded (upper tracing), a mechanical event (lower tracing) is also recorded.

approaches have had limited application in man, though electrodes have been placed on the human bowel, when a laparotomy has been done for other reasons.

In man, most attention has been given to recording from mucosal electrodes incorporated in oro-intestinal tubes (Christensen et al, 1966; Fleckenstein, 1978; Fleckenstein and Oigaard, 1978). Anatomical considerations however dictate that the mucosa is not the closest or most direct approach to the tunica muscularis, and few adequate electrical recordings from intact man are available. On the other hand, serosal electrodes have been used extensively in laboratory animals (Figure 2).

Studies in the several species have established the principle of the 'gradient of the small intestine'. First documented carefully by Alvarez (1928), this describes an intrinsic frequency of the slow wave which decreases distally; i.e. it is faster in the proximal than in the distal bowel. In the dog, this ranges from 14–18 per minute in the duodenum to 10–12 per minute in the ileum (Figure 2). Comparable values in man are, duodenum 11–13 and ileum 6–8 per minute. The human gradient was first described by electrical techniques (Christensen et al, 1966) and has been confirmed (Kerlin and Phillips, 1982) many times by mechanical tracings (Figure 3). The universality of this phenomenon among species has led most authors to conclude that the intrinsic capacity of the proximal gut to contract faster than the distal gut is important in the normal orad to distal transit of contents. A pacemaker has been localized in the duodenum of several species and, drawing an analogy from the conducting system in the heart, the faster proximal pacemaker is considered to be dominant. The mechanism whereby the faster rate captures and 'drives' the more distal bowel is thought to be by a series of 'relaxation oscillators' (Sarna et al, 1971; Sarna, 1985) though the precise cellular basis for this gradient of intrinsic, myogenic responses is uncertain.

Action Potentials and Slow Waves

Given that the slow wave acts as a 'pacesetter', the maximal rate at which contractions can occur is established for each level of the bowel by the frequency of the slow waves. This is borne out experimentally. When membrane depolarization occurs in association with a slow wave, an action potential (spike potential, electrical response activity— ERA) is recorded (Figures 1 and 2). When depolarization occurs in association with *all* slow waves, the small bowel contracts at its maximum rate and this shows the same gradient of frequency as does the slow wave (Figure 3). Alternatively, the bowel may contract in association with some or none of the slow waves (Figure 1). This capacity of the membrane potential (slow wave) *to react or not to react* (by 'firing' or not an action potential) provides the basis whereby muscular contraction varies widely in intensity, and subtle patterns of

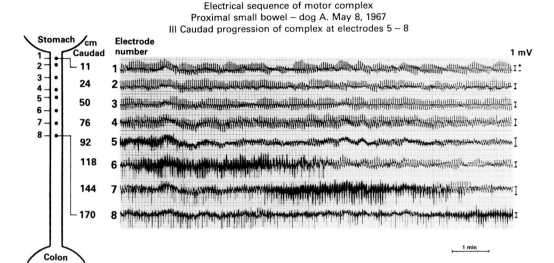

Figure 2. Electrical recording from the canine small bowel, from serosal electrodes at the loci indicated to the left. Slow waves are omnipresent in all recordings. A band of action potentials is ending at site 5, passes to sites 6 and 7 and is beginning at site 8. This is phase III of the interdigestive myoelectrical complex (see text for details).

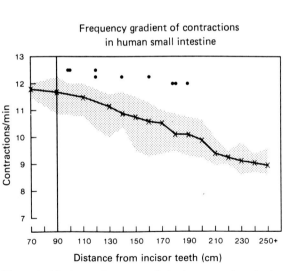

Figure 3. Maximum frequency of phasic contractions in the human small intestine, as recorded from perfused catheter pressure sensors. The maximum contractile frequency is equivalent to the frequency of slow waves at that locus; note the gradient of decreasing frequency along the small bowel. The mean and SEM are shown for a group of healthy subjects, the single symbols are from one subject who was outside the normal range. Reproduced from Kerlin and Phillips, 1982, with permission.

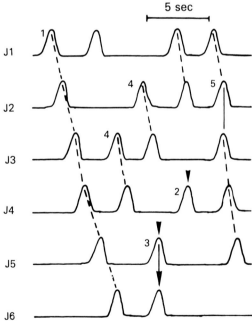

Figure 4. Mechanical contractions recorded from six strain gauges sewn to the circular muscle of the canine jejunum, four centimetres between successive gauges. Some mechanical events propagate aborally (dotted lines), others appear simultaneously at two sites (full lines) or are solitary (arrows). Reproduced from Schemann and Ehrlein, 1986a, with permission.

motility are established. Different patterns of motility or motor quiescence will be determined by the balance among local factors (e.g. luminal contents), extrinsic and intrinsic innervation, neuropeptides and other neurotransmitters.

Co-ordination or Propagation of Motility

In addition to the gradient of frequency for slow waves (and the maximal contractile frequency) along the bowel, a 'phase-lag' exists so that slow waves appear to move in an aborad direction. By progressing along the length of the bowel, slow waves not only 'set the pace' for contractile events at any one site but also offer the potential whereby mechanical activity may also be propagated. Further, it is logical to assume that mechanical activity which is propagated will be more likely to propel contents, whereas stationary contractile rings might be expected to move contents in both directions simultaneously. Moreover, the greater the length over which contractions are propagated, the greater should be the potential to propel. These questions have been approached by several investigators, the work of Schemann and Ehrlein (1986a, b) being a good example (Figure 4). Sophisticated computerized analysis of mechanical signals from strain gauges allowed them to correlate transit of contents (as assessed by simultaneous monitoring of radio-opaque chyme) with the numbers of motor events and the distances over which they propagated. Though the cellular and biochemical mechanisms whereby these degrees of co-ordination can be regulated are not known, herein presumably lies one of the keys to the wide range of transit rates achievable by the small intestine. Variations in degrees of co-ordination/propagation are demonstrable particularly in the postprandial state (see later).

The Interdigestive Complex

Prior to Szurszewski's description of a regular cycle of motility in the fasting small bowel (1969), many confusing and at times contradictory observations had been recorded. In particular, some authors reported minimal motor function when the small bowel was empty between meals, while others noted bursts of intense activity. When based only on short periods of recording, as most were, the fact that these were errors of sampling became obvious only when the cyclic nature of fasting motility was appreciated.

Though clearly conceived of by others, including Boldereff's observations in Pavlov's laboratory (for discussion, see Wingate 1981), Szurszewski's description of a migrating burst of intense spiking which passed from duodenum to ileum in the dog each 90–120 minutes during fasting first clearly identified this phenomenon (Figure 2). This is now recognized as a general property of the mammalian small intestine. In electrical terms, the interdigestive myoelectrical complex (IDMEC) is a short (several minutes) burst of spiking during which every slow wave shows an action potential. The complex migrates along the length of the small bowel, with a velocity and periodicity such that when one burst reaches the ileum, another commences in the duodenum. Code and Marlett (1975) subsequently divided the cycle of 90–120 minutes into four parts; phase I, a period of quiescence when spikes were absent, phase II, during which sporadic spiking was recorded, phase III, the 'front' or migrating motor complex (MMC), when the bowel contracted at its maximal frequency, and phase IV, a transition period back to quiescence. This sequence can be displayed neatly (Figure 5) to show the migration of the front. Note that the MMC migrates more slowly in the distal bowel, and that feeding interrupts the sequence. After a meal cycles are disrupted, to be replaced by random spiking and random contractions; this persists, as determined by the caloric load of the meal and its nutrient constituents, for up to three to four hours. Fat evokes a longer 'fed pattern' than do other nutrients (DeWever et al, 1978).

The IDMEC has its mechanical equivalent. During phase I very few contractions occur, sporadic mechanical activity is recorded during phase II (by either extraluminal strain gauges or sensors of intraluminal pressure) and phase III shows an intense burst of rhythmic mechanical events at the frequency of slow waves for that site (Figure 6). Designation of a phase IV, which is often poorly developed, has largely been discontinued.

Gastrointestinal interdigestive action potential pattern

Six hour period of recording in dog C

Three migrating complexes

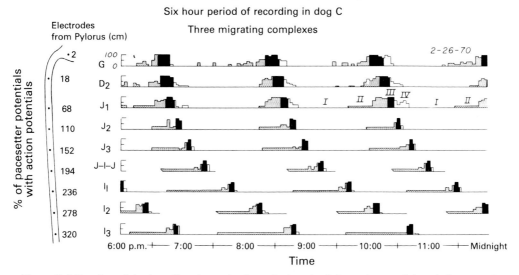

Figure 5. Migration of the interdigestive cycle along the length of the canine small bowel, from gastric antrum to distal ileum. Phases of the cycle (I–IV) are indicated and migration of phase III (black blocks) is evident. Note that passage of the front slows in the distal bowel. Reproduced from Code and Marlett, 1975, with permission.

Normal gastrointestinal motility

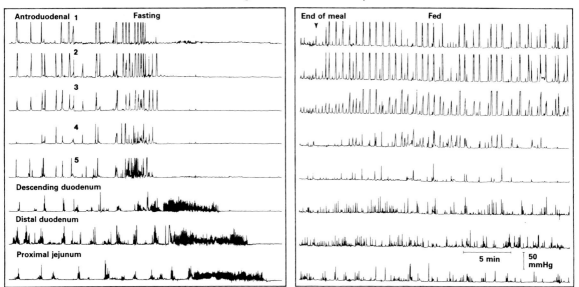

Figure 6. Intraluminal pressures from the antroduodenum of a healthy person. To the left is shown phases II, III, and I of a fasting cycle. Phase III consists of rhythmic contractions (3 per minute) in the antrum and duodenum (12–14 per minute). To the right is shown a typical postprandial pattern, sporadic contractions in the stomach and small bowel. Reproduced from Malagelada et al, 1986, with permission.

Code ascribed to the MMC the role of sweeping the fasting gut clear of accumulated interdigestive debris, in preparation for the anticipated next meal; the so-called 'house-keeper' function (Code and Schlegel, 1973). The concept has been modified somewhat by subsequent observations which suggest that transit rates are maximal *just before phase III*, in 'late phase II'; however, this interpretation does not negate the general principle that phase III may function as a 'back stop' for other propulsive sequences.

Variations on the MMC theme

Though the general phenomenon of the IDMEC has been recorded from most mammals, differences have been noted. In non-ruminants, the MMC is present only during fasting, but MMCs persist postprandially in ruminants. The pig has also been studied extensively, and it shows another variation; the MMC is present during fasting and after meals, but only when food is taken *ad libitum*. If the pig is fed only once a day, the pattern becomes that of non-ruminants, and meals disrupt the MMC cycle. The periodicity of the cycle varies widely; it can be correlated roughly with the size of the animal, and ranges from 15 to 120 minutes. In general, phase III is relatively brief, occupying 10% or less of the cycle; phase IV is brief and many investigators have ignored it. Phases I and II each comprise 30–50% of the cycle (Sarna, 1985). The proportions of phases I and II also vary with the conditions of recording; for example, most humans show longer periods of quiescence during overnight sleeping cycles than they do during the day. Rather than attempt a catalogue of multiple species, focus will be given to the human MMC, with note being made where the findings in man differ from those of the common experimental animals.

Our approach has been to use orocaecal tubes which are perfused by a low compliance system and we utilize the overnight period for prolonged fasting recordings (Kellow and Phillips, 1987; Quigley et al, 1984b). It is possible to incorporate 12 lumina in a tube of proportions acceptable to most volunteer subjects, and to utilize fluoroscopy and pattern recognition to localize the recording

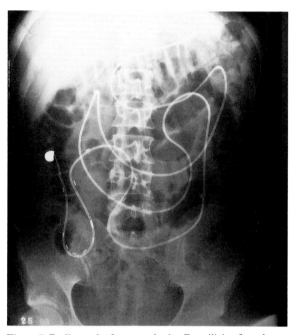

Figure 7. Radiograph of orocaecal tube. By utilizing four three-lumen pressure recording catheters in the composite assembly, recordings can be obtained from 12 sites along the bowel. A radio-opaque catheter helps localize the tube and recording sites are identified by small metallic slugs. See Borody et al, 1985, and Kellow et al, 1986, for details.

sites (Figures 7 and 8). In Table 1 are given the general characteristics of the MMC in healthy man; it highlights (a) the slowing of propagation velocity and (b) the lengthening of duration of the MMC with distal spread; (c) the rhythmic rate of contractions (equivalent to the frequency of the slow wave) is also given.

The distal oesophagus and stomach participate in the human interdigestive cycle (Figure 9), though not invariably; about 50% of cycles have an oesophageal and antral component, which often appear together. Conversely, in most species including man, a proportion of interdigestive cycles begins distally (e.g. in the proximal jejunum or even beyond). Thus, we found the maximal incidence in man to be in the proximal jejunum (Figure 10). An important and consistent human variant is that MMCs 'die out' in the ileum; less than 20% are recorded from the mid-ileum and even fewer from the ileocaecal junction (Figure 10). Occasionally, the MMC appears to progress

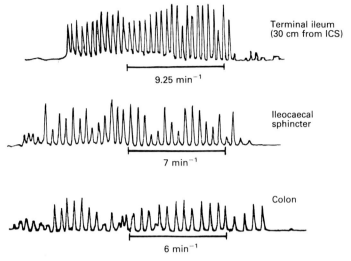

Figure 8. Different maximal rates of phasic contractions in the human bowel. See Quigley et al, 1984b, for details. Reproduced with permission.

into and be represented by a burst of acitivity in the caecum (Figure 11).

Periodicity of the cycle fluctuates widely within and between individuals; thus, care must be used when interpreting recordings in which inter-digestive cycling cannot be clearly demonstrated. Cycling as frequently as every 30 minutes is not uncommon in health, but intervals of three hours or more are also common (Kellow et al, 1986; Kerlin and Phillips, 1982). Vagotomy is often associated with a short interval between MMCs. Table 2 gives the mean and range for periodicities

of the MMC in health and in two groups of patients with irritable bowel syndrome (Kellow and Phillips, 1987). It emphasizes that MMCs are more frequent at night, except in patients with functional diarrhoea who maintain the shorter nocturnal cycle length during the day; the wide range of absolute values can also be appreciated from the table. Another feature of nocturnal MMCs is their slower rate of propagation (Kumar et al, 1986; Kellow et al, 1986) and the greater proportion of the cycle taken up by quiescence (phase I).

Table 1. General characteristics of the migrating motor complex (phase III of MMC) in the human upper gastrointestinal tract

Site	Velocity of propagation (cm min^{-1})	Maximum frequency of contractions (per minute)	Duration (minutes)
Duodenum	—	11.7±0.1	8.7±1.0
Jejunum 1	4.3±0.6	11.3±0.1	9.1±0.6
2	2.8±0.4	10.7±0.1	11.7±0.6
3	2.0±0.5	10.4±0.2	14.7±1.2
Ileum 1	1.3±0.2	9.8±0.2	15.6±1.6
2	0.9±0.1	9.3±0.2	15.3±1.0
3	0.7±0.2	8.9±0.2	13.9±1.1
4	0.6±0.2	8.5±0.2	13.8±1.5
Caecum	—	6.1±0.2	—

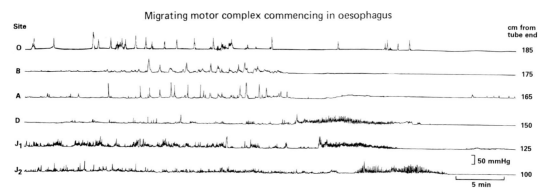

Figure 9. Human MMC beginning in the oesophagus, involving the body and antrum of the stomach, the duodenum and jejunum. The distances given are from the distal end of the tube which was in the proximal colon.

Phase II has received less attention than have the more immediately dramatic features of phase III. Thus, as shown in Figures 6 and 9 the features of phase III are visually striking. However, all apparently random activity of phase II *is not the same*. Within the sporadic contractions of phase II (and in the 'fed pattern' also) must be one of the keys to the major functions of the small intestine. Subtle differences within the patterns of phase II presumably determine that mixing, localized transit, absorption, and slow distal movement of contents will occur. Moreover, these fine variations on the basic theme provide mechanisms whereby contents are not inadvertently 'rushed' to the colon. The sophisticated techniques used by Ehrlein (Figure 4) and others to dissect phase

II (Schemann and Ehrlein, 1986a, b) are not easily applicable to intact man. However, even standard recording techniques in man illustrate variations on the usual patterns of phase II (see Figure 9); discrete groupings of phasic waves (Figure 12) are often seen, and they appear to migrate. These have been described (Fleckenstein and Oigaard, 1978) to occur regularly ('minute rhythm'), and should probably be considered to be normal for approximately 25% of the total duration of phase II. However, sequences such as these *are more commonly seen in patients with irritable bowel syndrome* (Kellow et al, 1987; Kellow and Phillips, 1987) and they are particularly prominent in patients with mechanical intestinal obstruction (Figure 13); they have also been noted

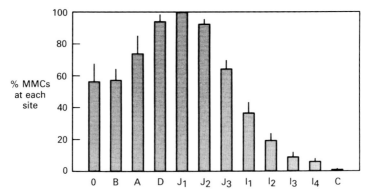

Figure 10. Incidence of MMCs at various sites in the human bowel. The maximum number was recorded from the proximal jejunum (J_1), designated as 100%. O is oesophagus, B and A the body and antrum, of stomach; J, I and C are jejunal, ileal and colonic sites. Reproduced from Kellow et al, 1986, with permission.

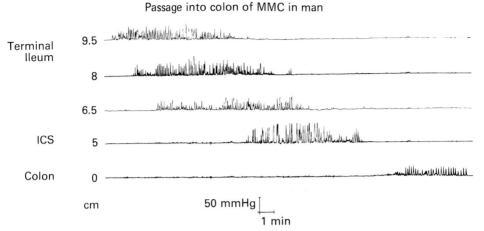

Figure 11. Tracings of intraluminal pressures from healthy man, showing the unusual occurrence of an MMC which appears to pass across the ileocaecal sphincter into the proximal colon. Distances of recording sites from the end of the tube are indicated (see Figure 7).

in the 'pseudo-obstruction syndromes' (Summers et al, 1983).

Postprandial Motility

Eating interrupts the interdigestive cycle, which is replaced by an apparently random occurrence of spikes or mechanical events. Figure 6 is a good example of the effect of food on the upper gut; the ileum behaves similarly except that, since MMCs are usually absent from the human ileum, the change is a less dramatic one. The literature is confusing as to whether or not the ileum has an immediate response to a meal, the so-called 'gastro-ileal reflex'. Our results (Kerlin et al, 1982, 1983) suggested that whether or not ileal motility was augmented after a meal depended on the level of motor activity immediately prior to the meal. However, in some persons an immediate and dramatic response may occur; Figure 14 shows an

Table 2. Periodicity of migrating motor complexes (MMC) in health and patients with irritable bowel syndrome (IBS)

	Periodicity of MMC (min, mean ± SEM, range)		
	Overall	Daytime (0400–2000 h)	Night-time (2000–0400 h)
Patients with IBS			
Predominantly diarrhoea	71 ± 6** (50–100)	77 ± 10† (43–117)	70 ± 7 (48–108)
Predominantly constipation	100 ± 7 (75–130)	118 ± 15 (81–208)	78 ± 6†† (57–106)
Control Subjects	108 ± 7 (66–174)	113 ± 10 (67–218)	91 ± 7 (51–143)

** $p < 0.01$ and $p < 0.05$ versus control and constipation predominant, respectively
 † $p < 0.05$ versus control and constipation predominant
†† $p < 0.05$ versus daytime periodicity

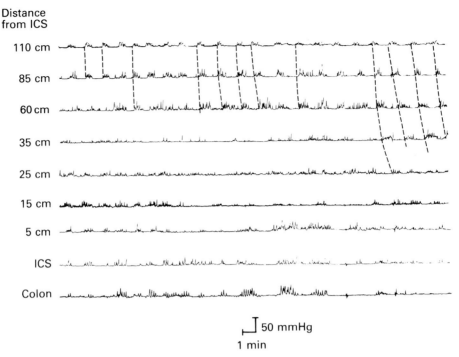

Figure 12. Intraluminal pressures from the jejunum and ileum of a healthy person from sites proximal to the ileocaecal sphincter. In this recording phase II consists mainly of short bursts of phasic waves which appear to migrate. These are presumed to be the mechanical equivalent of 'minute rhythm' recorded electrically by Fleckenstein, 1978 and Fleckenstein and Oigaard, 1978.

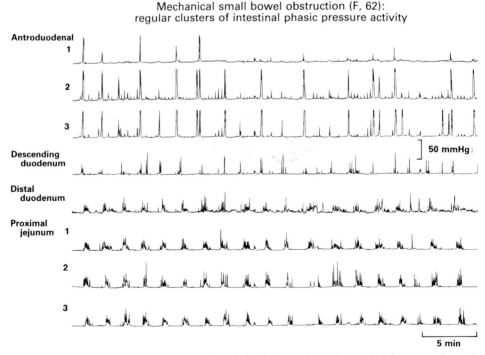

Figure 13. Regular clusters, an exaggeration of the 'minute rhythm' recorded from a patient with mechanical obstruction of the small bowel. Reproduced with permission from Malagelada et al, 1986.

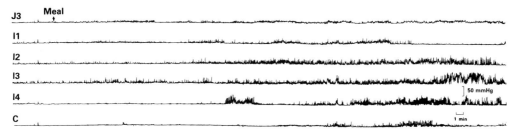

Figure 14. Intraluminal pressures from the jejunum, four ileal sites and caecum in a patient with irritable bowel syndrome. Ileal motility increases after the meal, the striking augmented motility to the right was accompanied by abdominal symptoms.

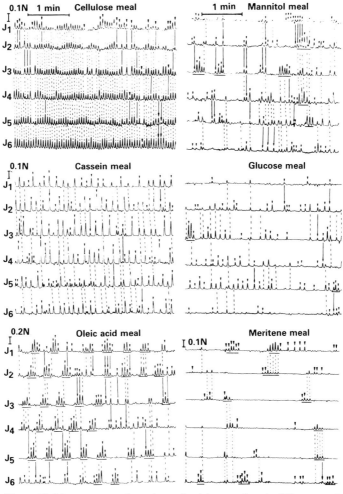

Figure 15. Motor patterns from the canine jejunum after six different meals, recorded from serosal strain gauges. Propagated contractions shown by dashed lines, simultaneous events by full lines and single events by arrows. Different nutrients induced different motor patterns and different rates of transit. Reproduced with permission from Schemann and Ehrlein (1986b).

exaggerated ileal response to food, accompanied by symptoms, in a patient with irritable bowel syndrome.

Postprandial motor patterns have received relatively little detailed analysis. Schemann and Ehrlein (1986b) examined the fed pattern in dogs given cellulose meals, to which were added a variety of nutrients. They analysed the mechanical response by methods described earlier in this chapter (see Figure 4) and reached several interesting conclusions. Firstly, the non-nutrient, control (cellulose) meal was associated with contractions which migrated for the longest distances and which produced the most rapid transit. Secondly, various nutrients induced different contractile patterns; some migrated for short, and others for intermediate or long distances. Rates of transit were variable and were best correlated with the mean distance of migration. Thirdly, since nutrients induced shorter patterns of migration and slower rates of transit, the findings offer an explanation as to how the small bowel slows the transit of chyme, and presumably optimizes digestion and absorption concomitantly (Figure 15).

Though fat is the most potent of the nutrients for inducing fed patterns in the dog (DeWever et al, 1978), we (Kellow et al, 1986) found that the duration of the fed pattern in man did not differ between isocaloric meals containing fat (395 calories total, 37% fat, fed pattern induced for 140 ± 25 minutes) and a no-fat meal (400 calories, 70% carbohydrate, 139 ± 20 minutes). After a meal, the human MMC returns usually first in the mid-jejunum.

Special Features of the Ileal Motility

The human ileum rarely displays phase III of the MMC (Figure 10) and phase II in the ileum shows features different from those of the duodenum and jejunum (Borody et al, 1985; Kellow et al, 1986, Quigley et al, 1984b). Motor activity tends to be more often grouped into bursts of phasic waves lasting 1–2 minutes, some of which migrate but others of which appear to be stationary or simultaneous (Figure 16). A second motor phenomenon occurs infrequently but predictably; we termed these 'prolonged propagated contractions' (PPCs, Figure 17). They are pressure waves of high amplitude (usually in excess of 50 mmHg, sometimes above 100 mmHg) and they last longer than the equivalent duration of the slow wave. Thus, they are probably *not* an event which is controlled by the slow wave. PPCs migrate very rapidly, so that at slow paper speed they may appear to be simultaneous; we even confused them

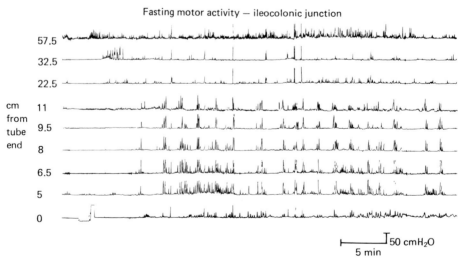

Figure 16. Motor patterns in the healthy human ileum, the recording assembly terminated in the proximal colon and the top eight tracings are from the ileum. No MMCs are recorded and the tracings show prominent clusters of phasic waves.

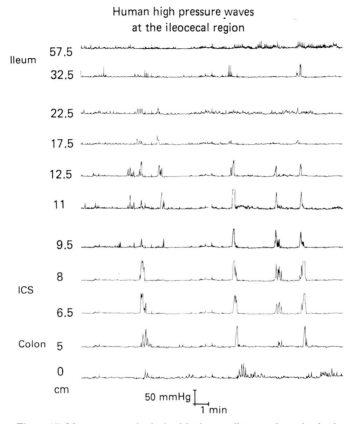

Figure 17. Motor patterns in the healthy human ileum and proximal colon. The striking feature is a series of broad-based ('prolonged', lasting 15–30 seconds) pressure waves which propagate rapidly through the ileum and into the proximal colon.

initially with mechanical artefacts. They are more commonly recorded from patients with irritable bowel syndrome (Kellow and Phillips, 1987) and are frequently concomitant with spontaneous complaints of abdominal pain (Figure 18).

We studied PPCs in the dog and found that they can be stimulated reproducibly by instilling into the ileum small boluses of a short-chain (or volatile) fatty acid solution (Kamath et al, 1987; Kruis et al, 1985); we used concentrations of short chain fatty acids (SCFA) similar to those recovered from canine stools (Figure 19). Thus, we proposed that PPCs may occur when SCFA reach the ileum as a result of colo-ileal reflux, since SCFA are universal constituents of colonic contents. Fatty acids reaching the ileum would then be a chemical

signal for a powerful motor response. In the dog, PPCs are propulsive; they rapidly empty liquid contents (Figure 20) from the ileum (Kruis et al 1985). In this way, perhaps, PPCs clear the ileum of reflux faecal materials. The proximal small bowel can also develop PPCs when exposed to an appropriate intraluminal stimulus (Sarna, 1984), but in normal dogs and man PPCs are rarely recorded from the duodenum and jejunum.

The Ileo-colonic Junction (ICJ)

The small intestine terminates in a specialized segment of bowel, the ileocolonic junction (or sphincter). Early anatomists recognized the possi-

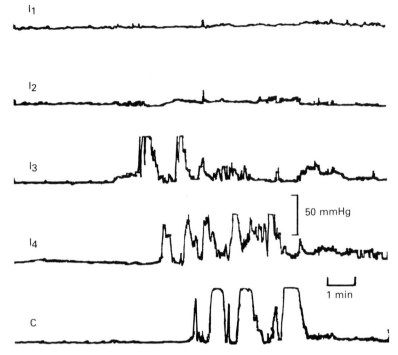

Figure 18. Pressure waves from the ileum (Il-4) and caecum (C) from a patient with irritable bowel syndrome. High pressure, broadly-based contractions (prolonged propagated contractions, PPCs) pass through the region and were accompanied by abdominal pain. Reproduced from Kellow and Phillips (1987) with permission.

Stimulation of PPCs by VFA

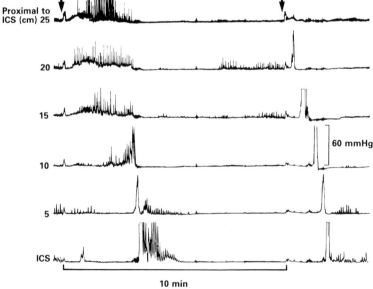

Figure 19. Pressure recordings from the canine ileum showing responses to boluses of volatile (short-chain) fatty acids (VFA). The first bolus elicited a phasic burst which also showed features of a single, large contraction at the ileocolonic sphincter (ICS). The second bolus elicited a prolonged propagated contraction.

Canine ileum: high pressure wave and ileal effluent

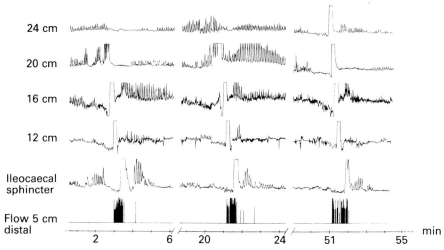

24 cm

20 cm

16 cm

12 cm

Ileocaecal
sphincter

Flow 5 cm
distal

2   6   20   24   51   55   min

Figure 20. Strain gauge recordings from the canine ileum. Three broad-based contractions migrate rapidly through the ileum as far as the ileo-caecal sphincter. Each is associated with a bolus outflow of fluid from the ileum into the colon.

Ileocaecal sphincter— anatomy and pressure profile

Sphincter

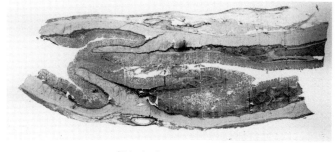

Side hole pressure

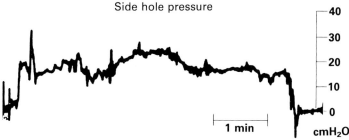

1 min

— 40
— 30
— 20
— 10
— 0
cmH₂O

Figure 21. Histological section of the canine ileocolonic junction showing a thickened band of circular muscle. Below is shown a pull-through pressure tracing illustrating the zone of sphincteric tone.

Distance from ICJ

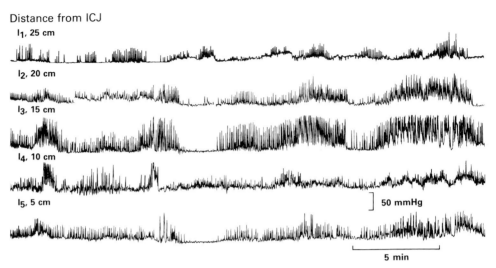

Figure 22. Pressure recordings from the canine terminal ileum after surgical reconstruction of the ileocolonic junction (ICJ), to produce colo-ileal reflux. Basal, fasting ileal motility was augmented. Reproduced with permission from Kumar et al, 1987.

bility that this region had the anatomical basis whereby it might function as a 'valve'. Surgeons have even based surgical procedures on its functional importance, devising restorative procedures to be used for 'incompetent' junctions (Gazet and Kopp, 1964). Later, properties of a physiological sphincter were identified, and attention swung more towards the importance of an ileocolonic sphincter (ICS). We have proposed that the junction region should be considered as including the terminal ileum, ICS and proximal colon, all of which act in concert (Quigley et al, 1983, 1984a, 1985).

Our studies confirm that the dog possesses a specialized band of muscle which has a resting tone (Figure 21); it relaxes in response to proximal distension and contracts when the proximal colon is stretched. However, studies in healthy man have not always confirmed that a comparable tonic sphincteric zone exists in man. Even under the influence of morphine, a pharmacological stimulus thought to elevate pressure at the ICS, no tonic zone could be clearly identified (Borody et al, 1985); others have also failed to demonstrate anything other than a low tonic pressure at the human ICS (Nasmyth and Williams, 1985). Perhaps, like other gastrointestinal 'gates' (e.g. pylorus, lower

oesophageal sphincter), the ileocolonic junction should be considered as an integrated functional unit, in which the terminal ileum, sphincter and proximal colon act together to control input to the colon and reflux from colon to ileum. Although a pathophysiological role for colo-ileal reflux has not been established, surgical manoeuvres which favour reflux (Kumar and Phillips, 1987; Kumar et al, 1987) have been shown to alter ileal motility (Figure 22).

Motility of the Small Intestine In Disease

The scope of this chapter permits only brief attention to pathophysiology; mention has already been made of several examples of dysfunction in the *irritable bowel syndrome*. One consistent finding has been the presence of bursts of rhythmic activity in the jejunum (Kellow and Phillips, 1987); these features occur in health (see Figure 12) but are more common in patients with functional abdominal pain (Figure 23). These findings have been confirmed using recording techniques that permit the study of ambulant patients in the home setting (Gill et al, 1987; Kellow et al, 1987).

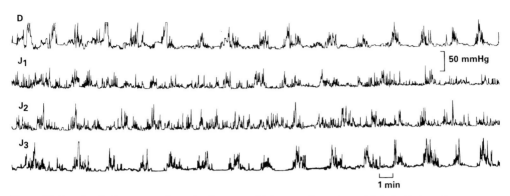

Figure 23. Intraluminal pressures from duodenum and jejunum of a patient with irritable bowel syndrome. Phase II shows prominent clusters of phasic bursts at all levels; these patterns occupy a greater proportion of phase II in irritable bowel syndrome than in controls (Kellow and Phillips, 1987).

The conditions of *mechanical obstruction* and *intestinal pseudo-obstruction* are associated with abnormal patterns of motility (see Figure 15), and Summers et al (1983) have drawn attention to the overlap of these motor features between mechanical and pseudo-obstruction. The pseudo-obstructions can be tentatively categorized into those with myopathic and those with neuropathic features (Figures 24 and 25).

Unusual motility patterns in the small intestine might be anticipated in diarrhoeal disease, and a variety of dysmotilities have been reported in clinical and experimental conditions (Vantrappen et al, 1986). At this time, a coherent picture has not emerged and it is still unclear whether the unusual motilities observed in diarrhoeal states are causative, or merely reflect the increased volume of intraluminal fluid in diarrhoea. The review of Vantrappen et al should be consulted for an overview of this area.

In summary, the most dramatic and reproducible facet of the small bowel's motor function in the MMC. Though a relatively constant finding among species, there are prominent variations of

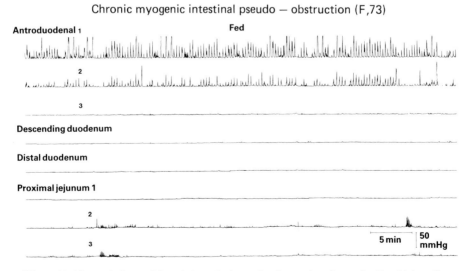

Figure 24. Myogenic form of chronic intestinal pseudo-obstruction, from a family with hereditary hollow viscus myopathy. In this postprandial recording antro-pyloric activity is within normal limits but there are very few, weak contractions in the small bowel. Reproduced from Malagelada et al, 1986, with permission.

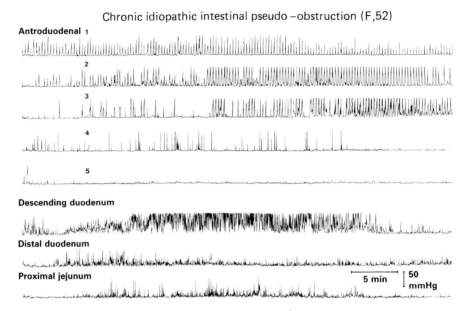

Figure 25. Chronic pseudo-obstruction in a patient with long-standing symptoms and no evidence of mechanical obstruction. This postprandial record shows antro-duodenal motility which is normal. The intestine shows a prolonged burst of intense phasic pressures with tonic change. The distal channels show abnormal waxing and waning of the fed pattern. The fasting recording was also abnormal. Reproduced from Malagelada et al, 1986, with permission.

this major theme; further, among individuals, wide differences are also seen. These must be kept in mind when small bowel motility is being recorded and analysed diagnostically. It is possible that abnormalities will be overdiagnosed if the wide range of normality is not fully appreciated. The more subtle patterns of phase II of the fasting cycle or of postprandial motility have received less attention, but are surely very important. It is also clear that abnormalities of motility can be recognized in some diseases, but closer pathophysiological correlations need to be established.

Acknowledgements

The work from the Mayo Gastroenterology Unit has been performed in conjunction with numerous research associates, whose contributions are acknowledged gratefully by extensive reference to their publications. This work was supported in part by grants from the National Institutes of Health, Bethesda, Maryland (AM32121, AM34988, RR585).

References

Alvarez, W. C., (1928), *The Mechanics of the Digestive Tract.* Hoeber, New York.

Borody, J. T., Quigley, E. M. M., Phillips, S. F., Weinbeck, M., Tucker, R. L., Haddad, A., and Zinsmeister, A. R., (1985), Effects of morphine and atropine on motility and transit in the human ileum. *Gastroenterology*, **89**:562–70.

Christensen, J., Schedl, H. P., and Clifton, J. A., (1966), The small intestinal basic electrical rhythm (slow wave) frequency gradient in normal man and in patients with a variety of diseases. *Gastroenterology*, **50**:309–15.

Code, C. F., and Marlett, J. A., (1975), The interdigestive myo-electric complex of the stomach and small bowel of dogs. *J. Physiol. (Lond.)*, **246**:289–309.

Code, C. F., and Schlegel, J. F., (1973), The gastrointestinal interdigestive housekeeper: motor correlates of the interdigestive myoelectric complex of the dog. In: *Proc. Fourth International Symposium on GI Motility* (Ed. Daniel, E. E.), Mitchell Press, Vancouver.

DeWever, I., Eeckhout, C., Vantrappen, G., and Hellemans, J., (1978), Disruptive effect of test meals on interdigestive motor complex in dogs. *Am. J. Physiol.*, **235**:661–5.

Fleckenstein, P., (1978), Migrating electrical spike activity in the fasting human small intestine. *Am. J. Dig. Dis.*, **23**:769–75.

Fleckenstein, P., and Oigaard, A., (1978), Electrical spike activity in the human small intestine. A multiple electrode study of fasting diurnal variations. *Am. J. Dig. Dis.*, **23**:776–80.

Gazet, J.-C., and Kopp, J., (1964), The surgical significance of the ileocecal junction. *Surgery*, **56**:565–73.

Gill, R. C., Kellow, J. E., and Wingate, D. L., (1987), The migrating motor complex at home (abstract). *Gastroenterology*, **92**: 1405.

Kamath, P. S., Hoepfner, M. T., and Phillips, S. F., (1987), Short chain fatty acids stimulate motility in the canine ileum. *Am. J. Phys.* (in press).

Kellow, J. E., Borody, T. J., Phillips, S. F., Tucker, R. L., and Haddad, A. C., (1986), Human interdigestive motility: variations in patterns from esophagus to colon. *Gastroenterology*, **91**:386–95.

Kellow, J. E., Gill, R. C., and Wingate, D. L., (1987), Proximal gut motor activity in irritable bowel syndrome patients at home and at work (abstract). *Gastroenterology*, **92**:1463.

Kellow, J. E., and Phillips, S. F., (1987), Altered small bowel motility in irritable bowel syndrome is correlated with symptoms. *Gastroenterology*, **92**:1885–93.

Kerlin, P., and Phillips, S. F., (1982), Variability of motility of the ileum and jejunum in healthy man. *Gastroenterology*, **82**:694–700.

Kerlin, P., Zinsmeister, A., and Phillips, S. F., (1982), Relationship of motility to flow of contents in the human small intestine. *Gastroenterology*, **82**:701–6.

Kerlin, P., Zinsmeister, A., and Phillips, S., (1983), Motor responses to food of the ileum, proximal colon, and distal colon of healthy humans. *Gastroenterology*, **84**:762–70.

Kruis, W., Azpiroz, F., and Phillips, S. F., (1985), Contractile patterns and transit of fluid in canine terminal ileum. *Am. J. Physiol.*, **249**:G264–70.

Kumar, D., Wingate, D., and Ruckebusch, Y. (1986), Circadian variation in the propagation velocity of the migrating motor complex. *Gastroenterology*, **91**:926–30.

Kumar, D., and Phillips, S. F., (1987), The contribution of external ligamentous attachments to function of the ileocecal junction. *Dis. Colon Rectum*, **30**:410–16.

Kumar, D., Phillips, S. F., and Brown, M. L., (1987), Coloileal reflux in the dog: role of external ligamentous attachments. *Dig. Dis. Sci.* (in press).

Malagelada, J.-R., Camilleri, M., and Stanghellini, V., (1986), *Manometric Diagnosis of Gastrointestinal Motor Disorders*. Thieme Inc., New York.

Nasmyth, D. G., and Williams, N. S., (1985), Pressure characteristics of the human ileocecal region—a key to its function. *Gastroenterology*, **89**:345–51.

Quigley, E. M. M., Phillips, S. F., Dent, J., and Taylor, B. M., (1983), Myoelectric activity and intraluminal pressure of the canine ileocolonic sphincter. *Gastroenterology*, **85**:1054–62.

Quigley, E. M. M., Phillips, S. F., and Dent, J., (1984a), Distinctive patterns of interdigestive motility at the canine ileocolonic junction. *Gastroenterology*, **87**:836–44.

Quigley, E. M. M., Borody, T. J., Phillips, S. F., Wienbeck, M., Tucker, R. L., and Haddad, A., (1984b), Motility of the terminal ileum and ileocecal sphincter in healthy humans. *Gastroenterology*, **87**:857–66.

Quigley, E. M. M., Phillips, S. F., Cranley, B., Taylor, B. M., and Dent, J., (1985), Tone of canine ileocolonic junction: topography and response to phasic contractions. *Am. J. Physiol.*, **249**: G350–7.

Sarna, S. K., Daniel, E. E., and Kingma, Y. J., (1971), Simulation of slow wave electrical activity of small intestine. *Am. J. Physiol.*, **221**:166–75.

Sarna, S. K., (1985), Cyclic motor activity: migrating motor complex. *Gastroenterology*, **89**:894–913.

Sarna, S. K., (1984), ECA independent 'giant migrating contractions' of small intestine (abstract). *Gastroenterology*, **86**:1232.

Schemann, M., and Ehrlein, H.-J., (1986a), Mechanical characteristics of phase II and phase III of the interdigestive migrating motor complex in dogs. *Gastroenterology*, **91**:117–23.

Schemann, M., and Ehrlein, H.-J., (1986b), Postprandial patterns of canine jejunal motility and transit of luminal content. *Gastroenterology*, **90**:991–1000.

Summers, R. W., Anuras, S., and Green, J., (1983), Jejunal manometry patterns in health, partial intestinal obstruction, and pseudo-obstruction. *Gastroenterology*, **85**:1290–300.

Szurszewski, J. H., (1969), A migrating electric complex of the canine small intestine. *Am. J. Physiol.*, **217**:1757–63.

Szurszewski, J. H., (1987), Electrophysiological basis of gastrointestinal motility. In: *Physiology of the Gastrointestinal Tract* (Ed. Johnson, L. R.), Raven Press, New York.

Vantrappen, G., Janssens, J., Coremans, G., and Jian, R., (1986), Gastrointestinal motility disorders: *Dig. Dis. Sci.*, **31** (Sept. Supplement): 5–25S.

Weisbrodt, N. T., (1987), Motility of the small intestine. In: *Physiology of the Gastrointestinal Tract* (Ed. Johnson, L. R.), Raven Press, New York.

Wingate, D. L., (1981), Backwards and forwards with the migrating complex. *Dig. Dis. Sci.*, **26**:641–4.

18
COLON

Michael Karaus, Martin Wienbeck
University Hospital, Dusseldorf, FRG

Colonic Motility

Colonic motility comprises different aspects of movements of the large intestine. Firstly, it describes the movements of contents within the large intestine and their characteristics which are called patterns of flow in the colon. Secondly, it describes the movements of the colonic wall called motor patterns. These are divided into contractile and myoelectrical patterns depending upon the methodology being used to record the motor activity. When two methods are combined and flow and motor activity are measured, it becomes possible to correlate colonic flow patterns with motor patterns. This will help us in understanding the role of colonic motor activity with respect to absorption, transport and evacuation.

Flow Patterns

Since the main function of the colon is storage and absorption, flow in the large intestine has to be slow and the contents have to be moved to and fro to provide optimal mixing.

Gross Movements and Storage

Retrograde migrating movements of contents were first observed by Cannon (1902) and Elliot and Barclay-Smith (1904). They studied, radiologically, colonic flow—using barium as radio-opaque marker—in different animal species. They stated that the normal movement in the proximal colon is antiperistalsis. The constrictions they described were moving toward the ileum rather than caudad

repelling the contents and temporarily preventing its caudad movement. Halls (1965)—using barium impregnated disks—confirmed these findings in part in man, showing free mixing of disks of different sizes throughout the colon but also suggesting that the main site of mixing was the right side of the colon. It remains, however, uncertain whether the proximal part of the colon is really the main site of storage. Recent transit studies by Metcalf et al (1987) using three distinct markers given on three successive days estimated segmental transit times for the right and left colon and the rectosigmoid. The results show no significant difference in transit time between the three sites of the colon. This is in agreement with the study of Martelli et al (1978) who also estimated segmental transit times by using radio-opaque markers. Figure 1 shows that these markers disappeared exponentially in each segment. That means that the markers are not repelled back into the right colon. The same conclusion can be drawn from a study of Krevsky et al (1986) using colonic transit scintigraphy to evaluate segmental transit times of the colon. In this study a small bolus containing a γ-radioisotope was instilled via a tube into the caecum and the emptying times of the different segments—divided by a computer into different regions of interest—could be calculated from the movement of the radioisotope as measured by a γ-camera. Figure 2 shows the different regions of interest for which the computer program analyses the activity separately and Figure 3 illustrates a typical serial colonic scintigram suggesting that the right colon empties within one to two hours whereas the transverse colon retains the contents for much longer (20–40 hours). The authors pro-

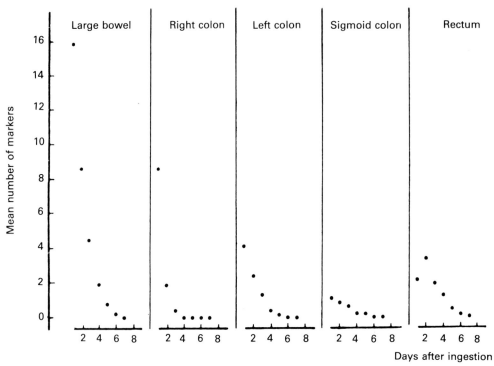

Figure 1. Transit of radio-opaque markers through the large intestine. Each colonic segment shows an exponential disappearance of markers. After a peak number of markers has been reached, there are never more markers than on previous days, indicating that there is no retrograde movement of markers (Martelli et al, 1978).

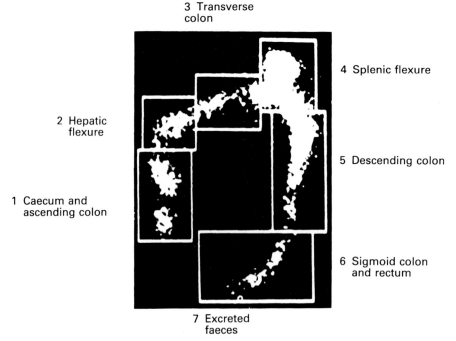

Figure 2. Illustration of computerized analysis of a colonic scintigram in order to measure colonic transit. The colon is divided into six regions of interest. Within each of them the counts depicted by the γ-camera are computerized (Krevsky et al, 1986).

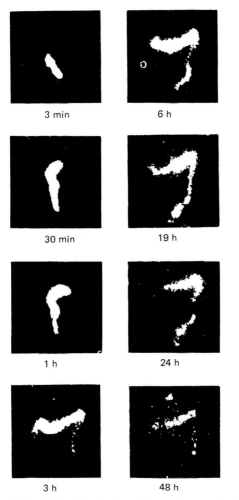

Figure 3. Typical serial colonic scintigram for transit time measurement in a human subject. The radionuclide moves fastest within the proximal colon and is stored for the longest time in the transverse colon (Krevsky et al, 1986).

posed that the transverse colon is the major site of storage within the colon.

These conflicting results might be due to species differences and to methodological problems. It seems possible that solid contents like those radio-opaque markers are moved differently from semi-solid or liquid contents which resemble normal ileal outflow. Both are certainly different from the flow of barium contrast media which is known to stimulate colonic motor activity (Williams, 1967). Using chromium sesquioxide as solid marker and PEG 4000 as liquid marker Findlay et al (1974) showed that normally solid and liquid phases of

contents pass the colon at the same rate. But the addition of bran to the diet changes this 'mixing' flow pattern into a 'streaming' pattern where the solid phase is passed more rapidly than the liquid phase, as shown in Figure 4 (Eastwood, 1975). This underlines the importance of the composition of contents on colonic flow. Because of these methodological problems the main site of storage in the colon remains uncertain at present.

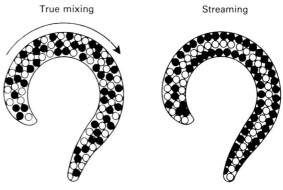

Figure 4. Schematic illustration of flow patterns in the colon. The left side shows the normal state where true mixing occurs and liquid and solid phases are moved with same velocity. As shown on the right side this pattern changes to a streaming pattern by adding bran to the diet. The solid phase is passed more rapidly than the liquid phase ($\bigcirc$ solid-chromium, $\bullet$ liquid-PEG 4000) (Eastwood, 1975).

Defined Flow Patterns

The above-mentioned studies described only gross movements of contents because of the great time lapse between serial pictures. In contrast, time-lapse-fluoroscopy takes pictures every minute. It reveals the underlying flow patterns in more detail. Ritchie et al defined slow and fast moving patterns of flow (Ritchie, 1968, 1971; Ritchie et al, 1971): individual haustral propulsion describes the displacement of the content of a single haustrum into the next segment. In contrast, the contraction of multiple segments as a co-ordinated unit is called multihaustral propulsion. This results in a spread of the contents over longer distances. Figure 5 shows a multihaustral propulsion on a series of cineradiographs taken two minutes apart after oral barium sulphate ingestion: a large volume of con-

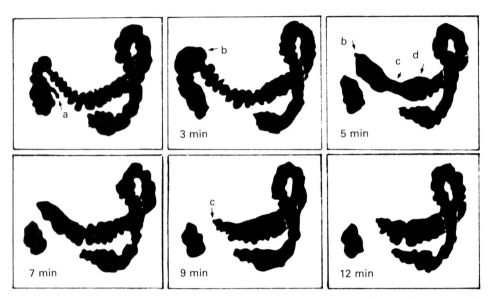

Figure 5. Schematic illustration of serial cineradiographic pictures showing multihaustral propulsion of contents in the human colon. On the upper left picture barium-impregnated contents entered the caecum and ascending colon (a). Three minutes later, a contraction of this part of the colon propelled a large part of the contents to distend the hepatic flexure (b). Another two minutes later, the contents were moved further into the transverse colon where the haustral markings disappeared. There was some narrowing of the mass in the middle segment (c). Contents propelled out of this region caused distension of the next four haustra (d). Four minutes later most of the proximal part of the transverse colon (b–c) also contracted and expelled the contents into the distal colon. The conical outline at (c) in the fifth picture is typical for multihaustral propulsion (adapted from Ritchie, 1968).

tents is moving slowly from the ascending colon up to the splenic flexure. The haustral indentations are temporarily lost when the faecal mass passes by. Most of these movements occurred as 'systolic' propulsion which means that the segments contracted more or less simultaneously. They were observed mainly in the ascending and transverse colon. Similar movements were seen to migrate in retrograde direction but these were less frequent.

A fast colonic flow pattern which Ritchie called mass propulsion had been previously described by Holzknecht (1909) and Hertz and Newton (1913). It consists of a very effective, but seldom occurring, movement of colonic contents which propels these contents within a few seconds over long distances. The original and nowadays accepted term for this pattern is 'mass movement'. Figure 6 shows schematically the original mass movement which Holzknecht (1909) described as follows: 'A long segment of the quiescent colon with deep rounded intrahaustral folds suddenly loses its haustra and is converted in a featureless tube. A constriction develops at the proximal end and a wave sweeps the contents rapidly into the next portion of the bowel.' The occurrence of these movements is often accompanied by an urge to defecate or sometimes even by the evacuation of faeces. This flow pattern can propel the contents over more than half of the colon. It has gained much interest in recent years and is believed to be one of the major propulsive forces within the colon (Holdstock et al, 1970). The motor correlate has now been defined in detail and will be discussed later.

The consistency of colonic contents becomes firmer during its transport along the large intestine which is due to the absorption of water. Thus, the descending and rectosigmoid colon have to handle rather solid contents which require a different type of motor activity for their transport. Here, systolic movements like the one described above are less

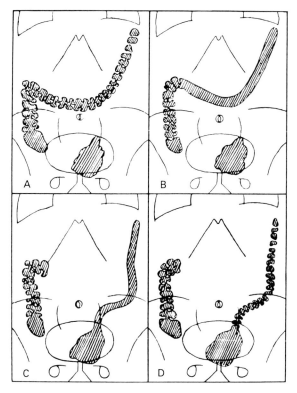

Figure 6. Drawings illustrating a mass movement as observed by Holzknecht in 1909. The rapid propulsion lasted only a few seconds as described in the text (Holzknecht, 1909).

effective because reduction of the gut diameter beyond a certain degree increases its resistance to flow of solid contents (Ritchie, 1968). Furthermore, there is no need for gross movements of contents in this area except for the time of defecation or for filling of the rectum. Therefore, flow in the descending and sigmoid colon seems to be very slow except for those peristaltic mass movements which occur only a few times a day. There are no specific flow patterns known for this part of the colon which might provide to and fro movements and mixing. Current thinking is that the hardened stool if not evacuated remains here and is stored. The angulation between the sigmoid colon and the rectum may act as a physical barrier and prevent the faeces from being propelled further into the rectum. In addition, it is speculated that the specific motor pattern of the rectosigmoid may play a role in hindering the flow into the rectum.

In summary, flow along the colon is generally very slow. It consists of to and fro movements of the contents which establish mixing of contents and, thus, optimize absorption. The contractions also provide net aboral propulsion. The main site of mixing and retrograde propulsion seems to be the proximal and middle colon although there is increasing evidence that no large retrograde movements occur within any part of the colon. It is believed that the distal colon stores the already hardened stools until evacuation takes place. From time to time a very rapid movement of colonic contents over long distances occurs which may cause an urge to defecate.

Motor Patterns in the Colon

Myoelectrical Patterns

Contractions in the colon are controlled as in other parts of the gut by electrical oscillations of the membrane potentials of the two muscle layers. However, this myogenic electrical control mechanism of colonic motility is different from that in the upper intestine. It is therefore essential to understand the specific myoelectrical activity of the longitudinal and circular muscle layer *in vitro* in order to be able to interpret the recordings of colonic myoelectrical activity *in vivo*.

Myoelectrical Activity in vitro

The stomach and the small intestine exhibit a well-defined electrical control activity which is stable in amplitude and frequency. It is also called slow waves. It sets the pace for the occurrence of electrical response activity or spikes and thus contractions. In the colon, similar types of slow waves were found to be generated by the circular muscle layer in several species (Christensen et al, 1969; Wienbeck and Christensen, 1971; El-Sharkawy, 1983). Figure 7 shows that this activity also controls the occurrence of spikes and contractions. The human colon also exhibits oscillations which resemble slow waves, but these oscillations show further differences: recordings from intracellular electrodes have shown that oscillations occur in the human circular muscle with a frequency

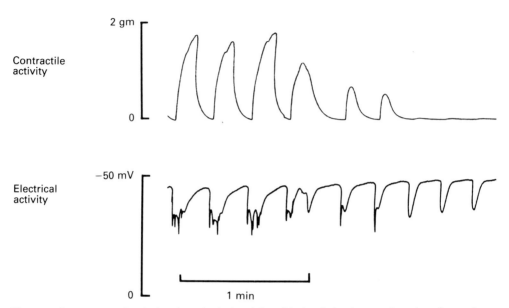

Figure 7. Spontaneous electrical and mechanical activity of isolated circular muscle strips of cat colon. Electrical activity was recorded by sucrose gap technique. Regular slow waves occurred with or without superimposed spikes. Spikes were accompanied by phasic contractions.

ranging from 4 to 60 cpm and in the longitudinal muscle ranging from 20 to 40 cpm (Kubota et al, 1983; Huizinga et al, 1985; Huizinga et al, 1986; Gill et al, 1986a). Thus, the frequency of the human colonic slow waves is variable in time. Another specific feature of human colonic myoelectrical activity is shown in Figure 8: the amplitude of the slow waves is variable and low in comparison to electrical potentials in other regions of the gut. Furthermore, colonic electrical activity

needs stimulation in order to occur, i.e. in the absence of an appropriate stimulus, like stretch, neural or humoral stimulation, the electrical oscillations decrease in amplitude to a level which make them not discernible from noise. This is shown in Figure 9. Thus, in the human colon electrical activity is not omnipresent. Furthermore, the high sensitivity of the human colon to stretch and other stimuli like cholinergic stimulation (Figure 10) observed *in vitro* underlines the importance of

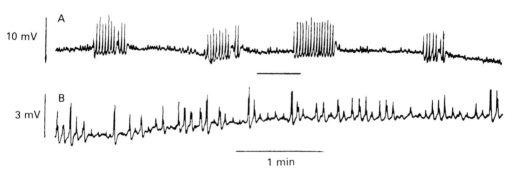

Figure 8. Spontaneous electrical activity of human colonic circular muscle strips measured with sucrose gap technique. A. Oscillations at 15 cpm occurred continuously, but the amplitudes increased periodically. Spikes occurred superimposed on high amplitude oscillations. B. Continuous oscillatory activity at 14 cpm with one or more spikes on each oscillation (Huizinga et al, 1985).

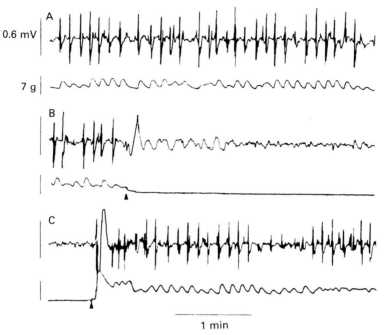

Figure 9. Stretch dependency of electrical activity in human circular muscle recorded by sucrose gap technique. A. Slow waves at 8 cpm with superimposed spikes associated with phasic contractions during stretch. B. After release of tension (arrow) all electrical activities ceased. C. Reintroduction of tension resulted in reappearance of electrical and mechanical activity (Huizinga et al, 1985).

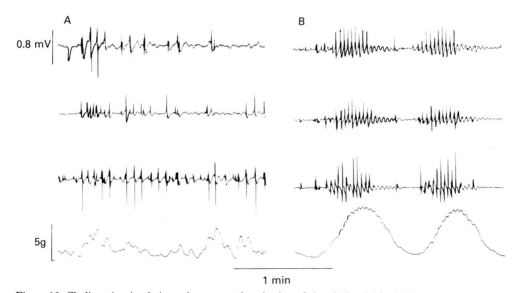

Figure 10. Cholinergic stimulation enhances synchronization of electrical activities in human circular colonic muscle. A. Spontaneous activity recorded by circumferentially placed suction electrodes was mainly uncoupled. B. 10^{-7} M carbachol induced simultaneous oscillating activity with superimposed spikes at each recording site resulting in co-ordinated contractile activity (Huizinga, 1986).

appropriate filling within the colon for normal motility to occur (Huizinga et al, 1985; Huizinga, 1986; Gill et al, 1968b).

When the myoelectrical characteristics of circular muscle are compared to those of the longitudinal muscle, as shown in Figure 11, it becomes evident that the circular layer can exhibit oscillations slower than 12 cpm whereas the longitudinal muscle cannot (Huizinga, 1986). The slow waves of the circular muscle control the occurrence of spikes and contractions as they do in other parts of the gut, i.e. one spike-burst is superimposed on one slow wave and results in one contraction. When the slow wave frequency reaches more than 12 cpm and spikes occur the contractions resulting from a series of individual oscillation-spike complexes may fuse together. Sustained contractions ensue (Figure 11) (Huizinga, 1986; Gill et al, 1986a). This means that colonic contractions can occur in different frequencies according to the underlying slow wave activity. Since high-frequency oscillation-spike

complexes vary in their duration and period of occurrence, it is conceivable that colonic motor activity *in vivo* is much more irregular than that of the small intestine and stomach.

This apparent irregularity of human colonic myoelectrical activity *in vitro* must caution against any overinterpretation of myoelectrical patterns *in vivo*. The fact that electrical slow waves may disappear if the colon is relaxed makes it very difficult to interpret any changes in frequency of this activity.

Myoelectrical Activity in vivo

Recording techniques. In most parts of the human gastrointestinal tract the recording of myoelectrical activity is difficult. The colon is not readily accessible and the methods used are prone to artefacts. Intraluminal electrodes usually render noisy signals which may prevent distinction of low amplitude slow waves. Better recordings are obtained from serosal electrodes

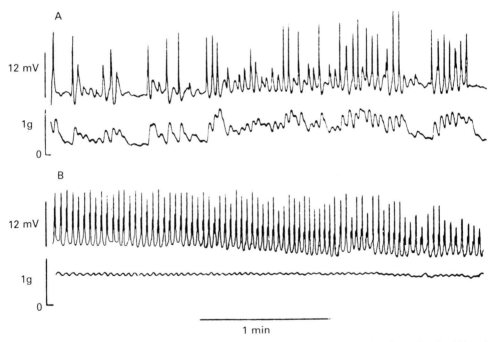

Figure 11. Spontaneous electrical activity of isolated human colonic muscle strips from circular (A) and longitudinal (B) layer. The circular muscle exhibited oscillations which were variable in frequency and amplitude. In the longitudinal muscle the oscillating frequency did not occur below 12 cpm. Oscillation-spike complexes of frequencies above 12 cpm caused sustained contractions in the circular layer (Huizinga, 1986).

Colon ascending

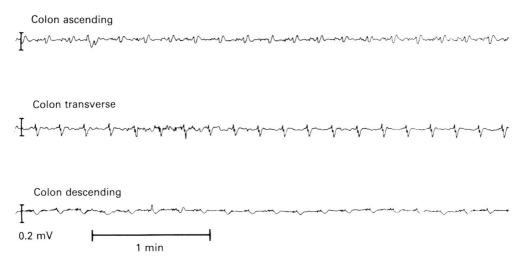

Colon transverse

Colon descending

0.2 mV |————————————|
                        1 min

Figure 12. Spontaneous electrical activity of cat colon *in vivo* recorded by implanted serosal electrodes. Slow waves occurred consistently and at a regular frequency at all recording sites.

implanted during intra-abdominal surgery such as cholecystectomy, but this procedure raises ethical problems. The electrodes have to be withdrawn at or before the tenth postoperative day, and, in addition, postoperative motor patterns may not be representative of the normal state (Sarna et al, 1981).

Thus, animal studies using chronically implanted bipolar electrodes are still indispensable for the study of certain aspects of the normal conditions and of the effects of intervening variables on the myoelectrical activity of the colon. Species differences have to be borne in mind.

Slow wave activity. The cat was the first and most extensively studied animal model of colonic myoelectrical activity. It exhibits omnipresent regular slow waves (Figure 12) (Wienbeck, 1972a, b). The frequency rises from 5.3 in the proximal colon to 5.6/min in the distal colon (Wienbeck et al, 1972).

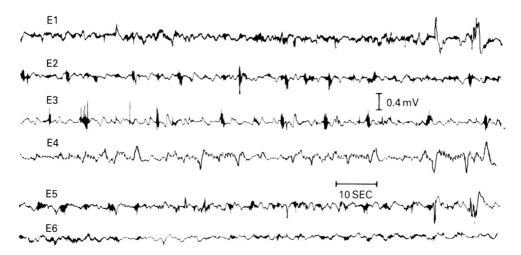

E1

E2

E3 $\mathbf{I}$ 0.4 mV

E4

                                    |——————|
E5   10 SEC

E6

Figure 13. Slow waves recorded postoperatively from transverse colon by serosal electrodes. Slow waves were largely phase-locked and hence they would not generally result in co-ordinated contractions (Sarna et al, 1980).

In dogs slow waves are more irregular than in cats: their frequency varies from 7 to 10 cpm (Kocylowski et al, 1979).

In the human colon, slow waves are even more variable in frequency and amplitude. Only very sensitive surgically implanted electrodes pick up slow waves continuously (Figure 13) (Sarna et al, 1980; Sarna, 1983). With intraluminal electrodes slow waves can be recognized only intermittently within the range of 25 to about 50% of the time (Taylor et al, 1975; Altaparmakow and Wienbeck, 1984). A frequency gradient is not apparent *in vivo*. The spectrum of frequencies of slow waves occurring in the human colon can be divided into a low frequency component and a high frequency component. Power spectrum analysis indicates that in the proximal and distal colon the overall dominant frequency is within a lower frequency range of 0–9 cpm as compared to a higher frequency range of 9–13 cpm in the transverse colon (Sarna et al, 1980). In contrast to the cat which exhibits slow waves coupled in a circumferential and axial direction, in man phase-locking of slow waves has been seen to occur only temporarily over short distances (Figure 13) (Sarna et al, 1983; Christensen and Hauser, 1971a, b).

Within the rectosigmoid area a downward frequency gradient of slow waves was described (Figure 14). The dominant frequency range is about 3 cpm in the rectum and this slow type of slow wave may be recorded more regularly in the rectum than in the upper colon (Taylor et al, 1975). This led to the hypothesis that it provides the electrical basis for the slowing of transit in the rectosigmoid area. One has to keep in mind, however, that the functional role of the different frequencies of slow waves within the large intestine is still unknown. In conclusion, the electrical mechanisms which control colonic contractions await further elucidation.

Spike activity and oscillations. In contrast to slow waves the functional role of spike activity of the colon and also that of oscillating activity is nowadays quite well understood.

Oscillating potentials are not unique in the human colon. They also occur in other species. The cat exhibits oscillations at a rate of 30–45 cpm

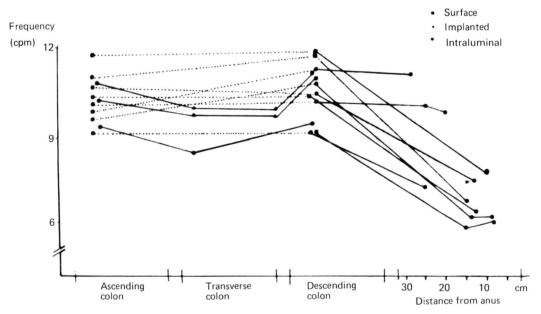

Figure 14. Mean frequency of slow waves throughout the human colon and rectum recorded by surface, implanted serosal and intraluminal electrodes. There was a tendency for a frequency gradient of slow waves in the distal colon and rectum (Taylor et al, 1975).

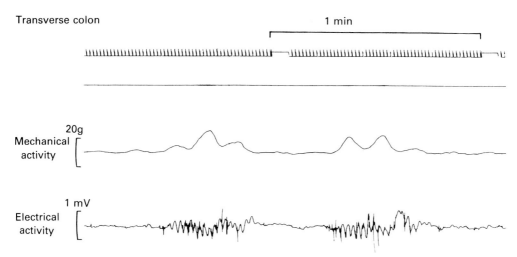

Figure 15. Spontaneous electrical and mechanical activities of feline transverse colon *in vivo* recorded by serosal electrodes and strain gauges. Oscillations (or contractile electrical complex) at 40 cpm were accompanied by sustained contractions consisting of a tonic component and superimposed phasic contractions.

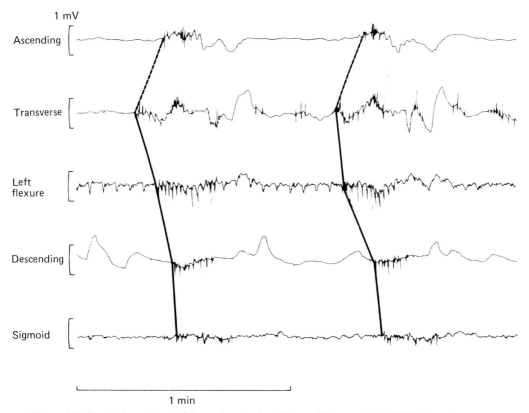

Figure 16. Electrical activity of feline colon *in vivo*. The oscillating activity (CEC) showed superimposed spike activity migrating in aborad direction (solid lines) and orad direction (broken lines).

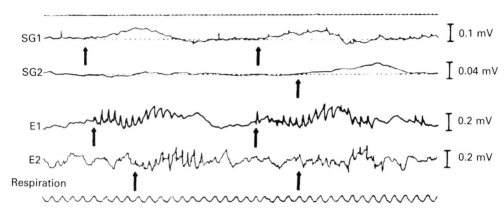

Figure 17. Electrical and mechanical activity of human descending colon recorded by an intraluminal recording tube mounted with two strain gauges (SG) and two electrodes. Two contractile electrical complexes occurred periodically and were associated with long duration contractions. The arrows indicate the onset of the CEC and show its migration pattern (Sarna et al, 1983).

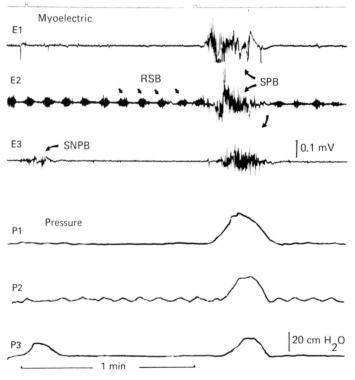

Figure 18. Spike activity of the sigmoid colon and corresponding mechanical activity recorded by intraluminal electromyography and manometry at three recording sites, 15 cm apart from each other. Slow electrical signals were eliminated through a filter (time constant 0.03 sec). Short spike bursts (= RSB, rhythmic sporadic bursts) occurred as stationary activity. Long spike bursts were either propagative (= SPB, sporadic propagating bursts) with associated propagating large amplitude contractions or stationary (= SNPB, sporadic nonpropagating bursts) also accompanied by a strong contraction (Schang et al, 1986).

with or without superimposed spikes and the dog at 25–45 cpm (Wienbeck, 1972a; Wienbeck et al, 1972; Sarna, 1986). Complexes of oscillations have been named the contractile electrical complex (CEC), because this activity is accompanied by long duration contractions (Figure 15). CECs may migrate along the colon (Figure 16). It is thought to represent in part the electrical equivalent of the colonic migrating motor complexes (see above) (Sarna, 1986). Migrating CECs may also be seen in man when serosal or intraluminal electrodes are used for recording (Figure 17) (Sarna et al, 1981, 1982; Sarna, 1983). The frequency of these oscillations in the human colon varies from 25 to 40 cpm. The CEC occurs either as a single event which may last up to several minutes, or it appears repeatedly with a duration of 12–40 sec. The period of these repeated CECs is about 1–2 min. The direction of migration of CECs varies (Sarna et al, 1981). CECs may arise from the circular as well as from the longitudinal muscle as discussed above.

Two patterns of spikes may be differentiated in the large intestine of man and other species: Long spike bursts (LSB) or continuous electrical response activity and short spike bursts (SSB) or discrete electrical response activity (Sarna et al, 1981; Sarna, 1986; Bueno et al, 1980; Frexinos et al, 1985).

The pattern of the short bursts corresponds to that of the spikes in the upper gut: the signals are superimposed on individual slow waves. Their duration is about 3 sec which is less than the cycle length of slow waves (Sarna et al, 1981). SSBs are likely to originate in the circular muscle layer (Huizinga et al, 1985). They are stationary, i.e. they do not migrate over longer distances (Figure 18). Thus, SSBs cannot be propulsive (Schang and Devroede, 1983). As a mechanical counterpart stationary phasic contractions of low amplitude can be recorded (Figures 18 and 19) (Sarna, 1986; Bueno et al, 1980; Schang et al, 1986).

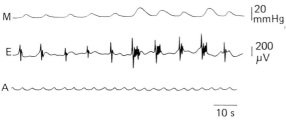

Figure 19. Electrical (E) and mechanical (M) activity of human rectosigmoid recorded intraluminally. (A) shows respiratory activity. Short spike bursts superimposed on slow waves were accompanied by single, low amplitude contractions.

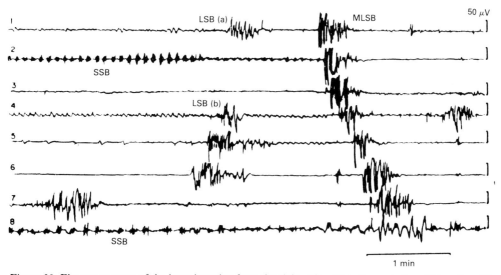

Figure 20. Electromyogram of the large intestine from the right colon (1) to the rectosigmoid junction (8) recorded by intraluminal electrodes showing the different types of spike activity: short spike bursts (SSB) are stationary, large spike bursts (LSB) are either stationary or propagating. Some of them migrate in orad direction (LSB (b)) and some in aboral direction (a). The migrating long spike burst (MLSB) shows one long spike burst which migrated from the right colon to the rectosigmoid (Frexinos et al, 1985).

Long spike bursts (LSB) last for 10–30 sec. They can originate in both muscle layers and they are associated with prolonged contractions. Since they last for more than one slow wave cycle, slow waves cannot be made responsible for their control. LSBs may be propagated or stationary. They are, therefore, also called propagating spike bursts or migrating long spike bursts as opposed to nonpropagating spike bursts (Figures 18 and 20) (Frexinos et al, 1985; Schang and Devroede, 1983; Schang et al, 1986). Propagated LSBs are more numerous than the nonpropagated ones. They usually migrate in the aboral direction, but occasionally they also migrate towards the caecum (Figure 20). Their occurrence varies with feeding and sleeping: LSBs increase during the three

hours following a meal and decrease during the night-time (Figure 21) (Frexinos et al, 1985). Propagated LSBs may be the electrical equivalent of the mass movements as seen radiologically.

In summary, the colon exhibits three distinct types of electrical activity. (1) Electrical control activity or slow waves with a frequency up to 13 cpm. This activity controls the occurrence of short spike bursts. In man it is not phase locked over long distances. Therefore, it is not associated with propulsive activity. (2) Complexes of electrical oscillating activity with a frequency of 20–45 cpm. Since it is accompanied by prolonged contractions, it is called contractile electrical complex (CEC). CECs occur with or without superimposed spikes and last up to several minutes. CECs may be isolated or repeated. Since, in general, CECs are propagated, they are thought to be the major control mechanism of propulsive motor activity. (3) Electrical response activity or spike activity which is superimposed either on slow waves or on CECs. The first is called short spike burst. This type of activity is stationary. The latter is called long spike burst. This type of activity is either stationary or, more frequently, propagated in an aboral direction, occasionally also in an orad direction. Stationary activity is associated with local contractions and probably provides mixing. Propagated activity is associated with migrating contractions and probably is the major force of propulsive movements.

Contractile Patterns

Recording Techniques

The relative inaccessibility of the colon makes recording of colonic mechanical activity almost as difficult as the recording of electrical activity. So far, most information has been gathered in the rectosigmoid because this area can be intubated more easily than others. Recently, several investigators succeeded in positioning probes for manometry into the proximal colon via endoscopy and via long swallowed tubes (Narducci et al, 1987; Spiller et al, 1986). For a detailed study of contractile patterns, however, implanted strain gauge transducers in animal models have been indispensable.

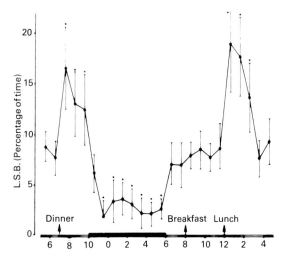

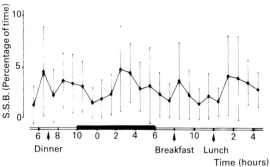

Figure 21. Circadian variation of spike activity in human transverse colon. Long spike bursts (LSB) increased during the three hours after the two meals and decreased during the night time (* indicates significance, p < 0.05). No significant fluctuation appeared for the short spike bursts (SSB) (Frexinos et al, 1985).

Total Motor Activity

Early studies of pelvic motor activity using balloon catheters or perfusion systems revealed that colonic motor activity consists of contractile states alternating with phases of motor quiescence (Connell, 1961, 1968). The colon in this region was active during slightly more than half the recording time. The percentage activity, however, was found to be very variable in different studies using different methods. It ranged from 13 to 59% of time (Connell, 1961; Deller and Wangel, 1965; Bloom et al, 1968). Moreover, marked alterations in the overall motor activity have been reported in diarrhoea, irritable bowel syndrome and other disorders (Connell, 1961; Waller and Misiewicz, 1972; Wangel and Deller, 1965; Sullivan et al, 1978). In addition, the total motor activity exhibits a circadian variation (Figure 22). An increase of activity was found after breakfast and after meals and a decrease during the night (Narducci et al, 1987).

Individual Contractions

Since recordings of intraluminal pressure changes within the sigmoid colon did not reveal specific spatial patterns of motor activity, attempts were made to classify individual contractions according to their morphology and to associate a functional role with them. The major type of pressure wave in the pelvic colon was called the 'principal wave'. It represent a tonic contraction of 20–30 sec duration, and it varies in amplitude (Figure 23). Its distribution is irregular. When the waves occur periodically the frequency of contractions is about 1–2 cpm (Connell, 1965).

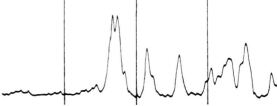

Figure 23. 'Principal waves' recorded by intraluminal balloons from the human sigmoid colon (Connell, 1965).

Only very few of these contractions appeared to be propagated. It was therefore concluded that the dominant type of motor activity in the colon is segmental, which may act as a resistance against flow. Inhibition of this activity was thought to facilitate transit through the colon by reducing the resistance against propulsive forces (Connell, 1965, 1968). The theory that inhibition of colonic motor activity is the major mechanism of acceleration of transit through the colon is still widely accepted, even though the distinction of different shapes of contraction waves, which was the basis for this theory, has been abandoned (Parks, 1973).

Migrating Motor Patterns

Recently, interest rose in spatial and temporal arrangements of colonic motor patterns. Since

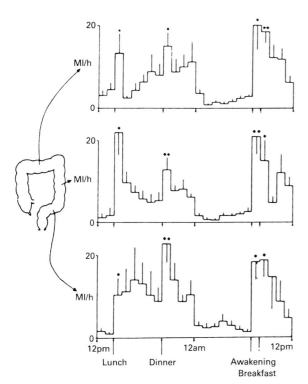

Figure 22. Total motor activity per hour of human transverse (upper), descending (mid) and sigmoid (lower diagram) recorded by intraluminal manometry. Significant increase of motor activity (⋆) occurred after lunch, after dinner and after awakening and breakfast. During the night-time the motor activity was reduced (Narducci et al, 1987).

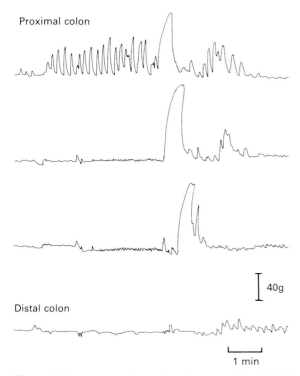

Figure 24. Spontaneous giant migrating contraction (GMC) in the dog colon recorded by implanted strain gauge transducers. The GMC migrated from the proximal to the mid-colon.

myoelectrical recordings showed well-defined migrating motor patterns, their mechanical counterpart was sought.

Giant migrating contractions. The main migrating motor pattern of the colon as described in animals and man is a single, large amplitude contraction which migrates over long distances in the aboral direction (Figure 24). In the dog colon these contractions occur regularly in the caecum and sporadically in the lower colon (Sarna et al, 1987; Karaus and Sarna, 1987). They are called giant migrating contractions (GMC). GMCs that migrate into the distal colon are often accompanied by an urge to defecate (Narducci et al, 1987; Karaus and Sarna, 1987). Similar contractions occurring sporadically during 24-hour manometric recordings in man are called high amplitude propagated contractions (Figure 25). The mean period of this motor pattern was found to be 4.4 hours. Most of the contractions were recorded in the morning after awakening, but some were seen in the late postprandial period (Narducci et al, 1987). In man these GMCs can be stimulated by balloon distension of the colon, thus providing evidence for the theory that co-ordinated colonic

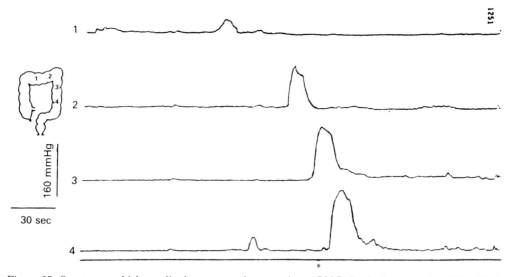

Figure 25. Spontaneous high amplitude propagated contractions (GMC) in the human colon. The GMC migrated from the proximal to the distal colon. The asterisk indicated that the subject felt an urge to defecate when the contraction reached the distal colon (Narducci et al, 1987).

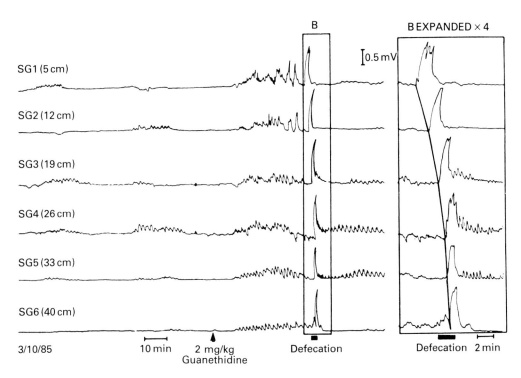

Figure 26. Giant migrating contraction in the dog colon induced by guanethidine, a ganglionic blocker. The GMC migrated over the entire colon and was associated with defecation. The insert on the right shows the migration characteristics expanded four times. Note the large amplitude of GMC in contrast to the regular activity before (Karaus and Sarna, 1987).

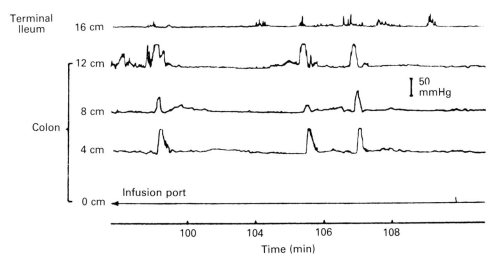

Figure 27. Giant migrating contractions in the human proximal colon recorded by intraluminal manometry via a long swallowed tube. GMCs were induced by the perfusion of oleic acid into the colon (Spiller et al, 1986).

motor activity requires stimulation by stretch (Narducci et al, 1985). In dogs, pharmacological agents such as neostigmine, guanethidine, hyperosmolar glucose solution, and castor oil stimulate GMCs. This is indicative of a neural control mechanism which may be turned on by drugs and mechanical stimuli (Figure 26) (Karaus and Sarna, 1987). In man GMCs can be induced by olive oil, bisacodyl and sennosides (Figure 27). They are accompanied by cramps and the urge to defecate (Spiller et al, 1986; Mann and Hardcastle 1970).

Migrating motor complexes. Since most of the myoelectrical patterns in the colon are propagated, it seems likely that more than just the GMCs would be found as migrating contractile patterns.

Indeed, a motor pattern consisting of a sequence of migrating contractions has been recorded from the dog colon (Sarna et al, 1984; Schuurkes and Tukker, 1980). This sequence of contractions (motor complex) lasts for 7–12 min. It recurs periodically at 20–50-min intervals. Motor com-

plexes may migrate in either direction. Those that migrate over at least half of the colon are called colonic migrating motor complexes (CMMC). CMMCs are propagated in the aborad more often than in orad direction. The others are called colonic nonmigrating motor complexes (CNMMC) (Sarna et al, 1984; Karaus et al, 1987). Figure 28 shows the characteristics of CMMCs and CNMMCs. In dogs, the mean amplitude of the strongest contractions within the motor complexes are in the range of one-half to one-quarter of the mean amplitude of GMCs (Karaus and Sarna, 1987). It therefore becomes unlikely that the contractions of the colonic motor complexes, in general, occlude the lumen of the large intestine. Figure 29 shows that the colonic motor complexes are independent of migrating motor complexes in the small intestine. The corresponding electrical event is the CEC with superimposed spikes (Sarna et al, 1984; Sarna, 1986). This motor pattern is thought to provide the basis for to and fro movements of colonic contents, resulting in a slow net propulsion. It is possible that they represent the

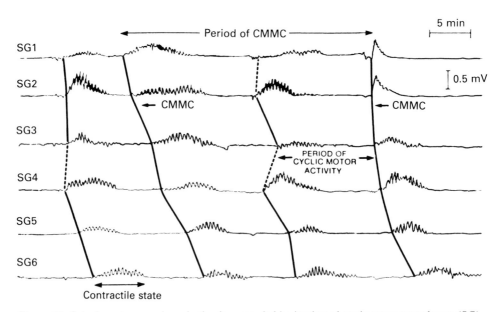

Figure 28. Colonic motor complexes in the dog recorded by implanted strain gauge transducers (SG). Each recording site showed bursts of contractions called contractile states followed by a period of quiescence. Solid lines connecting the onset of contractile states indicate aborad migration, broken lines orad migration. Two contractile states migrated over the entire length of the colon and were called colonic migrating motor complexes (CMMC). The remaining contractile states were non-migrating motor complexes (Karaus et al, 1987).

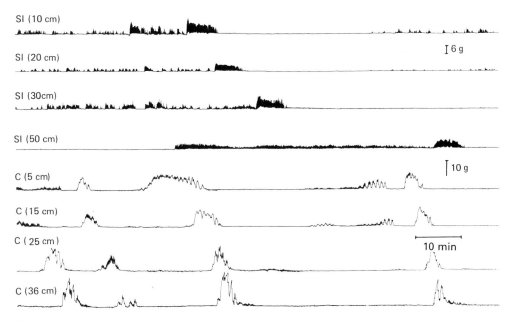

Figure 29. Colonic motor complexes and the migrating motor complex (MMC) of the small intestine. Motor complexes in the colon (C) are independent from the MMC. Their frequencies are different and the onset of colonic motor complexes is not related to any period of the MMC.

equivalent of multihaustral propulsion as described by Ritchie (1968).

Despite the similarity in the myoelectrical activity in the human and canine colon, manometric studies, so far, have not detected propagating motor patterns in man resembling the migrating motor complexes which are picked up by extraluminal strain gauge transducers in dogs. This may be due to the nonoccluding nature of the contractions which for physical reasons often

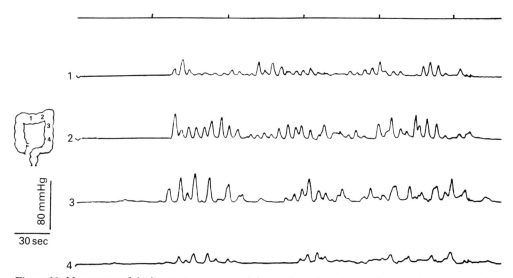

Figure 30. Manometry of the human transverse and descending colon. Bursts of contractions occurred almost simultaneously at the four recording sites. The frequency of individual contractions was about 8 cpm (Narducci et al, 1987).

do not cause an intraluminal pressure rise. Pressure changes within the lumen are required for a contraction to be detected by intraluminal manometry.

Long-term manometric studies in the human colon have shown that the contractile states which alternate with quiescent states comprise two types of contractions: (1) Contractions that occur at a frequency of 3 cpm, and (2) faster contractions at a rate of 8 cpm (Narducci et al, 1987). This corresponds well with the different types of contractions underlying the motor complexes in dogs (Sarna et al, 1984). Groups of contractions in man, however, do not show any migrating pattern. They often occur simultaneously (Figure 30). The physiological significance of these contractions with respect to propulsion and segmentation is unknown. Due to the inherent limitations of manometry, propagated contractions may be missed if they do not cause an intraluminal pressure rise. On the other hand, a small propagated contraction

may be recorded simultaneously at different sites if there is no pressure barrier in between (Connell, 1968). Simultaneous contractions may, thus, be erroneously diagnosed. The situation becomes clear only when lumen occluding propagated contractions such as the GMC occur.

Flow and Motor Patterns

So far, a combination of flow measurements and motor recordings has been applied only in studies of the fast moving contractions: the GMC which is recorded by intraluminal manometry and at the same time by cineradiography probably corresponds to fast propulsive movements of colonic contents which have been termed 'mass movement' by Holzknecht (1909) and Torsoli et al (1971) (Figure 31).

The slow flow patterns described by Ritchie in the human colon cannot yet be related to motor

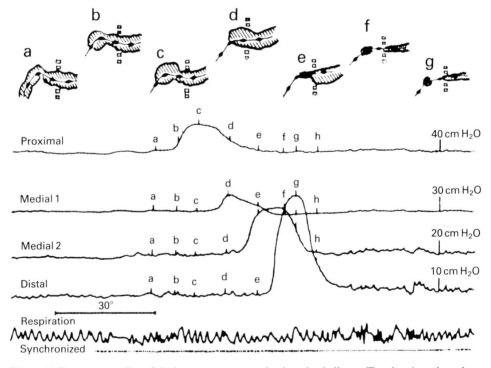

Figure 31. Pressure recording of the human transverse colon by microballoons. Top drawings show the corresponding cinefluorograms (a–g) at certain intervals which are also indicated on the pressure tracings. The strong propagating pressure rise resembled a giant migrating contraction and led to a fast propulsion of colonic contents similar to that described as 'mass movement' (Torsoli et al, 1971).

activity. In animals, however, acceleration of colonic transit has been found to be accompanied by an increase in the number of long spike bursts (Fioramonti et al, 1980). In dogs the flow within the colon seems to be related to contractile states and not to the periods of quiescence, suggesting that it is the contractile activity and not the loss of segmental activity which causes propulsion (Karaus et al, 1986).

References

Altaparmakov, I., and Wienbeck, M., (1984), Local inhibition of myoelectrical activity of human colon by loperamide. *Dig. Dis. Sci.,* 29:232–8.

Bloom, A. A., Lopresti, P., and Farrar, J. T., (1968), Motility of the intact human colon. *Gastroenterology,* 54:232–40.

Bueno, L., Fioramonti, J., Ruckebusch, Y., Frexinos, J., and Coulom P., (1980), Evaluation of colonic myoelectrical activity in health and functional disorders. *Gut,* 21:480–5.

Cannon, W. B., (1902), The movements of the intestines studied by means of the röntgen rays. *Am. J. Physiol.,* 6:251–77.

Christensen, J., Caprilli, R., and Lund, G. F., (1969), Electric slow waves in circular muscle of cat colon. *Am. J. Physiol.,* 217:771–6.

Christensen, J., and Hauser, R. L., (1971a), Longitudinal axial coupling of slow waves in proximal cat colon. *Am. J. Physiol.,* 221:246–50.

Christensen, J., and Hauser, R. L., (1971b), Circumferential coupling of electric slow waves in circular muscle of cat colon. *Am. J. Physiol.,* 221:1033–7.

Connell, A. M., (1961), The motility of the pelvic colon. I. Motility in normals and in patients with asymptomatic duodenal ulcer. *Gut,* 2:175–86.

Connell, A. M., (1965), Significance of the pressure waves of the sigmoid colon. *Am. J. Dig. Dis.,* 10:455–62.

Connell, A. M., (1968), Motor action of the large bowel. In: *Handbook of Physiology, Alimentary Canal IV,* (Ed. Code, C. F.) pp 2075–91. Waverly Press, Baltimore.

Deller, D. J., and Wangel, G., (1965), Intestinal motility in man. I. A study combining the use of intraluminal pressure recording and cineradiography. *Gastroenterology,* 48:45–57.

Eastwood, M. A., (1975), Medical and dietary management. In: *Clinics in Gastroenterology: Diverticular Disease.* (Ed. Smith, A. N.) pp 85–97. W.B. Saunders, London.

Elliott, T. R., and Barclay-Smith, E., (1904), Anti-peristalsis and other muscular activities of the colon. *J. Physiol.,* 31:272–304.

El-Sharkawy, T. Y., (1983), Electrical activities of the muscle layers of the canine colon. *J. Physiol.,* 342:67–83.

Findlay, J. M., Mitchell, W. D., Eastwood, M. A., Anderson, A. J. B., and Smith, A. N., (1974), Intestinal streaming patterns in cholerrhoeic enteropathy and diverticular disease. *Gut,* 15:207–12.

Fioramonti, J., Garcia-Villar, R., Bueno, L., and Ruckebusch, Y., (1980), Colonic myoelectrical activity and propulsion in the dog. *Dig. Dis. Sci.,* 25:641–6.

Frexinos J., Bueno, L., and Fioramonti, J., (1985), Diurnal changes in myoelectric spiking activity of the human colon. *Gastroenterology,* 88:1104–10.

Gill, R. C., Cote, K. R., Bowes, K. L., and Kingma, Y. J., (1986a), Human colonic smooth muscle: Electrical and contractile activity in vitro. *Gut,* 27:293–9.

Gill, R. C., Cote, K. R., Bowes, K. L., and Kinga, Y. J., (1986b), Human colonic smooth muscle: Spontaneous contractile activity and response to stretch. *Gut,* 27:1006–13.

Hall, J., (1965), Bowel content shift during normal defaecation. *Proc. Roy. Soc. Med.,* 58:859–60.

Hertz, A. F., and Newton, A., (1913), The normal movements of the colon in man. *J. Physiol., (Lond.),* 47:57–65.

Holdstock, D. J., Misiewicz, J. J., Smith, T., and Rowlands, E. N., (1970), Propulsion (mass movements) in the human colon and its relationship to meals and somatic activity. *Gut,* 11:91–9.

Holzknecht, G., (1909), Die normale Peristaltik des Kolon. *Münch. Med. Wschr.,* 56:2401–3.

Huizinga, J. D., Stern, H. S., Chow, E., Diamant, N. E., and El-Sharkawy, N. E., (1985), Electrophysiologic control of motility in the human colon. *Gastroenterology,* 88:500–11.

Huizinga, J. D., Stern, H. S., Chow, E., Diamant, N. E., and El-Sharkawy, T. Y., (1986), Electrical basis of excitation and inhibition of human colonic smooth muscle. *Gastroenterology,* 90:1197–1204.

Huizinga, J. D., (1986), Electrophysiology of human colon motility in health and disease. In: *Clinics in Gastroenterology: Pathophysiology of Non-neoplastic Colonic Disorders.* (Ed. Mendeloff, A. I.), pp 879–901. London: W. B. Saunders.

Karaus, M., Sarna, S. K., and Ammon, H. V., (1986), Relationship of colonic flow rate to colonic motor activity. *Gastroenterology,* 90:1483.

Karaus, M., and Sarna, S. K., (1987), Giant migrating contractions during defecation in the dog colon. *Gastroenterology,* 92:925–33.

Karaus, M., Sarna, S. K., Ammon, H. V., and Wienbeck, M., (1987), Effects of oral laxatives on colonic motor complexes in dogs. *Gut,* 28:1112–19.

Kocylowski, M., Bowes, K. L., and Kingma, Y. J.,

(1979), Electrical and mechanical activity in the ex vivo perfused total canine colon. *Gastroenterology*, 77:1021–6.

Krevsky, B., Malmud, L. S., D'Ercole, F., Maurer, A. H., and Fisher, R. S., (1986), Colonic transit scintigraphy. *Gastroenterology*, 91:1102–12.

Kubota, M., Ito, Y., and Ikeda, K., (1983), Membrane properties and innervation of smooth muscle cells in Hirschsprung's disease. *Am. J. Physiol.*, 7:G406–15.

Mann, C. V., and Hardcastle, J. D., (1970), Recent studies of colonic and rectal motor action. *Dis. Col. Rect.*, 13:225–30.

Martelli, H., Devroede, G., Arhan, P., Duguay, C., Dornic, C. D., and Faverdin, C., (1978), Some parameters of large bowel motility in normal man. *Gastroenterology*, 75:612–18.

Metcalf, A. M., Phillips, S. F., Zinsmeister, A. R., MacCarty, R. L., Beart, R. W., and Wolff, B. G., (1987), Simplified assessment of segmental colonic transit. *Gastroenterology*, 92:40–7.

Narducci, F., Bassotti, G., Gaburri, M., Solinas, A., Fiorucci, S., and Morelli, A., (1985), Distension stimulated motor activity of the human transverse, descending and sigmoid colon. *Gastroenterology*, 88:1515.

Narducci, F., Bassotti, G., Gaburri, M., and Morelli, A., (1987), Twenty-four-hour manometric recording of colonic motor activity in healthy man. *Gut*, 28:17–25.

Parks, T. G., (1973), Colonic motility in man. *Postgrad. Med. J.*, 49:90–9.

Ritchie, J. A., (1968), Colonic motor activity and bowel function. *Gut*, 9:442–56.

Ritchie, J. A., (1971), Movement of segmental constrictions in the human colon. *Gut*, 12:350–5.

Ritchie, J. A., Truelove, S. C., Ardran, G. M., and Tuckey, M. S., (1971), Propulsion and retropropulsion of normal colonic contents. *Dig. Dis.*, 16:697–704.

Sarna, S. K., Bardakjian, B. L., Waterfall, W. E., and Lind, J. F., (1980), Human colonic electrical control activity (ECA). *Gastroenterology*, 78:1526–36.

Sarna, S. K., Waterfall, W. E., Bardakjian, B. L., and Lind, J. F., (1981), Types of human colonic electrical activities recorded postoperatively. *Gastroenterology*, 81:61–70.

Sarna, S. K., Latimer, P., Campbell, D., and Waterfall, W. E., (1982), Electrical and contractile activities of the human rectosigmoid. *Gut*, 23:698–705.

Sarna, S. K., (1983), The control of colonic motility. In: *Functional Disorders of the Digestive Tract*. (Ed. Chey, W. Y.) pp 277–85. Raven Press, New York.

Sarna, S. K., Condon, R., and Cowles, V., (1984), Colonic migrating and nonmigrating motor complexes in dogs. *Am. J. Physiol.*, 246:G355–60.

Sarna, S. K., (1986), Myoelectric correlates of colonic motor complexes and contractile activity. *Am. J. Physiol.*, 250:G213–20.

Sarna, S. K., Prasad, K. R., and Lang, I. M., (1987), Giant migrating contractions of the canine cecum. *Gastroenterology*, 92:1614.

Schang, J. C., and Devroede, G., (1983), Fasting and postprandial myoelectric spiking activity in the human sigmoid colon. *Gastroenterology*, 85:1048–53.

Schang, J. C., Hémond, M., Hébert, M., and Pilote, M., (1986), Myoelectrical activity and intraluminal flow in human sigmoid colon. *Dig. Dis. Sci.*, 31:1331–7.

Schuurkes, J. A. J., and Tukker, J. J., (1980), The interdigestive colonic motor complex of the dog. *Arch. Int. Pharm. Ther.*, 247:329–34.

Spiller, R. C., Brown, M. L., and Phillips, S. F., (1986), Decreased fluid tolerance, accelerated transit, and abnormal motility of the human colon induced by oleic acid. *Gastroenterology*, 91:100–7.

Sullivan, M. A., Cohen, S., and Snape, W. J., (1978), Colonic myoelectrical activity in irritable-bowel syndrome. Effect of eating and cholinergics. *N. Engl. J. Med.*, 298:878–83.

Taylor, I., Duthie, H. L., Smallwood, R., and Linkens, D., (1975), Large bowel myoelectrical activity in man. *Gut*, 16:808–14.

Torsoli, A., Ramorino, M. L., Ammaturo, M. V., Capurso, L., Paoluzi, P., and Anzini, F., (1971), Mass movements and intracolonic pressures. *Dig. Dis.*, 16:693–6.

Waller, S., and Misiewicz, J. J., (1972), Colonic motility in constipation and diarrhea. *Scand. J. Gastroent.*, 7:93–6.

Wangel, A. G., and Deller, D. J., (1965), Intestinal motility in man. III. Mechanisms of constipation and diarrhea with particular reference to the irritable colon syndrome. *Gastroenterology*, 48:69–84.

Wienbeck, M., and Christensen, J., (1971), Cationic requirements of colon slow waves in the cat. *Am. J. Physiol.*, 220:513–19.

Wienbeck, M., (1972a), The electrical activity of the cat colon in vivo. I. The normal electrical activity and its relationship to contractile activity. *Res. Exp. Med.*, 158:268–79.

Wienbeck, M., (1972b), The electrical activity of the cat colon in vivo. II. The effects of bethanecol and morphine. *Res. Exp. Med.*, 158:280–7.

Wienbeck, M., Christensen, J., and Weisbrodt, N. W., (1972), Electromyography of the colon in the unanesthetized cat. *Dig. Dis.*, 17:356–62.

Williams, I., (1967), Mass movements (mass peristalsis) and diverticular disease of the colon. *Br. J. Radiol.*, 40:2–14.

19
ANORECTUM

N. R. Womack, N. S. Williams
The London Hospital, London, UK

Introduction

The motility of the anorectum is concerned with the maintenance of continence; it involves the processes of detection, discrimination, retention and finally controlled expulsion of the waste products of digestion. These functions require complex interactions between the visceral and somatic components of the region, co-ordinated by local reflex mechanisms and conscious will. Understanding of these processes is dependent on knowledge of the anatomy of the region.

Anatomy

The anorectal region comprises visceral and somatic components arranged one within the other (Figure 1). The visceral component, the terminal part of the alimentary tract, is tubular and consists of the rectum and upper part of the anal canal. Its wall is composed of outer longitudinal and inner circular layers of smooth muscle. The lowermost part of the circular muscle is thickened and embraces the proximal two-thirds of the anal canal as the internal anal sphincter. The tube is lined by a mucus-secreting columnar epithelium which extends half-way down the anal canal to the dentate line.

The somatic components of the anorectum are arranged around the visceral tube and comprise the voluntary muscles of the pelvic floor and external anal sphincter, and the epithelium of the anal canal below the dentate line. The somatic muscles divide into two anatomical groups. The proximal group, known collectively as the levator ani muscles, originate anteriorly from the pubic arch and side walls of the pelvis and insert posteriorly into a midline raphe and the coccyx to form a diaphragm that closes the pelvic outlet. This is penetrated in the midline by the 'effluent' viscera and the vagina in the female. The lower group of

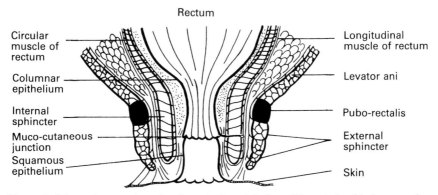

Figure 1. Schematic coronal section through the pelvic floor. The relationship between the visceral and somatic components is demonstrated.

muscles are arranged around the anal canal as the external anal sphincter. For descriptive purposes it is usual to divide them into three parts, subcutaneous, superficial and deep, but functionally they behave as one unit. The lower anal canal is lined by squamous epithelium which is richly supplied with sensory fibres that also extend a centimetre or so up the anal canal proximal to the dentate line (Duthie and Gairns, 1960).

As the rectum passes through the pelvis its course is not straight as its name suggests. Together with the anal canal it forms two angles of approximately 90° each (Figure 2). It has been suggested that the angle between the rectum and anal canal is of great functional importance in the maintenance of continence (see below). This angle results from the activity of the pelvic floor muscles and the puborectalis muscle is especially important in this respect. The puborectalis muscle is the most medial component of the levator ani group; it originates anteriorly from the pubic arch and loops behind the anorectal junction to unite in a raphe with its fellow from the opposite side. It overlaps the deep part of the external anal sphincter and on contraction pulls the anorectal junction upwards and forwards thus angulating the bowel.

The anorectum receives its innervation from the sacral segments of the spinal cord. The visceral structures are innervated by way of the autonomic nervous system. The rectum receives branches from the parasympathetic system via the pelvic splanchnic nerves (S2, S3), and also from the sym-

pathetic system with ganglion cells at L1 and L2. The sympathetic nerves have been shown to be excitatory, and the parasympathetic nerves inhibitory, to the activity of the internal anal sphincter. Both systems appear to be involved in conveying sensory information from the rectum. Somatic nerves supply the voluntary muscles, the levator ani muscles, including the puborectalis muscle, being innervated from their upper surface by a branch of S4 (Percy et al, 1981). The motor innervation of the external anal sphincter muscles and the sensory supply of the lower anal canal is via the pudendal nerve (S2, S3).

Anorectal Motility During the Resting State

The delivery of colonic contents into the rectum is intermittent and for long periods the rectum is empty. Under these circumstances continence is not immediately threatened but the sphincteric mechanisms are not inactive. Indeed even with an empty rectum there is continuous activity within both the internal and external sphincters (Floyd and Walls, 1953; Taverner and Smiddy, 1959; Kerremans, 1969).

Anal Canal Pressures at Rest

Withdrawal of a pressure-sensitive probe from the rectum reveals an area of high pressure in the anal canal even at rest. Figure 3 shows a system that uses a small diameter water-filled microballoon connected to a pressure transducer to measure pressure. By measuring the pressure at centimetre intervals (or stations) from the anal verge a pressure profile indicating the length and intensity of the pressure zone can be constructed. The pressure measured at rest in the anal canal is referred to as the basal anal canal pressure and the highest such pressure recorded along the anal canal as the maximum basal pressure (MBP). The basal pressure can be augmented by asking the subject to maximally contract the external sphincter at each station. The increment of pressure added by voluntary contraction is referred to as the squeeze pressure and the highest such increment as the

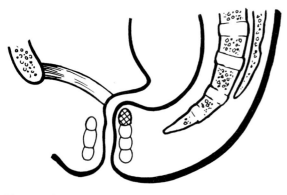

Figure 2. Schematic sagittal section through the pelvic floor. The angulations of the terminal rectum are demonstrated.

maximum squeeze pressure (MSP). The normal range for the MBP is 60–120 cm water and for MSP is 100–200 cm water (Read et al, 1979; Matheson and Keighley, 1981) (Figure 4).

The origin of the basal anal canal pressure has been the subject of much investigation. A contribution from the internal anal sphincter is indicated by the fact that the basal pressure undergoes regular fluctuations that coincide with periodic changes in the electrical activity within the internal anal sphincter (Kerremans, 1969). Demonstration of continuous electromyographic activity within the external anal sphincter at rest, and even during sleep (Floyd and Walls, 1953; Taverner and Smiddy, 1959), implies it also con-

tributes to the basal pressure. To determine the relative importance of their contributions to the resting pressure studies have been performed in which the external sphincter component was removed (Duthie and Watts, 1965; Frenckner and Von Euler, 1975). Local anaesthesia applied to the pudendal nerve abolished electromyographic activity in the external sphincter and resulted in a reduction of only 15% in the basal pressure. The major contributor to the basal anal canal pressure, therefore, appears to be the internal anal sphincter.

As was previously mentioned the basal pressure undergoes regular fluctuations. These have been termed slow waves and have a frequency of 10–20/min with an amplitude of 5–25 cm water (Figure 3B). They occur at a higher frequency in the distal anal canal and it has been postulated that they generate an inwardly directed force that empties the anal canal into the rectum (Kerremans, 1969; Pennickx et al, 1973; Hancock, 1975). Less commonly seen in normal subjects are ultra slow waves (amplitude 40–100 cm water, frequency less than 3/min); they tend to occur with high basal pressures in conditions such as fissure-in-ano and haemorrhoids (Hancock, 1977; Hancock and Smith, 1975).

The continuous, or tonic, activity demonstrated in the external anal sphincter by electromyography is unusual, since a skeletal muscle normally requires a conscious effort for contraction. It would seem that a postural stretch reflex liberates the subject from the necessity to continually direct his attention to the sphincters (Parks et al, 1966).

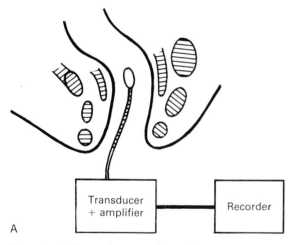

Figure 3. A. System for measuring anal canal pressure. The probe is a water-filled microballoon.

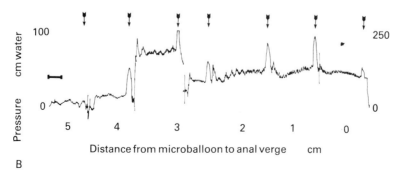

Figure 3. B. Measurement of anal canal pressure by the station pull-through technique. Slow waves are seen at 2 and 3 cm from the anal verge. (Note: Change of scale at 3 cm; arrows indicate voluntary contractions of the sphincters: time bar = 10 sec).

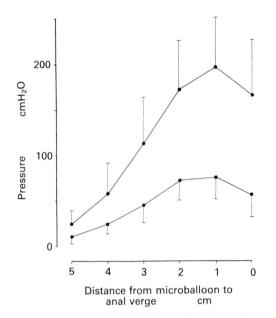

Figure 4. Anal canal pressure profile. The data are from 39 normal subjects. (Key: Squares = basal anal canal pressure, Circles = pressure during voluntary contraction of the sphincter. The values are plotted as means and SD.)

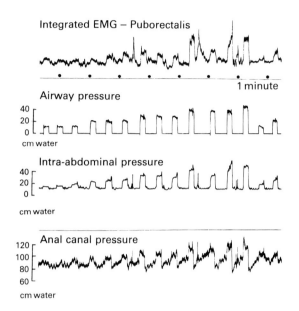

Figure 5. The response of the external anal sphincter to raised intra-abdominal pressure. Intra-abdominal pressure was raised by a series of forced expirations. The response of the puborectalis muscle was monitored via its EMG activity, this is displayed in integrated form in the upper trace. The superficial external and sphincter response was monitored by measuring the anal canal pressure. This is displayed in the lower trace.

The reflex is believed to operate via a simple arc between muscles and the spinal cord since it has been shown to persist intact below the level of the spinal injury in paraplegic subjects (Melzack and Porter, 1964). The sensory receptors for the reflex are thought to be muscle spindles that have been demonstrated in the pelvic floor and external sphincter muscles (Winckler, 1958). Afferent fibres from these receptors relay directly, or via interneurons, on the motorneurons of the anal sphincters. By this mechanism forces that tend to stretch the pelvic floor or sphincter muscles reflexly generate increased activity within them. The normal positive resting intra-abdominal pressure is responsible for the tonic activity within the muscles and when intra-abdominal pressure increases with activities such as lifting, coughing or walking there is rapid increase in activity (Taverner and Smiddy, 1959; Parks et al, 1966). This is illustrated in Figure 5. In this example a series of forced expirations of varying intensity produced rises in intra-abdominal pressure. These rises in intra-abdominal pressure resulted in increases in the electromyographic activity of the sphincteric muscles and corresponding increases in the anal

canal pressure. A plot of the increase in electromyographic activity in the puborectalis muscle in response to the increase in intra-abdominal pressure (Figure 6) indicates the sensitivity and precision of the mechanism.

In addition to the tonic activity of the external anal sphincter, voluntary effort may produce phasic increases in activity. Such phasic activity rapidly fatigues (Parks et al, 1966a; Read et al, 1979). It can only be sustained for periods of about one minute after which the activity fades. Contraction of the external sphincter raises the pressure throughout the anal canal but the effect is greatest distally which coincides with the situation of the largest part of the muscle, the superficialis.

Puborectalis Activity and the Anorectal Angle

Electromyographic studies of the puborectalis muscle have revealed a pattern of activity similar to that described above for the external anal sphincter (Taverner and Smiddy, 1959). The

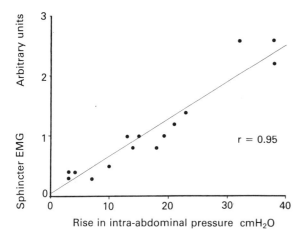

Figure 6. Plot of the puborectalis response to raised intra-abdominal pressure. The data for this plot were obtained from the study illustrated in Figure 5. There is a highly significant linear correlation between the increase in the puborectalis EMG activity (Y axis) and the rise in intra-abdominal pressure (X axis).

activity of the pelvic floor muscles opposes intra-abdominal pressure and prevents herniation of the pelvic viscera through the pelvic floor. The sling-like anatomical arrangement of the puborectalis muscle around the anorectal junction results in angulation of the bowel at this point as the muscle contracts. At rest the tonic activity within the puborectalis results in an angle of approximately 90° between the lower rectum and the anal canal (Kerremans, 1969; Hardcastle and Parks, 1970). This angle can be reduced by voluntary contraction of the pelvic floor muscles and made more obtuse by straining as if at stool.

Several authors have commented on the importance of the puborectalis muscle for the maintenance of continence. Milligan and Morgan (1934) reported that continence was preserved after fistula surgery involving sacrifice of the external anal sphincter provided the puborectalis remained intact. The importance of routing the rectum through the puborectalis sling in order for continence to be achieved after surgical correction of imperforate anus has been emphasized (Louw, 1962; Kieswetter, 1967; Swenson and Donnellan, 1967; Puri and Nixon, 1977). It is not surprising, therefore, that theories have been proposed that endow anorectal angulation with a role in the maintenance of continence. Having undertaken

radiological studies of the anal region Phillips and Edwards (1965) described rapid clearance of contrast from the segment of bowel at the anorectal junction. They concluded that this region was subjected to greater pressure than the surrounding bowel. They postulated that this indicated the pressure of a flutter valve created by apposition of the bowel walls as the latter passed through a slit-like opening in the pelvic floor (Figure 7). They argued that whenever intra-abdominal pressure increased such an arrangement would tend to oppose the walls more forcibly thus contributing to the maintenance of continence (Figure 7A).

A different type of valvular mechanism was suggested by Parks et al (1966b). They pointed out that, as a result of the right angle between the anal canal and rectum, the anterior rectal mucosa overlies the entrance to the anal canal. They sug-

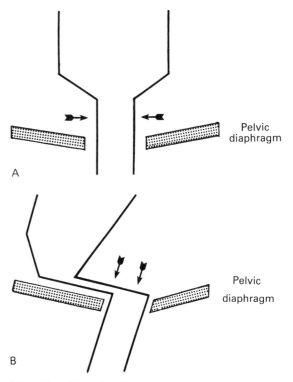

Figure 7. A. The principle of the flutter valve. It is suggested the increases of intra-abdominal pressure are transmitted to the walls of the anal canal, above the pelvic diaphragm, and contribute to its closure. B. The principle of the flap valve. It is suggested that increases of intra-abdominal pressure compress the anterior rectal wall mucosa onto the top of the anal canal and thereby occlude the rectal outlet.

gested that during periods of increased intra-abdominal pressure the rectal mucosa may be driven more forcibly onto the top of the anal canal, thus closing the rectal outlet (Figure 7B). This mechanism, which they described as a flap valve, could only work if rectal contents did not enter the terminal portion of the rectum and lift the rectal mucosa off the anal canal. In a recent radiological investigation, however, Bartolo et al (1986) demonstrated that rectal contents did occupy the terminal segment of the rectum, and yet continence was maintained when intra-abdominal pressure was raised. This has raised doubts about the value of a continence mechanism that can only function when the rectum is empty.

Rectal Filling: Detection and Discrimination of Rectal Contents

The precise nature of rectal filling is poorly understood, but for the purpose of studying anorectal motility it has frequently been simulated by the incremental distension, with air, of a balloon placed within the rectal ampulla (Melzack and Porter, 1964; Goligher and Hughes, 1951; Ihre, 1974) (Figure 8). Such distension gives rise to a feeling of fullness in the perineum or sacral area (Goligher and Hughes, 1951). In a normal subject a sensation of filling first occurs after approximately 30 ml of air has been introduced, this is referred to as the minimum perceived volume. The sensation changes to one of discomfort after approximately 300–350 ml of air have been introduced, this is the maximum tolerable volume. It was originally believed that the receptors responsible for the detection of rectal distension were present within the rectal wall. It has been shown, however, that similar sensations persist when a balloon is inflated in the 'neo-rectum' after a total resection of the rectum, with colo-anal anastomosis, has been performed (Lane and Parks, 1977). The receptors must, therefore, lie outside the bowel wall and it has been suggested that the muscle spindles within the pelvic floor muscles may fulfil this function.

Distension of a balloon placed in the rectum initiates reflex responses within the rectum itself and within the internal and external anal sphincters (Figure 8).

Rectal Response

When empty the rectum exhibits little spontaneous activity. Distension of a balloon initiates rectal contractions. These frequently occur after a bolus of air is introduced into the balloon and with a frequency of 5–10/min thereafter (Connell, 1961; Scharli and Kieswetter, 1970). Intrarectal pressure increases with the contraction that follows each bolus of air and then subsides to low levels as the rectum accommodates, over a period of about 45 seconds, to the increased volume. As the maximum tolerable volume is reached there is a failure of accommodation and the intrarectal pressure rises with associated discomfort (Ihre, 1974; Arhan et al, 1976).

Internal Anal Sphincter Response

To record the activity of the internal anal sphincter the anal pressure probe is placed within the anal canal at the position of the maximum basal pressure. This is usually 1–2 cm from the anal verge. With a low distending volume (50 ml) a rapid and short-lived reduction in the basal pressure is seen (Gowers, 1877; Denny-Browne and Robertson, 1935; Gaston, 1948; Schuster et al, 1963) (Figure 8). Over a period of about 30 sec the basal pressure returns to resting levels. Similar reductions in the basal pressure are seen with subsequent inflations, but as the distending volume increases the decrease in pressure becomes greater and it does not return to resting levels (Schuster et al, 1965). During these reductions in anal canal pressure the normal fluctuations in anal canal pressure (slow waves) and the associated oscillations in the electrical activity within the internal anal sphincter are abolished (Bouvier and Gonella, 1981). The decrease in pressure appears, therefore, to be due to relaxation of the internal sphincter. This internal anal sphincter response is probably mediated through an intramural neural pathway the activity of which is modulated by spinal cord activity (Meunier and Mollard, 1977).

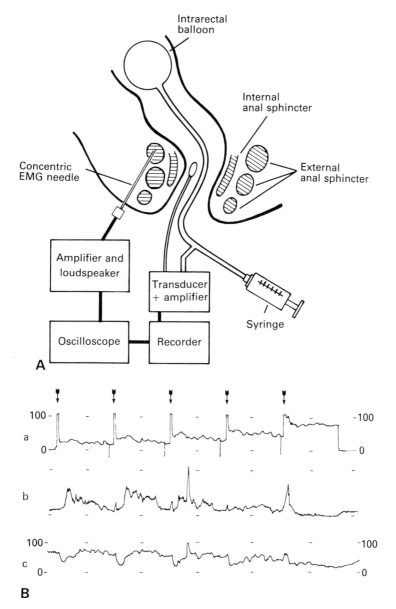

Figure 8. A. Method of measuring the effects of rectal distension. The microballoon records summated internal and external anal sphincter activity, but when placed at the site of maximal basal pressure it records predominantly internal sphincter function. An EMG needle placed within the external anal sphincter records its activity. The rectal balloon was inflated, in increments, using a syringe. B. An example of the response to rectal distension.
Key: a, pressure within the rectal balloon; b, integrated sphincter EMG (external sphincter); c, anal canal pressure (predominantly internal sphincter). The arrows indicate inflations of the balloon with 50 ml of air at minute intervals. Note: Trace a, Rectal accommodation until maximum tolerable volume (MTV) is reached. Trace b, Phasic and tonic components of external sphincter response, the tone in the sphincter is at first increased from resting tone but then decreases at MTV. Trace c, The inhibitory recto-anal reflex, seen after the first four inflations; at MTV the inhibition of the internal anal sphincter persists while the balloon remains inflated.

External Anal Sphincter Response

The activity of the external anal sphincter can be monitored by the insertion of a concentric electromyography needle into the superficialis muscle. The inflation of a balloon in the rectal ampulla causes an increase in the activity of the external sphincter at low volumes (Porter, 1962). This increased activity has phasic and tonic components (Ihre, 1974); the phasic component immediately follows inflation and has a duration of approximately 20 sec. It coincides with the reduction of activity that occurs in the internal anal sphincter. A pressure probe placed in the distal centimetre of the anal canal may register an increase in pressure during this response. The tonic component follows the phasic component and persists while the balloon remains inflated. As rectal distension proceeds the level of increased activity within the external sphincter gradually decreases (Ihre, 1974; Porter, 1962) (Figure 8). As the distending volume approaches the maximum tolerable volume there is, frequently, electrical silence within the external sphincter and the balloon may escape from the rectum. It is thought that these responses are mediated by spinal reflexes. Preservation of the responses after proctectomy and colo-anal anastomosis implies that the receptors involved are located in the pelvic walls or floor (Lane and Parks, 1977).

The 'Sampling Reflex'

Awareness of the complex response to rectal filling, together with knowledge of the distribution of sensory perception in the anal canal, led Duthie and Bennett (1964) to postulate a mechanism for the fine discrimination of rectal contents. This has become known as the sampling reflex. They determined the proximal level in the anal canal at which normal subjects could discriminate light touch. By measuring the pressure profile of the anorectum at rest they concluded that this sensitive area would be inaccessible to rectal contents because of the higher pressure in the anal canal than in the rectum. They argued that relaxation of the internal anal sphincter with reduction of pressure in the proximal anal canal, in response to

rectal filling, would allow the rectal contents to come into contact with the sensitive mucosa and facilitate discrimination.

Thus anal canal sensation has an important role in normal anorectal function and a potential role in the aetiology of anorectal disease. In order to investigate this a method to quantify sensory function at specified points along the anal canal has been developed (Roe et al, 1986). The method determines the sensory threshold of an electrical stimulus delivered to the anal canal via a specially designed probe. This technique has demonstrated decreased sensation in the proximal anal canal in subjects with haemorrhoids, and decreased sensation throughout the anal canal in subjects with faecal incontinence. The significance of these findings is, however, difficult to determine since the sensory abnormality in these conditions is usually only one of several abnormalities that can be demonstrated. A cautious interpretation is indicated as a result of another study, in which the effect of anaesthetizing the anal canal with local anaesthetic in normal subjects was investigated (Read and Read, 1982). The amplitude and duration of voluntary contractions of the anal sphincters were reduced but anal continence was retained despite absent anal canal sensation.

Defecation

Propulsion of colonic contents into the rectum results in rectal distension. By the mechanisms described above their presence and nature is perceived allowing a decision to be made about the timing of rectal evacuation. If defecation is to be deferred a voluntary contraction of the pelvic floor and external anal sphincter muscles reinforces the sphincteric mechanisms and returns rectal contents to the rectal ampulla from the upper anal canal (Phillips and Edwards, 1965). If the situation is opportune defecation may proceed.

Investigation of the act of defecation presents the investigator with several difficulties. Foremost of these is reproduction of the natural state during the investigation. The fact that the subject is aware that he is being monitored during a normally personal and private function means that all results must be interpreted in the light that they were recorded in at best a close approximation to the natural state. The study of spontaneous defecation imposes difficulties in the timing of investigation and this is one reason why workers have often substituted models of defecation for the natural act in their investigations (Kerremans, 1969; Bartolo et al, 1986; Porter, 1962; Fry et al, 1966; Preston et al, 1974; Womack et al, 1985; Mahieu et al, 1984). Various methodologies have been employed; these have included radiology (Kerremans, 1969; Bartolo et al, 1986; Fry et al, 1966; Preston et al, 1984; Womack et al, 1985; Mahieu et at, 1984), manometry (Bartolo et al, 1986), radiotelemetry (Womack et al, 1985) and electromyography (Kerremans, 1969; Bartolo et al, 1986; Porter, 1962; Womack et al, 1985). It has been usual to study only one modality at a time and the interpretation of results has, therefore, frequently involved inference and extrapolation of results, often between studies that employed different models of defecation. This situation was obviously unsatisfactory from a scientific point of view; and suggestions that certain anorectal conditions result from abnormal defecation (Porter, 1962; Rutter, 1974; Preston and Lennard-Jones, 1985) necessitated an integrated system of investigation of rectal voiding to enable accurate diagnosis. We have, therefore, developed a method to visualize the anorectum during voiding, whilst simultaneously measuring the electromyographic activity of the puborectalis and superficial parts of the external anal sphincter, and the intrarectal pressure by radiotelemetry (Womack et al, 1985).

The method (Figure 9) entails the use of a semisolid contrast medium made from rolled oats, barium sulphate and water which simulates a soft stool to be voided. Apart from outlining the anorectum it offers the advantages of consistency of texture of the rectal contents and the ability to control the timing of the investigation. It is performed without bowel preparation, the contrast being introduced into the rectum, via a proctoscope, using a wide-tipped syringe. Approximately 300 ml of contrast is used and this produces the sensation of a call to stool. Intrarectal pressure is measured by a pressure-sensitive radiotelemetry capsule. This is pre-calibrated against a water manometer, at 37°C, before it is introduced into the rectum prior to the contrast. The radio signal emitted by the capsule is detected by an omnidirectional aerial strapped over the subject's sacrum.

The electromyographic activity of the superficial and puborectalis components of the external

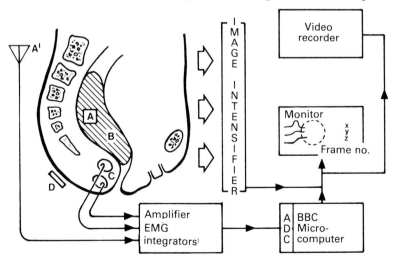

Figure 9. Method for dynamic assessment of rectal voiding. (Key: A, pressure-sensitive radiotelemetry capsule; A^1, omnidirectional antenna; B, Semisolid radio-opaque contrast medium; C, Wire electrodes in puborectalis and superficial external anal sphincter; D, 3 cm metal marker on the skin.) A composite image of the radiological, EMG and pressure data is produced. This is stored on video tape for later play back and analysis.

anal sphincter is recorded by the insertion of fine stainless steel wire electrodes into the muscles (Basmajamian and Stecko, 1963). The ends of these wire electrodes are hooked to prevent displacement from the muscle despite the movement caused by contraction. The wires are so fine that within a few seconds of their introduction the subjects become unaware of their presence. The signal recorded from the electrodes is integrated to allow comparison of the degree of activity of the muscle from time to time. With the patient seated on a radiolucent commode the anorectum is visualized during voiding by lateral fluoroscopy. A microcomputer is used to store the pressure and electromyographic data. It also produces a graphic display of the data that is synchronized and mixed with the video image produced by the image intensifier thereby producing a composite picture that contains pressure, electromyographic and radiological data (Figure 10).

From the results of this and the previous methods of investigation we know that during defecation intrarectal pressure rises and the pelvic floor descends. The anorectal angle becomes more obtuse as the distal rectum opens out into a funnel that extends into the anal canal as voiding starts. The rise in intrarectal pressure results, at least in part, from transmission of increased intra-abdominal pressure caused by voluntary contraction of the abdominal wall musculature against a closed glottis. A contribution from contraction of the rectal musculature has been postulated but as yet remains unproven. Descent of the pelvic floor results from a combination of the rise in intra-abdominal pressure and inhibition of the pelvic floor muscles. This inhibition may commence immediately as the intra-abdominal pressure rises, or it may follow one or two seconds after the rise in pressure, after a transient increase in sphincter activity (Kerremans, 1969; Womack et al, 1987a). In a minority of normal subjects straining is accompanied by increased sphincter activity which persists throughout voiding (Kerremans, 1969; Womack et al, 1987a); this pattern is frequently observed in patients who complain of various anorectal symptoms and it may be related to their aetiology (Rutter, 1974; Preston and Lennard-Jones, 1985; Womack et al, 1985, 1987a, b). At the end of defecation a contraction of the sphincteric and pelvic floor musculature, the closing reflex, returns the pelvic floor to the rest position and reconstitutes the resting anorectal angle (Kerremans, 1969; Porter, 1962; Womack et al, 1985).

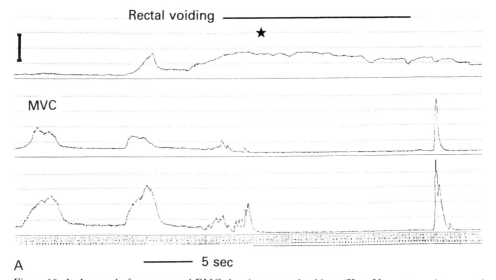

Figure 10. A. A record of pressure and EMG data in a normal subject. (Key: Upper trace, intra-rectal pressure (bar = 100 cm H_2O); Middle trace, puborectalis EMG activity; Lower trace, superficial external anal sphincter EMG activity. Maximal voluntary contraction is of the anal sphincters.) The frame numbers (below the lower trace) allow the record to be correlated with the radiological data.

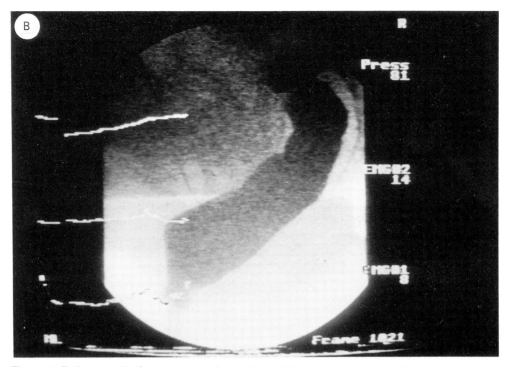

Figure 10. B. An example of a proctogram taken during voiding in a normal subject. This is from the same investigation as that illustrated in Figure 10A; the asterisk marks the position of the photograph on that record.

References

Arhan, P., Faverdin, C., Persoz, B., Devroede, G., Dubois, F., Dornic, C., and Pellerin, D., (1976), Relationship between viscoelastic properties of the rectum and anal pressure in man. *J. Appl. Physiol.*, 41:677–82.

Bartolo, D. C. C., Roe, A. M., Locke Edmonds, J. C., Virgee, J., and Mortensen, N. J. McC., (1986), Flap-valve theory of anal continence. *Br. J. Surg.*, 73:1012–14.

Basmajamian, J. V., and Stecko, G., (1963), A new bipolar indwelling electrode for electromyography. *J. Appl. Physiol.*, 17:849.

Bouvier, M., and Gonella, J., (1981), Nervous control of the internal anal sphincter of the cat. *J. Physiol.*, 310:457–69.

Connell, A. M., (1961), The motility of the pelvic colon. *Gut*, 2:175–86.

Denny-Browne, D., and Robertson, E. G., (1935), An investigation of the nervous control of defaecation. *Brain*, 58:256–310.

Duthie, H. L., and Gairns, F. W., (1960), Sensory nerve endings and sensation in the anal region of man. *Br. J. Surg.*, 47:585–95.

Duthie, H. L., and Watts, J. M., (1965), Contribution of the external anal sphincter to the pressure zone in the anal canal. *Gut*, 6:64–8.

Duthie, H. L., and Bennett, R. C., (1964), The relation of sensation in the anal canal to the functional anal sphincter: a possible factor in anal continence. *Gut*, 4:179–82.

Floyd, W. F., and Walls, E. W., (1953), Electromyography of the sphincter and externum in man. *J. Physiol.*, 122:599–609.

Frenckner, D., and Von Euler, C., (1975), Influence of pudendal block on the function of the anal sphincters. *Gut*, 16:482–9.

Fry, I. K., Griffiths, J. D., and Smart, P. J. G., (1966), Some observations on the movement of the pelvic floor and rectum with special reference to rectal prolapse. *Br. J. Surg.*, 53:784–7.

Gaston, E. A., (1948), The physiology of faecal incontinence. *Surg. Gynec. Obstet.*, 87:280–90.

Goligher, J. C., and Hughes, E. S. R., (1951), Sensibility at the rectum and colon: its role in the mechanism of anal continence. *Lancet*, i:543–8.

Gowers, W. R., (1877), The autonomic action of the sphincter ani. *Proc. R. Soc. (Lond.)*, 26:77–84.

Hancock, B. D., (1975), Measurement of anal pressure and motility. *Gut*, 17:645–51.

Hancock, B. D., (1977), The internal sphincter and anal fissure. *Br. J. Surg.*, **64**:92–5.

Hancock, B. D., and Smith, K., (1975), The internal anal sphincter and Lord's procedure for haemorrhoids. *Br. J. Surg.*, **62**:833–6.

Hardcastle, J. D., and Parks, A. G., (1970), A study of anal incontinence and some principles of surgical management. *Proc. R. Soc. Med.*, **63**:Suppl., 116–18.

Ihre, T., (1974), Studies on anal function in continent and incontinent patients. *Scand. J. Gastroent.*, **9**:Suppl. 25.

Kerremans, R., (1969), *Morphological and Physiological Aspects of Anal Continence and Defecation.* Editions Arscia, Brussels.

Kieswetter, W. B., (1967), Imperforate anus. II. The rationale and technique of sacro-abdomino-perineal operation. *J. Ped. Surg.*, **2**:106–11.

Lane, R. H. S., and Parks, A. G., (1977), Function of the anal sphincters following colo-anal anastomosis. *Br. J. Surg.*, **64**:596–9.

Louw, J. H., (1962), Some observations on the musculature of the pelvic floor, and anal sphincters, and rectal continence. *S. African J. Clin. Med.*, **8**:54–8.

Mahieu, P., Pringot, J., and Bodart, P., (1984), Defecography; I. Description of a new procedure and results in normal patients. *Gastrointestinal Radiol.*, **9**:247–51.

Matheson, D. M., and Keighley, M. R. B., (1981), Manometric evaluation of rectal prolapse and faecal incontinence. *Gut*, **22**:126–9.

Melzack, J., and Porter, N. H., (1964), Studies of the reflex activity of the external sphincter ani in spinal man. *Paraplegia*, **1**:277–96.

Meunier, P., and Mollard, P., (1977), Control of the internal anal sphincter (manometric study with human subjects). *Pflugers Archiv für die gesamte Physiologie des Menschen und der Tierre*, **370**:233–9.

Milligan, E. T. C., and Morgan, C. N., (1934), Surgical anatomy of the anal canal with special reference to anorectal fistulae. *Lancet*, **ii**:1150–6.

Parks, A. G., Porter, N. H., and Melzack, J., (1966a), Experimental study of the reflex mechanism controlling the muscles of the pelvic floor. *Proc. R. Soc. Med.*, **59**: 477–82.

Parks, A. G., Porter, N. H., and Hardcastle, J. D., (1966b), The syndrome of the descending perineum. *Proc. R. Soc. Med.*, **59**: 477–82.

Penninckx, F., Kerremans, R., and Beckers, J., (1973), Pharmacological characteristics of the non-rectal musculature in cats. *Gut*, **14**:393–8.

Percy, J. P., Neill, M. E., Swash, M., and Parks, A. G., (1981), Electrophysiological study of motor nerve supply of pelvic floor. *Lancet*, **i**:16–17.

Phillips, S. F., and Edwards, D. A. W., (1965), Some aspects of anal continence and defecation. *Gut*, **6**:396–405.

Porter, N. H., (1962), Physiological study of the pelvic floor in rectal prolapse. *Ann. R. Soc. Med.*, **286**:379–404.

Preston, D. M., Lennard-Jones, J. E., and Thomas, B. M., (1984), The balloon proctogram. *Br. J. Surg.*, **71**:29–32.

Preston, D. M., and Lennard-Jones, J. E., (1985), Anismus in chronic constipation. *Dig. Dis. Sci.*, **30**:413–18.

Puri, P., and Nixon, N. H., (1977), The results of treatment of anorectal anomalies: a 13–20-year follow up. *J. Ped. Surg.*, **12**:27–32.

Read, N. W., Harford, W. V., Schmulen, A. C., Read, M. G., Santa Ana, C., and Fordtran, J. S., (1979), A clinical study of patients with faecal incontinence and diarrhoea. *Gastroenterology*, **76**:747–56.

Read, M. G., and Read, N. W., (1982), Role of anorectal sensation in preserving continence. *Gut*, **23**:345–7.

Roe, A. M., Bartolo, D. C. C., and Mortensen, N. J. McC, (1986), New method for assessment of anal sensation in various anorectal disorders. *Br. J. Surg.*, **73**:310–12.

Rutter, R. P., (1974), Electromyographic changes in certain pelvic floor abnormalities. *Proc. R. Soc. Med.*, **67**:53–6.

Scharli, A. F., and Kieswetter, W. B., (1970), Defaecation and continence: some new concepts. *Dis. Colon. Rect.*, **13**:81–107.

Schuster, M. M., Hendrix, T. R., and Mendeloff, A. I., (1963), The internal anal sphincter response: manometric studies on its normal physiology, neural pathways, and alteration in bowel disorders. *J. Clin. Invest.*, **42**:196–207.

Schuster, M. M., Hookman, P., Hendrix, T. R., and Mendeloff, A. J., (1965), Simultaneous manometric recording of internal and external sphincter responses. *Bull. Johns Hopkins Hosp.*, **116**:79–88.

Swenson, O., and Donnellan, W. L., (1967), Preservation of the puborectalis sling in imperforate anus. *Surg. Clin. N. America*, **47**:173.

Taverner, D., and Smiddy, F. G., (1959), An electromyographic study of the normal function of the external anal sphincter and pelvic diaphragm. *Dis. Colon Rectum*, **2**:153–60.

Williams, N. S., Price, R., and Johnston, D., (1980), The long term effect of sphincter preserving operations for rectal carcinoma on the function of the anal sphincter in man. *Br. J. Surg.*, **67**:203–8.

Winckler, G., (1958), Remarques sur la morphologie et l'innervation du muscle releveur de l'anus. *Archives Anatomie et Histologie et Embryologie* (Strasbourg) **41**:77–95.

Womack, N. R., Williams, N. S., Holmfield, J. H. M., Morrison, J. F. B., and Simpkins, K. C., (1985), New method for the dynamic assessment of anorectal function in constipation. *Br. J. Surg.*, **72**:994–8.

Womack, N. R., Williams, N. S., Holmfield, J. H. M., and Morrison, J. F. B., (1987a), Anorectal function in the solitary rectal ulcer syndrome. *Dis. Colon Rectum*, **30:**319–23.

Womack, N. R., Williams, N. S., Holmfield, J. H. M., and Morrison, J. F. B., (1987b), Pressure and prolapse—the cause of solitary rectal ulceration. *Gut*, **28:**1228–33.

20
SPHINCTERIC REGIONS

K. Schulze-Delrieu

University of Iowa Hospitals and Clinics, Iowa, USA

The Sphincters of the Mammalian Gastrointestinal Tract

Six sphincteric segments can be recognized in the mammalian gastrointestinal tract. From the pharynx to the anus these include the following organ junctions and muscular sphincters: (1) pharyngo-oesophageal junction with the upper oseophageal sphincter (UOS, cricopharyngeal muscle), (2) gastro-oesophageal junction and lower oesophageal sphincter (LOS), (3) gastroduodenal junction and pylorus, (4) chole-

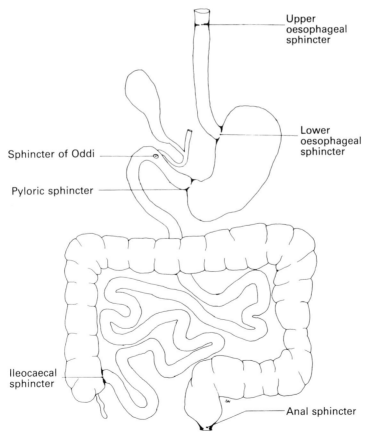

Figure 1. The sphincters of the gastrointestinal tract. The diagram shows the location of sphincteric regions at the boundaries of the oesophagus, stomach, biliary tract, and the small and large intestine.

dochoduodenal junction and sphincter of Oddi, (5) ileocolonic junction and Bauhin's valve, and (6) anorectal junction and anal sphincter.

The sphincteric regions of the gastrointestinal tract are located at organ boundaries; the organs on the opposite ends of the sphincters are often of different size and serve different functions; the sphincteric segments separate the luminal contents of these two organs. Whether a junctional segment restricts antegrade or retrograde flow depends primarily on the timing of the contraction of its sphincter in relation to the contractile activity of the adjacent gut segments.

Two sphincter regions form an end-to-side connection between organs, the sphincter of Oddi between the bile duct and duodenum, and Bauhin's valve between the ileum and colon. These sphincters are therefore partially intramural structures. Most sphincter segments join organs end to end, but many enter the distal organ obliquely, and are curved in themselves. This arrangement is thought to help closure of the segment by a 'flap' or 'flutter valve' mechanism.

The lumen of all sphincter regions is narrow. An increased thickness of the circular muscle forms a muscular ring which protrudes into the lumen. Further occlusion of the lumen may be produced by the puckering of the mucosa (mucosal rosette or plug), and by large vascular plexuses in the submucosa. The walls of sphincteric segments may be rendered rigid by the relatively great development of connective tissue. Sometimes the connective tissue forms rings or septae that separate the sphincteric segment proper from the adjacent gut segment.

Individual sphincter regions vary considerably in their structure and function. While sphincters throughout most of the gut are composed of smooth muscle, the sphincters at its proximal and distal end (UOS and external anal sphincter), are made up of striated muscle, and controlled by somatic rather than by autonomic nerves. Some sphincteric regions demonstrate a single, discrete thickening of the circular muscle (i.e. cricopharyngeus muscle), others are composed of separate muscle loops (proximal and distal pyloric loops, inner and outer anal sphincter). In most sphincteric segments, and particularly in the LOS,

the gut lumen is obliterated completely at rest. The sphincters of these junctional regions relax when peristalsis approaches, and their lumens are opened by the approaching bolus. After the bolus has passed, the segment collapses, and the sphincter resumes its constricting action. In contrast, the gastroduodenal junction in several species, including man, is patent at rest. The pylorus contracts rather than relaxes when gastric peristalsis moves a bolus towards it. The bolus is entrapped by the closing pylorus, and is wholly or in part retained and retropelled into the stomach (Code, 1970). Thus, the timing between peristaltic and sphincteric activity at the gastro-oesophageal junction facilitates antegrade flow and prevents reflux; timing at the gastroduodenal junction provides a variable resistance to outflow from the stomach (Pröve and Ehrlein, 1982; Schulze-Delrieu and Wall, 1983).

The Gastro-oesophageal Junction and the LOS

The gastro-oesophageal junction is a short segment between the tubular oesophagus and the saccular stomach. It enters the stomach on its lesser curvature side in an oblique direction. Within the segment there are several anatomical landmarks. Some of these landmarks are fixed while others vary in their positions with respect to each other and with time. One such landmark is the junction of the squamous epithelium of the oesophagus with the columnar epithelium of the stomach. The margin of this squamocolumnar junction is slightly irregular around the circumference of the gastro-oesophageal junction, and so this is also called the *Z line*. Its location varies between individuals, with contractions of the gastro-oesophageal junction, and with disease. At some point distal to the squamocolumnar junction, the longitudinal folds of the tubular oesophagus and gastro-oesophageal junction terminate, and the more transversely orientated folds of the stomach start. In between these two mucosal surfaces there is an indentation (Liebermann-Meffert et al, 1979).

Unlike in the remainder of the oesophagus, the

mucosal folds in the gastro-oesophageal junction are covered by transverse ridges. These transverse ridges may provide added surface to fill the lumen of the gastro-oesophageal junction, and thereby enhance its continence. Also, within the segment of the gastro-oesophageal junction, the circular muscle layer thickens over a segment of about 3 cm to about double its normal width. This muscular ring is the anatomical counterpart of the physiological LOS (Figure 2).

The proximal end of the gastro-oesophageal junction serves also as the point of insertion for the phreno-oesophageal membrane. The phreno-oesophageal membrane is a continuation of the thoracic and especially the abdominal fascia of the diaphragm, which enfolds and suspends the distal oesophagus (Eliŝka, 1973). This suspension permits the gastro-oesophageal junction to change its position with regard to the diaphragmatic hiatus. With swallowing and inspiration, the gastro-oesophageal junction moves up into the hiatus.

Special formations of the circular oesophageal muscle and of the third gastric muscle layer (the oblique gastric fibres) contribute to the anatomical LOS. Along the lesser curvature, circular muscle fibres of the distal oesophagus and proximal stomach form semicircular bundles ('muscle clasps'). The ends of these muscle bands insert in the anterior and posterior midline of the gastro-oesophageal junction (Figure 3). On the greater curvature side of the gastro-oesophageal junction, oblique fibres of the gastric type occur in the oesophagus well above the angle of His (the indentation between the oesophagus and gastric fundus). These oblique fibres encircle the gastric fundus and form the gastric sling fibres anterior and posterior to the lesser curvature (Liebermann-Meffert et al, 1979).

One characteristic of sphincter regions of the gut is that they generate higher luminal pressures than adjacent gut segments. The pressures generated depend on factors such as the diameter of the pressure-sensing probe. In the illustrated pressure tracing (Figure 4), four pressure sensors at the same level of the probe but separated by a 90° angle were drawn from the stomach into the oesophagus. As the probe approaches the gastro-oesophageal junction, each inspiration leads at first to a brief pressure peak. Subsequently, there is an elevation of the baseline pressure. Further withdrawal of the probe leads to a sudden increase in the baseline pressure and a drop in pressures with inspiration. Further withdrawal leads to a complete disappearance of the high pressure, but the anterior sensor subsequently records pressure

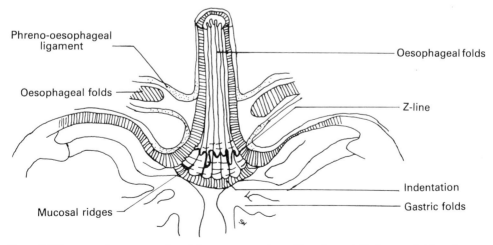

Figure 2. Diagrammatic representation of the gastro-oesophageal junction and diaphragmatic hiatus in man. Note that the junction of the squamous and the columnar epithelium (Z-line) is proximal to the point of identation where the longitudinal oesophageal folds are replaced by transverse gastric folds. The mucosal folds of the distal oesophagus have characteristic transverse mucosal ridges (after Liebermann-Meffert et al, 1979).

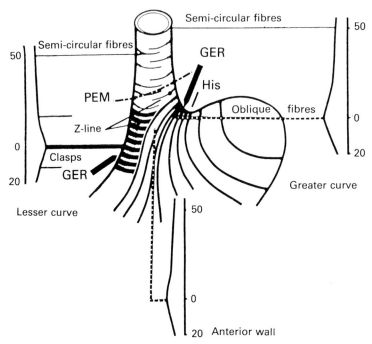

Figure 3. Synopsis of arrangement of the oesophageal and gastric musculature across the gastro-oesophageal junction of man. Projections of longitudinal gut through the anterior wall and the lesser and greater curvatures show that the muscular walls of the gastro-oesophageal junction are eccentric (from Liebermann-Meffert et al, 1979).

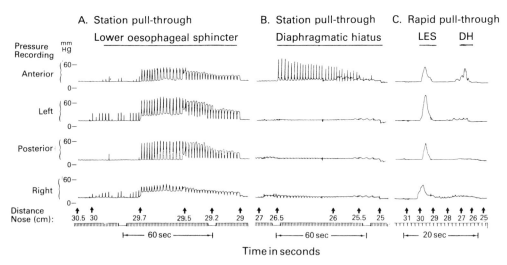

Figure 4. Manometric demonstration of high pressure zone at the gastro-oesophageal junction. This particular tracing was obtained in the American opossum, a popular model for the study of oesophageal physiology. In this species, the sphincter region is located well below the diaphragmatic hiatus, making it easy to separate intrinsic from extrinsic components of the gastro-oesophageal high pressure zone (from Schulze et al, 1977).

peaks generated by the diaphragm. The baseline luminal pressure drops from slightly positive once the thoracic cavity is entered. Presumably because of the above described peculiarities in the muscular anatomy of the LOS, the pressure profile generated by the gastro-oesophageal junction is asymmetrical. The highest pressures are generated on the greater curvature side (left), where the gastric sling fibres enter.

Sphincter muscle generates a particularly high degree of baseline tension (Christensen et al, 1973). This baseline tension can be seen as the tendency of the muscle to develop a high tension when stretched or to shorten when not stretched. It is this type of tone of the sphincter muscle together with the narrowness of the lumen of sphincter regions that accounts for the finding of high luminal pressures on manometry. In Figure 5, the circular muscle from the anatomical LOS develops at each degree of stretch a higher isometric tension than circular muscle from the proximal stomach or from the oesophagus. Furthermore, when an electrical stimulus is applied to stimulate the intramural nerves, the oesophagus and the stomach contract, and the LOS relaxes. Thus, another prominent feature of sphincter segments is that their muscle is inhibited by the local nerves (Christensen et al, 1973).

In the LOS, all tension is abolished when the muscle is inhibited. Thus, LOS tension development is entirely due to myogenic tone. In some sphincters, notably the pylorus, a large component of the baseline tension is generated by passive forces, and therefore relates to connective tissue.

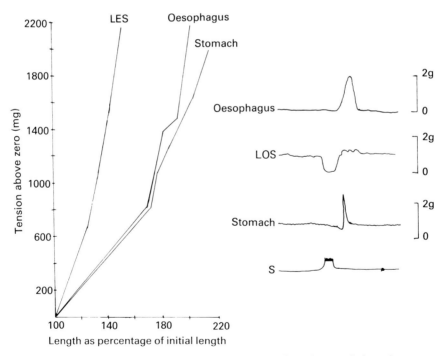

Figure 5. Response to stretch and to nervous stimulation of circular muscle from the gastro-oesophageal junction. In the left figure, it is shown that for each relative degree of stretch, lower oesophageal sphincter (LOS) muscle generates more force than muscle from the stomach and the oesophagus. In the right panel it is shown that LOS muscle relaxes when intrinsic nerves are stimulated. The oesophagus contracts and the stomach shows a biphasic response to stimulation (modified from Christensen et al, 1973).

The Gastroduodenal Junction and the Pylorus

The Neuromuscular Components of the Pylorus

The gastroduodenal junction connects the funnel-shaped gastric antrum to the tubular duodenum (Figure 6). The pyloric segment begins with a proximal pyloric loop on the gastric side, and terminates with the distal pyloric loop on the duodenal side. The muscle loops are clearly separated from one another only on the greater curvature, where they have a groove between them. On the lesser curvature, the pyloric loops converge to form a muscle knob known as the pyloric torus. During pyloric contraction, the pyloric torus is wedged into the pyloric groove (Torgersen, 1942; Keet, 1957).

The proximal and the distal pyloric loops differ in their structures and neuromuscular properties. The proximal loop is a flat muscle bundle which in the relaxed state is not easy to distinguish from the adjacent antral muscle; like the circular muscle of the gastric antrum, muscle in the proximal pyloric loop generates phasic contractions but no baseline tension when stretched or stimulated. The distal muscle loop forms a discrete ridge that protrudes into the lumen of the gastroduodenal junction. The distal loop generates a baseline tension when stretched, and relaxes when stimulated. Only part of the baseline tension generated by the distal loop is due to active muscle contraction (Schulze-Delrieu and Shirazi, 1983).

The configuration of the gastroduodenal junction varies with the activity of the pyloric sphincter (Williams, 1962). If both sphincter loops are relaxed, the gastroduodenal junction is patent and its mucosa flat. The lumen is narrowest at the level of the distal pyloric loop (Torgersen, 1942; Keet, 1957). This point of the gastroduodenal junction is known as the pyloric orifice or pyloric ring and easily identified on radiographic studies as a waist-like indentation between the antrum and the duodenum (Figure 7).

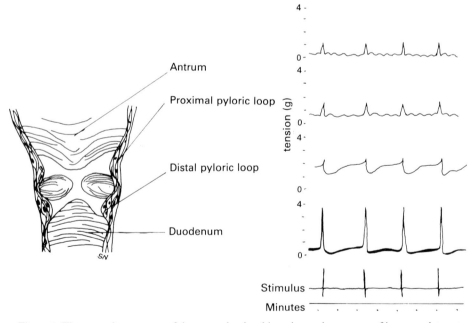

Figure 6. The muscular anatomy of the gastroduodenal junction and responses of its musculature to nervous stimulation. The pyloric musculature forms two discrete loops which have a butterfly configuration. The mechanical activity of the proximal loop resembles circular muscle of the antrum. It generates contractions spontaneously and in response to stimulation. The distal loop generates baseline tension, and relaxes in response to nervous stimulation (modified from Schulze-Delrieu and Shirazi, 1983).

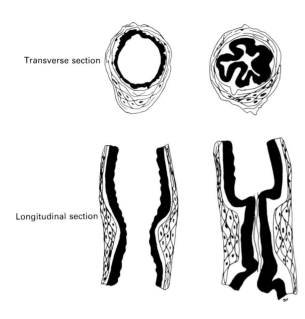

Transverse section

Longitudinal section

Figure 7. Transverse and longitudinal sections through the relaxed (left panel) and the contracted (right panel) gastroduodenal junction. In the longitudinal sections, the upper end corresponds to the duodenal side, the lower end to the gastric side. At rest, the distal pyloric loop produces a waist-like indentation of the outline of the gastroduodenal junction, the pyloric ring or pyloric orifice. When both pyloric loops contract, a several cm long segment proximal to the pyloric orifice is obliterated. Its mucosa is thrown up in folds (modified from Williams, 1962 and Biancani et al, 1980).

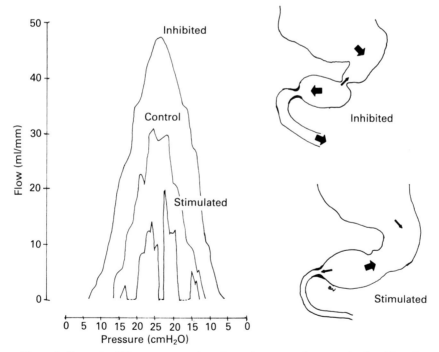

Figure 8. Synopsis of flow pattern and configuration across the gastroduodenal junction. The left panel shows flow rates across the pylorus as a function of pressure. If the pyloric musculature is inhibited, flow starts at low pressures, and for a given pressure occurs at high rates and is steady. If the pyloric muscle is contracting, flow starts at high pressures only and is minimal for a given pressure and often interrupted. The sketch on the right shows that in the intact animal, rapid flow across the gastroduodenal junction occurs when the pyloric and duodenal diameters are wide, and antral contractions are deep. The reverse is true with inhibition of gastric outflow (modified from Schulze-Delrieu and Wall, 1983, and Pröve and Ehrlein, 1982).

If both sphincter loops contract, the lumen of a segment extending several centimetres proximal from the pyloric orifice is completely obliterated. This formation is variously known as the pyloric canal or the terminal antral contraction. At the end of pyloric closure, the entire gastroduodenal junction between the pyloric muscle loops is narrower than it is at its narrowest point (the pyloric orifice) at rest. The contraction of the pyloric segment leads to a throwing up of the mucosal folds inside the gastroduodenal junction. With complete pyloric closure, the mucosal folds are arranged strictly in the longitudinal axis of the junctional segment, and on cross-section leave only a star-like slit in place of the lumen (Williams, 1962; Biancani et al, 1980).

Even though pyloric closure is an intermittent process, occurring whenever gastric peristaltic contractions spread all the way into the distal antrum, it is conventionally described as a segmental rather than as a peristaltic contraction. This is because pyloric contraction leads very rapidly to complete closure of a segment, and this closure is maintained for some time (Code, 1970; Pröve and Ehrlein, 1982). Also, the intermediate stages of closure of the gastroduodenal junction can be recognized as the lumen narrows first at the level of the proximal pyloric loop, and the pyloric groove bulges to form a pseudodiverticulum (Torgersen, 1942; Keet, 1957).

Flow across the gastroduodenal junction is determined by the phasic mechanical activity as generated by the proximal pyloric loop, and the tonic activity as generated by the distal loop (Schulze-Delrieu and Wall, 1983; Schulze-Delrieu and Shirazi, 1983). If the pyloric muscle is inhibited, the gastroduodenal junction is widely patent, little force is needed to initiate flow across the gastroduodenal junction and the flow is steady. If the pyloric muscle is stimulated, the junctional segment is narrow, considerable force is needed to force flow through it, and the flow is pulsatile (Figure 8).

Modulation of pyloric activity occurs during gastric emptying, and may be dependent on the nature of the meal. The pylorus appears to be inhibited in the presence of aqueous, noncaloric solutions, and the pylorus seems stimulated by viscous and caloric meals. There is also an inverse relationship beween the pyloric diameter and the diameter of the antral contraction wave. If antral waves are deep (as they are with noncaloric, acqueous solutions), the diameter of the pylorus is wide and the bulk of the antral contents is delivered into the duodenum. If antral contractions are shallow, as occurs with highly viscous and caloric gastric contents, the pylorus is set at a narrow diameter. Only a small fraction of the antral contents escapes into the duodenum, and the

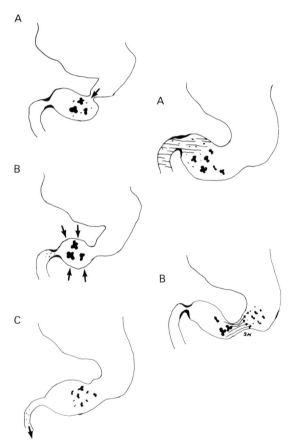

Figure 9. Two views of the processes of gastric sieving and grinding. In the panel on the left, particles are swept into the distal stomach; only small particles escape through the narrow pylorus, the large ones are smashed by the contraction of the distal antrum and pylorus. In the right panel, fluid and small particles are swept over the ridge formed by the pylorus. The larger particles sediment to the bottom of the stomach. They are retropelled into the proximal stomach through the antral contractions that occur against the closed pylorus. The resulting jet-effect grinds the particles down.

remainder is retropelled into the stomach (Pröve and Ehrlein, 1982).

The normal stomach 'sieves and grinds' its contents. It selectively empties aqueous solutions while retaining solid components until they have been broken down into tiny particles. The pylorus and the antrum act in concert to achieve this mechanical digestion (Hinder, 1983). The hydromechanical events responsible for sieving and grinding are only partially understood. One view is that the phenomenon is similar to what occurs in a garlic press: gastric contents are entrapped between the closing pylorus and the approaching antral contraction. Only liquids escape through the narrow pyloric opening. Solids are crushed by the tight squeeze developed by the powerful pyloric musculature (Figure 9). Another view is that this separation of solid and liquid material resembles the process of decanting: liquids are swept over the pyloric ridge as the gastric contraction wave approaches. Solids sediment to the bottom of the stomach and are thereby retained. Antral and pyloric contractions sweep remaining solids away from the pyloric orifice back into the stomach. According to this view, mixing and grinding occurs when the solid contents are retropelled through the orifice of the advancing antral contraction. This retropulsion is accompanied by a powerful jet effect.

References

Biancani, P., Zabinski, M. P., Kerstein, M. D., and Behar, J., (1980), Mechanical characteristics of the cat pylorus. *Gastroenterology*, **78**:301–9.

Christensen, J., Freeman, B. W., and Miller, J. K., (1973), Some physiologic characteristics of the esophagogastric junction in the opossum. *Gastroenterology*, **64**:1119–25.

Code, C. F., (1970), The mystique of the gastroduodenal junction. *Rendic. Rev. Gastroenterol.* **2**:20–37.

Eliška, O., (1973), Phreno-oesophageal membrane and its role in the development of hiatal hernia. *Acta. Anat. (Basel)*, **86**:137–50.

Hinder, R., (1983), Individual and combined roles of the pylorus and the antrum in the canine: gastric emptying of a liquid and digestible solid. *Gastroenterology*, **84**:281–6.

Keet, A. D., Jr., (1957), The prepyloric contractions in the normal stomach. *Acta. Radiol.*, **48**:413–24.

Liebermann-Meffert, D., Allgöwer, M., Schmid, F., and Blum, A. L., (1979), Muscular equivalent of the lower esophageal sphincter. *Gastroenterology*, **76**:31–8

Pröve, J., and Ehrlein, H. J., (1982), Motor function of gastric antrum and pylorus for evacuation of low and high viscosity meals in dogs. *Gut*, **23**:150–6.

Schulze, K., Dodds, W. J., Christensen, J., and Wood, J., (1977), Esophageal manometry in the opossum. *Am. J. Physiol.*, **233**:E152–9.

Schulze-Delrieu, K., and Shirazi, S. S. (1983), Neuromuscular differentiation of the human pylorus. *Gastroenterology*, **84**:287–92.

Schulze-Delrieu K., and Wall, J., (1983), Determinants of flow across isolated gastroduodenal junction of cats and rabbits. *Am. J. Physiol.*, **245**:G257–64.

Torgerson, J., (1942), The muscular build and the movements of the stomach and the duodenal bulb. *Acta Radiol. (Suppl.)*, **45**:1–187.

Williams, I., (1962), Closure of the pylorus. *Br. J. Radiol.*, **35**:653–70.

IV
EFFECT OF STRESS, DRUGS AND SURGERY ON GASTROINTESTINAL MOTILITY

21
STRESS AND GASTROINTESTINAL MOTILITY

David L. Wingate, Devinder Kumar
The London Hospital Medical College, London, UK

Introduction

For the layman as much as for the clinician, there is nothing unexpected in the notion that stress may affect gastrointestinal motility. It is gastrointestinal motor activity that is responsible for the propulsion of the contents of the digestive tube, and there can be few individuals who are unaware of the possibility of unusual propulsion—or, as commonly perceived, expulsion—of contents under conditions of stress. Such a concept has anecdotal and therefore qualitative validity; the problems arise in quantifying the relationship. Subjective evidence is only reliable under extreme conditions; diarrhoea may be experienced under conditions of extreme physical or emotional stress, but that does not exclude the possibility that lesser degrees of stress provoke more subtle, and hence less obvious, changes in propulsive activity.

This, in turn, leads to the problem not only of quantifying stress but even of defining stress with any precision. For the scientist there is the additional problem of translating stress as a subjective experience accessible only through human communication to animal models. Given these problems it is less than surprising that there has been relatively little progress in the objective study of the effects of stress on gastrointestinal motility.

General Considerations

Stress: Definition, Classification, and Measurement

It is no easy matter to classify a modality that defies accurate definition. A dictionary definition is a useful starting point; stress has been defined as:

> 'A physical, chemical, or psychological factor or combination of factors that pose a threat to the homeostasis or well-being of an organism, and that produces a defensive response, as, for example, physical or emotional trauma or infection' (Landau, 1986).

This definition requires some manipulation for the purposes of human biology. Many would not agree that 'physical, chemical, and psychological' are useful distinctions. It is also obvious that stress involves not only threat but also actual disturbance of well-being or homeostasis. Nevertheless the definition embodies the important concept that it is the homeostasis of the whole organism that is involved, and implicit in this is the role of the central nervous system (CNS). Immersion of the hand in hot water is only a stress in the presence of an intact CNS; if the noxious stimulus cannot be conveyed to the CNS, as happens in denervation syndromes, local damage can be inflicted without any central effect and is not therefore a source of stress. For higher organisms, including mammals, it is obvious that a stimulus can only be a source of stress, or more particularly a stressor, through mediation by the CNS.

If it is accepted that stress is a phenomenon that requires neural input, it is most easily classified by the receptor populations involved, rather than by the crude distinctions of 'physical, chemical, and psychological'. These receptor populations may be considered under three headings:

Somatosensory

Somatosensory receptors produce afferent information on all noxious stimuli affecting the body surface, physical or chemical, as well as from deep structures such as skeletal muscle, such as tetanic pain.

Visceral

Visceral receptors convey afferent information on adverse conditions within viscera, for example the pain of visceral distension or ischaemia.

Special Senses

The special senses convey stressors that come under the general classification of 'psychological'. Mental stress is the result of information or phenomena that are perceived through the senses of sight, hearing, and smell, but the same receptors may also respond to stimuli that are directly noxious. For example, conditioning is not required for a blinding white light, or deafening white noise to be perceived as unpleasant, but for an image to be perceived as unpleasant depends upon the prior conditioning, or training, of the organism.

These classifications illustrate the difficulty of devising stressors that are uniform in their effect between subjects, or that have single effects. Theoretically, a sudden painful blow to the periphery should be a uniform noxious stimulus, but actually its effect will depend very much upon the context in which it was delivered; was it, for example,

expected or unexpected or was the subject preconditioned or not to tolerate pain? Most physical stressors have a psychic component; the converse is also often true if only in the sense of the restraint, boredom, and discomfort involved in subjection to mental stressors.

Nevertheless, the classification of stressors in the simple schema above is important because it corresponds to major different groups of neural inputs to the CNS. If we are to make sense of the effects of stress, it must be in terms of objective neurobiology (Wingate, 1985).

The Brain–Gut Axis

Given that a stimulus becomes a stressor only by virtue of transmission through the central nervous system, the next point to be considered is how perturbation of the central nervous system in this way can modulate motor activity in the digestive tract. Concepts of brain–gut interaction have evolved in three stages.

Originally, it was the discovery of the autonomic nervous system that led to a biological model of central neural control of the gut. This model was dominated by the idea of the parasympathetic and sympathetic systems as efferent outflows from the CNS with opposing actions—the Ying and Yang of neurophysiology—with the gut as a passive effector system. The digestive tube assumed a greater prominence with the discovery of multiple peptides which were assumed to have a hormonal action; physiological modulation of gut function was ascribed to humoral agents relased from the mucosa of the digestive tract in response to specific local physicochemical stimuli. The hormonal hypothesis enjoyed a considerable vogue in the 1970s and also stimulated a considerable volume of research activity, but it became increasingly untenable when it became apparent that the new 'gut hormones' were not confined to the mucosa of the gut, or indeed to the gut itself, but were widely distributed throughout the body and, in particular, within nerve networks. These discoveries, based on advances in immunohistochemistry, undermined the assumption that an increase in the circulating plasma level of a 'gut hormone' was due to release of that peptide from mucosal cells in the gut responding to a specific stimulus.

The current view of the brain–gut axis depends heavily upon the re-evaluation of the function of the nervous system. First, it has now been appreciated that the vagus nerve is largely a sensory nerve, relaying information from visceral receptors to the brain (Ewart, 1985). Estimates of the afferent component of the vagus nerve vary, but it is generally agreed that approximately 90% of vagal fibres are afferent. In man, this implies that there are only about 5000 vagal efferent fibres compared with 45 000 vagal afferents. The latter innervate sensory endings in the gut, have cell bodies in the nodose ganglia, and synapse within the nucleus of the solitary tract in the brain stem. There is evidence that there is a degree of sensory integration at the brain stem level, but more important, it is now also known that the 'vago–vagal arc' is not a simple monosynaptic reflex; communication between sensory and motor vagal nuclei is polysnaptic via interneurons.

The second component in the revised hypothesis of brain–gut interaction is an appreciation of the size, complexity, and functional importance of the enteric nervous system (ENS). In man, this consists of about 5 000 000 neurons grouped largely into two major plexuses, the myenteric (Auerbach) and submucous (Meissner), that surround the entirety of the digestive tube. It is the ENS that provides the motor neurons that govern the effector cells, such as smooth muscle, in the digestive tract. Neural inputs into the ENS are from gut sensory receptors, but also from the CNS via vagal efferents and spinal efferents via the prevertebral ganglia (Wood, 1984). The ENS does not merely provide the final common effector pathway; it also has a major information processing and programming function. The relationship between ENS and CNS has been compared to that of an intelligent computer terminal connected to a mainframe computer (Figure 1).

In particular, it is now clear that much, if not all, of the programmed motor activity of the digestive tract is organized at the level of the ENS (Figure 2); this applies not only to simple stereotypic activity such as peristalsis, but also to the complex sequence of the migrating motor complex (MMC). Input from CNS efferents may modulate ENS-programmed activity, and may also determine which programme is selected (Figure 3). As an example, one can consider the effect of feeding on small bowel motor activity, which is the replacement of periodic MMCs by a long sequence of apparently irregular contractions. The arrival of food in the gut stimulates vagal receptors; this information is conveyed by the afferent vagus to the brain stem, and from the brain stem to the ENS by the efferent vagus, whereupon the ENS reponds by a programmed change of output to

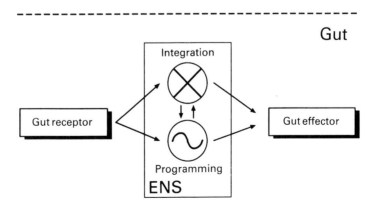

The "Gut Brain"

Figure 1. Heuristic model of the enteric nervous system as an integrative and programming entity.

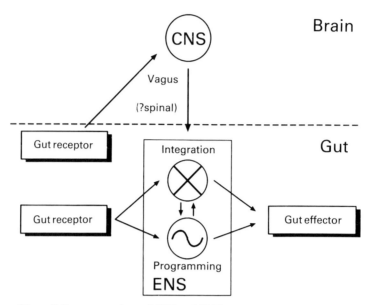

Figure 2. Interconnections of CNS and ENS (see text).

the musculature. However, stressors affecting the CNS may influence the output from the vagal motor nucleus, thereby changing the motor response to food.

It has to be remembered that CNS modulation of ENS activity is not merely confined to the effect of stressors. During the waking state, ENS activity is continually modulated by the CNS, as shown by the marked differences between sleeping and waking ENS cycles (Gill et al, 1987). Presumably such modulation is a normal requirement of overall homeostasis or well-being; it could be argued that wakefulness is by definition stressful, but such a definition is not clinically helpful. CNS modulation through stressors should only be postulated when the presence of the stress can be

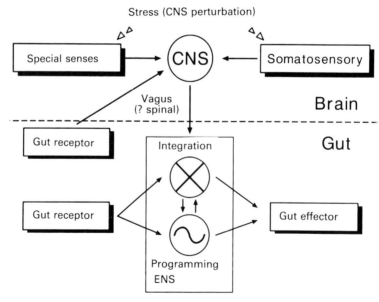

Figure 3. Major inputs of stress into ENS via CNS (see text).

confirmed by the existence of accepted stress responses.

The Identification and Measurement of Stress

In the definition of stress situations, a degree of pragmatism is required. It is possible to argue, in philosophical terms, that the conscious state can at all times be equated with stress, but as discussed earlier this is not a useful definition. Stress is therefore best considered in terms of stressors and stress responses.

Stressors can be defined as identified, and preferably controlled stimuli that evoke subjective and/or stress responses. An experimenter may apply a stimulus that he considers stressful to a subject, but if that stimulus does not evoke a stress response, it is not a stressor. A stress response is a significant deviation from the average value of a biological variable during the application of a stressor.

Objective stress responses include alterations in cardiovascular performance, as indicated by heart rate and systolic blood pressure, alterations in respiratory rate, and alteration in plasma levels of chemical substances such as catecholamines and endorphins. Subjective stress responses are indicated by altered hedonistic ratings in scales of well-being/discontent and pleasure/displeasure, and also affective changes including increased levels of anxiety and depression. On the face of it, the measurement of stress ought to be easy, but it isn't. The effect of a stressor may depend upon context. For example, the physical stress on a long-distance swimmer is similar whether he is taking part in an escorted distance swim, or escaping from a shipwreck, but the psychological stress is very different. To complicate matters further, the circumstances of stress may make it difficult to measure stress responses. Subjective stress is often measured by asking subjects to score affective states on visual analogue scales; this is easily done by a subject sitting subjected to acoustic stressors, but very difficult for someone who happens to be running hard at the time.

Since a standard stimulus will have a stressor effect that depends upon its context, it is apparent that stressors must be defined for each study, and equivalence between stressors cannot be assumed. Nor, since our objective measures of stress response are relatively crude, can it be assumed that stressors that produce an apparently similar stress response are equivalent.

Stress and 'Functional Disorders'

In the absence of identified pathology, it is sometimes assumed that patients with functional disorders of the gut have (a) disorders of motility that (b) are induced by stress. Such assumptions are unwarranted unless supported by data; relevant studies on this point have rarely been performed. It is equally probable that in many such patients motility is normal, and there is no reason to suppose, without proof, that such patients are more exposed to stressors than those without functional syndromes.

Local Gut Motor Responses to Stress

Stress and Oesophageal Motility

Controlled studies of the effect of stressors on the oesophagus are generally lacking. There is indirect evidence that stress may have some modulatory effect on the upper oesophageal sphincter. Upper oesophageal pressure has been shown to be markedly decreased during stable sleep and elevated on arousal from sleep (Kahrilas et al, 1987). A recent study, however, has shown that acute emotional stress, in the form of a dichotic listening test, increases upper oesophageal sphincter pressure (Cook et al, 1987).

Stress and Gastric Motility

Many individuals are familiar with sensations suggesting abnormal gastric motility under stress. Some objective basis for this was first provided by Wolf and Wolff (1943) on their patient 'Tom'; through his gastrostomy, they were able to observe increased gastric movements during periods of emotional stress. Evidence of diminished emptying under cold pain stress was obtained by Thompson et al (1982; 1983), and the phenom-

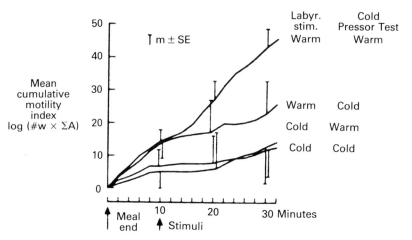

Figure 4. Effect of the two centrally acting stimuli on antral pressure activity. This plot illustrates the mean ($\pm$ SE) cumulative motility index for each combination of stimuli, beginning at the time individuals finished eating their meals. Stimuli were applied 10 min later. The linear trend in this cumulative (log) motility index was used for analysis. Both active stimuli, alone or in combination, inhibited the cumulative increase in antral phasic pressure activity, which remained unchanged after control stimulation (warm, warm). Reproduced with permission from Stanghellini et al, 1983).

enon is associated with—but not necessarily caused by—catecholamine and endorphin release (Stanghellini et al, 1983). No good description of the pattern of gastric motor activity under stress has so far been published, but Gue et al (1987) have shown suppression of gastric activity fronts in dogs under acoustic stress. Stanghellini et al (1983) studied the effect of cold pain and laby-rinthine stimulation on the motor response to feeding and showed that the motility index in the gastric antrum was significantly reduced under stress (Figure 4).

Stress and Small Bowel Motility

Studies to date on the effect of small bowel contractile and propulsive activity give a striking illustration of how the effects found are dependent upon the nature of the experimental paradigm. In 1969 Sadler and Orton studied a human subject with a Thiry-Vella loop who 'earned his living as a human laboratory'. From their studies, they concluded that anger, rage and aggression caused hypermotility, whereas sadness diminished

motility and paralysing fear abolished it. The latter conclusion was to some extent supported by Granata et al (1972), who found that canine intestinal motility was diminished by confrontation with a cat. Recent studies by McRae et al (1982) (Figure 5), and subsequently by Valori et al (1986) have used standardized psychological stressors to demonstrate that mental stress diminishes the incidence of MMCs (Figures 6 and 7). Kumar and Wingate (1985) studied the effect of standardized laboratory stress on normal human controls and patients with inflammatory disease and showed a similar reduction in the incidence of MMCs under stress (Figure 8).

The paraxodical effects of differing stressors are illustrated by studies on small bowel transit. Cann et al (1983), using breath hydrogen estimation, found that psychological stress accelerates mouth-to-caecum transit (Figure 9). In contrast, O'Brien et al (1986) used cold pain stress to study the same variable, and found that pain stress retards small bowel transit; this effect is mediated via the beta-1 adrenergic receptors, as it is blocked by propranolol.

Control period   Stress period

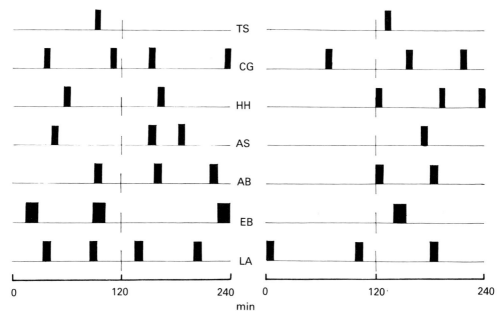

Figure 5. Incidence of MMCs (vertical bars) over two periods of 4 hours in seven volunteers. During the stress-free control period (left), MMCs were evenly distributed over the period. Under stress (right), MMCs were markedly diminished during the first 2 hours, but although the stressor was maintained, MMCs occurred normally during the second 2 hours, indicating adaptation to stress by the subjects. Reproduced with permission from McRae et al, 1982.

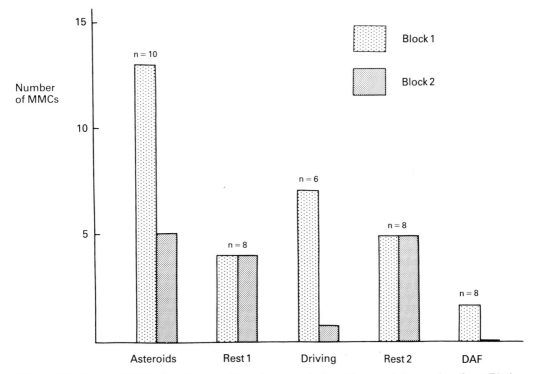

Figure 6. Incidence of MMCs in volunteer subjects during equivalent 7-hour periods on a day of rest (Block 1) and a day of intermittent stress (Block 2). The stressors were a video arcade game 'Asteroids' (2 hours), driving a car (1 hour), and delayed audio feedback (1 hour); the rest periods between each stressor were each 1 hour. Reproduced with permission from Valori et al, 1986.

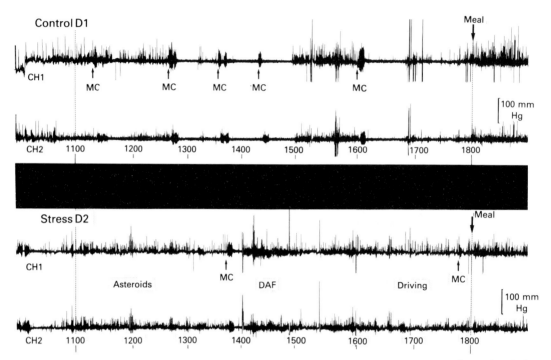

Figure 7. Contractile activity recorded from distal duodenum (Channel 1) and proximal jejunum (Channel 2) during a day of rest (D1) and a day of stress (D2) in a healthy volunteer. During the second day, shaded areas indicate the duration of stressors. Note the suppression of motor complexes (MC) during the day of stress in comparison with the equivalent time period on the previous day. Reproduced with permission from Valori et al, 1986.

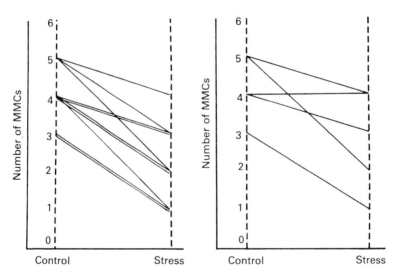

Figure 8. Frequency of MMCs during control and stress periods in healthy subjects (left) and inflammatory bowel disease patients (right). Each line joins aggregate number of MMCs in control period for one subject to aggregate number in stress period. Reproduced with permission from Kumar and Wingate, 1985.

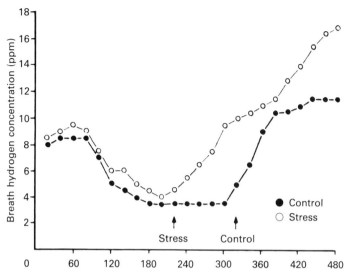

Figure 9. Two graphs show the mean breath hydrogen levels for all subjects during control and stress studies respectively. Note similarity in profile of curves, but also that there was 'shift to the left' during stress studies with rise in breath hydrogen level occurring well before rise during control studies. Reproduced with permission from Cann et al, 1983.

Stress and the Colon

A classic experiment by Almy (1951) provided anecdotal evidence of increased sigmoid motility induced by fright in a human volunteer. Objective appraisal of the effects of stress on colonic motility requires techniques for recording colonic motility that are able to discriminate normal from abnormal motility in conscious volunteers without requiring constraints and discomforts which are in themselves stressors; such techniques have not yet been validated. There have been some reports of altered colonic motor activity in patients with the irritable bowel syndrome; not only are the results contradictory but also, as pointed out above, IBS is not, of itself, a stressor. In a recent study, Narducci et al (1985), reported the effect of three standardized stressful conditions (ice water immersion, stoop stimulus differentiation test and ball sorting) on human colon and showed that motility increased after the first exposure to each of the three stressors used. However, repeat exposures to stress did not stimulate colonic motility.

References

Almy, T. P., (1951), Experimental studies on irritable colon. *Am. J. Med.*, **10**:60–7.

Cann, P. A., Read, N. W., Cammack, J., Childs, H., Holden, S., Kashman, R., Longmore, J., Nix, S., Simms, N., Swallow, K., and Weller, J., (1983), Psychological stress and the passage of a standard meal through the stomach and small intestine in man. *Gut*, **24**:236–40.

Cook, I. J., Dent, J., Shannon, S., and Collins, S. M., (1987), Measurement of upper esophageal sphincter pressure: effect of acute emotional stress. *Gastroenterology*, **93**:526–32.

Ewart, W. R., (1985), Sensation in the gastrointestinal tract. *J. Comp. Physiol. Biochem.*, **82A**:489–93.

Gill, R. C., Kellow, J. E., and Wingate, D. L., (1987), The migrating motor complex at home. *Gastroenterology*, **92**:1405 (abstract).

Granata, L., Leone, D., Paccione, F., and Ruccia, D., (1972), Changes in jejunal motility during emotional reaction. *Arch. Sci. Biol. (Bologna)*, **57**:87–97.

Gue, M., Fioramonti, J., Frexinos, J., Alvinerie, M., and Bueno, L., (1987), Influence of acoustic stress by noise on gastrointestinal motility in dogs. *Dig. Dis. Sci.*, **32**:1411–17.

Kahrilas, P. J., Dodds, W. J., Dent, J., Haeberle, B.,

Hogan, W. J., and Arndorfer, R. C., (1987), The effect of sleep, spontaneous gastro-oesophageal reflux, and a meal on upper oesophageal sphincter pressure in normal human volunteers. *Gastroenterology*, **92**:446–71.

Kumar, D., and Wingate, D. L., (1985), The irritable bowel syndrome: a paroxysmal motor disorder. *Lancet*, **ii**:973–7.

Landau, S. J., (Ed), (1986), *International Dictionary of Medicine and Biology*, John Wiley & Sons, New York.

McRae, S., Younger, K., Thompson, D. G., and Wingate, D.L., (1982), Sustained mental stress alters human jejunal motor activity. *Gut*, **23**:404–9.

Narducci, F., Snape, W. J., Battle, W. M., London, R. L., and Cohen, S, (1985), Increased colonic motility during exposure to a stressful situation. *Dig. Dis. Sci.* **30**:40–4.

O'Brien, J., Thompson, D. G., Walker, E., Holly, J., and Burnham, R., (1986), Stress disturbs human gastrointestinal transit via a beta-1 adrenoceptor mediated pathway. *Gut*, **26**:559.

Sadler, H. H., and Orton, A. U., (1969), The complementary relationship between the emotional state and the function of the ileum in the human subject. *Am. J. Psychiatry*, **124**:1375–84.

Stanghellini, V., Malagelada, J. R., Zinsmeister, A. R., Go, V. L. W., and Kao, P. C., (1983), Stress-induced gastroduodenal motor disturbances in humans: possible humoral mechanisms. *Gastroenterology*, **85**:83–91.

Thompson, D. G., Richelson, E., and Malagelada, J. R., (1983), Perturbation of upper gastrointestinal function by cold stress. *Gut*, **24**:277–83.

Thompson, D. G., Richelson, E., and Malagelada, J. R., (1982), Perturbation of gastric emptying and duodenal motility via the central nervous system. *Gastroenterology*, **83**:1200–6.

Valori, R. M., Kumar, D., and Wingate, D. L., (1986), Effects of different types of stress and of 'prokinetic drugs' on control of the fasting motor complex in humans. *Gastroenterology*, **90**:1890–900.

Wingate, D. L., (1985), The brain-gut link. *Viewpoints on Dig. Dis.*, **17**:17–20.

Wolf, S., and Wolff, H. G., (1943), *Human Gastric Function*. Oxford University Press, New York.

Wood, J. D., (1984), Enteric neurophysiology. *Am. J. Physiol.*, **247**:G585–98.

22

PHARMACOLOGICAL AGENTS

A.

DRUG DELIVERY IN THE GASTROINTESTINAL TRACT

S. S. Davis, J. G. Hardy

University of Nottingham, Nottingham, UK and Queen's Medical Centre, Nottingham, UK

Oral Administration of Drugs

This chapter will consider drug delivery to the gastrointestinal tract. Drug delivery systems taken orally can take many different forms; the simplest being liquids and suspensions, while the more complex can be controlled release matrices, osmotic pumps and, more recently, devices to deliver drugs to specific sites (e.g. the colon). Hence some of these systems are intended to release the drug rapidly to permit early appearance of the active compound in the systemic circulation, while others should provide a more controlled release. The latter may be desired in order to protect the drug from a hostile environment (usually the stomach) or to give a modified plasma level–time profile, usually with an extended duration of action and a reduced frequency of dosing and possibly lowered side-effects. The science of the design and evaluation of drug delivery systems is termed biopharmaceutics and space does not permit more than a brief overview. Detailed treatments can be found in various monographs (Blanchard et al, 1979; Notari, 1980; Gibaldi, 1984; Gibaldi and Perrier, 1982).

The important stages that can affect the appearance of the drug in the systemic circulation (biological availability) are in the sequence, disintegration of the dosage form, release of the drug (dissolution), absorption across the gastrointestinal mucosa and metabolism (perhaps in the gut wall or in the liver (first pass effect)). Not all these processes may be relevant. For example, a controlled release tablet may need to maintain its integrity in the gastrointestinal tract in order to provide the appropriate blood level–time profile. The release of drugs (dissolution) and their subsequent absorption in the different regions of the gastrointestinal tract will be influenced not only by the nature of the delivery system but also by the local environment (e.g. agitation conditions and, particularly, pH) and the properties of the drug substance (Nelson and Miller, 1979).

Drug Release and Absorption

The dissolution of a drug can be altered by changing its particle size (surface area), salt form and crystal type (polymorphism). Many drugs are either weak acids or weak bases and therefore their solubility will be greatly affected by the local pH conditions and the ionization characteristics of the compound itself (pKa). Consequently, weak bases will usually be soluble in the stomach and weak acids soluble in the intestines. Drug absorption is largely dictated by the converse, in that the non-ionized lipid soluble form of a drug will usually be well absorbed by a process of passive diffusion so that weak acids should be well absorbed from the intestines. This physicochemical basis for drug absorption has been summarized by the well-known pH-partition (lipid solubility) hypothesis (Houston and Wood, 1980). However, since one is dealing with a diffusional process, not only is the concentration of the diffusing (non-ionized) species important but also the available surface area. Consequently, a weak acid such as aspirin is better absorbed from the small intestine than from the stomach even though in the latter, its state of non-ionization is far greater (perhaps 80% or more) than that in the intestines (10% or less). Indeed, few drugs are believed to be absorbed significantly from the stomach.

Since drugs are normally foreign materials (xenobiotics) they are not absorbed by active or facilitated transport processes. Notable exceptions are the vitamins and the aminopenicillins. The latter can take advantage of the absorption pathways for dietary di- and tripeptides present in the proximal small intestine. The presence of a specific absorption mechanism in a limited region of the gastrointestinal tract has given rise to a so-called 'absorption window' concept (Houston and Wood, 1980).

Drug absorption from the colon has usually been dismissed as being insignificant. This may be true for 'immediate release' delivery systems since the major part of the dose should have been absorbed well before it reaches the large intestine. However, in the case of controlled release formulations, where the objective is to achieve twice (or even once) daily dosing, absorption from the colon could be an important factor in maintaining satisfactory blood levels for therapeutic effect. Recent studies using intubation and colonoscopy, and those described below following the transit of controlled release formulations, have revealed that colonic absorption of drugs can be far more efficient than thought hitherto (Gleiber et al, 1985). Some have even suggested that the colon could be a suitable site for the absorption of the products of biotechnology, namely bio-active polypeptides (Saffran et al, 1986).

Gastrointestinal Transit of Dosage Forms

In many situations, it is of importance to have objective information about the transit of a delivery system within the gastrointestinal tract, especially when dealing with the more sophisticated controlled release systems. Indeed, in our recent studies we have been faced with answering a series of questions concerning the fate of drug delivery systems (Table 1). The available literature was either unhelpful or even misleading. For example, on the question of small intestinal transit (of tablets) one anecdotal report suggested a transit time of eight hours. We have found this to be a two- to three-fold overestimation (Davis et al, 1986a).

In our studies, normally conducted in healthy volunteers, we have employed the non-invasive technique of gamma scintigraphy. In some of these investigations, we have administered placebo delivery systems and have been concerned solely with integrity and/or transport, while in others we have used active drug and have measured not only transit but also blood levels for subsequent pharmacokinetic evaluation (Wilson et al, 1984; Boertz et al, 1987; Hardy et al, 1987a). In these latter studies we have related the position of the dosage form to absorption behaviour. Attempts to change gastrointestinal transit characteristics based upon pharmaceutical strategies such as dosage form size and density (Davis et al, 1986b), putative adhesive coatings (Khosla and Davis, 1987) have been largely unsuccessful save for the exploitation of the known difference in the behaviour of the stomach in the fed and fasted (interdigestive) modes and the ability of small objects to empty from a fed stomach and for larger objects to await clearance by phase III of the migrating myolectric complex ('housekeeper wave') (Davis et al, 1984b).

Table 1. Questions relevant to the gastrointestinal transit of drug delivery systems

(Bechgaard et al, 1985; Christensen et al, 1985; Daly et al, 1982; Davis, 1983, 1985, 1986; Davis et al, 1984a, b, c, 1986a, b, c, 1987; Hardy et al, 1985, 1986a, b, 1987a, b; Khosla and Davis, 1987; Ollerenshaw et al, 1987; O'Reilly et al, 1987; Wilson and Hardy, 1985; Wilson et al, 1984).

General

Do enteric coatings work properly? How rapidly do capsules/tablets disintegrate? How does the release of a labelled marker *in vivo* compare with the situation *in vitro*? Do single non-disintegrating units retain their integrity *in vivo* if designed to do so? Can position in the gastrointestinal tract be related to a pharmacokinetic profile? Do osmotic devices pump *in vivo* at the same rate as found *in vitro*?

Oesophagus

Do dosage forms get stuck or lodge?

Stomach

How is gastric emptying influenced by physiological factors (e.g. food, age, time, position, exercise), pathological factors, co-administered drugs and pharmaceutical strategies (e.g. size, density, shape, bioadhesives)?

Small intestine

What is the transit time in the small intestine and is it affected by physiological, pathological and pharmaceutical factors? Do multiple unit systems spread in the small intestine? Do dosage forms get 'stuck' in the small bowel?

Ileocaecal junction

What is the role of the ileocaecal valve in controlling transit from small to large bowel and how is it affected by pharmaceutical, physiological and pathological factors?

Large intestine

What is the transit behaviour of dosage forms in the different regions and are there periods of stagnation (e.g. in the caecum and at hepatic and splenic flexures)? Do large single units and small multiple units have differential transit behaviour?
How well do multiparticles spread in the large bowel?
How do pathological conditions such as the irritable bowel syndrome and inflammatory bowel disease affect the transit of delivery systems?
Is it possible to achieve site specific delivery to the colon or to designated regions thereof?
What is the total transit time for different novel delivery systems?

Studies Using Gamma Scintigraphy

Gamma scintigraphy provides a means of monitoring the distributions of pharmaceutical preparations in the gastrointestinal tract under normal physiological conditions. The preparations are radiolabelled with appropriate gamma-emitting radionuclides, such as ^{99m}Tc and ^{111}In, which result in relatively low radiation doses to the subjects. The main limitaton of this technique is that few drug molecules can be readily labelled with a suitable radionuclide. It is usual, therefore, to incorporate into the formulation a non-absorbable tracer, for example radiolabelled ion exchange resin powder in a tablet matrix. Following administration, frequent or even continuous monitoring with a gamma camera provides information about the preparation, such as its location, transit rate, integrity and extent of dispersion.

The main factor influencing the gastric emptying of pharmaceutical preparations is the presence of food in the stomach (Davis et al, 1986a). Dosing after an overnight fast results in most preparations emptying from the stomach within one hour. Administration after a meal delays gastric emptying. In general, liquids empty faster than solids. Small particles up to a few millimetres in diameter, empty along with food particles (O'Reilly et al, 1987), whilst larger, non-disintegrating capsules and tablets are retained in the stomach until the digestible components have emptied. Consumption of food at regular intervals throughout the day can result in large units being retained in the stomach for many hours; gastric emptying eventually takes place during the night when the stomach has emptied of food. Dosing after a meal with a large unit from which the active ingredient is slowly released, provides a means of prolonging drug infusion into the small intestine. In contrast, preparations designed to prevent drug release in the stomach, such as enteric coated tablets, are best dosed on an empty stomach to ensure predictable times of drug delivery.

The transit of pharmaceutical preparations through the small intestine is the same for both liquids and solids and typically takes 3–4 hours (Davis et al, 1986a). Thus for drugs principally absorbed from the small intestine, controlled release preparations have only a relatively short duration of action once they have left the stomach. The constancy of small intestinal transit times allows products to be designed to release drugs at particular sites in the intestine. The timing of the dispersion of tablets and capsules can be controlled by varying the thickness of enteric coatings, which dissolve slowly at about pH6 but are insoluble in the more acidic environment in the stomach (Figure 1) (Hardy et al, 1987a). Tablets with coatings that take four hours to dissolve in the intestine will mainly release their drugs to the colon. This may be appropriate for the delivery of topically active drugs to the large bowel; for example mesalazine, which is readily absorbed from the small intestine (Hardy et al, 1987c).

The time taken for a preparation to pass from the terminal ileum into the colon is highly variable (Ollerenshaw et al, 1987). Care must be exercised in the interpretation of gamma camera images when measuring the time of transit across the ileocaecal junction. It is necessary to continue the monitoring until the morphology of the colon is well defined. Otherwise images, such as that in Figure 2 recorded at 8.0 h, could be mistakenly interpreted as showing the preparation in the caecum and ascending colon.

Transit through the colon is characterized by propulsive phases separated by prolonged periods of stasis (Hardy et al, 1985). Transit times vary considerably even in healthy subjects with regular bowel habits. Large units pass through the colon faster than liquids or small particles (Hardy et al, 1985, 1986b) as illustrated in Figure 3. Solutions and particles tend to disperse extensively within the colon (Figures 1 and 2).

The extent of penetration of rectally administered preparations into the large bowel is dependent on the dosing volume. Suppositories (Hardy et al, 1987b) and foam enemas (Wood et al, 1985) tend to remain within the rectum and sigmoid colon. Enema solutions of 50–200 ml, in general, spread into the descending colon but only infrequently into the ascending colon (Wood et al, 1985; Hardy et al, 1986a).

The information obtained by gamma scintigraphy provides a useful adjunct in the interpretation of pharmacokinetic data. For example, the

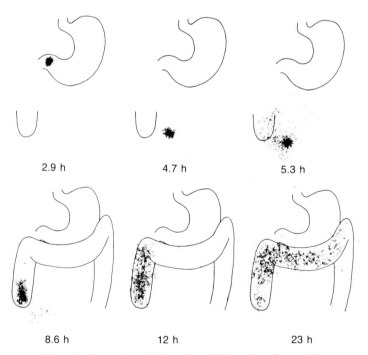

2.9 h   4.7 h   5.3 h

8.6 h   12 h   23 h

Figure 1. Gastrointestinal transit and dispersion of an enteric coated tablet dosed after a meal.

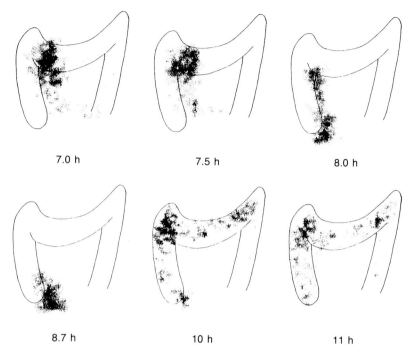

7.0 h   7.5 h   8.0 h

8.7 h   10 h   11 h

Figure 2. Transit of a preparation from the ileum into the colon.

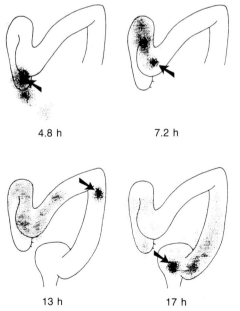

4.8 h   7.2 h

13 h   17 h

Figure 3. Transit of a capsule (arrowed) and small particles through the colon.

time of disintegration of enteric coated tablets determined by gamma camera imaging correlates closely with the time of initial detection of drug in the plasma (Figure 4). Dosing after a meal results in a wide range of disintegration times, due mainly to differences in gastric emptying rates (Hardy et al, 1987a). Pharmacokinetic data become more readily intelligible if the blood concentrations of the drug are related to the times after gastric emptying rather than after tablet administration. Similarly, the inclusion of gamma scintigraphy in a pharmacokinetic study of a sustained release preparation provides an explanation for variations in the plasma drug concentration profiles as illustrated in Figure 5. The drug is absorbed throughout the intestines and the duration of the plateau of the plasma concentration is greatly influenced by the transit rate of the delivery system through the colon and its subsequent excretion.

The physiological factors affecting the behaviour of pharmaceutical preparations in the gas-

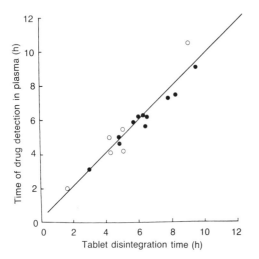

Figure 4. Relationship between the times of disintegration of enteric coated tablets and drug absorption (○ naproxen, ● mesalazine).

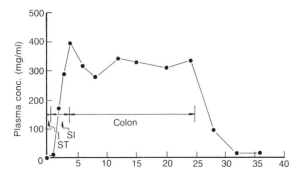

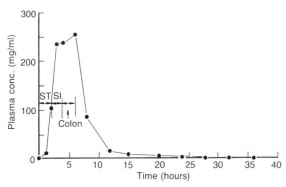

Figure 5. Plasma drug concentration profiles for a sustained release oxprenolol formulation in two subjects.

trointestinal tract can be readily appreciated using the technique of gamma scintigraphy. Interpretation of the images in conjunction with pharmacokinetic data is proving useful in the development of more efficacious pharmaceutical products.

References

Bechgaard, H., Christensen, F. N., Davis, S. S., Hardy, J. G., Taylor, M. J., Whalley, D. R., and Wilson, C. G., (1985), Gastrointestinal transit of pellet systems in ileostomy subjects and the effect of density. *J. Pharm. Pharmacol.*, **37**:718–21.

Blanchard, J., Sawchuk, R. J., and Brodie, B. B., (Editors) (1979), *Principles and Perspectives in Drug Bioavailability*, Basel, Karger.

Boertz, A., Cawello, W., Cordes, G., Davis, S. S., Fischer, W., and Sandrock, K., (1987), Gastrointestinal transit investigation and the in vivo drug release of isosorbide-5-nitrate. *Pharm. Res.* (in press).

Christensen, F. N., Davis, S. S., Hardy, J. G., Taylor, M. J., Whalley, D. R., and Wilson, C. G., (1985), The use of gamma scintigraphy to follow the gastrointestinal transit of pharmaceutical formulations. *J. Pharm. Pharmacol.*, **37**:91–5.

Daly, P. B., Davis, S. S., Frier, M., Hardy, J. G., Kennerley, J. W., and Wilson, C. G. (1982), Scintigraphic assessment of the in vivo dissolution rate of a sustained release tablet. *Int. J. Pharm.*, **10**:17–24.

Davis S. S., (1983), The use of scintigraphic methods for the evaluation of drug dosage forms in the gastrointestinal tract. In: *Topics in Pharmaceutical Sciences* (Eds Breimer, D. D., and Speiser, P.), pp 205–15. Elsevier, Amsterdam.

Davis, S. S., (1985), The design and evaluation of controlled release delivery systems for the GI tract. *J. Controlled Release*, **2**:27–38.

Davis, S. S., (1986), Studies on the gastrointestinal transit of dosage forms in human subjects using the technique of gamma scintigraphy. *STP Pharma*, **2**:1015–22.

Davis, S. S., Hardy, J. G., Taylor, M. J., Whalley, D. R., and Wilson, C. G., (1984a), A comparative study of the gastrointestinal transit of a pellet and a tablet formulation. *Int. J. Pharm.*, **21**:167–77.

Davis, S. S., Hardy, J. G., Taylor, M. J., Whalley, D. R., and Wilson, C. G., (1984b), The effect of food on the gastrointestinal transit of pellets and an osmotic device (Osmet). *Int. J. Pharm*, **21**:331–40.

Davis, S. S., Hardy, J. G., Taylor, M. J., Stockwell, A., Whalley, D. R., and Wilson, C. G., (1984c), The in vivo evaluation of an osmotic device (Osmet) using gamma scintigraphy. *J. Pharm. Pharmacol.*, **36**:740–2.

Davis, S. S., Hardy, J. G., and Fara, J. W., (1986a), Transit of pharmaceutical dosage forms through the small intestine. *Gut*, **27**:886–92.

Davis, S. S., Hardy, J. G., Wilson, C. G., Feely, L. C., and Palin, K. J., (1986b) Gastrointestinal transit of a controlled release naproxen tablet formulation. *Int. J. Pharm.*, **32**:85–90.

Davis, S. S., Stockwell, A., Taylor, M. J., Hardy, J. G., Whalley, D. R., Wilson, C. G., Bechgaard, H., and Christensen, F. N., (1986c), The effect of density on the gastrointestinal transit time of single and multiple unit dosage forms. *Pharm. Res.*, **3**:208–13.

Davis, S. S., Khosla, R., Wilson, C. G., and Washington, N., (1987), The gastrointestinal transit of a controlled release pellet formulation of tiaprofenic acid. *Int. J. Pharm.*, **35**:253–8.

Gibaldi, M., (1984), *Biopharmaceutics and Clinical Pharmacokinetics*, 3rd edn, Lee and Febiger, Philadelphia.

Gibaldi, M., and Perrier, D., (1982), *Pharmacokinetics*, 2nd edn, Dekker, New York.

Gleiber, C. H., Antonin, K.-H., Bieck, P., Godbillon, J., Schonleber, W., and Malchow, H., (1985), Colonoscopy in the investigation of drug absorption in healthy volunteers. *Gastrointest. Endosc.*, **31**:71–3.

Hardy, J. G., Wilson, C. G., and Wood, E., (1985), Drug delivery to the proximal colon. *J. Pharm. Pharmacol.*, **37**:874–7.

Hardy, J. G., Lee, S. W., Clark, A. G., and Reynolds, J. R., (1986a) Enema volume and spreading. *Int. J. Pharm.*, **31**:151–5.

Hardy, J. G., Wood, E., Clark, A. G., and Reynolds, J. R., (1986b), Whole bowel transit in patients with the irritable bowel syndrome. *Eur. J. Nucl. Med.*, **11**:393–6.

Hardy, J. G., Evans, D. F., Zaki, I., Clark, A. G., Tønnesen, H. H., and Gamst, O. N., (1987a), Evaluation of an enteric coated naproxen tablet using gamma scintigraphy and pH monitoring. *Int. J. Pharm.* (in press).

Hardy, J. G., Feely, L. C., Wood, E., and Davis, S. S., (1987b), The application of gamma scintigraphy for the evaluation of the relative spreading of suppository bases in rectal hard gelatin capsules. *Int. J. Pharm.* (in press).

Hardy, J. G., Healey, J. N. C., Lee, S. W., and Reynolds, J. R., (1987c), Gastrointestinal transit of an enteric-coated delayed-release 5-aminosalicylic acid tablet. *Aliment. Pharmacol. Therap.* (in press).

Houston, J. B., and Wood, S. G., (1980), Gastrointestinal absorption of drugs and other xenobiotics. *Drug Metab.*, **4**:57–125.

Khosla, R., and Davis, S. S., (1987), The effect of polycarbophil on the gastric emptying of pellets. *J. Pharm. Pharmacol.*, **39**:47–9.

Nelson, K. G., and Miller, K. W., (1979), *Principles of Drug Dissolution and Absorption Related to Bioavailability* pp 20–58.

Notari, R. E., (1980), *Biopharmaceutics and Clinical Pharmacokinetics: an introduction*, 3rd edn., Dekker, New York.

Ollerenshaw, K. J., Norman, S., Wilson, C. G., and Hardy, J. G., (1987), Exercise and small intestinal transit. *Nucl. Med. Commun.*, **8**:105–10.

O'Reilly, S., Wilson, C. G., and Hardy, J. G., (1987), The influence of food on the gastric emptying of multi-particulate dosage forms. *Int. J. Pharm.*, **34**:213–16.

Saffran, M., Kumar, G. S., Savariar, C., Burnham, J. C., Williams, F., and Neckers, D. C., (1986), A new approach to the oral administration of insulin and other peptide drugs. *Science*, **223**:1081–4.

Wilson, C. G., and Hardy, J. G., (1985), Gastrointestinal transit of an osmotic tablet drug delivery system. *J. Pharm. Pharmacol.*, **37**:573–5.

Wilson, C. G., Parr, G. D., Kennerley, J. W., Taylor, M. J., Davis, S. S., Hardy, J. G., and Rees, J., (1984), Pharmacokinetics and in vivo scintigraphic monitoring of a sustained release acetylsalicylic acid formulation. *Int. J. Pharm.*, **18**:1–8.

Wood, E., Wilson, C. G., and Hardy, J. G., (1985), The spreading of foam and solution enemas. *Int. J. Pharm.*, **25**:191–7.

22B.

ACTIONS OF PHARMACOLOGICAL AGENTS ON GASTROINTESTINAL FUNCTION

Thomas F. Burks

University of Arizona, Health Sciences Center, Tucson, Arizona, USA

Diverse types of drugs are capable of causing changes in patterns of contraction of gastrointestinal smooth muscle (Table 1). Often, a change in gastrointestinal motility is the intended effect of the drug. However, in many cases, changes in gastrointestinal motility are undesired side-effects of drug therapy. For example, tricyclic antidepressant drugs used for therapy of affective disorders or histamine H_1 antagonists given for relief of allergic symptoms may induce undesired changes in motility because of intrinsic anticholinergic actions of these classes of drugs. Whether drugs are considered as therapeutic agents intended to bring about relief from a disease process, as experimental tools to probe gastro-intestinal biology, or simply as sources of annoying side-effects, it is essential to consider their cellular mechanisms of action to utilize their therapeutic or experimental value optimally or to minimize their gastrointestinal side-effects. Drug actions are generally explicable in terms of increasing or decreasing functions of one or more specific influences that regulate smooth muscle excitability or contractility. In most cases, the actions of the drugs may be relatively simple and straight-forward. The complexity encountered in their actions results from the confusing array of multiple systems that regulate smooth muscle contractions.

Mechanisms of Drug Actions

Sites of Action

The usual first step in defining the mechanism of motility action of a particular drug requires identification of the site(s) of action. Established sites of action of drugs that affect gastrointestinal motility include gastrointestinal smooth muscle, intrinsic nerves of the gut, autonomic ganglia, the spinal cord, and the brain (Figure 1).

A number of drugs, hormones and neurotransmitter chemicals act directly upon smooth muscle. In the laboratory, drugs that act directly on gastrointestinal smooth muscle can be studied by a variety of techniques, such as use of tetrodotoxin (TTX) or by use of dispersed smooth muscle cells. These and other types of preparations have been employed to demonstrate that gastrointestinal smooth muscle cells can respond directly to a large number of chemicals.

Many drugs can exert their pharmacological actions within the wall of the bowel by effects on

Table 1. General classification of drugs that increase gastrointestinal contractions ('stimulatory') or inhibit contractions ('inhibitory').

Stimulatory	Inhibitory
Cholinergic agonists	Adrenergic agonists
Acetylcholinesterase inhibitors	Dopamine[+]
	Anticholinergics[†]
Prokinetic agents	Phenothiazines
Opioid agonists[*]	Tricyclic antidepressants
Adrenergic blockers	
Ergotamine	Histamine H_1 antagonists
Vasopressin	
Cholecystokinin	Calcium blockers
Gastrin	Progestins
Bile salts	Oestrogens
	Xanthines
	Papaverine
	Glucagon
	Nitrates
	Iron

[*] Decrease contractions of antrum
[+] Increases contractions of colon
[†] Includes both muscarinic and nicotinic antagonists

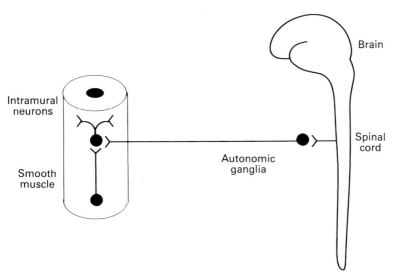

Figure 1. Diagrammatic representation of potential sites of actions of drugs that influence gastrointestinal motility. Drugs may act in the brain, spinal cord, at autonomic ganglia, gut intramural neurons, or upon gut smooth muscle.

the enteric nervous system rather than by, or in addition to, direct actions on the smooth muscle. The enteric nervous system, containing two ganglionated plexuses (myenteric plexus and submucous plexus), is a complex neuronal network embedded in the wall of the digestive tube (Costa et al, 1987). The enteric nervous system contains a number of neurons approximately equal to the number in the spinal cord and may be considered to represent a third component of the autonomic nervous system, along with the sympathetic and parasympathetic divisions. The enteric nervous system contains both afferent and efferent neurons and is responsible for co-ordination of motility to bring about carefully controlled transit of luminal contents through the digestive tract. The rich network of nerve cell bodies and fibres offers an array of possibilities for drug action that can increase or decrease release of excitatory or inhibitory neurotransmitters in the smooth muscle layers (Figure 2).

The ganglia of the sympathetic division of the autonomic nervous system provides an extramural target of drug, hormone and neurotransmitter action. It is becoming increasingly apparent that both paravertebral and prevertebral sympathetic

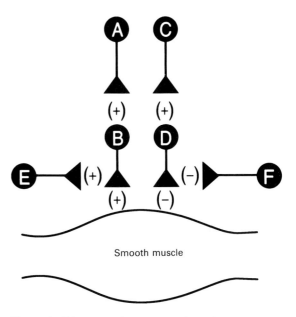

Figure 2. Diagrammatic representation of neural control systems that regulate gastrointestinal smooth muscle. Neural pathway A–B represents an excitatory (+) neural system. Pathway C–D represents an inhibitory (−) neural system. Neuron E can produce an excitatory effect by facilitation of pathway A–B. Neuron F can produce excitation by inhibition of pathway C–D (disinhibition). The excitability of the smooth muscle at any moment will be influenced by the net excitatory or inhibitory effects of these nerve pathways.

ganglia are important information integration and processing stations that participate in regulation of gastrointestinal motility. The ganglia receive sensory information from the digestive organs and motor (efferent) signals from the spinal cord; this information is processed through local neural circuits and is relayed to the enteric nerves by postganglionic sympathetic fibres.

The spinal cord was only recently identified as a site of drug action of importance in regulation of gastrointestinal motility (Porreca et al, 1983; Porreca and Burks, 1983). Drugs and neurotransmitter substances can act within the spinal cord both in ascending (afferent) and descending (efferent) pathways to alter autonomic outflow to the gastrointestinal tract.

It has been known for many years that the brain can influence gastrointestinal motility. Even the ancients recognized the connection between strong emotions and bowel function. However, recognition that drugs can act in the brain to influence gastrointestinal motility has come more recently (Burks, 1978). It is now evident that the brain is an important site of action for several types of drugs that influence gastrointestinal motility.

It is often difficult to determine the relative importance of individual sites of drug action when the drug in question acts at multiple sites. However, understanding of its action at each site contributes greatly to overall understanding of the drug's mechanism of action.

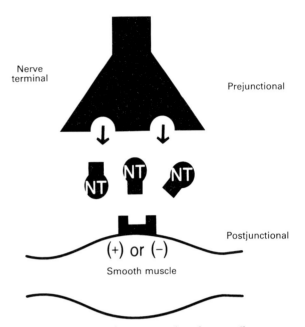

Figure 3. Diagrammatic representation of neuro-effector communication between a nerve terminal and gastrointestinal smooth muscle. Neurotransmitter molecules released from the prejunctional nerve terminal act at postjunctional smooth muscle receptors to produce excitation (+) or inhibition (−), depending on the type of receptor.

Receptors

Most drugs that affect gastrointestinal motility do so by means of actions at specific cellular receptors. The receptors may exist physiologically for the purpose of receiving messages from endogenous neurotransmitters, hormones, paracrine and autocrine chemicals (Figure 3). Most neural and smooth muscle receptors of importance in gastrointestinal motility occur on the outer side of the cell's plasma membrane and penetrate through the membrane to the interior of the cell. Great progress has occurred recently in understanding the structure and functions of membrane receptors. Chemically, receptors that have been char-acterized consist of complex proteins or glycoproteins.

Each receptor consists of three major components (Figure 4): a recognition site, a transduction mechanism, and an amplifier system. The

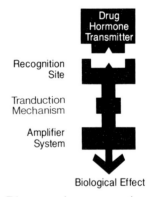

Figure 4. Diagrammatic representation of the principal elements of drug receptor systems. The receptor consists of a recognition site coupled by means of a transduction mechanism to an intracellular amplifier system. The drug, hormone or neurotransmitter molecule combines with the recognition site to activate the transduction mechanism and produce a biological effect by means of the amplifier system.

recognition site is that component of the transmembrane receptor that resides on the extracellular surface of the cell and binds to the drug, hormone or neurotransmitter molecules it recognizes. The receptor recognition site presents a specific array of physical and chemical features complementary to those of the messenger molecules it binds. There is thus a mutual chemical attraction between the messenger molecule and the corresponding receptor recognition site. Once binding between the drug, hormone or neurotransmitter molecule and the receptor recognition site has occurred, the binding may lead to activation of the transduction mechanism. It is the ability to activate the transduction mechanism that separates agonists from antagonists. The best characterized of the transducer systems involves proteins that bind guanosine triphosphate (GTP), and the proteins are thus called 'G proteins'. The importance of the transducer G proteins is the interesting way they are connected to the amplification system to provide either positive or negative regulatory influences (Figure 5).

Three major types of receptor-coupled cellular amplification systems have been identified: ion channels, cyclic nucleotides, and phosphoinositide metabolites. Some receptors, such as the nicotinic cholinergic receptor, are coupled directly to membrane ion channels. Other membrane receptors may be coupled to adenylate cyclase, which generates cyclic adenosine monophosphate (cyclic AMP), or to guanylate cyclase, which generates cyclic guanosine monophosphate (cyclic GMP). Receptors that are positively coupled to adenylate cyclase, such as beta adrenergic receptors, are linked to a stimulatory G protein (G_s) which is, in turn, linked to the cyclase. Binding of agonist drugs to the beta adrenergic receptor activates the stimulatory G protein, which increases adenylate cyclase activity. As a result, more adenosine triphosphate (ATP) is converted by the cyclase to cyclic AMP. Through a series of chemical steps, the cyclic AMP results in activation of intracellular protein kinase. Other receptors, such as delta opioid receptors and some muscarinic cholinergic receptors, may be negatively coupled to adenylate cyclase by means of an inhibitory G protein (G_i). In this case, binding of the agonist to the recognition site activates the inhibitory G protein, which inhibits enzymic activity of the coupled adenylate cyclase and decreases the amount of cyclic AMP generated. The third major type of amplification system of importance in gastrointestinal smooth muscle is inositol triphosphate (IP_3). Membrane receptors, such as those for cholecystokinin and some muscarinic cholinergic receptors, are coupled through a regulatory G protein to phospholipase C, which mobilizes the membrane lipid, phosphatidylinositol 4,5-biphosphate, which is hydrolysed to yield inositol 1,4,5-triphosphate and diacylglycerol. In terms of contraction of gastrointestinal smooth muscle, all three types of amplifier systems act to increase or decrease availability of calcium to the contractile proteins (Hartshorne, 1987). The practical significance of the transducer and amplification systems is the potential ability to develop totally new drugs that influence motility by acting on these mechanisms. For example, calcium entry blocking drugs alter motility by decreasing the influx of calcium required by many agents for generation of contractions.

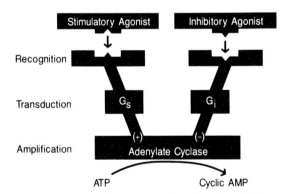

Figure 5. Diagrammatic representation of coupling of different receptors to a single intracellular amplifier system. The recognition site for the cellular receptor for the stimulatory agonist is coupled by means of a G_s protein to the intracellular enzyme, adenylate cyclase. The recognition site of the cellular receptor for the inhibitory agonist is coupled by means of a G_i protein to intracellular adenylate cyclase. Binding of the stimulatory agonist to its receptor activates G_s, which in turn activates adenylate cyclase and results in production of cyclic AMP. Binding of the inhibitory agonist activates G_i, which in turn inhibits adenylate cyclase activity and decreases production of cyclic AMP.

Characteristics of Drugs

Drugs that act at smooth muscle or neural membrane receptors may be classified as 'agonists' or 'antagonists'. Agonists are molecules that bind to receptors (possess 'affinity') and, once bound, can activate the transducer mechanism to which the receptor is coupled (possess 'efficacy'). Thus, interaction of an agonist with its corresponding cellular receptors will bring about a change in cellular function. The specific change, an increase or a decrease in function, depends on the type of transducer mechanism and amplifier system coupled to the receptor. For example, activation of an intestinal smooth muscle muscarinic cholinergic receptor leads to contraction of the muscle cell. Conversely, activation of a smooth muscle beta adrenergic receptor leads to relaxation of the smooth muscle cell. In both cases, the respective receptors were activated by agonist molecules. However, the amplifier system connected to the smooth muscle muscarinic cholinergic receptor (IP_3) increases availability of calcium to smooth muscle and generates contraction. Activation of the beta adrenergic receptor increases production of intracellular cyclic AMP and decreases availability of calcium to the contractile proteins, thus causing relaxation. Most smooth muscle cells contain many individual types of receptors. For example, an individual gastrointestinal smooth muscle cell may possess receptors for acetylcholine, 5-hydroxytryptamine, histamine, cholecystokinin, substance P, and angiotensin, each of which leads to smooth muscle contraction, and receptors for norepinephrine and glucagon, which generally cause relaxation. Multiple receptors coupled by different mechanisms to the contractile machinery provide both a large number of mechanisms for physiological regulation of contractile activity and potential sites of drug action.

Antagonists are drugs that have affinity for receptor recognition sites, but lack the ability to activate the transduction mechanism. Thus, antagonists are molecules lacking in efficacy. Because they do not activate receptor-linked transduction mechanisms, pure antagonists cannot directly influence cellular function. Their effect is to block actions of agonists. When administration

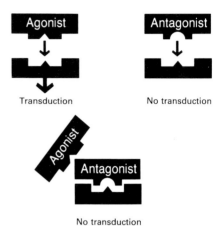

Figure 6. Diagrammatic representation of cellular actions of receptor agonists and antagonists. Binding of the agonist to the receptor recognition sites activates the transduction mechanism leading to a biological response. Binding of an antagonist to the receptor recognition sites does not bring about transduction. The antagonist occupies the recognition site and competes with agonist molecules for binding.

of an antagonist results in a change in contractile activity, it is because the antagonist blocked receptor activity of an agonist (Figure 6).

Antagonists are generally classified according to whether they act through competitive or non-competitive mechanisms. Competitive antagonists bind reversibly to receptors and thereby compete with agonist molecules for occupancy of the recognition site. The antagonism produced by competitive antagonists can be overcome by the addition of more agonist (Figure 7), that is, the effect of a competitive antagonist is surmountable. Non-competitive antagonists, on the other hand, do not simply compete with agonist molecules for the receptor recognition site. Some, such as phenoxybenzamine or chlornaltrexamine, produce essentially permanent alkylation of the receptor recognition site. This type of blockade cannot be overcome by the addition of more agonist. Typically, competitive antagonists cause a shift in the agonist dose-response curve parallel to the right (Figure 7). When sufficient amounts of agonist are added in the presence of the competitive antagonist, a full reponse to the agonist can be achieved. It is characteristic that the dose of agonist required for a half-maximal response (D_{50}) is increased in the presence of a competitive

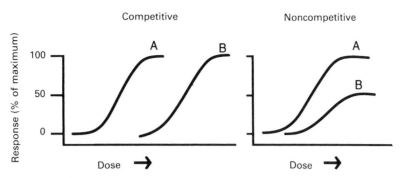

Figure 7. Conceptual dose-response curves illustrating actions of competitive and non-competitive antagonists. In both panels, curve A shows the response to the agonist alone. Curve B shows the response to the same agonist in the presence of an antagonist. A competitive antagonist shifts the agonist dose-response curve parallel to the right with the same maximal response attained even in the presence of the antagonist. A non-competitive antagonist displaces the agonist dose-response curve downward, decreasing the maximum response to the agonist that can be attained.

antagonist. By contrast, non-competitive antagonists generally reduce the maximum response that can be produced by the agonist with relatively little change in the agonist D_{50} values.

Indirectly Acting Drugs

Some drugs can produce biological effects indirectly by promoting release of neurotransmitter or neurohormone that in turn interacts with the cellular receptor. For example, tyramine can release norepinephrine from the terminals of adrenergic nerves. The norepinephrine released by tyramine can then interact with neural or smooth muscle norepinephrine receptors. Actions of tyramine may be blocked pharmacologically in two ways. A treatment may be given that blocks ability of tyramine to release norepinephrine. For example, treatment of the preparation with cocaine prevents neural uptake of tyramine and thus blocks its ability to release norepinephrine. Another approach is to block norepinephrine receptors by use of alpha or beta adrenergic antagonists.

In vivo, drugs may act at remote sites to promote release of an intermediate mediator. For example, drugs may release catecholamines from the adrenal medulla or promote formation of angiotensin. These effects may be brought about by direct drug action or can be secondary to an unrelated phar-

macological action, such as drug-induced decreases in blood pressure.

Another indirect way that drugs can act is by altering catabolism of neurotransmitter chemicals. For example, acetylcholinesterase inhibitors may produce indirect cholinergic actions by preventing enzymatic hydrolysis of neurally secreted acetylcholine. Uptake inhibitors, such as cocaine, desipramine or fluoxetine, can prevent inactivation of norepinephrine and 5-hydroxytryptamine that occurs by neural uptake.

Drug Actions

Cholinergic Drugs

Acetylcholine has been recognized as an important neurotransmitter since the early years of this century (Dale, 1914). In the digestive tract, acetylcholine generally induces smooth muscle contraction by direct actions at smooth muscle muscarinic receptors or at neural nicotinic cholinergic receptors. The excitatory response to activation of smooth muscle muscarinic receptors is thought to result from activation of phospholipase C, resulting in intracellular formation of inositol triphosphate, which releases calcium ion that activates contractile proteins (Harden et al, 1986). Acetylcholine is rarely used for therapeutic purposes becaue of its lack of receptor selectivity and its rapid hydrolysis by acetylcholinesterase and plasma cholinesterase. Many synthetic analogues of acetylcholine have been synthesized that exhibit selectivity for muscarinic cholinergic receptors and resistance to hydrolysis by acetyl-cholinesterase and plasma cholinesterase. The best known of the directly acting selective acetyl-choline-like drugs is bethanechol (Figure 8). While both are choline esters, bethanechol differs chemically from acetylcholine in two important ways. In bethanechol, a methyl group is sub-stituted in the beta position relative to the ammonium function. The beta-methyl sub-stitution confers selectivity for muscarinic chol-inergic receptors. Also, an amide group is substituted for the methyl function of the acetate portion of the molecule. The resulting carbamyl ester of choline is resistant to hydrolysis by both acetylcholinesterase and plasma cholinesterase. Bethanechol is thus a selective muscarinic receptor agonist with a relatively long duration of action. It is related chemically and pharmacologically to carbachol, which also possesses the carbamyl ester function, and to methacholine, which contains a beta-methyl function. Because of its muscarinic selectivity and resistance to enzymatic hydrolysis, bethanechol is the directly acting cholinergic agonist most often used in gastroenterology and serves as the prototype of this class of drugs.

Bethanechol and other muscarinic cholinergic agonists produce contractions of gastrointestinal smooth muscle. The excitatory effects of muscar-inic agonists on isolated muscle cells from longi-tudinal and circular muscle layers of the small intestine of various species, including the

human, have been demonstrated (Bitar et al, 1982; Makhlouf, 1987). In *in vitro* preparations of gastrointestinal smooth muscle, muscarinic cholinergic agonists produce increases in smooth muscle tone and amplitude of contractions. In animals and humans, ongoing cholinergic neuro-transmission to gastrointestinal smooth muscle is of importance in maintaining normal contractility and propulsion of intestinal contents (Galligan and Burks, 1986; Nowak et al, 1986; Borody et al, 1985). Subcutaneous administration of bethane-chol induces contractions of smooth muscle in the body of the oesophagus, lower oesophageal sphincter, stomach, small intestine, large intes-tine, and the internal anal sphincter (Nostrant et al, 1986; Burks, 1987; Burleigh and D'Mello, 1983; Roman and Gonella, 1987). Co-ordination of contractile activity is important in gastric emptying and propulsion of contents through the small intestine (Camilleri et al, 1986a; Meyer, 1987). Bethanechol and related muscarinic chol-inergic agonists produce co-ordinated, aborally moving contractions that greatly increase gastric emptying and intestinal propulsion (Figure 9).

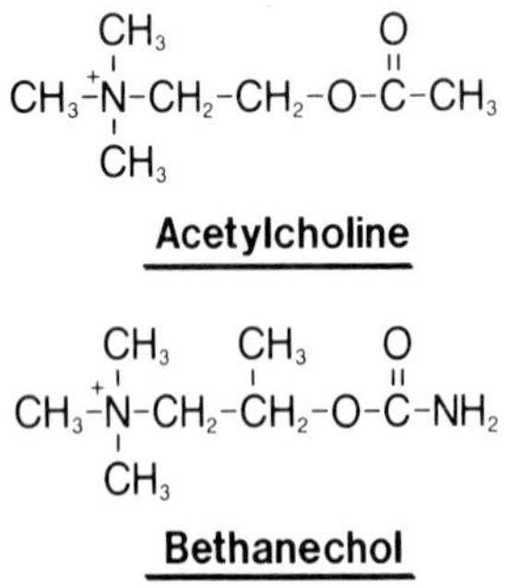

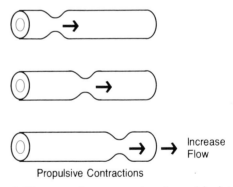

Propulsive Contractions

Figure 9. Diagrammatic representation of propulsive intestinal contractions typical of those induced by cholinergic agonists.

$$CH_3 \quad\quad\quad O$$
$$CH_3\text{-}\overset{+}{N}\text{-}CH_2\text{-}CH_2\text{-}O\text{-}\overset{\|}{C}\text{-}CH_3$$
$$CH_3$$

Acetylcholine

$$CH_3 \quad CH_3 \quad O$$
$$CH_3\text{-}\overset{+}{N}\text{-}CH_2\text{-}\overset{|}{CH}\text{-}CH_2\text{-}O\text{-}\overset{\|}{C}\text{-}NH_2$$
$$CH_3$$

Bethanechol

Figure 8. Chemical structures of acetylcholine and bethane-chol.

Bethanechol can be of clinical utility in the treat-ment of certain cases of gastroparesis and post-operative abdominal distension (Taylor, 1985a). Careful use of bethanechol can increase gastric emptying and promote intestinal propulsion. Because it can increase oesophageal motility and lower oesophageal sphincter pressure, bethane-chol can decrease gastro-oesophageal reflux (Thanik et al, 1982). Bethanechol causes contractions of the human gall-bladder and promotes gall-bladder emptying (Fisher et al, 1985).

Bethanechol and other cholinergic agonists can produce a wide variety of distressing and serious side-effects. In the gastrointestinal tract, muscarinic cholinergic agonists stimulate gastric and pancreatic secretion, and can produce abdominal cramps and watery diarrhoea. These drugs also slow the heart and can produce vasodilatation and hypotension. Because of the possibility of serious adverse cardiovascular effects, bethanechol should not be administered intravenously. The muscarinic agonists produce contraction of the urinary bladder and induce urination. They also act at the sweat glands to induce sweating. Bethanechol and other muscarinic agonists can produce bronchial constriction, especially in patients with asthma. Contraindications to the use of muscarinic agonists include peptic ulcer disease, heart block, and reactive or obstructive pulmonary disease. Whenever bethanechol is given by injection, atropine should be available as an antidote in the event of serious adverse effects.

Experimental evidence has recently been provided for subtypes of muscarinic receptors, termed M_1 and M_2. The muscarinic receptor subtypes are differentiated primarily by the actions of antagonists (Watson et al, 1986). Gastrointestinal smooth muscle receptors contain primarily the M_2 subtype of receptors, whereas gastric acid secretion is stimulated primarily by the M_1 subtype of muscarinic receptors. Agonist and antagonist drugs selective for M_1 and M_2 muscarinic receptors should eventually become available.

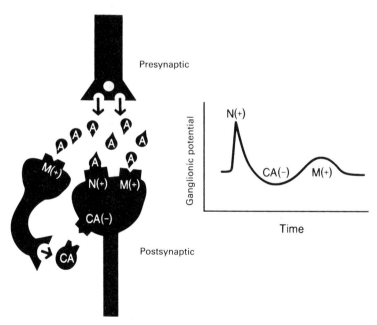

Figure 10. Diagrammatic representation of the components of sympathetic ganglionic neurotransmission. Acetylcholine (A) released from the presynaptic nerve terminal interacts with principal ganglion cell nicotinic (N) excitatory receptors (+) and with muscarinic (M) excitatory receptors. Acetylcholine also interacts with excitatory muscarinic receptors in ganglionic interneurons that release catecholamines (CA). The catecholamine released from the ganglionic interneuron interacts with inhibitory (−) receptors (CA) on the principal ganglion cell. The panel on the right illustrates the ganglionic electrical potentials generated by each component of the transmission process. Acetylcholine activation of nicotinic receptors causes a rapid depolarization, activation of catecholamine receptors causes a late hyperpolarization, and activation of ganglion cell muscarinic receptors causes late depolarization.

Nicotinic Cholinergic Receptors

Nicotinic cholinergic receptors of importance to gastrointestinal motility are located primarily on autonomic ganglion cells in the wall of the bowel or in sympathetic ganglia. Sympathetic ganglionic transmission is much more complex than is generally appreciated. Recording of ganglionic electrical potential during stimulation of preganglionic fibres yields a complex wave form characterized by a rapid depolarization, a slow hyperpolarization, and a late depolarization (Figure 10). The initial depolarization results from actions of neurally secreted acetylcholine at ganglion cell nicotinic cholinergic receptors. The slow hyperpolarization is mediated by catecholamines released from small ganglionic interneurons that are activated by the neurally secreted acetylcholine acting at muscarinic cholinergic receptors. The late depolarization results from actions of neurally secreted acetylcholine at ganglion cell muscarinic cholinergic receptors. Nerve impulses are initiated in the ganglion cells and postganglionic fibres by the nicotinic receptor-mediated rapid depolarization. The actions of acetylcholine at the ganglionic nicotinic receptors can be mimicked by other chemicals, including nicotine. As illustrated in Figure 11, nicotine can combine with the enteric nervous system ganglion cell nicotine cholinergic receptor to generate a nerve action potential and release of acetylcholine from the terminals of the postganglionic fibres. In the gastrointestinal tract, many postganglionic cholinergic fibres terminate near the smooth muscle layers and the neurally secreted acetylcholine acts at smooth muscle muscarinic cholinergic receptors to cause contractions. Thus, nicotine and other ganglionic nicotinic agonists can produce contraction of smooth muscle by activating cholinergic neurons in the wall of the gut. In some species, stimulation of

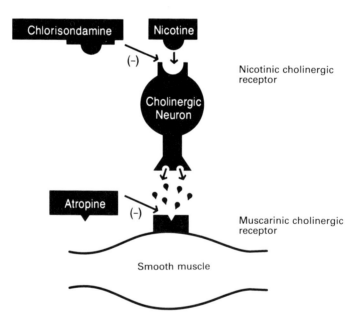

Figure 11. Diagrammatic representation of excitatory actions of nicotine on gastrointestinal smooth muscle. Nicotine acts at ganglionic nicotinic receptors of cholinergic neurons, causing them to release acetylcholine from their nerve terminals. The acetylcholine interacts with smooth muscle muscarinic cholinergic receptors. The interaction of nicotine with the nicotinic receptor can be blocked by ganglion blocking drugs, such as chlorisondamine. Acetylcholine actions on smooth muscle can be blocked by the muscarinic antagonist, atropine.

nicotinic cholinergic receptors results in intestinal inhibition, presumably as a result of activating inhibitory neural pathways (Burks et al, 1974).

Ganglionic stimulants are not employed as therapeutic agents.

Acetylcholinesterase Inhibitors

Acetylcholinesterase is the enzyme responsible for terminating synaptic and neuro-effector actions of acetylcholine. Drugs that inhibit actions of acetylcholinesterase allow a local accumulation of acetylcholine that can act as postsynaptic acetylcholine receptors. Acetylcholinesterase inhibitors are examples of indirectly acting cholinergic drugs.

The classical acetylcholinesterase inhibitor is physostigmine, also known as eserine. However, physostigmine can cross the blood–brain barrier and produce undesired effects in the central nervous system. For this reason, neostigmine (Figure 12) is more useful therapeutically. Neostigmine is a quaternary amine and does not effectively cross the blood–brain barrier. Edrophonium is related chemically to neostigmine, but exhibits a shorter duration of action. The organophosphate drugs, insecticides and nerve gases, such as diisopropylfluorophosphate, malathion and tabun, are extremely potent, irreversible acetylcholinesterase inhibitors. Organophosphate acetylcholinesterase inhibitors are rarely used in gastroenterology.

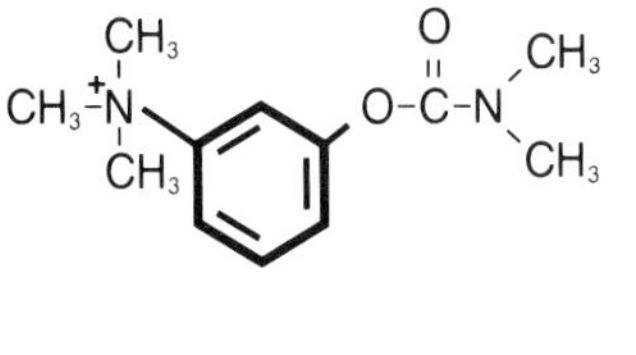

Neostigmine

Figure 12. Structure of neostigmine.

Neostigmine and other reversible acetylcholinesterase inhibitors release the motor activity of the stomach, small intestine, and large intestine. Muscle tone, amplitude of phasic contractions, and gastrointestinal propulsion are stimulated.

The overall stimulatory effect of acetylcholinesterase inhibitors on gastrointestinal motility represents a combination of actions within the myenteric plexus and in the muscle layers. Cholinesterase inhibitors can be useful for management of abdominal distension and paralytic ileus (Taylor, 1985b).

The major shortcoming of acetylcholinesterase inhibitors as therapeutic agents is their relative lack of selectivity in that they indirectly activate both nicotinic and muscarinic cholinergic receptors at all sites of cholinergic neurotransmission. Gastrointestinal symptoms of side-effects may include nausea and vomiting, abdominal cramps, and diarrhoea. Other side-effects can include excess salivation, hypotension, sweating, urination, and lacrimation. Atropine is an effective antidote.

Cholinergic Antagonists

Atropine is the prototype of the selective muscarinic cholinergic receptor antagonists. Atropine and scopolamine, which are pharmacologically similar, are natural plant alkaloids. A number of synthetic congeners of atropine have been prepared. The synthetic muscarinic receptor antagonists include methantheline (Figure 13), propantheline, tridihexethyl, anisotropine, clidinium, and numerous others. In general, the synthetic drugs possess quaternary ammonium structures and are somewhat more specific than the natural compounds for the gastrointestinal tract. Atropine and related compounds are competitive antagonists at muscarinic cholinergic receptors.

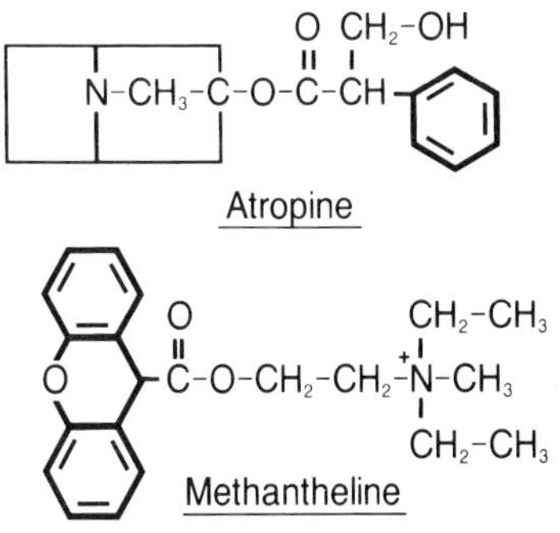

Figure 13. Structures of atropine and methantheline.

That is, they compete with acetylcholine for the receptor recognition site, but, lacking ability to activate the transducer mechanism, simply occupy the binding site to prevent access of acetylcholine to the receptor. Because of the importance of ongoing cholinergic neurotransmission in regulation of gastrointestinal contractions and propulsion, the muscarinic receptor antagonists can significantly reduce the incidence and amplitudes of contractions and inhibit gastrointestinal propulsion (Borody et al, 1985; Nowak et al, 1986).

While muscarinic receptor antagonists can decrease gastrointestinal motility and transit, their use is generally associated with uncomfortable side-effects such as dry mouth, difficulty in urination, and constipation. In sufficient doses, atropine and other antimuscarinic drugs can decrease gastric acid secretion and pancreatic secretion. Pirenzepine, an antagonist at the M_1 subtype of muscarinic receptors, can decrease gastric secretion with minimal effects on smooth muscle (Watson et al, 1986). Another experimental drug, AF-DX 116, is a selective antagonist at the M_2 subtype of muscarinic receptors. It is probable that new drugs with selectivity for individual subtypes of muscarinic cholinergic receptors will become useful therapeutic agents in the future.

Ganglion blocking drugs are neural nicotinic receptor antagonists. High (toxic) doses of nicotine alone can cause varying degrees of ganglionic blockade. Drugs that act selectively as ganglion blockers include chlorisondamine, hexamethonium, mecamylamine, and trimethaphan. These drugs are all competitive antagonists at ganglionic nicotinic receptors. Ganglionic blocking drugs decrease gastrointestinal contractions and transit, mainly by actions at ganglion cells of the myenteric plexus. The ganglion blocking drugs are rarely used in modern medicine. Because they block both sympathetic and parasympathetic ganglionic transmission (Figure 11) these drugs are non-specific and produce many troublesome side-effects. In particular, they lower blood pressure and frequently cause postural hypotension.

It should be noted that certain neuromuscular blocking agents, such as d-tubocurarine, can also block ganglionic neurotransmission.

Adrenergic and Anti-adrenergic Drugs

Adrenergic receptor agonists and antagonists are seldom used in therapy of disorders of gastrointestinal motility, but can produce profound motility effects. Actions of this class of drug are complex because of multiple types of adrenergic receptors (adrenoceptors). Adrenergic receptors were originally divided into two types, alpha and beta (Ahlquist, 1948). Subsequently, subtypes were identified (Lands et al, 1967; Langer, 1974). Postsynaptic (postjunctional) norepinephrine alpha receptors are mainly classified as the alpha$_1$ subtype. Alpha$_2$ receptors are mainly located at presynaptic (prejunctional) neural sites and are responsible for negative feedback inhibition of neural transmitter release. Postjunctional alpha$_2$ receptors have been identified in vascular smooth muscle. Beta$_1$ adrenergic receptors occur primarily in the heart, whereas beta$_2$ adrenergic receptors occur in smooth muscle of the gastrointestinal tract, bronchi, and blood vessels. Dopamine receptors occur on neurons and in some vascular smooth muscle. In the gastrointestinal tract, the wall of the stomach, small intestine, and large intestine is relaxed by activation of alpha and beta receptors. Activation of dopamine receptors generally causes relaxation in the small intestine, and contraction in the large intestine. Activation of alpha$_1$ adrenergic receptors causes contraction of the ileocaecal junction. The inhibitory effects of alpha$_1$ and beta$_1$ receptors result primarily from neural actions in the myenteric plexus. Activation of alpha$_2$ prejunctional receptors can also cause inhibition of the intestine by decreasing release of excitatory neural transmitter. Activation of smooth muscle beta adrenergic receptors causes smooth muscle relaxation (Makhlouf, 1987). The smooth muscle component of the relaxation may occur primarily from activation of beta$_2$ adrenergic receptors (Ek et al, 1986).

The receptor types and subtypes activated by natural and synthetic adrenergic agonists are shown in Table 2. Most of the agonists shown decrease gastrointestinal motility. The structures of norepinephrine, phenylephrine and isoproterenol are given in Figure 14. The gastrointestinal actions of the adrenergic agonists

Table 2. Receptor preferences of selected adrenergic and dopamine (DA) agonists.

Drugs	Receptor types				
	α_1	α_2	β_1	β_2	DA
Natural					
Epinephrine	+	+	+	+	
Norepinephrine	+	+	+		
Dopamine	+		+		+
Synthetic					
Phenylephrine	+				
Clonidine		+			
Isoproterenol			+	+	
Dobutamine			+		
Metaproterenol				+	

+ = Significant agonist activity

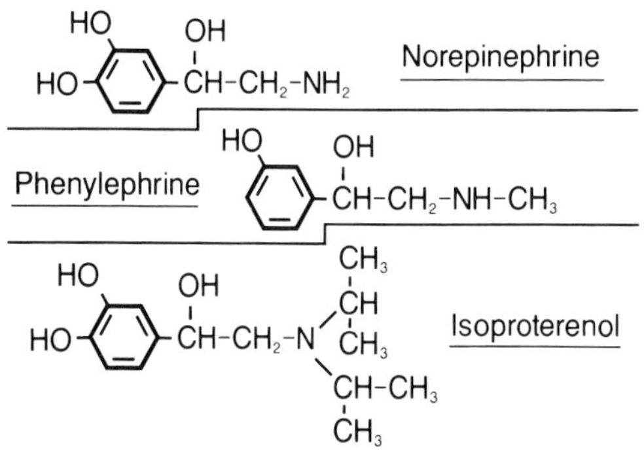

Figure 14. Structures of norepinephrine (noradrenaline), phenylephrine and isoproterenol (isoprenaline).

tend to be transient and gastrointestinal side-effects, other than nausea and vomiting, are rare.

Some adrenergic drugs can act indirectly by promoting release of norepinephrine from its storage sites in adrenergic nerve terminals. The prototype indirectly acting adrenergic drug is tyramine. Tyramine acts almost exclusively by release of endogenous norepinephrine. Ephedrine and amphetamine produce their adrenergic actions partly by release of neural norepinephrine. Norepinephrine uptake inhibitors, such as cocaine and desipramine, can produce norepinephrine-like effects by preventing neural uptake of norepinephrine.

Adrenergic receptor antagonists are slightly less complex than the agonists. The receptor

selectivities of prototypic adrenergic and dopamine receptor antagonists are given in Table 3.

Under certain circumstances, administration of alpha and beta adrenergic receptor antagonists may be associated with increased gastrointestinal motility and transit. Because adrenergic agonists generally inhibit gastrointestinal motility, it is assumed that blockade of endogenous catecholamines is responsible for the intestinal stimulation that can occur after alpha or beta blockade. However, certain adrenergic antagonists, such as phentolamine, may possess intrinsic intestinal stimulatory activity.

Table 3. Receptor preference of selected adrenergic and dopamine (DA) antagonists.

Drugs	Receptor types				
	α_1	α_2	β_1	β_2	DA
Phenoxybenzamine	+	+			
Phentolamine	+	+			
Prazosin	+				
Yohimbine		+			
Labetalol	+		+	+	
Propranolol			+	+	
Nadolol			+	+	
Metoprolol			+		
Atenolol			+		
Tolamolol			+		
Butoxamine*				+	
Droperidol		+			+
Haloperidol					+

+ = Significant auto-agonist activity
* = Experimental compound

Prokinetic Drugs

The so-called 'prokinetic drugs' can be divided into two general categories: those with pronounced dopamine receptor antagonist properties (e.g. metoclopramide and domperidone) and those that possess no dopamine receptor blocking activity (e.g. cisapride). The potential role of dopamine receptor blockade in the mechanism of prokinetic action is yet to be established (Lombardi et al, 1986). A number of drugs with pronounced dopamine receptor antagonist activity have relatively little effect on gastrointestinal transit. However, nearly all of the prokinetic drugs related to metoclopramide and cisapride appear to increase release of acetylcholine from neurons of the myenteric plexus, and possibly induce cholinergic stimulation of gastrointestinal smooth muscle (Hay and Man, 1979).

Metoclopramide (Figure 15), domperidone and cisapride increase gastric motility and promote gastric emptying (Schulze-Delrieu, 1981). The effect of prokinetic drugs on gastric emptying is of therapeutic value in the treatment of diabetic gastroparesis and dystrophia myotonia (Snape et al, 1982; Horowitz et al, 1987; Stacher et al, 1987; Feldman and Smith, 1987). Cisapride has been shown effective in reducing delayed intestinal transit in some patients with chronic intestinal pseudo-obstruction (Camilleri et al, 1986b). Metoclopramide, in particular, possesses significant central nervous system dopamine receptor antagonist activity. The central dopamine antagonist actions may contribute significantly to the pronounced anti-emetic effects of metoclopramide. However, a number of related agents with relatively little central dopamine receptor antagonist activity also possess anti-emetic properties. Domperidone and related agents exert only slight effects on the central nervous system, yet display anti-emetic activity and promote gastric motility and emptying.

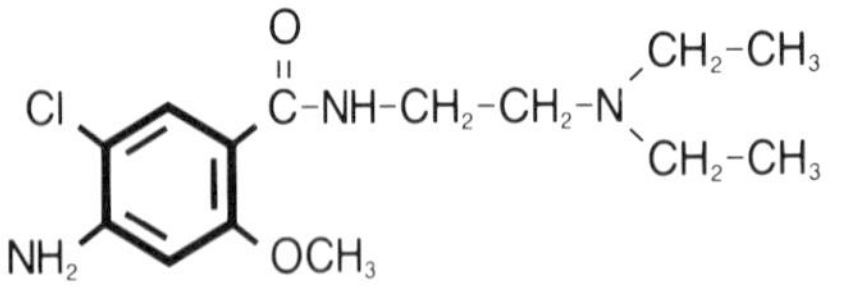

Metoclopramide

Figure 15. Structure of metoclopramide.

It is possible that peripheral dopamine receptor antagonist actions somehow contribute to the enhancement of cholinergic neural transmission by certain prokinetic drugs. It is now established that there are multiple types of dopamine receptors (Burks, 1987) and the roles of different types of dopamine receptors in regulation of gastro-intestinal motility may dictate responses to prokinetic drugs. For example, dopamine-induced relaxation of the lower oesophageal sphincter, mediated by DA_1 receptors, is not blocked by metoclopramide or domperidone (Lombardi et al, 1986). On the other hand, dopamine-induced stimulation of the colon was attenuated by domperidone (Wiley and Owyang, 1987). Other actions of the prokinetic drugs, such as interactions with 5-hydroxytryptamine receptors, may be of importance (Nemeth et al, 1985).

Opioid Drugs

Opium and opium-derived drugs have been used in medicine for literally thousands of years, mainly for their effects on gastrointestinal function and as analgesics. The motility effects of opioids have been studied extensively in modern times (Burks et al, 1982). One of the most striking pharmacological features of opioid drugs is their ability to produce constipation. The mechanism of the constipating action of opioids has been explored in detail.

It has been evident since the 1960s that morphine and other opioid drugs must act at specific pharmacological receptors to produce their biological effects (Martin, 1967). Saturable, stereospecific opioid binding sites in brain and intestine were described in 1973 (Pert and Snyder, 1973). Within two years, endogenous opioid peptides, [Met5]enkephalin and [Leu5]enkephalin, were discovered (Hughes, 1975). Discovery of other brain, pituitary, gut and adrenal opioid peptides followed. It is now apparent that the endogenous opioid peptides are derived from three families of precursor peptides: pro-opiomelanocortin, proenkephalin, and prodynorphin (Table 4). As studies of the endogenous opioid peptides progressed, the concept of multiple types of opioid receptors was reinforced. Three major types of opioid receptors can be demonstrated in a variety of mammalian tissues: mu, delta and kappa opioid receptors. Morphine, methadone, meperidine (pethidine), codeine and other opioid drugs produce their effects by means of agonist actions at receptors for the endogenous opioids. Different opioid ligands display different pre-

Table 4. Receptor preferences of selected opioid agonists.

Ligands	Receptor types		
	μ	δ	κ
Nonpeptides			
Morphine	+ +	+	+
Sufentanyl	+ +		
U-50 488			+ +
Peptides			
Pro-opiomelanocortin family			
β-Endorphin	+ +	+	
Pro-enkephalin family			
[Met⁵]enkephalin		+	+ +
[Leu⁵]enkephalin		+	+ +
Peptide E	+ +	+	
Prodynorphin family			
Dynorphin-(1–17)		+	+ +
α-Neoendorphin		+	+ +
Synthetic peptides			
DAGO	+ +		
PLO17	+ +		
DPDPE		+ +	

+ + = Preferred receptor type
+ = Significant agonist activity

ferences for the multiple types of opioid receptors (Table 4). For example, morphine is mu-receptor preferring but can act also at delta and kappa opioid receptors. Sufentanyl and the experimental peptides, DAGO and PLO17 (Figure 16), act almost exclusively at mu opioid receptors (James and Goldstein, 1984). The experimental peptide, DPDPE (Figure 16), acts selectively at delta opioid receptors (Mosberg et al, 1983). U-50488 acts selectively at kappa opioid receptors (Von Voigtlander et al, 1983). However, most peptide

[Met⁵]enkephalin

Try-Gly-Gly-Phe-Met

DAGO

Tyr-D-Ala-Gly-N-MePhe-Gly-ol

PLO17

Tyr-Pro-MePhe-D-Pro-NH₂

DPDPE

Tyr-D-Pen-Gly-Phe-D-Pen

Figure 16. Amino acid sequences of [Met⁵]enkephalin, DAGO, PLO17 and DPDPE.

and non-peptide ligands interact with more than one type of receptor. The gastrointestinal functional significance of multiple types of opioid receptors has revealed a rich complexity. Opioid drugs can affect gastrointestinal motility by actions in the brain, spinal cord, intrinsic neurons, and directly on smooth muscle (Stewart et al, 1977, 1978). The different anatomical sites of action often involve different types of opioid receptors (Burks et al, 1987). Motility responses to opioid agonists appear to involve primarily mu and delta opioid receptors (Hirning et al, 1985; Vaught et al, 1985).

Systemic administration of morphine results in characteristic changes in gastrointestinal motility. Typically, gastric emptying is inhibited, small bowel transit is delayed, and colonic transit is prolonged. When contractile activity is measured, morphine is generally found to increase the incidence and amplitudes of randomly distributed segmenting contractions similar to phase III of the migrating myoelectric complex. The segmenting, non-propulsive contractions increase resistance to flow and decrease the transit of intestinal contents (Figure 17). Morphine has also been found to initiate 'premature' phase III migrating complex activity (Borody et al, 1985; Matsumoto et al, 1986). Like synthetic opioids, human beta-endorphin decreases antral contractions and delays gastric emptying (Camilleri et al, 1986c).

Presently available opioid agonist drugs, such as morphine (Figure 18), produce changes in gastrointestinal motility and contractions of the sphincter of Oddi, inhibit outflow of bile, promote intestinal absorption of fluid and electrolytes, and induce constipation. Several synthetic opioids related chemically to meperidine (pethidine) are employed in therapeutics primarily as anti-

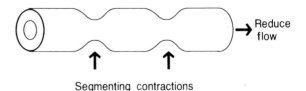

Segmenting contractions

Figure 17. Diagrammatic representation of the effects of opioids on intestinal motility. Opioids increase segmenting contractions that increase intraluminal pressure and thereby increase resistance to flow. Intestinal flow is thereby decreased.

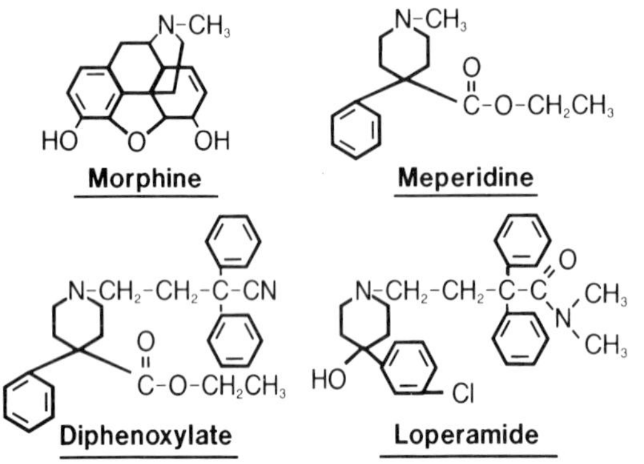

Figure 18. Structures of morphine, meperidine, diphenoxylate and loperamide.

CCK-8

Asp-Tyr-Met-Gly-Trp-Met-Asp-Phe-NH$_2$
           SO$_3$

Substance P

Arg-Pro-Lys-Pro-Gln-Gln-Phe-Phe-Gly-Leu-Met-NH$_2$

Bombesin

Glp-Gln-Arg-Leu-Gly-Asn-Gln-Trp-Ala-Val-Gly-His-Leu-Met-NH$_2$

Figure 19. Amino acid sequences of cholecystokinin octapeptide (CCK-8), substance P and bombesin.

diarrhoeal drugs. The two best known synthetic antidiarrhoeal opioids are diphenoxylate and loperamide (Figure 18). These drugs produce naloxone-reversible changes in gastrointestinal motility and delay of intestinal transit (Basilisco et al, 1987; Kachel et al, 1986). While diphenoxylate and loperamide resemble meperidine chemically, meperidine itself is relatively non-constipating. The antidiarrhoeal properties of loperamide may result in part from non-opioid mechanisms (Reynolds et al, 1984).

Special care must be taken in use of opioids as nonspecific antidiarrhoeal drugs, since opioids may exacerbate enteric infections by invasive organisms (DuPont and Hornick, 1973). Opioids are generally considered only for short-term use, as tolerance to the motility effects can occur (Burks and Long, 1976) and opioids that cross the blood–brain barrier (morphine, codeine and other alkaloid-type opioids) can induce dependence. The major hazard associated with acute medical use of opioids is respiratory depression. Naloxone is an effective antagonist.

Peptides

Cholecystokinin (CCK) is a brain–gut peptide that serves both neurotransmitter and hormonal functions. It is released after meals from endocrine cells in the mucosa of the upper small intestine. CCK exists in multiple molecular forms, but the principal smaller form is the carboxyl-terminal octapeptide known as CCK-8 (Figure 19). CCK

is a potent stimulant of gall-bladder contraction and of sphincter of Oddi relaxation (Walsh, 1987). CCK induces contractions of gall-bladder both by direct actions on smooth muscle CCK receptors and indirectly by increasing neural release of acetylcholine (Behar and Biancani, 1987; Harada et al, 1986). CCK also induces contractions of intestinal smooth muscle, both by direct actions at smooth muscle CCK receptors and indirectly by release of acetylcholine (Stewart and Burks, 1977; Grider and Makhlouf, 1987). Pharmacological doses of CCK inhibit gastric emptying and postprandial delay of gastric emptying has often been ascribed to physiological actions of CCK (Liddle et al, 1986). However, the availability of potent and selective CCK antagonists, such as L-346 718 (Pendleton et al, 1987), fail to block postprandial inhibition of gastric emptying and call into question a physiological role of CCK in regulation of gastric emptying. CCK may serve as a sensory neurotransmitter in ganglionic reflex pathways regulating gastrointestinal motility (Schumann and Kreulen, 1986).

The tachykinins, also known as neurokinins, are neurotransmitters in peripheral sensory pathways (Buck and Burks, 1986). Substance P (Figure 19) and substance K (also known as neurokinin alpha and neuromedin L) and neurokinin beta (also known as neuromedin K) occur in neurons associated with both sensory and motor function (Mantyh et al, 1984). Multiple types of tachykinin receptors occur in gastrointestinal nerves and smooth muscle (Mantyh et al, 1984; Burcher et al,

1986). Evidence has been put forward that substance P or a related tachykinin is responsible for initiation of intestinal reflexes responsible for postoperative ileus and ileus produced by peritoneal irritation (Holzer et al, 1986).

A number of other gastrointestinal hormones produce motility effects when administered exogenously (Walsh, 1987). Somatostatin, gastrin, motilin, and other hormones produce changes in motility that may eventually be of therapeutic value. Gastrin-releasing peptide, the mammalian equivalent of bombesin, produces striking changes in gastrointestinal motility and transit after peripheral or central administration in animals (Koslo et al, 1986). Interestingly, the actions of bombesin may result primarily from effects in sensory neural pathways.

Conclusions

A great deal has been learned about the motility effects of drugs in the past few years. With increasing recognition of the importance of disorders of gastrointestinal motility in a number of disease states, additional new drugs will be introduced for therapeutic use in regulation of motility. Likewise, new approaches will be available to eliminate or combat the motility side-effects of drugs directed at other therapeutic endpoints.

Acknowledgements

Supported by US Public Health Service grants DA02163 and AM36289. The assistance of Ms. Rita Sainz is gratefully acknowledged.

References

Ahlquist, R. P., (1948), A study of the adrenotropic receptors. *Am. J. Physiol.*, **153**:586–600.

Basilisco, G., Camboni, G., Bozzani, A., Paravicini, M., and Bianchi, P. A., (1987), Oral naloxone antagonizes loperamide-induced delay of orocecal transit. *Dig. Dis. Sci.*, **32**:829–32.

Behar, J., and Biancani, P., (1987), Pharmacologic characterization of excitatory and inhibitory chole-

cystokinin receptors of the cat gallbladder and sphincter of Oddi. *Gastroenterology*, **92**:764–70.

Bitar, K. N., Saffouri, B., and Makhlouf, G. M., (1982), Cholinergic and peptidergic receptors on isolated human antral smooth muscle cells. *Gastroenterology*, **82**:832–7.

Borody, T. J., Quigley, E. M. M., Phillips, S. F., Wienbeck, M., Tucker, R. L., Haddad, A., and Zinsmeister, A. R., (1985), Effects of morphine and atropine on motility and transit in the human ileum. *Gastroenterology*, **89**:562–70.

Buck, S. H., and Burks, T. F., (1986), The neuropharmacology of capsaicin: review of some recent observations. *Pharmacol. Rev.*, **38**:179–226.

Burcher, E., Buck, S. H., Lovenberg, W., and O'Donohue, T. L., (1986), Characterization and autoradiographic localization of multiple tachykinin binding sites in gastrointestinal tract and bladder. *J. Pharmacol. Exp. Ther.*, **236**:819–31.

Burks, T. F., (1978), Central sites of action of gastrointestinal drugs. *Gastroenterology*, **74**:322–4.

Burks, T. F., (1987), Actions of drugs on gastrointestinal motility. In: *Physiology of the Gastrointestinal Tract*, Second Edition (Ed Johnson, L. R.), pp 723–43, Raven Press, New York.

Burks, T. F., Galligan, J. J., Hirning, L. D., and Porreca, F., (1987). Brain, spinal cord and peripheral sites of action of enkephalins and other endogenous opioids on gastrointestinal motilty. *Gastroenterol. Clin. Biol.*, **11**:44B–51B.

Burks, T. F., Hirning, L. D., Galligan, J. J., and Davis, T. P., (1982), Motility effects of opioid peptides in dog intestine. *Life Sci.*, **31**:2237–40.

Burks, T. F., Jaquette, D. L., and Grubb, M. N., (1974), Motility responses of dog and monkey isolated perfused intestine to morphine 5-hydroxytryptamine and cholinergic stimulants. *Gen. Pharmacol*, **5**:213–16.

Burks, T. F., and Long, J. P., (1976). Responses of isolated dog small intestine to analgesic agents. *J. Pharmacol. Exp. Ther.*, **158**:264–71.

Burleigh, D. E., and D'Mello, A., (1983), Neural and pharmacologic factors affecting motility of the internal anal sphincter. *Gastroenterology*, **84**:409–17.

Camilleri, M., Brown, M. L., and Malagelada, J.-R., (1986a), Relationship between impaired gastric emptying and abnormal gastrointestinal motility. *Gastroenterology*, **91**:94–9.

Camilleri, M., Brown, M. L., and Malagelada, J.-R., (1986b), Impaired transit of chyme in chronic intestinal pseudoobstruction-correction by cisapride. *Gastroenterology*, **91**:619–26.

Camilleri, M., Malagelada, J.-R., Stanghellini, V., Zinsmeister, A. R., Kao, P. C., and Li, C. H., (1986c), Dose-related effects of synthetic human β-endorphin and naloxone on fed gastrointestinal motility. *Am. J. Physiol.*, **251**:G147–54.

Costa, M., Furness, J. B., and Llewellyn-Smith, I. J., (1987), Histochemistry of the enteric nervous system. In: *Physiology of the Gastrointestinal Tract*, Second Edition (Ed Johnson, L. R.), pp 1–40, Raven Press, New York.

Dale, H. H., (1914), The actions of certain esters and ethers of choline, and their relation to muscarine. *J. Pharmacol. Exp. Ther.*, 6:147–90.

DuPont, H. L., and Hornick, R. B., (1973), Adverse effects of Lomotil therapy in shigelloisis. *J. Am. Med. Assoc.*, 226:1525–8.

Ek, B. A., Bjellin, L. A. C., and Lundgren, B. T., (1986), β-Adrenergic control of motility in the rat colon. I. Evidence for functional separation of the β_1- and β_2-adrenoceptor-mediated inhibition of colon activity. *Gastroenterology*, 90:400–7.

Feldman, M., and Smith, H. J., (1987), Effect of cisapride on gastric emptying of indigestible solids in patients with gastroparesis diabeticorum—a comparison with metoclopramide and placebo. *Gastroenterology*, 92:171–4.

Fisher, R. S., Rock, E., and Malmud, L. S., (1985), Cholinergic effects on gallbladder emptying in humans. *Gastroenterology*, 89:716–22.

Galligan, J. J., and Burks, T. F., (1986), Cholinergic neurons mediate intestinal propulsion in the rat. *J. Pharmacol. Exp. Ther.*, 238:594–8.

Grider, J. R., and Makhlouf, G. M., (1987), Regional and cellular heterogeneity of cholecystokinin receptors mediating muscle contraction in the gut. *Gastroenterology*, 92:175–80.

Harada, T., Katsuragi, T., and Furukawa, T., (1986), Release of acetylcholine mediated by cholecystokinin receptors from the guinea pig sphincter of Oddi. *J. Pharmacol. Exp. Ther.*, 239:554–8.

Harden, T. K., Tanner, L. I., Martin, M. W., Nakahata, N., Hughes, A. R., Hepler, J. R., Evans, T., Masters S. B., and Brown, J. H., (1986), Characteristics of two biochemical responses to stimulation of muscarinic cholinergic receptors. In: *Subtypes of Muscarinic Receptors II* (Eds Levine, R. R., Birdsall, N. J. M., Giachetti, A., Hammer, R., Iverson, L. L., Jenden, D. J., and North, R. A.), pp 14–18, Elsevier, Amsterdam.

Hartshorne, D. J., (1987), Biochemistry of the contractile process in smooth muscle. In: *Physiology of the Gastrointestinal Tract*, Second Edition. (Ed Johnson, L. R.), pp 432–82, Raven Press, New York.

Hay, A. M., and Man, W. K., (1979), Effect of metoclopramide on guinea pig stomach. *Gastroenterology*, 76:492–6.

Hirning, L. D., Porreca, F., and Burks, T. F., (1985), Mu, but not kappa, opioid agonists induce contractions of the canine small intestine, ex vivo. *Eur. J. Pharmacol.*, 109:49–54.

Holzer, P., Lippe, I. T., and Holzer-Petsche, U., (1986), Inhibition of gastrointestinal transit due to

surgical trauma or peritoneal irritation is reduced in capsaicin-treated rats. *Gastroenterology*, 91:360–3.

Horowitz, M., Maddox, A., Maddern, G. J., Wishart, J., Collins, P. J., and Shearman, J. C., (1987), Gastric and esophageal emptying in dystrophia myotonica—effect of metoclopramide. *Gastroenterology*, 92:570–7.

Hughes, J., (1975), Isolation of an endogenous compound from the brain with pharmacological properties similar to morphine. *Brain Res.*, 88:295–308.

James, I. F., and Goldstein, A., (1984), Site-directed alkylation of multiple opioid receptors. I. Binding selectivity. *Mol. Pharmacol.*, 25:337–42.

Kachel, G., Ruppin, H., Hagel, J., Barina, W., Meinhardt, M., and Domschke, W., (1986), Human intestinal motor activity and transport: effect of a synthetic opiate. *Gastroenterology*, 90:85–93.

Koslo, R. J., Burks, T. F., and Porreca, F., (1986), Centrally administered bombesin affects gastrointestinal transit and colonic bead expulsion through supraspinal mechanisms. *J. Pharmacol. Exp. Ther.*, 238:62–7.

Lands, A. M., Luduena, F. P., and Buzzo, H. J., (1967), Differentiation of receptors responsive to isoproterenol. *Life Sci.*, 6:2241–9.

Langer, S. Z., (1974), Presynaptic regulation of catecholamine release. *Biochem. Pharmacol.*, 23:1793–800.

Libet, B., (1970), Generation of slow inhibitory and excitatory postsynaptic potentials. *Fed. Proc.*, 29:1945–56.

Liddle, R., Morit, E., Conrad, C., and Williams, J., (1986), Regulation of gastric emptying in humans by cholecystokinin. *J. Clin. Invest.*, 77:992–6.

Lombardi, D. M., Grous, M., Fine, C. F., Barone, F. C., Fowler, P. J., Phyall, W. B., Rush, J. A., and Ormsbee, H. S., (1986), DA$_1$ Receptor mediates dopamine-induced relaxation of opossum lower esophageal sphincter in vitro. *Gastroenterology*, 91:533–9.

Makhlouf, G. M., (1987), Isolated smooth muscle cells of the gut. In: *Physiology of the Gastrointestinal Tract*, Second Edition (Ed Johnson, L. R.), pp 555–69, Raven Press, New York.

Mantyh, P. W., Goedert, M., and Hunt, S. P., (1984), Autoradiographic visualization of receptor binding sites for substance P in the gastrointestinal tract of the guinea pig. *Eur. J. Pharmacol.*, 100:133–4.

Martin, W. R., (1967), Opioid antagonists. *Pharmacol. Rev.*, 19:463–521.

Matsumoto, T., Sarna, S. K., Condon, R. E., Cowles, V. E., and Frantzides, C., (1986), Differential sensitivities of morphine and motilin to initiate migrating motor complex in isolated intestinal segments. *Gastroenterology*, 90:61–7.

Meyer, J. H., (1987), Motility of the stomach and gastroduodenal junction. In: *Physiology of the Gas-*

trointestinal Tract, Second Edition (Ed Johnson, L. R.), pp 613–29. Raven Press, New York.

Mosberg, H. I., Hurst, R., Hruby, V. J., Gee, K., Yamamura, H. I., Galligan, J. J., and Burks, T. F., (1983), Bis-penicillamine enkephalins possess highly improved specificity towards delta opioid receptors. *Proc. Natl. Acad. Sci., USA*, **80**:5871–4.

Nemeth, P. R., Ort, C. A., Zafirov, D. H., and Wood, J. D., (1985), Interactions between serotonin and cisapride on myenteric neurons. *Eur. J. Pharmacol.*, **108**:77–83.

Nostrant, T. T., Sams, J., and Huber, T., (1986), Bethanechol increases the diagnostic yield in patients with esophageal chest pain. *Gastroenterology*, **91**:1141–6.

Nowak, T. V., Harrington, B., Kalbfleisch, J. H., and Amatruda, J. M., (1986), Evidence for abnormal cholinergic neuromuscular transmission in diabetic rat small intestine. *Gastroenterology* **91**:124–32.

Pendleton, R. G., Bendesky, R. J., Schaffer, L., Nolan, T. E., Gould, R. J., and Clineschmidt, B. V., (1987), Roles of endogenous cholecystokinin in biliary, pancreatic and gastric function: studies with L-364,718, a specific cholecystokinin receptor antagonist. *J. Pharmacol. Exp. Ther.*, **241**:110–16.

Pert, C. B., and Snyder, S. H., (1973), Opiate receptor: demonstration in nervous tissue. *Science* (Washington), **179**:1011–14.

Porreca, F., and Burks, T. F., (1983), The spinal cord as a site of opioid effects on gastrointestinal transit in the mouse. *J. Pharmacol. Exp. Ther.*, **227**:22–7.

Porreca, F., Filla, A., and Burks, T. F., (1983), Spinal cord-mediated opiate effects on gastrointestinal transit in mice. *Eur. J. Pharmacol.*, **86**:135–6.

Reynolds, I. J., Gould, R. J., and Snyder, S. H., (1984), Loperamide: blockade of calcium channels as a mechanism for antidiarrheal effects. *J. Pharmacol. Exp. Ther.*, **231**:628–32.

Roman, C., and Gonella, J., (1987), Extrinsic control of digestive tract motility. In: *Physiology of the Gastrointestinal Tract*, Second Edition, (Ed Johnson, L. R.), pp 507–53, Raven Press, New York.

Schulze-Delrieu, K., (1981), Metoclopramide. *N. Engl. J. Med.*, **305**:28–33.

Schumann, M. A., and Kreulen, D. L., (1986), Action of cholecystokinin octapeptide and CCK-related peptides on neurons in inferior mesenteric ganglion of guinea pig. *J. Pharmacol. Exp. Ther.*, **239**:618–25.

Snape, W. J., Battle, W. M., Schwartz, S. S., Braunstein, S. N., Goldstein, H. A., and Alavi, A., (1982), Metoclopramide to treat gastroparesis due to diabetes mellitus. *Ann. Int. Med.*, **96**:444–6.

Stacher, G., Bergmann, H., Wiesnagrotzki, S., Kiss, A., Schneider, C., Mittelbach, G., Gaupmann, G.,

and Hobart, J., (1987), Intravenous cisapride accelerates delayed gastric emptying and increases antral contraction amplitude in patients with primary anorexia nervosa. *Gastroenterology*, **92**:1000–6.

Stewart, J. J., and Burks, T. F., (1977), Actions of cholecystokinin octapeptide on smooth muscle of isolated dog intestine. *Am. J. Physiol.*, **232**:E306–10.

Stewart, J. J., Weisbrodt, N. W., and Burks, T. F., (1977), Centrally mediated intestinal stimulation by morphine. *J. Pharmacol. Exp. Ther.*, **202**:174–81.

Stewart, J. J., Weisbrodt, N. W., and Burks, T. F., (1978), Central and peripheral actions of morphine on intestinal transit. *J. Pharmacol. Exp. Ther.*, **205**:547–55.

Taylor, P., (1985a), Cholinergic agonists. In *Goodman and Gilman's The Pharmacological Basis of Therapeutics*, Seventh Edition (Eds Gilman, A. G., Goodman, L. S., Rall, T. W., and Murad, F.), pp 100–9, Macmillan, New York.

Taylor, P., (1985b), Anticholinesterase agents. In *Goodman and Gilman's The Pharmacological Basis of Therapeutics*, Seventh Edition (Eds Gilman, A. G., Goodman, L. S., Rall, T. W., and Murad, F.), pp 110–29, Macmillan, New York.

Thanik, K., Chey, W. K., Shak, A., Hamilton, D., and Nadelson, N., (1982), Bethanechol or cimetidine in the treatment of symptomatic reflux esophagitis. *Arch. Intern. Med.*, **142**:1479–81.

Vaught, J. L., Cowan, A., and Jacoby, H. I., (1985), μ and δ, but not κ, opioid agonists induce contractions of the canine small intestine in vivo. *Eur. J. Pharmacol.*, **109**:43–8.

Von Voigtlander, P. F., Lahti, R. A., and Ludens, J. H., (1983), U-50,488H: a selective and structurally novel non-mu (kappa) opioid agonist. *J. Pharmacol Exp. Ther.*, **24**:7–12.

Walsh, J. H., (1987), Gastrointestinal hormones. In: *Physiology of the Gastrointestinal Tract*, Second Edition (Ed Johnson, L. R.), pp 181–253, Raven Press, New York.

Watson, M., Roeske, W. R., Vickroy, T. W., Smith, T. L., Akiyama, K., Gulya, K., Duckles, S. P., Serra, M., Adem, A., Nordberg, A., Gehlert, D. R., Wamsley, J. K., and Yamamura, H. I., (1986), Biochemical and functional basis of putative muscarinic receptor subtypes and its implications. In: *Subtypes of Muscarinic Receptors II* (Eds Levine, R. R., Birdsall, N. J. M., Giachietti, A., Hammer, R., Iverson, L. L., Jenden, D. J., and North, R. A.), pp 46–55, Elsevier, Amsterdam.

Wiley, J., and Owyang, C., (1987), Dopaminergic modulation of rectosigmoid motility: action of domperidone. *J. Pharmacol. Exp. Ther.*, **242**:548–51.

23
EFFECT OF GASTRIC AND SMALL BOWEL OPERATIONS ON GASTROINTESTINAL MOTILITY

Sven Gustavsson, Keith A. Kelly

University Hospital, Uppsala, Sweden and the Mayo Clinic, Rochester, Minnesota, USA

Evaluation of gastrointestinal motility in the post-surgical patient requires a knowledge of the effects of surgical procedures and rearrangements on motor function. In this chapter we review the motility alterations that can follow commonly performed operations on the stomach and small bowel. Due to an incredible capacity of the stomach and small intestine to normalize function following operation, such alterations are usually well tolerated by the patients. However, sometimes severe postoperative symptoms occur which require careful evaluation, including motility studies.

Gastric Operations

All operations on the stomach produce some change in gastric motility. The type of change and the symptoms resulting from it depend on the nature of the operation and the region of stomach involved. Disorders of gastric motility resulting from operations on the proximal stomach differ from those produced by operations on the distal stomach.

This section will review the motor disorders produced by gastric operations, indicate how the disorders can lead to symptoms, and suggest possible treatments for the disorders.

Gastrectomy

The gastrectomies commonly performed today are proximal gastrectomy, distal gastrectomy, and total gastrectomy. Most are performed in the treatment of gastric malignancies, but gastrectomies are occasionally done in peptic ulcer disease, stress ulcers and Menetrier's disease and in other benign conditions.

Proximal Gastrectomy

Resections of the proximal stomach reduce the area of the gastric reservoir and impair receptive relaxation and gastric accommodation. Because of the impaired accommodation, patients often complain of a small gastric capacity and early satiety. Gastric distension produces a greater increase in intragastric pressure, with the result that gastric emptying occurs more rapidly. This rapid gastric emptying may lead to the 'dumping' syndrome, especially when hyperosmolar liquids are ingested. In this syndrome, the rapid entry of large quantities of hyperosmolar gastric content into the small intestine produces distension, nausea, cramps, borborygmi, diarrhoea, and sometimes even hypotension.

Resection of the mid-gastric corpus removes the

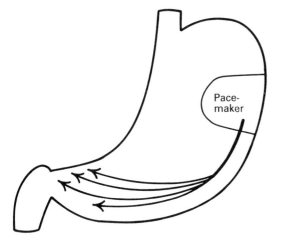

Figure 1. Site of the gastric pacemaker and pathways of propagation of the gastric pacesetter potentials (arrows).

natural gastric pacemaker, the site at which the gastric electrical waves are generated that phase the onset of peristaltic contractions (Figure 1). A new pacemaker arises just distal to the site of resection, but it generates pacesetter potentials, hence

peristaltic waves, at a lower frequency. The decrease in frequency is likely to affect the gastric emptying of solids, although this point has not been carefully studied.

Distal Gastrectomy

In distal gastrectomy, a variable portion of the distal stomach including the pylorus is excised, and the proximal gastric remnant is then anastomosed to the duodenum (Billroth I) or to the jejunum (Billroth II) (Figure 2). Antrectomy is a special type of distal gastrectomy, where care is taken to excise only the gastrin-producing area and leave the parietal-cell-bearing area intact. Because resections of the antrum and pylorus abolish antral propulsion and retropulsion, they greatly impair the antral mixing and grinding of solids.

Antrectomy causes only a slight increase in the rate at which liquids are emptied from the stomach. The increase that does occur may be due to the fact that the anastomosis offers less resistance to the flow of liquids than does the

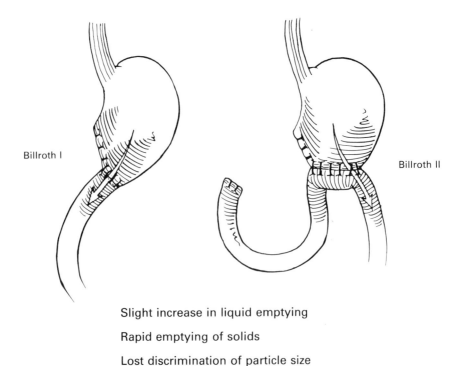

Billroth I

Billroth II

Slight increase in liquid emptying

Rapid emptying of solids

Lost discrimination of particle size

Figure 2. Gastric emptying after subtotal gastrectomy—schematic.

Billroth I

Roux–en–y

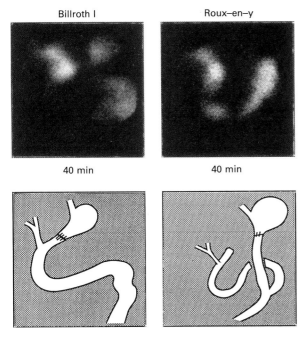

40 min

40 min

Figure 3. Scintiphotographs showing duodenogastric reflux in a patient with Billroth I gastrectomy 40 minutes after injection of ^{99m}Tc-HIDA intravenously (left). After Roux-en-Y reconstruction, reflux does not occur (right).

normal gastroduodenal junction. Another factor is removal of the source of antral gastrin. The resulting impairment of the gastrin-enhanced accommodation in the proximal stomach results in greater increases in intragastric pressure as the stomach fills and thus speeds the gastric emptying of liquids. Finally, distal gastrectomy followed by reconstruction of the Billroth II-type allows gastric chyme to bypass the receptors in the mucosa of the duodenum and proximal jejunum that slow gastric emptying. When the receptors are bypassed, this braking effect is lost or greatly impaired and gastric emptying is faster. Gastric emptying of solids is enhanced after distal gastrectomy, and the discrimination of particle size is lost. Distal gastrectomy also results in reflux of small intestinal contents into the stomach, because it excises or bypasses the pylorus (Figure 3). In the intact stomach, a small resting pressure is present at the pylorus. When acid or a fatty meal enters the duodenum, or when cholecystokinin or secretin is released, the pylorus contracts strongly, thus preventing reflux of duodenal contents into the stomach. Excision of the distal antrum and

Modes of reconstruction after total gastrectomy

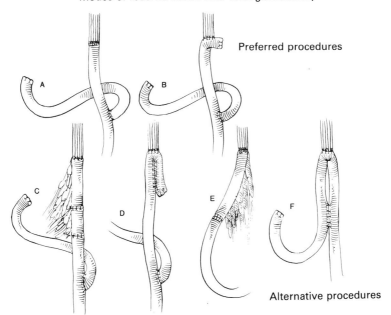

Preferred procedures

Alternative procedures

Figure 4. Methods of reconstruction after total gastrectomy. Preferred (A + B) and alternative (C − F) procedures.

pylorus removes the mechanism that prevents reflux. The increased duodenal-gastric reflux can result in vomiting of bile and alkaline gastritis.

Total Gastrectomy

In total gastrectomy, the entire stomach is excised, following which the oesophagus is usually anastomosed to the end of a Roux-en-Y jejunal limb (Figure 4). Nowadays, total gastrectomy is performed almost exclusively in the treatment of gastric cancer.

The major motor functions ordinarily performed by the stomach—storage of ingesta, trituration of solids, mixing of content with digestive juices, and emptying of chyme into the small intes-

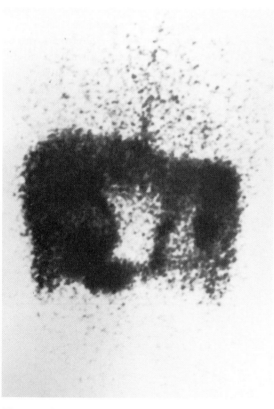

Figure 5. Gamma camera scintiphoto showing reflux into the oesophagus extending to the upper border of the camera at the suprasternal notch. The patient had had a total gastrectomy and an end-to-side oesophagojejunostomy with a long entero-anastomosis, which clearly does not protect against reflux. Reprinted with permission from Donovan et al, 1982.

tine—are abolished or greatly impaired by total gastrectomy. The loss of the pylorus results in entero-oesophageal reflux and its attendant risk of oesophagitis. The loss of the gastro-oesophageal sphincter leads to reflux of enteric content back into the oesophagus which adds to the inflammatory reaction in the oesophagus. The risk of oesophagitis after total gastrectomy is especially pronounced if the oesophagus is anatomosed to the side of the intact small intestine or directly to the duodenum. In a scintigraphic study, Donovan et al (1982) found that the end-to-side oesophago-jejunostomy was not successful in diverting bile from the oesophagus and reflux was always associated with severe symptoms (Figure 5). Anastomosing the oesophagus to the end of a 45-cm jejunal Roux-en-Y limb has decreased the incidence of reflux alkaline oesophagitis.

The interposition of a pouch made of small bowel between the oesophagus and the small bowel after total gastrectomy has been described (Huguier et al, 1976). One type of pouch reconstruction has an isoperistaltic inlet to prevent reflux and an antiperistaltic outlet to slow emptying. Another uses a variation of the Roux-en-Y reconstruction, in which the Roux limb and end-to-side oesophagojejunostomy is anastomosed side-to-side to itself at two sites (Lygi-dakis, 1984). In spite of theoretical advantages, such pouches are not obviously so superior to simple end-to-end oesophagojejunostomy that their routine use is warranted. Generally speaking, Roux-en-Y anastomosis with the leading of duodenal secretions into the digestive tract at a point at least 45 cm below the oesophagus is the most attractive procedure.

Scintigraphic studies after total gastrectomy and Roux-en-Y reconstruction have shown that solid food passes rapidly from the oesophagus through the Roux limb and becomes uniformly distributed through long segments of small bowel (Pellegrini et al, 1986) (Figure 6). Patients with gastrectomy actually have a prolonged transit time through the small bowel in comparison with healthy people. The proximal jejunum does not act as a reservoir, but because the transit time through the small bowel is prolonged and because the Roux limb empties itself rapidly, a meal of

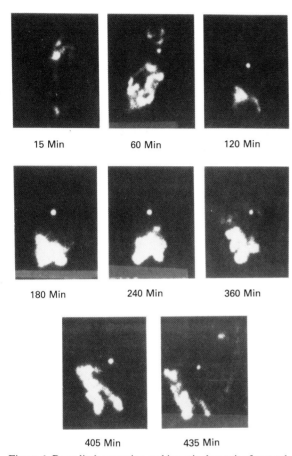

15 Min   60 Min   120 Min

180 Min   240 Min   360 Min

405 Min   435 Min

Figure 6. Roux limb emptying and intestinal transit after total gastrectomy. Reprinted with permission from Pellegrini et al, 1986.

a normal size can usually be consumed. These findings further support the idea that artificial gastric pouches are not important after total gastrectomy.

There are limited data from humans as to the effect of gastric resection on the motility of the small bowel. As mentioned above, Pellegrini and colleagues (1986) have shown that the small intestinal transit may be prolonged after total gastrectomy. However, in experiments in dogs (Heppel et al, 1984), the migrating motor complexes were retained even after total gastrectomy, but the initiation of a fed pattern came more promptly after the operation, probably as a consequence of the early entrance of food into the small bowel (Figure 7). Normal interdigestive migrating motor complexes have also been observed after subtotal gastrectomy in man (Malagelada et al, 1986).

Vagotomy

Three types of vagotomy are in use today: proximal gastric vagotomy, selective gastric vagotomy and truncal vagotomy (Figure 8). In proximal gastric vagotomy, the vagal branches to the gastric fundus and corpus are divided, while those to the antrum and pylorus (the nerves of Latarjet) and to the remaining abdominal viscera are left intact. Selective gastric vagotomy consists of division of

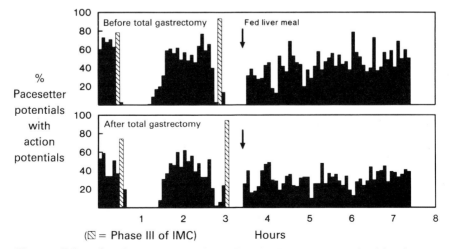

Figure 7. Effect of total gastrectomy and oesophagoduodenostomy on canine jejunal myoelectric activity during fasting and after feeding a 200 g liver meal. Reprinted with permission from Heppell et al, 1984.

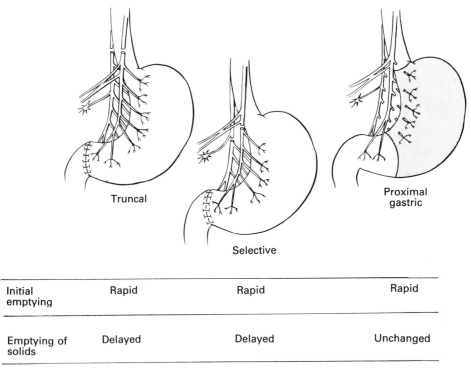

	Truncal	Selective	Proximal gastric
Initial emptying	Rapid	Rapid	Rapid
Emptying of solids	Delayed	Delayed	Unchanged

Figure 8. Three different types of gastric vagotomy. Effect on gastric motility is schematically outlined.

the vagal nerves to the entire stomach, but not those to the other abdominal viscera. In truncal vagotomy not only the vagal nerves to the stomach are divided but also those to other abdominal viscera are severed. The latter two vagotomies are usually combined with a so-called 'drainage' operation, such as pyloroplasty or gastroenterostomy. In contrast, proximal gastric vagotomy does not require a drainage procedure. All three types of vagotomy have been widely employed in the surgical treatment of peptic ulcer.

Proximal Gastric Vagotomy

Proximal gastric vagotomy abolishes the receptive relaxation and impairs the accommodation of the proximal stomach. Receptive relaxation occurs with the onset of swallowing. The proximal stomach relaxes to receive the bolus, keeping intragastric pressure low as the stomach fills. Accommodation to distension also occurs with gastric filling. Both receptive relaxation and

accommodation are vagally mediated functions. Both are impaired by vagotomy. After vagotomy, intragastric pressure increases to larger values with eating and gastric distension compared to before vagotomy. As a consequence, the ability of the stomach to store chyme is diminished.

The larger increases in intragastric pressure that occur with gastric filling after the vagotomy lead to early satiety and more rapid gastric emptying of liquids (Wilbur and Kelly, 1973; Lavigne et al, 1979). The speeding of gastric emptying occurs mainly in the first 10 minutes after a liquid meal is introduced, with about 50% of the meal emptying in this period. The initial rapid gastric emptying is followed by a nearly normal rate of emptying, despite the fact that a large volume of fluid may still be present in the stomach. Fortunately, proximal gastric vagotomy seldom accelerates the rate of gastric emptying sufficiently to cause dumping and diarrhoea.

Proximal gastric vagotomy does not greatly disturb the motor properties of the distal stomach.

After the operation, the oral corporal gastric pace-maker continues to generate cyclic changes in potential at a regular rhythm and with a frequency of about 3 cycles/minute (Hinder and Kelly, 1977). These cycles, which are called pacesetter potentials, sweep distally through the gastric wall from the pacemaker to the pylorus, phasing the onset of action potentials and hence of contractions.

These cycles are still propagated in a distal direction after proximal gastric vagotomy. The rate of propagation is unchanged. Moreover, the strength of antral peristaltic contractions is not greatly altered. Gastric trituration and emptying of digestible solids and gastric emptying of indigestible solids are delayed slightly in the immediate postoperative period, but return to normal within a few weeks or months (Wilkinson and Johnston, 1973; Lopasso et al, 1982). Also, the distal gastric and pyloric mechanisms that maintain gastric continence for solids and prevent duodenogastric reflux are not impaired by the operation. Thus, duodenogastric reflux is seldom found after proximal gastric vagotomy.

Truncal Vagotomy and Selective Gastric (Total Gastric) Vagotomy

In contrast to proximal gastric vagotomy, truncal vagotomy and selective gastric vagotomy alter the electrical and motor patterns of the distal stomach. The stabilizing effect of the vagal nerves on the pattern of the gastric pacesetter potentials is removed, allowing ectopic pacemakers to appear in the distal stomach (Kelly and Code, 1977). These pacemakers, firing at rapid rates of 4–10 cycles/minute (tachygastria), may suppress the natural gastric pacemaker, capture the gastric smooth muscle, and destroy the usual orderly pattern of aborally directed gastric peristalsis (Figure 9). These potentials are propagated orally as well as aborally. During such dysrhythmias, co-ordinated gastric peristalsis cannot occur, and gastric emptying of solids is slowed. Gastric stasis, distension, nausea and vomiting result. Furtunately, these disturbed patterns are uncommon, especially after the first postoperative week.

Truncal and selective vagotomy also disrupt the

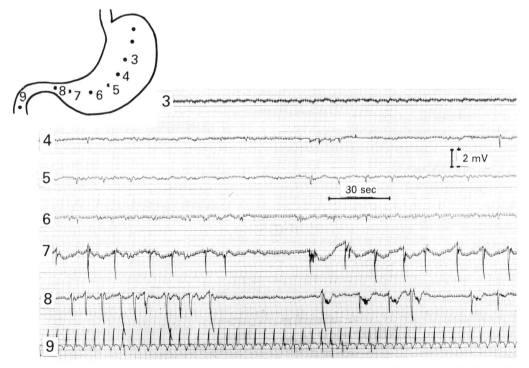

Figure 9. Disorganized canine gastric myoelectric activity one week after transthoracic vagotomy. Reprinted with permission from Kelly and Code, 1977.

initiation of action potentials, usually brought about by vagal stimuli during the fed state. Action potentials are the electrical counterpart of contractions. With fewer action potentials after vagotomy, fewer and weaker contractions occur. Impaired antral trituration of gastric solids results, so that the time required for gastric trituration and emptying of solids is prolonged.

Indigestible solids are also emptied poorly after truncal and selective gastric vagotomies (Mroz and Kelly, 1977). Materials left after meals, such as indigestible fibre, are ordinarily moved distally by cyclically recurring bursts of contractions that appear in the stomach at about 3-hour intervals during fasting. The vagal nerves have a role in regulating these cycles (Marik and Code, 1975). After truncal vagotomy, the cycles are more irregular in rhythm, the periods are shorter, and the bursts of contractions briefer or even absent (Diamant et al, 1980; Malagelada et al, 1980). As a consequence, gastric emptying of debris left over after a meal is slowed or abolished. Patients may note that indigestible portions of foods can be regurgitated from the stomach days after their ingestion.

The gastric stasis of digestible and indigestible solids after selective gastric or truncal vagotomy requires that an additional manoeuvre be done with the vagotomies to speed gastric emptying. Pyloroplasty and gastroenterostomy have been the two procedures usually employed in this situation. They decrease resistance to outflow from the stomach and so usually speed gastric emptying of solids. However, the size of solid particles allowed to empty after the drainage operation is greater than the size that empties from the intact stomach. The intact stomach retains solids greater than 1 mm in diameter for continued trituration by antral peristalsis. After the drainage operations, particles larger than 1 mm are allowed to empty prematurely. Moreover, the loss of the pyloric barricade allows reflux of enteric contents into the stomach.

Parasympathetic nervous interruption to the small bowel brought about by truncal vagotomy has no obvious effect on resting small bowel motility during fasting. Malagelada et al (1986) have observed frequent although normally propa-

gated phase III activity during fasting and also that the phase II activity after vagotomy is often shortened or even absent.

After vagotomy, the physiological rearrangement of the motility after feeding is not as prompt and induction of a fed state requires a higher caloric load in comparison with nonvagotomized individuals (Marik and Code, 1975). It is a matter of speculation whether or not this alteration is responsible for the postvagotomy diarrhoea.

Other Gastric Operations

Exposure and Handling of Stomach

Exposure and palpation of the stomach at surgery slow the frequency and disorganize the rhythm of the gastric pacesetter potentials, and temporarily abolish action potentials, and hence contractions. These changes, which last 6–24 hours, are probably responsible for the slow gastric emptying noted after operation.

Gastrotomy

When incising the stomach, the surgeon needs to consider the gastric pacemaker and the fact that the longitudinal muscle of the stomach propagates the gastric pacesetter potentials. Because incisions that cut across the longitudinal muscle disrupt propagation temporarily, they are more likely to disturb gastric peristalsis and gastric emptying of solids than would incisions parallel to the longitudinal muscle.

Pyloroplasty

Pyloroplasty disturbs gastric emptying in much the same way as distal gastrectomy or antrectomy.

Gastrojejunostomy, side-to-side

After gastrojejunostomy, gastric contents leave the stomach by two routes. Some are discharged through the stomach into the efferent jejunal limb, whence they proceed into the small intestine. If there is no obstruction at the gastric outlet, however, more of the content exits via the gastroduodenal junction into the duodenum. The chyme discharged into the duodenum is propelled into the proximal jejunum, whence it can re-enter the stomach through the stoma. This re-entrance of gastric contents into the stomach accounts for the fact that the net rate of gastric emptying of liquids may be slower after gastro-jejunostomy than before. Since bile and pancreatic juice, as well as chyme, can enter the stomach through the stoma, bilious vomiting and alkaline gastritis may occur.

Entero-enteroanastomosis

The side-to-side entero-enteroanastomosis according to Braun is commonly performed in Europe between the afferent and efferent loop after a gastrojejunostomy (Figure 10). The reason given is that this connection between the loops should protect against obstruction of the afferent loop (so called afferent loop syndrome). Because bile and pancreatico-duodenal juice can flow in both directions through the anastomosis, it does not, however, protect against bile reflux to the stomach.

Gastrojejunostomy, Roux-en-Y

In the Roux-en-Y anastomosis, the proximal jejunum is divided about 20 cm distal to the ligament of Treitz. The distal cut end is brought into the epigastrium, where it is anastomosed end-to-side or end-to-end to the gastric remnant. The proximal cut end is anastomosed to the side of the mid-jejunum 40 cm distal to the gastro-jejunostomy (Figure 11). The procedure is designed to prevent reflux of duodenal content into the stomach. Since there is a risk of jejunal ulceration adjacent to the stoma, a vagotomy is often added to the Roux-en-Y reconstruction.

Combining vagotomy with Roux-en-Y gastrectomy usually speeds gastric emptying of liquids, but the speeding is less in magnitude than that following the Billroth II anastomosis. Controversy surrounds the emptying of solids after the operation. Some have claimed that solids empty unduly slowly after vagotomy and Roux gastrectomy, because of a hold-up in the stomach and the Roux limb as a result of the vagotomy (Hocking et al, 1981; Vogel et al, 1983). Mathias et al (1985) described seven Roux patients, all of whom had chronic abdominal pain, persistent nausea and

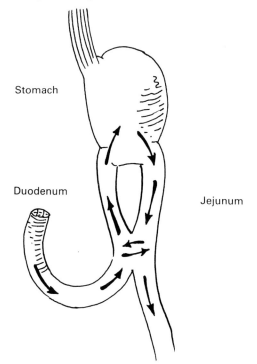

Figure 10. The entero-enteroanastomosis between afferent and efferent jejunal limbs does not protect against bile reflux into the stomach after distal gastrectomy and gastrojejunostomy.

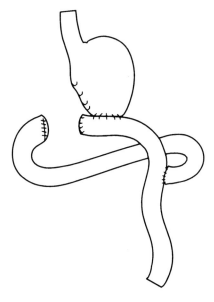

Figure 11. Distal gastrectomy with Roux-en-Y gastro-jejunostomy. The distance between the gastrojejunostomy and the end-to-side jejuno-jejunostomy should be around but not more than 40 cm.

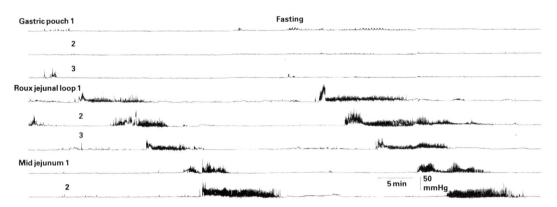

Figure 12. Pressure patterns in a 46-year-old man who had vagotomy and partial gastrectomy with Roux-en-Y gastrojejunal anastomosis. Fasting tracing shows frequent episodes of phase III activity in the efferent loop which migrate normally but have no preceding phase II activity. Reprinted with permission from Malagelada et al, 1986.

intermittent vomiting, leading to a definition of a 'Roux-stasis syndrome'. In a careful evaluation of 234 Roux patients, Gustavsson et al (1987) found Roux-stasis in 30% of patients after gastro-jejunostomy and the development of this syndrome was related to the construction of an especially long limb. Probably the ideal length is around but not over 40 cm.

The slower emptying of solids with the Roux gastrectomy, as compared to the Billroth gas-trectomies, may be due to the appearance of ectopic pacemakers in the Roux limb after the operation. The pacemakers would drive the con-tractions of the limb, or a portion of them, in an oral direction, and, hence, slow gastric emptying. In addition, the incidence and amplitude of jejunal contractions may be increased when the jejunum is positioned as a Roux limb after the gastrectomy (Figure 12). The enhanced contractility would augment resistance to gastric outflow and so slow gastric emptying, especially if the Roux limb is made longer than 40 cm. Further, jejunal con-tractions in the Roux limb may be unco-ordinated.

Treatment

Can the disturbed patterns of gastric motor and electrical activity brought about by surgery be restored to normal? To date, there is little evidence that they can, despite attempts to do so by dietary, medical, and surgical measures.

Patients with rapid gastric emptying due to impaired receptive relaxation and accommodation may be helped by eating slowly, by taking four or five small meals a day, and by ingesting solids and liquids at different times. Such patients should avoid hyperosmolar foods like concentrated sweets, which can precipitate the dumping syn-drome.

The only drugs that are currently showing promise in the treatment of postoperative gastric disorders are the prokinetic drugs, meto-clopramide being the best evaluated example. In some patients who have gastric stasis after oper-ations on the stomach, such drugs speed gastric emptying.

Operations that interpose a segment of jejunum between the stomach and the small bowel (Roux-en-Y) can prevent bile from entering the stomach when duodenal-gastric reflux is present. Jejunal interpositions have also occasionally been used to slow rapid gastric emptying. It is difficult, however, to determine the length and polarity of the jejunal segment that will slow gastric emptying sufficiently without obstructing the stomach.

Recent experiments in dogs offer hope for patients with postoperative abnormalities of gastric motility. Electrical stimuli delivered to electrodes implanted in the canine stomach have generated pacesetter potentials, so that the fre-quency of peristaltic contractions was speeded or slowed at will (Kelly and Code, 1977). By means of these implanted electrodes, the direction of gastric peristalsis can be reversed and gastric emptying of liquids and solids can be slowed. Pacing of Roux limbs in dogs in a backward direction will delay gastric emptying and could provide a basis for treating humans with postgastrectomy dumping (Cranley et al, 1983).

These exciting experiments suggest the possibility of using electric pacing to control abnormal gastric electrical and motor patterns in human patients. Such pacing could be used either alone or in combination with gastrointestinal hormones known to inhibit or stimulate gastric motility.

Intestinal Operations

This section will describe the motor disorders produced by operations on the small intestine, indicate how the disorders can lead to symptoms, and suggest possible treatments for the disorders.

Transection and Anastomosis

Interruption of intestinal continuity disturbs the myogenic and intrinsic neural activity within the bowel wall. The coupling of the slow waves in the small bowel is disrupted so that entrainment of distal bowel segments by proximal oscillations of higher frequency is lost. The slow wave frequency distal to an anastomosis decreases to a lower value (Sarna et al, 1971a, 1971b). Since the slow wave frequency determines the maximum frequency of contractions, the segment of gut distal to an anastomosis contracts at a lower maximum frequency.

The magnitude of the decrease depends upon the site of transection. A transection in the proximal small intestine results in a greater decrease than a transection in the distal small intestine because the intrinsic frequency gradient is steeper in the proximal small intestine than more distally. The inderdigestive migrating motility complex will pass an anastomosis relatively unhindered.

The effect of transection and re-anastomosis with end-to-end technique on intestinal transit has not been studied in man. From a theoretical point, it should increase because of the decreased maximum frequency of contraction but clinical

experience speaks against any important disturbance.

Resection

Resection of a part of the small bowel is a common procedure in the treatment of small bowel disease like Crohn's disease, benign and malignant tumours and incarcerated bowel due to adhesions or irreducible hernias. Often, a small bowel resection has to be done due to small bowel fistulas or severe adhesions after previous surgical procedures. Usually the resection involves only a small part of the small intestine so that the resorptive reserve capacity will cover the loss completely. After massive small bowel resection, however, the assimilation of nutrients might be disturbed leading to the short bowel syndrome.

Jejunal resections are usually tolerated better than ileal resections. This may be, in part, because the ileum can slow transit through the jejunum by neurally mediated and hormonally mediated inhibitory mechanisms, the so-called ileal brake. The net result is that small bowel transit, hence small bowel digestion and absorption, may be only slightly impaired after jejunectomy. In contrast, with ileal resections, the ileal braking mechanism is lost, leading to more rapid small intestinal transit and impaired digestion and absorption.

With extensive resections of jejunum-ileum, transit from mouth to colon is greatly speeded. The rapid transit plus the loss of absorbing surface leads to malabsorption, diarrhoea, weight loss, nutritional deficiencies, and inanition, the so-called short bowel syndrome. Reversal of segments of small intestine slows transit in the small bowel (see below) and so may improve absorption in subjects with the short bowel syndrome.

Ileal Pouches

Construction of a pouch out of the terminal ileum is a common procedure to create a reservoir for luminal contents. When connected to the skin through an out-flow nipple, the patient can empty the pouch at regular intervals and avoids having an incontinent ileostomy. When connected to the dentate line of the anus, most patients can empty the pouch the normal way with retained continence.

Pouch motility has been evaluated by manometry and by scintigraphy and by the barostat.

As evaluated by manometry, the jejuno-ileal motility is not greatly altered by construction of the pouch (Stryker et al, 1985a). Large amplitude waves were observed and they were considered secondary to the increased demands of the small bowel to store content.

Pouch Distensibility and Capacity

In health, the rectum adapts or accommodates to intraluminal distension. Only small increases in intraluminal pressure occur as intraluminal volume is gradually expanded (Figure 13). The mean ± SEM change in volume per change in pressure among seven healthy volunteers was 16.8 ± 2 ml/cm H_2O (Heppell et al, 1982a). A volume of 400 ml was usually readily accepted.

The goal with an ileal pouch is to create a 'neorectum' that would be as distensible and capacious as the healthy rectum. Initially, a straight ileal segment was used to form the neorectum (Beart et al, 1982), rather than the ileal pouch we use today. Many patients with the straight ileo-anal anastomosis had daytime continence, but experienced soiling at night. Stool frequency was great, initially six to 12 stools per day and four to six at

night. A gradual reduction in frequency and an improvement in continence took place over the early months after operation. These improvements were found in association with some dilatation of the distal ileum as it formed a larger reservoir. A detailed physiological study of 12 adult patients four months or more after the straight ileo-anal anastomosis, however, showed that the capacity and distensibility of the neorectum were still considerably less than those of the healthy rectum. An inverse relationship was found between stool frequency and both the capacity and distensibility (Heppell et al, 1982a). The larger the capacity and the greater the distensibility, the fewer the number of stools per day. Patients with a small capacity and poor distensibility had upwards of 20 stools per day. A longer term clinical follow-up of 50 adult patients with a straight ileo-anal anastomosis disclosed an eventual failure rate of 32% usually because of excessive stooling and incontinence (Telander and Dozois, 1984).

To facilitate the early development of the neorectum with the straight ileo-anal anastomosis, some of our paediatric patients were instructed to use balloon dilatation of the distal bowel during the interval between ileo-anal anastomosis and ileostomy closure. This procedure did reduce stool frequency at both three and six months after ileostomy closure (Telander and Perrault, 1981).

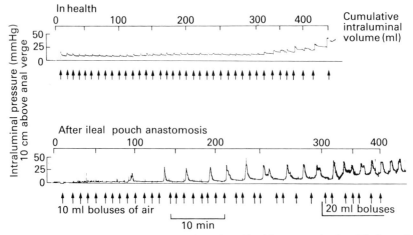

Figure 13. Pattern of pressure waves on distension of healthy rectum (top) and ileal pouch after ileal pouch-anal anastomosis (bottom). Reprinted with permission from Kelly and Pemberton 1987.

These observations, coupled with the physiological results showing the poor capacity and compliance of the undilated straight ileo-anal anastomosis, suggested that the incorporation of an ileal pouch to provide a faecal reservoir above the ileo-anal anastomosis would improve results.

Experience with the Kock pouch in the 1970s had confirmed that an ileal pouch could be constructed with a capacity sufficient to hold one-third or one-fourth of the daily faecal volume. Such pouches required intubation three to four times per day (Kock, 1969). Follow-up of patients with a Kock pouch showed few long-term metabolic consequences (Nilsson et al, 1979), despite bacterial overgrowth in both the pouch (Brandberg et al, 1972) and jejunum (Kelly et al, 1983). Absorption from the pouch was similar to that of the ileum proximal to a conventional ileostomy (Gadacz et al, 1977). The construction of a pouch did not appreciably alter the patterns of ileal electrical or motor activity (Akwari et al, 1980), but the distensibility of the pouch was greater than that of normal ileum. It seemed, thus, that an ileal pouch could be combined successfully with the ileo-anal anastomosis.

A commonly used ileal pouch is the J-shaped ileal pouch made by a side-to-side anastomosis of the distal 30 cm of ileum. The distensibility of the J pouch is similar to the distensibility of the healthy rectum (Figure 13). In our studies, the slope of the pressure–volume curve of the pouch patients during gradual pouch distension was nearly identical to the slope obtained from healthy subjects (O'Connell et al, 1987). The capacity of the pouch (approximately 400 ml) was also similar to the capacity of the healthy rectum.

The satisfactory distensibility and capacity of the ileal pouch are reflected in improved clinical results. Patients with the pouch had fewer stools and less incontinence than those with the straight ileo-anal anastomosis (Taylor et al, 1983a). Again, the more distensible the pouch, the fewer the stools passed per day. Also, pouch distensibility prior to ileostomy closure correlated well with the postclosure stool frequency, the ability of the pouch to distend being reflected in a lower stool frequency (Heppell et al, 1983). Thus, the J pouch provides a distensible, compliant, and capacious neorectum, a factor contributing to satisfactory postoperative faecal continence.

Pouch Motility

In health, the rectum exhibits only infrequent and small amplitude (mean ± SEM amplitude, 10 ± 3 cm H_2O) contractions, even when distended

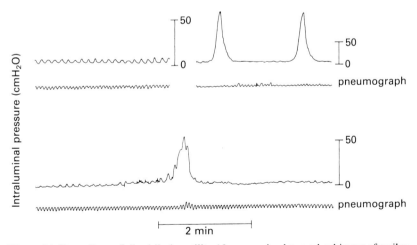

Figure 14. Recordings of distal ileal motility 10 cm proximal to anal sphincter after ileo-anal anastomosis in man. Top left: Changes in intraluminal pressure of small amplitude and duration. Top right: Pressure changes of large amplitude and duration. Bottom: Pressure changes of both small and large amplitude. (Reprinted with permission from Heppell et al, 1982b).

to volumes as large as 400 ml. Motility in the ileum differs. Code et al (1957) studied ileal motility in subjects with a conventional ileostomy, and Heppell et al (1982b), who studied ileal motility after straight ileo-anal anastomosis, described two types of ileal motor waves. The first type was a wave of small amplitude and short duration, while the second type had a large amplitude and a long duration (Figure 14). The large waves propagated distally and were associated with the expulsion of ileal content. The stimulus for large waves was luminal distension. While similar large waves have been identified in Kock pouches, the construction of a reservoir greatly increased the amount of content accommodated before they appeared (Akwari et al, 1980; Berglund et al, 1984).

To compare the contractile pattern of ileal pouches in patients to that of the healthy rectum, we studied the motility of the ileal pouch using open-tipped perfusion catheters and a flaccid, pressure-sensitive, distending bag placed in the pouch. It seemed possible that the differences in continence among patients were related to differences in the motility of the reservoirs. We (Taylor et al, 1983b; Stryker et al, 1986; O'Connell et al, 1987) and others (Rabau et al, 1982) found that large waves (mean ± SEM amplitude, 49 ± 2 cm H_2O) appeared in the pouches in response to distension (Figure 13). Pressures achieved in the pouch during the large waves sometimes even exceeded the resting anal sphincteric tone. When the large waves were present, our patients experienced the desire to evacuate. Voluntary squeeze contraction of the external anal sphincter was then required to maintain continence. Nonetheless, leakage of stool occasionally occurred. The frequency and amplitude of the large waves were found to increase with time during fasting and following a meal, presumably as the pouch filled. With evacuation, the large waves promptly subsided (Stryker et al, 1985a). It seemed, therefore, that the threshold volume at which the waves appear in the ileal pouch may be an important determinant of postoperative stool frequency (O'Connell et al, 1987). As the threshold is a function of pouch capacity and distensibility, it would explain why both of these functions are also determinants of clinical outcome.

Clearly, the presence of large amplitude contractions in the ileal pouch with pouch distension contrasts markedly with the absence of such contractions in the healthy rectum distended to the same degree. The large amplitude ileal pouch contractions are one factor that leads to less than perfect continence in the patients after operation.

Pouch Evacuation

Healthy individuals can evacuate the distal bowel voluntarily and spontaneously. Most use the Valsalva manoeuvre during faecal discharge to enhance the rate of faecal flow.

After operation, evacuation also occurred spontaneously and voluntarily; none of our patients with a J-shaped pouch required intubation for evacuation. As in the healthy rectum, no obstruction to defecation by a segment of bowel distal to the reservoir was present. The pouch itself was anastomosed to the anal canal. The apex of the pouch lay partly within the pelvis and partly below the pelvic diaphragm within a short, 3–5 cm distal rectal muscular cuff.

Another type of pouch is the triple loop, S-shaped, ileal pouch, described by Parks et al (1980). The Parks-type pouch had been previously attempted in dogs, but was abandoned because of an unacceptable mortality from sepsis (Valiente and Bacon, 1955). The initial results that Parks' group described in patients were generally good, all patients having daytime continence and an acceptable stool frequency. However, pouch emptying was a major problem; only half of the patients could evacuate spontaneously, the remainder having to use intermittent catheterization to evacuate. Long-term follow-up of these patients revealed that only 40% continued to evacuate spontaneously (Nicholls et al, 1984). Fonkalsrud (1981) experienced similar difficulties in five patients with an S pouch. We have used the S pouch on seven patients; one patient requires a catheter to empty the pouch. Animal studies of the S pouch indicated that the length of the efferent limb leading from the pouch to the anus was critical to efficient emptying (Rosemurgy et al, 1983). Evaluation of S-pouch function using fluoroscopy confirmed that a shorter efferent limb

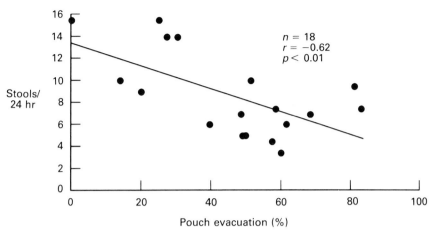

Figure 15. Relationship of the completeness of ileal pouch evacuation to stool frequency after ileal pouch-anal anastomosis. Reprinted with permission from Stryker et al, 1986.

was associated with a more efficient evacuation of the pouch (Pescatori et al, 1983). Nonetheless, the presence of an efferent ileal limb of any length interposed between an ileal pouch and the anal canal has the potential of impeding evacuation of the pouch.

The lateral-lateral pouch of Fonkalsrud (1982) was also considered as a means of creating a neo-rectum. This technique requires a mid-ileal transection during its construction, a manoeuvre that might possibly impair the blood supply to the distal portion of the pouch. We were also concerned about the efficiency of evacuation of the lateral-lateral pouch. This pouch also has an efferent limb connecting the pouch to the anal canal. For these reasons, we decided against using this approach.

As stated above, incomplete evacuation of the

S pouch has been found to be a cause of poor postoperative results (Parks et al, 1980). Therefore, it was of interest to study the completeness of pouch emptying in our J-pouch patients. Incomplete evacuation of any type of pouch would reduce the volume of stool required to again distend the pouch to its threshold volume, when large pressure waves and an urge to defecate would then appear. Using recovery of a semi-solid artificial stool instilled into the pouch to estimate efficiency of evacuation, we found that patients who emptied their pouch less completely had a greater daily stool frequency than those with more complete pouch emptying (Figure 15) (Stryker et al, 1986). However, most patients studied could evacuate their pouches nearly as completely as could healthy persons. Patients evacuated $57 \pm 3\%$ of a semi-solid, artificial stool instilled per rectum

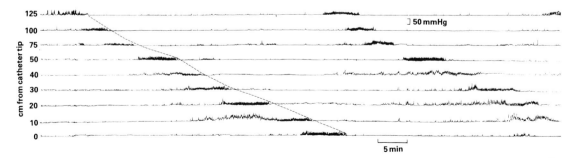

Figure 16. Small intestinal migrating motor complexes during fasting in a patient after ileal pouch-anal anastomosis. The catheter tip is in the distal ileum. The broken line indicates distal propagation of the complex. Reprinted with permission from Stryker et al, 1985a.

compared to $73 \pm 7\%$ evacuated by healthy volunteers ($P > 0.05$) (O'Connell et al, 1987). Moreover, the voluntary onset of evacuation, the rate of faecal flow, and the use of the Valsalva manoeuvre to facilitate evacuation were in general similar to what was found in health. Thus, the fact that faecal evacuation is not greatly disturbed after ileal J pouch-anal anastomosis likely contributes to the satisfactory faecal continence present after operation.

Enteric Motility Proximal to Pouch

In health, migrating motor complexes sweep distally through the jejuno-ileum during fasting at about two-hourly intervals. These complexes are abolished by feeding, which induces intermittent contractions in the small intestine. Large pressure waves, similar to those observed in the ileal pouch in response to distension, have been observed in the distal 20–30 cm of healthy ileum (Quigley et al, 1984). They sometimes propagate across the ileocaecal valve. After operation, the migrating motor complexes were still present in the jejuno-ileum (Figure 16), and they were readily abolished by feeding. Large ileal pressure waves similar to those found in health were also present after ileal pouch-anal anastomosis, but they arose more proximally, perhaps because chyme is stored in more proximal bowel after the operation. Unlike the large amplitude waves generated *de novo* in the ileal pouch, these more proximal waves did not result in a desire to defecate (Stryker et al, 1985b). The abnormalities described by Summers et al (1983) in mechanical small bowel obstruction were not seen in our studies. Overall, both fasting and fed motor patterns in the proximal small bowel remained largely undisturbed after the operation.

Nonetheless, the pattern of ileal contractions after ileo-anal anastomosis must differ from the pattern of contractions in the descending colon and sigmoid colon in health. The ileum may develop more propulsive waves when distended than does the distal colon. Such ileal propulsion could stress the mechanisms for continence more than would the colonic waves. This may be a factor leading to impaired continence after ileo-anal anastomosis.

Treatment

Decreasing the fat content of the diet in subjects with intestinal hurry after small intestinal operations may decrease diarrhoea. The opioid drugs, codeine, Lomotil and Imodium, also slow transit, improve absorption and decrease diarrhoea.

Insertion of an antiperistaltic segment has been

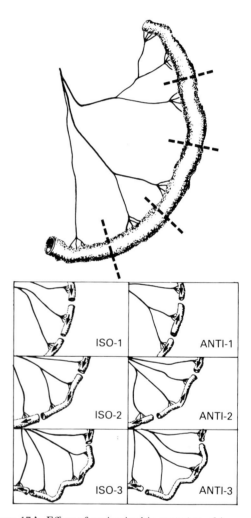

Figure 17A. Effect of antiperistaltic segments of increasing length on small bowel propulsion in rats. The interpolated segments were made 2, 4 or 6 cm long and the propulsion in antiperistaltic segments (ANTI-1, ANTI-2, ANTI-3) was compared with that isoperistaltic segments (ISO-1, ISO-2, ISO-3).

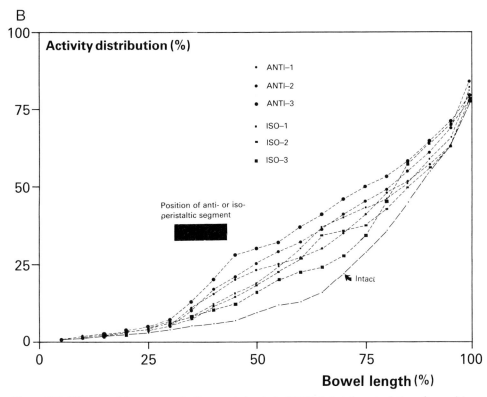

Figure 17B. The propulsion was markedly retarded only in ANTI-3, but the retardation of propulsion through the segment was fully compensated for by a faster transport rate through the distal small bowel. Reproduced with permission from Gustavsson, 1979.

tried in an attempt to improve absorption from a critically short small bowel after massive small bowel resection. The length of the interposed segment has to be chosen accurately so that a retardation of intestinal propagation is achieved without provoking an ileus or subileus state. In humans, the optimum length of small bowel is between 10 and 15 cm. Experimental studies have been performed to clarify the mechanisms for the remedial effect of this operation in the clinical setting (Gustavsson, 1979). In rats, the small bowel length corresponding to the human length of 10–15 cm is about 2 cm based on the relation between length and width (Figure 17). This length did not, however, affect the propagation of a radioactive test substance. The test segment had to be made 6 cm long before a clear-cut reduction in intestinal propulsion could be noted. Astonishingly enough, the slow propagation proximal and through the interposed antiperistaltic segment was fully compensated by increased transport rate through the more distally located segments.

Pacing a segment of intestine may have a role in treatment of these disorders in the future. Pacing is accomplished by applying suitable electrical stimuli to the muscularis propria greater than the natural pacesetter potential frequency recorded at the locus of the stimulating electrode. Most information of intestinal pacing has been obtained from experiments in the dog. Entrainment of pacesetter potentials in the intact canine small bowel is possible only in the proximal part where the frequency is high (19 cycles/min).

The myoelectric properties of the human intestine appear similar to those of the dog, although the pacesetter potentials appear with slower frequency (12 cycles/min) in comparison with the dog. However, Richter and Kelly (1986) were able

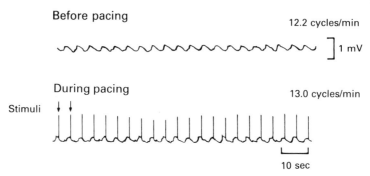

Figure 18. Effect of pacing on human jejunal pacesetter potentials in a patient with intact jejunum. Cycles/min = PP frequency. Reprinted with permission from Richter and Kelly, 1986.

to entrain jejunal pacesetter potentials of only one out of nine patients in whom pacing was undertaken with similar techniques as that used in dogs (Figure 18).

Transplantation of the small bowel will likely have an increasing role in the future. Dogs with autotransplanted jejuno-ileum have lived for periods beyond one year with an apparently healthy life-style. Diarrhoea, noted in the first week after transplantation, subsides after two to three months. Once the rejection phenomenon is resolved and the graft-versus-host response is controlled, transplantation of small bowel in humans can begin.

Acknowledgement

Supported in part by United States Public Health Service, National Institutes of Health Grants DK18278 and DK34988.

References

Akwari, O. E., Kelly, K. A., and Phillips, S. F., (1980), Myoelectric and motor patterns of continent pouch and conventional ileostomy. *Surg. Gynecol. Obstet.*, **150**: 363–71.

Beart, R. W., Dozois, R. R., and Kelly, K. A., (1982), Ileoanal anastomosis in the adult. *Surg. Gynecol. Obstet.*, **154**: 826–8.

Berglund, B., Kock, N. G., and Myrvold, H. E., (1984), Volume capacity and pressure characteristics of the continent ileostomy reservoir. *Scand. J. Gastroenterol.*, **19**: 683–90.

Brandberg, A., Kock, N. G., and Philipson, B., (1972), Bacterial flora in intraabdominal ileostomy reservoir. *Gastroenterology*, **63**: 413–16.

Code, C. F., Rogers, A. G., Schlegel, J., Hightower, N. C., and Bargen, J. A., (1957), Motility patterns in the terminal ileum: studies on two patients with ulcerative colitis and ileal stomas. *Gastroenterology*, **32**: 651–65.

Cranley, B., Kelly, K. A., Go, V. L., and McNichols, L. A., (1983), Enhancing the anti-dumping effect of Roux gastrojejunostomy with intestinal pacing. *Ann. Surg.*, **198**: 516–24.

Diamant, N. E., Hall, K., Mui, H., and El-Sharkawy, T. Y., (1980), Vagal control of the feeding motor pattern in the lower esophageal sphincter, stomach, and small intestine of dog. In: *Gastrointestinal Motility* (Ed. Christensen, J.) pp. 365–70. Raven Press, New York.

Donovan, I. A., Fielding, J. W. L., Bradley, H., Sorgi, M., and Harding, L. K., (1982), Bile diversion after total gastrectomy. *Br. J. Surg.*, **69**: 389–90.

Fonkalsrud, E. W., (1981), Endorectal ileal pullthrough with lateral ileal reservoir for benign colorectal disease. *Ann. Surg.*, **194**: 761–6.

Fonkalsrud, E. W., (1982), Endorectal ileal pullthrough with ileal reservoir for ulcerative colitis and polyposis. *Am. J. Surg.*, **144**: 81–7.

Gadacz, T. R., Kelly, K. A., and Phillips, S. F., (1977), The continent ileal pouch: absorptive and motor features. *Gastroenterology*, **72**: 1287–91.

Gustavsson, S., (1979), Transport of small bowel contents after interposition of an antiperistaltic jejunal segment in the rat. *Eur. Surg. Res.*, **11**: 381–91.

Gustavsson, S., Ilstrup, D. M., Morrison, P., and Kelly, K. A., (1987), The Roux-stasis syndrome after gastrectomy. *Am. J. Surg.* (in press).

Heppell, J., Kelly, K. A., Phillips, S. F., Beart, R. W., Telander, R. L., and Perrault, J., (1982a), Physiologic aspects of continence after colectomy, mucosal proctectomy, and endorectal ileo-anal anastomosis. *Ann. Surg.*, **195:** 435–43.

Heppell, J., Pemberton, J. H., Kelly, K. A., and Phillips, S. F., (1982b), Ileal motility after endorectal ileo-anal anastomosis. *Surg. Gastroenterol.*, **1:** 123–7.

Heppell, J., Taylor, B. M., Beart, R. W., Dozois, R. R., and Kelly, K. A., (1983), Predicting outcome after endorectal ileoanal anastomosis. *Canad. J. Surg.*, **26:** 132–4.

Heppell, J., Taylor, B. M., and Kelly, K. A., (1984), Gastric influences of canine small intestinal myoelectric activity. *Dig. Dis. Sci.*, **29:** 849–52.

Hinder, R. A., and Kelly, K. A., (1977), Human gastric pacesetter potential. Site of origin, spread and response to gastric transection and proximal gastric vagotomy. *Am. J. Surg.*, **133:** 29–33.

Hocking, M. P., Vogel, S. B., Falasca, C. A., and Woodward, E. R., (1981), Delayed gastric emptying of liquids and solids following Roux-en-Y biliary diversion. *Am. Surg.*, **194:** 494–501.

Huguier, M., Lancret, J. M., Bernard, P. F., Baschet, C., and LeHernand, F., (1976), Functional results of different reconstructive procedures after total gastrectomy. *Br. J. Surg.*, **63:** 704–8.

Kelly, K. A., and Code, C. F., (1977), Duodenal-gastric reflux and slowed gastric emptying by electrical pacing of the canine duodenal pacesetter potential. *Gastroenterology*, **72:** 429–33.

Kelly, K. A., and Pemberton, J. H., (1987), Mechanisms of fecal continence: alterations with ileal pouch-anal anastomosis. In: *Cellular Physiology and Clinical Studies of Gastrointestinal Smooth Muscle.* (Ed. Szurszewski, J. H.) pp. 399–418. Elsevier, Amsterdam.

Kelly, D. G., Phillips, S. F., Kelly, K. A., Weinstein, W. M., and Gilchrist, M. J., (1983), Dysfunction of the continent ileostomy: clinical features and bacteriology. *Gut*, **24:** 193–201.

Kock, N. G., (1969), Intraabdominal 'reservoir' in patients with permanent ileostomy. *Arch. Surg.*, **99:** 229–31.

Lavigne, M. E., Wiley, Z. D., Martin, P., Way, L. W., Meyer, J. H., Sleisenger, M. H., and MacGregor, I. L., (1979), Gastric, pancreatic and biliary secretion and the rate of gastric emptying after parietal cell vagotomy. *Am. J. Surg.*, **138:** 644–51.

Lopasso, F. P., Bruno de Mello, J., Meneguetti, J., Gama-Rodrigues, J., and Pinotti, H. W., (1982), Study of gastric emptying in patients with duodenal ulcer before and after proximal gastric vagotomy. The use of solid and digestible particles labelled with ^{99m}Tc. *Surg. Gastroenterology*, **1:** 321–6.

Lygidakis, N. J., (1984), Long term results of a new method of reconstruction for continuity of the alimentary tract after total gastrectomy. *Surg. Gynecol. Obstet.*, **158:** 335–8.

Malagelada, J. R., Rees, W. D. W., Mazzotta, L., and Go, V. L. W., (1980), Gastric motor abnormalities in diabetic and postvagotomy gastroparesis: effect of metoclopramide and bethanechol. *Gastroenterology*, **78:** 286–93.

Malagelada, J. R., Camilleri, M., and Stanghellini, V., (1986), *Manometric Diagnosis of Gastrointestinal Motility Disorders*. Thieme Inc, New York.

Marik, F., and Code, C. F., (1975), Control of the interdigestive myoelectric activity in dogs by the vagus nerves and pentagastrin. *Gastroenterology*, **69:** 387–95.

Mathias, J. R., Fernandez, A., Sninsky, C. A., Clench, M. H., and Davis, R. H., (1985), Nausea, vomiting and abdominal pain after Roux-en-Y anastomosis: motility of the jejunal limb. *Gastroenterology*, **88:** 101–7.

Mroz, C. T., and Kelly, K. A., (1977), The role of the extrinsic antral nerves in the regulation of gastric emptying. *Surg., Gynecol. Obstet.*, **145:** 369–77.

Nicholls, R. J., Pescatori, M., Motson, R. W., and Pezim, M. E., (1984), Restorative proctocolectomy with a three loop ileal reservoir for ulcerative colitis and familial adenomatous polyps. *Ann. Surg.*, **199:** 383–8.

Nilsson, L. O., Andersson, H., Hultén, L., Jagenberg, R., Kock, N. G., Myrvold, H. E., and Philipson, B., (1979), Absorption studies in patients six to 10 years after construction of ileostomy reservoirs. *Gut*, **20:** 499–503.

O'Connell, P. R., Pemberton, J. H., Brown, M. L., and Kelly, K. A., (1987), Determinants of stool frequency after ileal 'J' pouch-anal anastomosis. *Am. J. Surg.*, **153:** 157–64.

Parks, A. G., Nicholls, R. J., and Belliveau, P., (1980), Proctocolectomy with ileal reservoir and anal anastomosis. *Br. J. Surg.*, **67:** 533–8.

Pellegrini, C. A., Deveney, C. W., Patti, M. G., Devine, M., and Way, L. W., (1986), Intestinal transit of food after total gastrectomy and Roux-Y esophagoojejunostomy. *Am. J. Surg.*, **151:** 117–24.

Pescatori, M., Manhire, A., and Bartram, C. I., (1983), Evacuation pouchography in the evaluation of ileoanal reservoir function. *Dis. Colon Rectum*, **26:** 265–368.

Quigley, E. M. M., Borody, T. J., Phillips, S. F., Wienbeck, M., Tucker, R. L., and Haddad, A., (1984), Motility of the terminal ileum and ileocecal sphincter in healthy humans. *Gastroenterology*, **87:** 857–66.

Rabau, M. Y., Percy, J. P., and Parks, A. G., (1982), Ileal pelvic reservoir: a correlation between motor patterns and clinical behaviour. *Br. J. Surg.*, **69:** 391–5.

Richter, H. M. III, and Kelly, K. A., (1986), Effect of

transection and pacing on human jejunal pacesetter potentials. *Gastroenterology*, **91**: 1380–5.

Rosemurgy, A. S., Schraut, W. H., and Block, G. E., (1983), The physiologic effects of ileal reservoirs and efferent conduits complementing ileoanal anastomosis: an experimental study in dogs. *Surgery*, **94**: 697–703.

Sarna, S. K., Daniel, E. E., and Kingma, Y. J., (1971a), Stimulation of the electrical control activity of stomach by array of relaxation oscillators. *Am. J. Dig. Dis.*, **17**: 299–310.

Sarna, S. K., Daniel, E. E., and Kingma, Y. J., (1971b), Stimulation of slow wave electrical activity of small intestine. *Am. J. Physiol.*, **221**: 161–75.

Stryker, S. J., Borody, T. J., Phillips, S. F., Kelly, K. A., Dozois, R. R., and Beart, R. W., Jr., (1985a), Motility of the small intestine after proctocolectomy and ileal pouch-anal anastomosis. *Ann. Surg.*, **201**: 351–6.

Stryker, S. J., Daube, J. R., Kelly, K. A., Telander, R. L., Phillips, S. F., Beart, R. W., and Dozois, R. R., (1985b), Anal sphincter electromyography after colectomy, mucosal rectectomy, and ileoanal anastomosis. *Arch. Surg.*, **201**: 713–16.

Stryker, S. J., Kelly, K. A., Phillips, S. F., Dozois, R. R., and Beart, R. W., (1986), Anal and neorectal function after ileal pouch-anal anastomosis. *Ann. Surg.*, **203**: 55–61.

Summers, R. W., Anuras, S., and Green, J., (1983), Jejunal manometry pattern in health, partial intestinal obstruction, and pseudoobstruction. *Gastroenterology*, **85**: 1290–300.

Taylor, B. M., Beart, R. W., Dozois, R. R., Kelly, K. A., and Phillips, S. F., (1983a), Straight ileoanal anas-tomosis vs ileal pouch-anal anastomosis after colectomy and mucosal proctectomy. *Arch. Surg.*, **118**: 696–701.

Taylor, B. M., Cranley, B., Kelly, K. A., Phillips, S. F., Beart, R. W., and Dozois, R. R., (1983b), A clinico-physiological comparison of ileal pouch-anal and straight ileoanal anastomoses. *Ann. Surg.*, **198**: 462–8.

Telander, R. L., and Perrault, J., (1981), Colectomy with rectal mucosectomy and ileoanal anastomosis in young patients: its use in ulcerative colitis and familial polyposis. *Arch. Surg.*, **116**: 623–9.

Telander, R. L., and Dozois, R. R., (1984), Endorectal ileoanal anastomosis. *Problems in General Surgery*, **1**: 39–50.

Valiente, M. A., and Bacon, H. E., (1955), Construction of pouch using 'pantaloon' technique for pull-through of ileum following total colectomy. *Am. J. Surg.*, **90**: 742–50.

Vogel, S. B., Hocking, M. P., and Woodward, E. R., (1983), Radionuclide evaluation of gastric emptying in patients undergoing Roux-Y biliary diversion for alkaline reflux gastritis and postgastrectomy dumping. *Surg. Forum*, **34**: 173–5.

Wilbur, B. G., and Kelly, K. A., (1973), Effect of proximal gastric, complete gastric, and truncal vagotomy on canine gastric electrical activity, motility and emptying. *Ann. Surg.*, **128**: 295–302.

Wilkinson, A. R., and Johnston, D., (1973), Effect of truncal vagotomy, selective vagotomy and highly selective vagotomy in man on gastric emptying and transit of a food-barium meal in man. *Ann. of Surg.*, **178**: 190–3.

V
GASTROINTESTINAL MOTILITY DISORDERS

24
OESOPHAGUS

A.
OESOPHAGEAL DISORDERS

G. Vantrappen, J. Janssens
University Hospital Leuven, Leuven, Belgium

The normal oesophageal motility pattern, consisting of peristaltic contractions in the body of the oesophagus and sphincteric closing and opening mechanisms at both ends of the gullet, may be disordered in several ways. The peristaltic nature of the contractions may be lost, often to be replaced by segmental or simultaneous tertiary contractions. On manometric examination these contractions may be of normal amplitude and duration, may be weak or may be of abnormally high amplitude and long duration. Monophasic pressure waves may be replaced by double peaked waves or by repetitive contractions (several contractions in response to a single swallow). Lower oesophageal sphincter relaxations may be absent or incomplete, so that stasis develops. The sphincter may be hypertensive or may be hypotensive and allow excessive reflux. In most cases of disordered motility, combinations of these abnormalities occur. A clear distinction must be made between manometric or contraction abnormalities and clinical motility disorders of the oesophagus (Cohen, 1987). With the currently available manometric techniques various contraction abnormalities can be identified but their relation to symptoms such as dysphagia, chest pain and heartburn is not always clear. Moreover, pressure changes only reflect the final step of a chain of events—the contraction—but do not give direct information on the central and peripheral neural mechanisms nor the smooth or striated muscle activity that leads to the contraction. Moreover, longitudinal muscle contractions are not picked up by intraluminal pressure measurements. Therefore, in the present state of our understanding of oesophageal motility disorders, it would seem wise to develop a way of describing and classifying the manometric abnormalities of oesophagus and lower oesophageal sphincter (LOS). The final clinical diagnosis would then be based upon these laboratory data and upon the results of other investigations (clinical, radiological, scintigraphic, pH measurements, pharmacological). Such an approach could form a data base for studies on the nature and mechanism of oesophageal motility disorders.

Primary Oesophageal Motility Disorders

These disorders, in which the oesophagus is the major site of involvement, constitute a spectrum of conditions composed of achalasia, diffuse oesophageal spasm and intermediate types (Figure 1). This is particularly true in patients with severe functional dysphagia. In a series of 156 consecutive patients with a severe degree of dysphagia

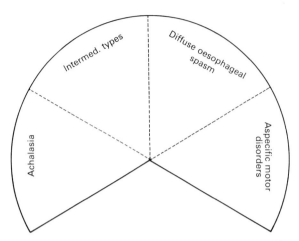

Figure 1. Primary oesophageal motility disorders probably constitute a spectrum of conditions.

that required treatment by pneumatic dilatation, the nature of the motility disorder was analysed on the basis of simple manometric criteria, i.e. the presence or absence of peristaltic contractions and the presence or absence of normal sphincteric relaxations (Vantrappen et al, 1979). Theoretically four different combinations are possible in these patients: absence of both peristalsis and LOS relaxation (achalasia); severe oesophageal motor disorders with preservation of some peristalsis and some LOS relaxation (diffuse oesophageal spasm); and two intermediate types in which either some peristalsis or some LOS relaxation is preserved. In this series of 156 patients, typical achalasia was found in 70%, typical diffuse oesophageal spasm in 11% and intermediate types in 19%. The boundary between achalasia and diffuse oesophageal spasm, therefore, is vague; equally difficult is the distinction, on the basis of manometric data, between diffuse oesophageal spasm and so-called non-specific motility disorders, i.e. changes in the progression characteristics of the contractions (e.g. simultaneous waves) and changes in the number of contractions in response to a single swallow. The correct interpretation of these abnormalities often requires additional information that can be obtained by endoscopy, pH measurements, combined 24-hour pH and pressure recording, radiology and provocative tests.

Secondary Motor Disorders

In secondary disorders the oesophageal abnormalities are due to more generalized neural, muscular or systemic diseases, to metabolic disturbances or to inflammatory or new growth lesions of the oesophageal wall.

This chapter will focus on three main motility disorders of the oesophagus: achalasia, diffuse oesophageal spasm, the irritable oesophagus, and systemic sclerosis.

Achalasia

The motility disorders that characterize achalasia are (1) absence of peristalsis in the body of the oesophagus and (2) failure of a frequently hypertonic lower oesophageal sphincter to relax in a normal way in response to swallowing (Figure 2a). Loss of propulsive peristaltic contractions and, particularly, the defective sphincter relaxations result in stasis of food in a progressively dilating gullet. This oesophageal stasis forms the basis for most symptoms and complications of achalasia.

The symptoms of achalasia are schematically presented in Figure 3 (Vantrappen and Hellemans, 1974). The dysphagia varies from day to day but is present from the beginning, both for liquids and solids. Regurgitation occurs not only in relation to meals but also in the recumbent position and may then result in coughing spells and bronchopulmonary complications. Cramplike chest pain is often unrelated to meals. On manometric examination the deglutitive pressure peaks occur simultaneously throughout the oesophageal body and begin shortly after swallowing. If the oesophagus is not fully decompensated peristaltic contractions may be seen to progress over 2–4 cm in the striated muscle portion of the gullet. The resting pressure of the LOS is often increased and the relaxation of the sphincter upon swallowing is absent or incomplete (Cohen and Lipschutz, 1971). The residual pressure ($\pm 70\%$ of the basal pressure) is probably responsible for the functional obstruction at the cardia.

In the course of the disease the oesophagus becomes progressively more dilated, with stasis of

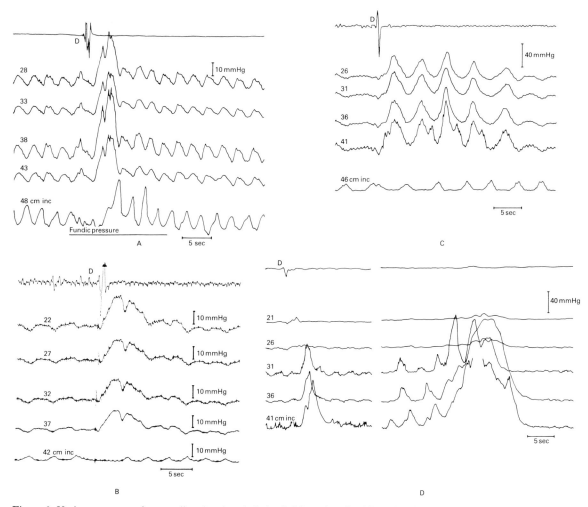

Figure 2. Various patterns of motor disorders in achalasia: A. Normal peristalsis replaced by simultaneous pressure peaks with early onset, and normal amplitude and duration; relaxations incomplete. B. As (A) but pressure waves become broader. C. Vigorous achalasia, with multiple pressure peaks in response to a single swallow (repetitive contractions). D. Spontaneous activity, not induced by swallowing.

food and secretions. Because the LOS fails to open normally following deglutition, the distal end of the barium column takes a typical, smoothly tapered 'bird's beak' appearance (Figure 4A). In about 20% of cases, there is symmetrical or asymmetrical dilatation in the narrowed sphincter zone. When the oesophagus becomes wide, the pressure peaks tend to become broader and of lower amplitude (Figure 2B). Eventually the oesophagus becomes elongated and tortuous (Figure 5A). The retained food and fluids may fill most of the oeso-

phagus, with an air-fluid level high up in the gullet. In some patients with otherwise typical achalasia, the disordered motility is characterized by a pattern of repetitive pressure peaks, which may be of relatively high amplitude, a condition that has been termed vigorous achalasia (Sanderson et al, 1967) (Figure 2C). Spontaneous contractions, not induced by swallowing, may be seen. Attacks of cramp-like pain in these patients are probably related to strong long-lasting spontaneous contractions (Figure 2D). Although

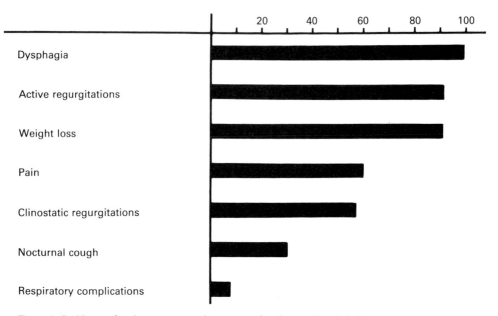

Figure 3. Incidence of various symptoms in a group of patients with achalasia.

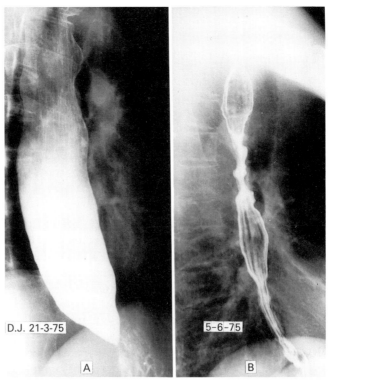

Figure 4. Typical X-ray picture of achalasia, before (A) and after (B)
pneumatic dilatation.

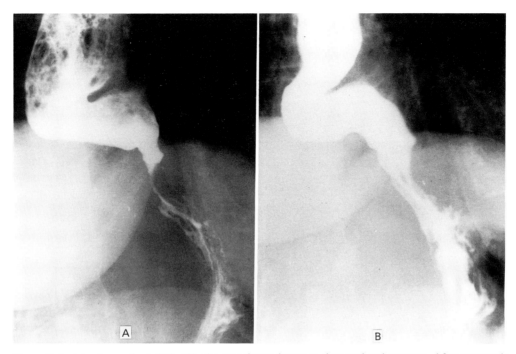

Figure 5. In late stages of achalasia (A), the oesophagus becomes elongated and tortuous. After pneumatic dilatation (B) the narrow distal segment opens.

radiological examination in these cases may show a curling picture, the typical achalasia picture is often seen on routine X-rays.

Repeated pneumatic dilatations with balloons of progressively larger diameter yield good results in 77% of the patients, whereas 7% are not improved (Vantrappen and Hellemans, 1980). The dilatations with balloons of increasing size (3 cm, 3.5 cm, 4 cm; Figure 6) are continued on separate days until the pressure in the LOS has decreased to ± 8 mmHg. Myotomy with or without an anti-reflux procedure is only carried out if this treatment fails.

After treatment the oesophagus empties much better (Figure 4B). Patients may become asymptomatic, even if there is still some degree of stasis. The diameter of the oesophagus normalizes or decreases and the narrow distal segment becomes wider (Figure 5B). Occasional peristaltic contractions, progressing over a distance of at least 10 cm, reappear in nearly one-third of the patients (Vantrappen et al, 1979) (Figure 7).

Diffuse Oesophageal Spasm

Diffuse oesophageal spasm is characterized by chest pain and/or dysphagia, accompanied by abnormal non-peristaltic contractions on oesophageal manometry, in a patient who has no demonstrable organic lesion of the oesophagus (Castell, 1976; Cohen, 1979; Vantrappen and Hellemans, 1976). The pain may be precipitated by swallowing and result in painful dysphagia (odynophagia) in some patients, but in others it may mimic pain of coronary origin. The dysphagia lacks the severity and persistence seen in achalasia or organic stenoses. The motility disorders of diffuse spasm are less severe than those of achalasia. The disease affects mainly the distal half or two-thirds of the oesophageal body. The oesophagus has not completely lost its capability to produce peristaltic contractions and LOS relaxations. Two-thirds of the patients have normal LOS function (DiMarino and Cohen, 1974). Many deglutitions, however, result in non-

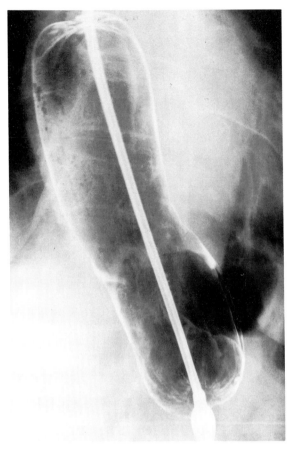

Figure 6. Pneumatic dilatation, with inflated balloon positioned at the gastro-oesophageal junction.

contractions (Figures 8C and D). Amplitude and duration of the pressure peaks are often increased in diffuse spasm. This does not mean that every simultaneous or repetitive deglutition complex necessarily consists of giant waves; in the same subject some of these pressure waves may have a normal or a markedly increased amplitude and duration.

There are no uniform, generally accepted criteria for the manometric diagnosis of diffuse oesophageal spasm. The following criteria have been proposed.

1. Thirty percent of the deglutitive responses consist of simultaneous waves of high amplitude (± 100 mmHg or more) and long duration (> 7.5 sec) (DiMarino and Cohen, 1974; Clouse and Staiano, 1983; Mellow, 1977).
2. Repetitive waves occur in 56–95% of the patients (Gillies et al, 1967; Roth and Fleshler, 1964). Spontaneous activity, not induced by swallows, is seen in more than 50% (Mellow, 1977).
3. Interrupted peristalsis was observed in seven out of 12 patients with diffuse oesophageal spasm (Kaye, 1981) (Figure 9).

The diagnosis of diffuse oesophageal spasm, therefore, is not based on a single well-defined motility pattern, but on the combination of clinical symptoms and a poorly defined complex of manometric abnormalities.

Irritable Oesophagus

One of the main problems in diagnosing diffuse spasm is the relation between this disorder and the disorders associated with gastro-oesophageal reflux (Brand et al, 1977). This is particularly true in patients with chest pain. The best way to determine whether gastro-oesophageal reflux or motor disorders or both play a role in the production of chest pain of non-cardiac origin are the combined pH and pressure recordings in the oesophagus over a period of 24 hours or more, using a device that allows the patient to signal his typical pain episodes on the tracing (Janssens et al, 1986, Vantrappen et al, 1981). If this investigation

sequential, mostly simultaneous pressure peaks of high amplitude and long duration (giant contractions). The abnormal deglutitive response may begin as a peristaltic wave progressing normally down the upper third or half of the oesophagus and change suddenly into a simultaneous contraction of the distal gullet without necessarily affecting LOS relaxation (Figure 8A). The abnormal deglutitive response in the lower part of the oesophagus may also consist of two or more pressure peaks in response to a single swallow. Whereas M-shaped peaks may be found in normal subjects, triple peaked responses are definitely abnormal (Clouse and Staiano, 1983) (Figure 8B). Other motility patterns seen in diffuse spasm are interrupted peristalsis (Figure 9) and segmental

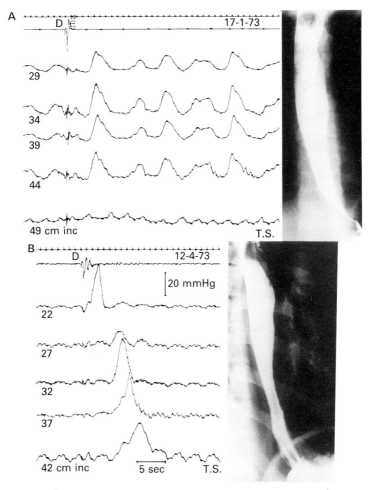

Figure 7. Vigorous achalasia before (A) and after (B) pneumatic dilatation.

shows that the spontaneous pain episodes are associated with reflux and unaccompanied by motor disorders, it is very likely that reflux is the cause of the pain (Figure 10). If, however, the pain episodes are preceded by severe motor disorders, not present during the 15-minute periods preceding and following the pain, motor disorders may be considered as the cause of the pain (Figure 11). Provocative tests do not allow this distinction, because a Bernstein test may be positive in a patient having motor disorders without reflux at the time of the spontaneous pain attack (Vantrappen et al, 1987). Similarly, the edrophonium test may be positive (causing pain and

motility disorders) in patients having reflux without motor disorders at the time of their spontaneous pain attacks. A positive Bernstein test does not indicate that reflux is the cause of the patient's spontaneous pain, and a positive edrophonium test does not mean that the pain is due to oesophageal motor disorders.

24-hour pH and pressure recordings also contribute to the diagnosis of irritable oesophagus (Vantrappen et al, 1987). In this condition identical attacks of chest pain can be elicited by two or more independent factors, i.e. chemical stimulation by acid due to spontaneous gastro-oesophageal reflux or to iatrogenic acid perfusion of

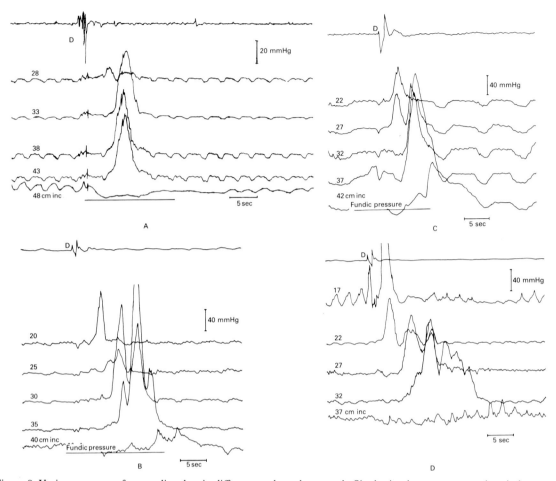

Figure 8. Various patterns of motor disorders in diffuse oesophageal spasm: A. Single simultaneous contractions in lower two-thirds of the oesophagus with almost normal relaxation of LOS. B. Repetitive simultaneous contractions of high amplitude and normal relaxation of LOS in response to single swallow. C and D. Segmental contractions.

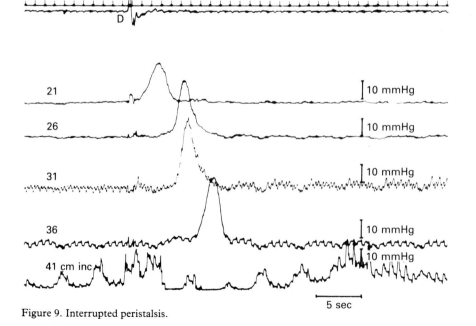

Figure 9. Interrupted peristalsis.

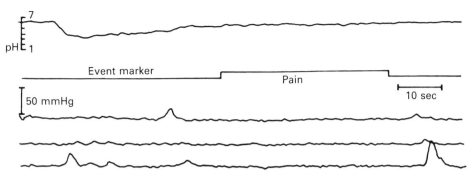

Figure 10. Segment of 24-hour pH and pressure recording showing episodes of chest pain accompanied by gastro-oesophageal reflux (upper trace) without oesophageal motor disorders (lower three traces).

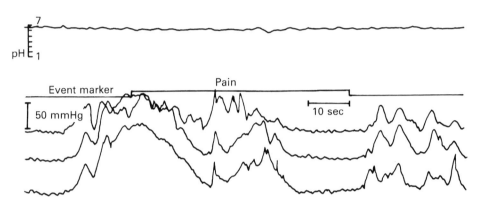

Figure 11. Segment of 24-hour pH and pressure recording showing episodes of chest pain accompanied by severe oesophageal motor disorders (lower three traces), without gastro-oesophageal reflux (upper trace).

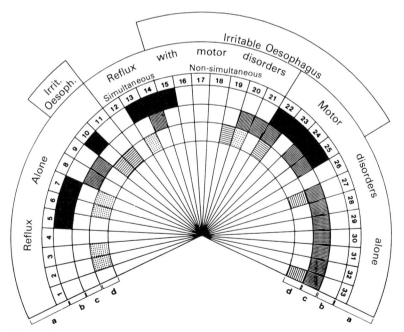

Figure 12. Diagram to show results in 33 patients with angina-like chest pain of oeso-phageal origin. (a) 24-hour pH and pressure measurements; (b) acid-perfusion tests; (c) conventional manometry; and (d) edrophonium-stimulation test (n = 12). ■ = positive related acid-perfusion test; ▥ = severe motor disorders on conventional manometry; ▤ = positive edrophonium-stimulation test; ▦ = negative edrophonium test.

the oesophagus, and mechanical stimulation by spontaneously developing or edrophonium-induced motor disorders or by balloon distension of the oesophagus. We studied a series of 31 patients with non-cardiac chest pain by means of 24-hour pH and pressure measurements, and several provocative tests (acid perfusion, edrophonium, balloon distension, conventional manometry). In 13 patients it could be shown that sometimes the chest pain episodes were related to acid, without motor component, and on other occasions to mechanical factors without acid involvement. This condition may be termed irritable oesophagus (Figure 12).

The role of motor blocking agents such as calcium entry blockers (nifedipine, dicetel) in the treatment of diffuse oesophageal spasm and related motility disorders is not yet well established. Both good and poor results have been reported. This may be due to the heterogeneous nature of the patient population in some studies (Richter et al, 1987; Janssens et al, to be published). It is very unlikely indeed that sphincter relaxing drugs are helpful in patients with pain due to gastro-oesophageal reflux. When dysphagia is the most prominent symptom in patients with pure motor disorders (not accompanied by reflux) and LOS function is abnormal, pneumatic dilatation may yield good results. If neither drugs nor dilatation relieve the pain, a long cardiomyotomy may have to be performed.

Systemic Sclerosis

Motor disorders of the oesophagus are seen in 50–80% of patients with scleroderma (Hellemans and Vantrappen, 1974). The disease usually does not

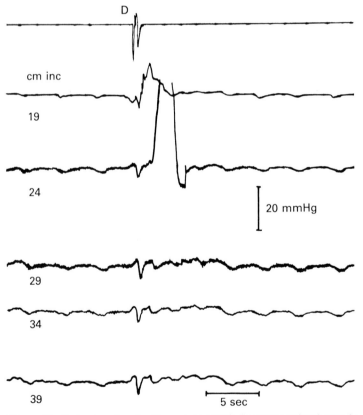

Figure 13. Systemic sclerosis. Normal peristalsis in upper striated muscle portion of the oesophagus, absence of deglutitive contractions in distal oesophagus.

affect the striated muscle portion of the gullet where the muscle fibres are remarkably well preserved and peristalsis is normal. In the more distal part of the oesophagus, where smooth muscle fibres are atrophied with some fibrous replacement, the deglutitive contractions are often non-peristaltic, weak and may eventually disappear completely (Figure 13). It is unlikely that muscle atrophy is responsible for the motor disturbances in the early stages of the disease. Probably neural dysfunction has a role. The LOS pressure is frequently lower than normal, which leads to gastro-oesophageal reflux and eventually to oesophagitis, due to the poor clearing function of the oesophagus.

References

Brand, D. L., Martin, D., and Pope, C. E., (1977), Esophageal manometries in patients with angina-like chest pain. *Dig. Dis. Sci.*, **22:** 300–4.

Castell, D. O., (1976), Achalasia and diffuse esophageal spasm. *Archs. Intern. Med.*, **136:** 571–9.

Clouse, R. E., and Staiano, A., (1983), Contraction abnormalities of the esophageal body in patients referred for manometry. *Dig. Dis. Sci.*, **28:** 784–91.

Cohen, S., (1979), Motor disorders of the esophagus. *New Engl. J. Med.*, **301:** 184–92.

Cohen, S., (1987), Esophageal motility disorders and their response to calcium channel antagonists. *Gastroenterology*, **93:** 301–3.

Cohen, S., and Lipshutz, W., (1971), Lower esophageal sphincter dysfunction in achalasia. *Gastroenterology*, **61:** 814–20.

DiMarino, A. J. Jr., and Cohen, S., (1974), Characteristics of lower esophageal sphincter function in symptomatic diffuse esophageal spasm. *Gastroenterology*, **66:** 1–6.

Gillies, M., Nicks, R., and Skyring, A., (1967), Clinical, manometric and pathological studies in diffuse oesophageal spasm. *Br. Med. J.*, **ii:** 527–30.

Hellemans, J., and Vantrappen, G., (1974), Motor disorders due to collagen diseases. In: *Diseases of the Esophagus* (Eds. Vantrappen, G., and Hellemans, J.), pp. 383–90, Springer-Verlag, Berlin, Heidelberg, New York.

Janssens, J., Vantrappen, G., and Ghillebert, G., (1986), 24-hour recording of esophageal pressure and pH in patients with noncardiac chest pain. *Gastroenterology*, **90:** 1978–84.

Janssens, J., Vantrappen, G., and Ghillebert, G., (1988), Letter to the editor. *Gastroenterology*, **94:** 553–4.

Kaye, M. D., (1981), Anomalies of peristalsis in idiopathic diffuse oesophageal spasm. *Gut*, **22:** 217–22.

Mellow, M., (1977), Symptomatic diffuse esophageal spasm. Manometric follow-up and response to cholinergic stimulation and cholinesterase inhibition. *Gastroenterology*, **73:** 237–40.

Richter, J. E., Dalton, C. B., Bradley, L. A., and Castell, D. O., (1987), Oral nifedipine in the treatment of noncardiac chest pain in patients with the nutcracker esophagus. *Gastroenterology*, **93:** 21–8.

Roth, H. P., and Fleshler, B., (1964), Diffuse esophageal spasm. *Ann. Intern. Med.*, **61:** 914–23.

Sanderson, D. R., Ellis, F. H. Jr., Schlegel, J. F., and Olsen, A. M., (1967), Syndrome of vigorous achalasia: clinical and physiologic observations. *Dis. Chest*, **52:** 508–17.

Vantrappen, G., and Hellemans, J., (1974), Achalasia In: *Diseases of the Esophagus* (Eds. Vantrappen, G., and Hellemans, J.), pp. 287–341, Springer-Verlag, New York, Heidelberg, Berlin.

Vantrappen, G., and Hellemans, J., (1976), Diffuse muscle spasm of the oesophagus and the hypertensive lower oesophageal sphincter. *Clin. Gastroenterol.*, **5:** 59–72.

Vantrappen, G., and Hellemans, J., (1980), Treatment of achalasia and related motor disorders. *Gastroenterology*, **79:** 144–54.

Vantrappen, G., Janssens, J., and Ghillebert, G., (1987), The irritable esophagus—a frequent cause of angina-like chest pain. *Lancet*, **May 30:** 1232–4.

Vantrappen, G., Janssens, J., Hellemans, J., and Coremans, G., (1979), Achalasia, diffuse esophageal spasm, and related motility disorders. *Gastroenterology*, **76:** 450–7.

Vantrappen, G., Servaes, J., and Peeters, T., (1981), A 24-hour pH and pressure monitoring device for outpatients. *Zeitschr. Gastroenterol.*, **19:** 422–3.

24B.

GASTRO-OESOPHAGEAL REFLUX DISEASE

Giovanni Zaninotto, Tom R. DeMeester
Creighton University School of Medicine, Omaha, Nebraska, USA

Gastro-oesophageal reflux disease accounts for approximately 75% of oesophageal pathology and is among the most challenging diagnostic and therapeutic problems in benign oesophageal disease. A major factor contributing to this challenge is the lack of a universally accepted definition of the disease.

It is difficult to define the disease by symptoms indicative of gastro-oesophageal reflux such as acid regurgitation and heartburn for three reasons. First, these symptoms are very common in the population (5–7%) (Nebel et al, 1976, Tibbling, 1982), but in the absence of oesophagitis they are not absolutely specific and can be caused by other diseases such as achalasia, diffuse spasm, oesophageal carcinoma, pyloric stenosis, cholelithiasis, gastritis, gastric or duodenal ulcer, and coronary artery disease. Second, a symptomatic definition fails to incorporate the whole clinical spectrum of the disease. Gastro-oesophageal reflux is often associated with other disorders of the foregut such as duodenogastric reflux (Kaye and Showalter, 1974) and oesophagopharyngeal reflux (Pellegrini et al, 1979). The symptoms of the former are more gastric in character: epigastric pain, nausea, vomiting, postprandial fullness and belching. The latter are more respiratory in character: choking, chronic cough, wheezing, and hoarseness. The severity of these symptoms can override or modify the typical symptoms of heartburn and regurgitation that are necessary to diagnose gastro-oesophageal reflux disease on a symptomatic basis. Because gastro-oesophageal reflux can have such a varied symptomatic presentation, no one symptom complex can be depended upon to indicate its presence. Third, a symptomatic definition of the disease does not provide the incentive to further evaluate patients who do not present with typical complaints. Consequently, patients with poorly understood symptoms are dismissed as not having the disease when they should be further evaluated for the presence of the disease. A symptomatic definition of the disease excludes this possibility and encourages the use of nonspecific or shotgun therapy.

An alternative definition for gastro-oesophageal reflux disease is the presence of oesophagitis on endoscopy. Based on this definition, only those symptomatic patients with endoscopic oesophagitis have the disease. There are problems with this definition as well. First, it assumes that all patients who have oesophagitis have excessive regurgitation of gastric juice into their oesophagus. Data indicate that this is true in 90% of patients, but in 10% the oesophagitis is caused by other aetiologies, the most common being unrecognized chemical injury from drug ingestion (DeMeester et al, 1980; Bonavina et al, 1987). Second, the definition leaves undiagnosed those patients who have symptoms of gastro-oesophageal reflux, but do not have endoscopic oesophagitis. Data indicate that this occurs in 40% of patients with typical symptoms of gastro-oesophageal reflux (DeMeester et al, 1980). Obtaining an oesophageal biopsy is of little help since the sensitivity and specificity of an epithelial biopsy in the absence of endoscopic oesophagitis is 0.75 and 0.9 respectively (DeMeester and Johnson, 1976) and depends on an interested pathologist for proper reading. Consequently, a large number of patients with complaints of sufficient severity to seek medical advice are treated expectantly. Third, the definition characterizes the gastro-oesophageal reflux on the basis of a complication of the disease. Oesophagitis is a tissue injury that can occur as a consequence of gastro-oesophageal reflux, but is not synonymous with the presence of the disease. Defining the disease by its complication is not a workable solution.

A third approach to defining gastro-oesophageal

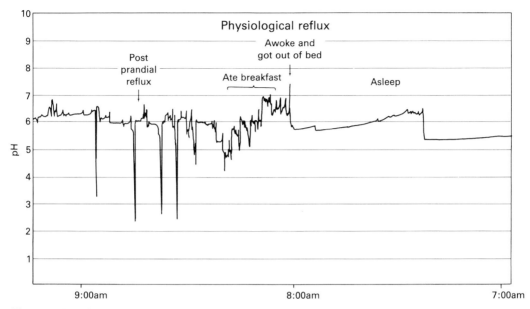

Figure 1. A 24-hour oesophageal pH record showing physiological gastro-oesophageal reflux. Note the rapid clearing occurring during the postprandial period and the lack of reflux during the sleep period.

reflux disease is measuring the basic patho-physiological abnormality accountable for the disease, that is the presence of more than normal oesophageal exposure to gastric juice. This can be done by monitoring the oesophageal pH during a 24-hour period and assuming that changes in pH below a certain level (pH 4) are due to the reflux of acid gastric juice, provided the subject excluded acid food or drink from his diet. The problem with this approach is that acid gastric juice regurgitates occasionally into the oesophagus in the healthy individual as shown by 24-hour pH monitoring in asymptomatic subjects. This 'physiological reflux' occurs mostly during the postprandial period and rarely during sleep. It is uncommon to find more than three episodes of physiological reflux lasting longer than five minutes, and the longest episode usually does not last more than 13 minutes. Physiological reflux results when the lower oeso-phageal sphincter relaxes on swallowing and the expected peristaltic sequences in the body of the oesophagus do not occur (DeMeester et al, 1980). Swallowing occurs at a rate of seven times per hour when asleep compared to 72 times per hour

Table 1. Oesophageal exposure to gastric juice in healthy volunteers (n = 50) using pH 4 as an indicator of gastric juice.

	Mean	S.D.	Median	Max	Min	95 percentile	97.5 percentile
% Total reflux time	1.57	1.47	1.1	6.0	0.0	4.8	5.8
% Reflux in upright	2.35	2.42	1.7	9.3	0.0	8.4	9.1
% Reflux in supine	0.55	1.02	0.0	4.0	0.0	3.4	3.9
Number of episodes of reflux	23.87	22.96	20.0	126.0	0.0	51.0	76.0
Number of episodes longer than 5 min	0.95	1.27	0.0	5.0	0.0	4.0	0.0
Longest reflux episode	6.82	8.25	3.2	46.0	0.0	20.0	40.0

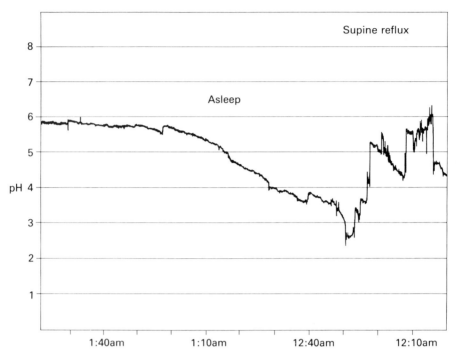

Figure 2. A 24-hour oesophageal pH record showing a reflux episode with slow clearing, occurring while the patient is asleep. The delayed clearing is due to the loss of gravity in the supine position and the lack of oesophageal contractions during sleep.

while awake. Consequently, physiological reflux is more common when awake than during sleep. Belching also causes reflux in healthy individuals. During the awake hours each pharyngeal swallow results in ingestion of air which collects in the stomach, causing gastric dilatation. A belch occurs when the dilatation becomes excessive and is often associated with the regurgitation of acid gastric juice as well as air. The typical pattern of physiological reflux in normal subjects is illustrated in Figure 1. Twenty-four hour oesophageal exposure to gastric juice can be measured by pH monitoring of the oesophagus. To obtain a global assessment of the 24-hour oesophageal exposure to gastric juice, six parameters have been measured using the pH of 4 as a tag for the presence of gastric juice. They are: the percentage time the pH was 4 or less for the total period and time spent in the upright and supine position; the total number of reflux episodes, i.e., the number of times the pH of the oesophagus dropped below pH 4; the number of episodes lasting five minutes or more;

and the duration (in minutes) of the longest reflux episode. Table 1 shows the values measured for these six parameters in 50 healthy volunteers.

In patients these parameters are not uniformly abnormal. For instance, the most common abnormality is acid exposure during sleep, that is when the patient is supine. Reflux episodes during this period are of long duration due to the lack of gravity and oesophageal contraction to clear the oesophagus (Figure 2). On the other hand, such patients commonly have a normal number of reflux episodes. For this reason, the definition of abnormal oesophageal acid exposure is based on a scoring system that integrates the values for all six parameters, whether normal or abnormal, and weighs each parameter according to its standard error of measurement (Johnson and DeMeester, 1986; Johnson and Harmony, 1986). The resulting score reflects the severity and pattern of oesophageal acid exposure compared to normal subjects.

The pathophysiology of gastro-oesophageal

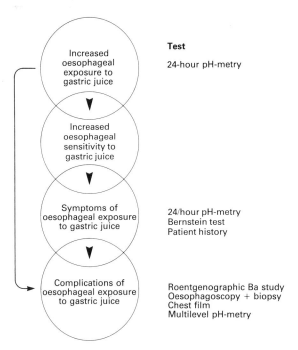

	Test
Increased oesophageal exposure to gastric juice	24-hour pH-metry
Increased oesophageal sensitivity to gastric juice	
Symptoms of oesophageal exposure to gastric juice	24/hour pH-metry Bernstein test Patient history
Complications of oesophageal exposure to gastric juice	Roentgenographic Ba study Oesophagoscopy + biopsy Chest film Multilevel pH-metry

Figure 3. Pathophysiological sequence of gastro-oesophageal reflux disease: an increased exposure to gastric juice is the basic pathophysiological abnormality which leads to an increased sensitivity of the oesophageal mucosa to the gastric juice, resulting in symptoms and complications from tissue damage.

reflux disease is illustrated in Figure 3. The increased oesophageal exposure to gastric juice leads to an increased sensitivity of the oesophagus to the refluxed material which in turn gives rise

to the symptoms of the disease. If the increased exposure to gastric juice persists, complications can occur such as oesophagitis, stricture, the development of Barrett's oesophagus, and progressive pulmonary fibrosis or recurrent pneumonia from repetitive pulmonary aspiration. Usually, but not always, the development of oesophagitis or a stricture is preceded by symptoms. A few patients, however, can develop these complications without going through the sensitivity and symptom stages.

There are three known causes of increased oesophageal exposure to gastric juice in patients with gastro-oesophageal reflux disease. The first is a mechanically incompetent distal oesophageal sphincter. This accounts for about 60% of the causes of reflux. It is identified by oesophageal manometry and is the one aetiology that antireflux surgery can correct. The other two causes are inefficient oesophageal clearance of reflux gastric juice and abnormalities of the gastric reservoir which augment physiological reflux such as increased gastric pressure, excessive gastric dilatation, delayed gastric emptying, and/or increased gastric acid secretion.

The resistance to gastro-oesophageal reflux provided by the lower oesophageal sphincter is dependent on the integrated effects of its pressure, overall length and the length exposed to the pressure environment of the abdomen (Bonavina et al, 1986). Figure 4 shows the manometric recording

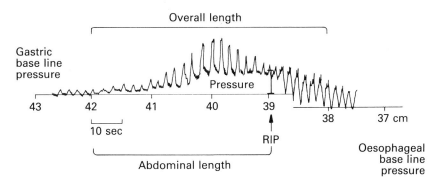

RIP = Respiratory inversion point

Figure 4. Manometric recording of the lower oesophageal sphincter (see explanation in the text).

Sphincter pressure

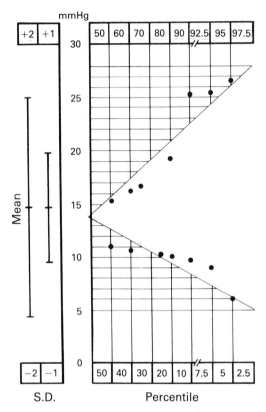

Figure 5. Nomogram for lower oesophageal sphincter pressure. To obtain the percentile value, locate the pressure on the vertical axis and follow the horizontal line to its intersection with the best fit line. Mean and ± one or two standard deviations (SD) are on the left.

of the lower oesophageal sphincter. The end respiratory gastric baseline is used as a zero reference; a persistent rise in pressure exceeding 2 mmHg above the gastric baseline marks the distal border of the sphincter. The proximal border is marked by the point where sphincter pressure drops to end inspiratory oesophageal baseline pressure. The distance between these two points represents the overall length of the sphincter. The point at which the end inspiratory pressure changes from a positive to a negative deflection represents the respiratory inversion point (RIP). The distance between the RIP and the distal border of the sphincter, that is the part of the sphincter that

reflects positive excursions with respiration, represents the abdominal length of the sphincter. Sphincter pressure is measured as the difference between the gastric baseline and the pressure at the respiratory inversion point during the middle of the respiratory cycle. Sphincter pressure, overall length and abdominal length in an asymptomatic population are not dependent on age, sex, height, and weight (Zaninotto et al, in press). The nomograms for these values are shown in Figures 5, 6, and 7. A deficiency in one or a combination of these manometric measurements of the sphincter can result in increased oesophageal exposure to gastric juice.

Sphincter overall length

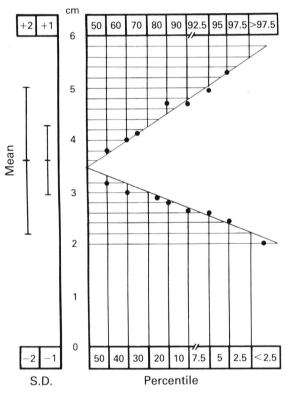

Figure 6. Nomogram for the abdominal length of lower oesophageal sphincter pressure. To obtain the percentile value, locate the pressure on the vertical axis and follow the horizontal line to its intersection with the best fit line. Mean and ± one or two standard deviations (SD) are on the left.

Sphincter abdominal length

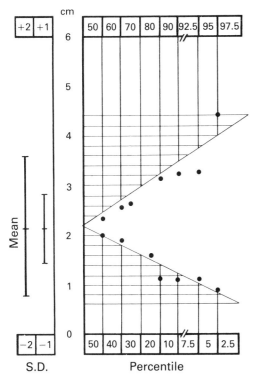

Figure 7. Nomogram for the overall length of lower oesophageal sphincter pressure. To obtain the percentile value, locate the pressure on the vertical axis and follow the horizontal line to its intersection with the best fit line. Mean and ± one or two standard deviations (SD) are on the left.

Table 2 shows the normal values of the lower oesophageal sphincter pressure, overall length and abdominal length obtained from 50 healthy subjects (Zaninotto et al, 1988). The manometric definition of a mechanically incompetent distal oesophageal sphincter was developed by comparing the normogram value to a population of

620 patients with symptoms of gastro-oesophageal reflux disease, 324 of whom had increased oesophageal exposure to acid gastric juice on 24-hour pH monitoring. From the data shown in Figures 8, 9 and 10 a sphincter presence of 6 mmHg or less (below the 2.5th percentile of normal), an abdominal length of less than 1 cm (below the 5th percentile of normal), and an overall length of less than 2 cm (below the 2.5th percentile of normal) have an incidence of 79.2, 80 and 79.4 respectively for increased oesophageal exposure to acid gastric juice.

Patients with a low sphincter pressure (less than 6 mmHg) or with a short abdominal length (less than 1 cm) are unable to prevent the reflux caused by an increase in intragastric pressure resulting from increases in intra-abdominal pressure. Patients with a short overall sphincter length (2 cm or less) are also less able to protect against reflux caused by progressive gastric dilatation. This is due to the further shortening of the sphincter with gastric dilatation, similar to the shortening of the neck of a balloon on inflation. In this situation, reflux occurs when the overall length decreases below that necessary for the sphincter pressure present to maintain competency. Figures 11 and 12 illustrate the different motility recordings of a mechanically incompetent lower oesophageal sphincter. Figure 11 shows a patient with low sphincter pressure, although the overall and abdominal length are normal. Figure 12 shows a patient with normal sphincter pressure, but with short abdominal and overall length. Both patients were symptomatic and had abnormal acid exposure at 24-hour pH monitoring.

In 60% of the 324 patients with proven gastro-oesophageal reflux disease, the cause for increased oesophageal exposure to acid gastric juice was a mechanically incompetent cardia, as defined

Table 2. Lower oesophageal sphincter in healthy volunteers (n = 50).

	Mean	S.D.	Median	Max	Min	5 percentile	2.5 percentile
Pressure (mmHg)	14.87	5.14	13.8	25.6	5.2	8	6.1
Abdominal length (cm)	2.18	0.72	2.2	5	0.8	1.1	0.89
Overall length (cm)	3.65	0.68	3.6	5.5	2.4	2.6	2.4

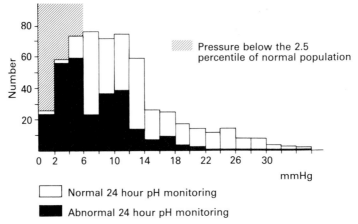

Figure 8. Distribution of lower oesophageal sphincter pressure in 622 symptomatic patients. The 79.2% of patients with a pressure of 6 mmHg or less (shaded area) had an abnormal oesophageal exposure to acid gastric juice.

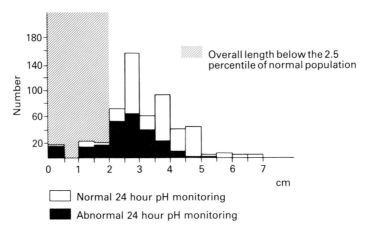

Figure 9. Distribution of the abdominal length of the lower oesophageal sphincter in 622 symptomatic patients. Of the patients with an abdominal length less than 1 cm (shaded area) 80% had an abnormal oesophageal exposure to acid gastric juice.

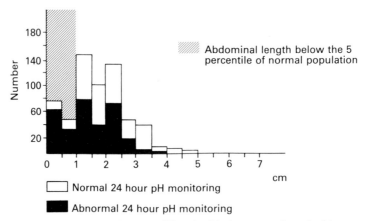

Figure 10. Distribution of the overall length of the lower oesophageal sphincter in 622 symptomatic patients. Of the patients with an abdominal length less than 2 cm (shaded area) 79.4% had an abnormal oesophageal exposure to acid gastric juice.

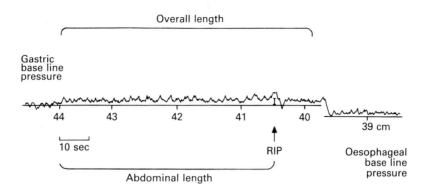

RIP = Respiratory inversion point

Figure 11. Lower oesophageal sphincter manometric recording in a patient with increased acid exposure in the distal oesophagus at the 24-hour pH monitoring: the sphincter pressure measured at the respiratory inversion point was 5 mmHg.

above, while 40% had a normal oesophageal sphincter at manometry indicating that the abnormal gastro-oesophageal reflux was due to gastric or oesophageal pathology. The most common manometric defect of the sphincter was an isolated low pressure, accounting for about 30% of all the defects. A combination of a low pressure and short

abdominal length was second, and an isolated short abdominal length third (Figure 13). When the three manometric defects of the sphincter are simultaneously present, the chances that the patient has abnormal oesophageal acid exposure are more than 98%.

If no mechanical abnormalities of the lower

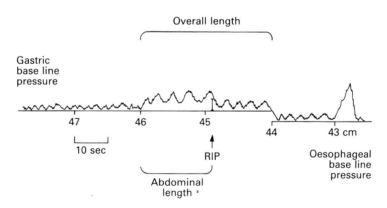

RIP = Respiratory inversion point

Figure 12. Lower oesophageal sphincter manometric recording in a patient with increased acid exposure in the distal oesophagus. A normal pressure of 10 mmHg is measured at the RIP, but the overall length and the length of the sphincter exposed to the abdominal pressure environment are abnormally short. Consequently, the sphincter cannot maintain its competence when challenged by an increase of abdominal pressure or gastric dilatation.

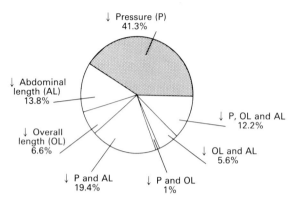

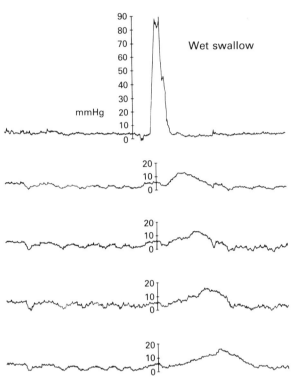

Figure 13. Specific manometric abnormalities in 196 patients with increased oesophageal exposure to acid gastric juice and abnormal sphincter manometry.

oesophageal sphincter are found at manometry, a gastric or oesophageal cause for increased oesophageal exposure to gastric juice should be considered. The gastric factors are increased gastric dilatation, increased gastric pressure and increased acid secretion. Of these, the latter is most

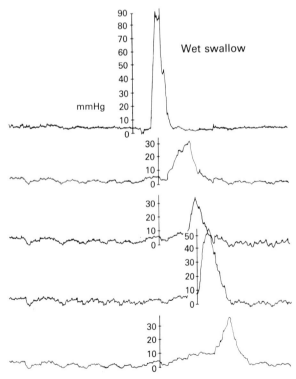

Figure 14. Normal peristaltic sequence in a healthy volunteer. The first channel records the pressure 1 cm below the upper oesophageal sphincter. The subsequent channels record pressure at 5 cm intervals in the oesophageal body.

Figure 15. Oesophageal body motility in patients with a stricture secondary to gastro-oesophageal reflux disease: a marked reduction of the amplitude of the waves is observed, especially in the lower third of the oesophageal body.

important and has been reported in 67% of patients with gastro-oesophageal reflux disease (Johansson and Tibbling, 1986). In this situation, increased oesophageal exposure to gastric juice is due to physiological reflux of more concentrated gastric secretion.

Oesophageal causes for increased oesophageal exposure to gastric juice are related to the capacity of the organ to clear physiological amounts of refluxed gastric juice. This is related to the efficiency of the oesophageal peristalsis and salivary secretion. In healthy subjects, 95% of reflux episodes are cleared to above pH 4 in less than 5 minutes. The oesophageal clearance is a two-step phenomenon: in the first step almost the entire volume of the refluxed acid is propelled out of the oesophagus by the advancing peristaltic wave (Longhi and Jordan, 1971) (Figure 14). The minimal residue of acid is then neutralized by swallowed saliva (Helm et al, 1984). Since the frequency of a swallow-induced primary oeso-phageal contraction, i.e., the predominant motor activity of the oesophagus required for acid clear-ance, is coupled to the flow of saliva, an efficient flow of saliva is necessary for an efficient oeso-phageal clearance (Dent et al, 1980).

Although any contraction amplitude within the broad range of normal is sufficient to obliterate the oesophageal lumen and strip almost all the lumen contents from the oesophagus, an abnormal wave progression or an amplitude below the 2.5th per-centile of the normal will result in ineffective clear-ance and gastric acid juice can remain in the oesophagus despite several swallows (Helm et al, 1985). Motility abnormalities characterized by low amplitude waves have been reported in patients with peptic stricture (Atharidis et al, 1979). Whether such peristaltic dysfunction is secondary to the oesophagitis or a primary predisposing

factor to the development of the stricture is unclear (Figure 15). Patients with a primary oesophageal motility abnormality and incompetent lower oeso-phageal sphincter usually tend to develop severe oesophagitis and/or stricture due to their inability to clear the refluxed gastric juice (Figure 16). They represent one of the more difficult challenges for the surgeon and may require an oesophageal resec-tion to relieve their reflux symptoms.

References

Atharidis, G., Snape, W., and Cohens, S., (1979), Clini-cal and manometric findings in benign peptic stric-tures of the esophagus. *Dig. Dis. Sci.*, **24**: 858–61.

Bonavina, L., DeMeester, T. R., McChesney, L., Schwizer, W., Albertucci, M., and Bailey, R. T., (1987), Drug induced esophageal strictures. *Ann. Surg.*, **206**: 173–83.

Bonavina, L., Evanders, A., DeMeester, T. R., Walther, B., Cheng, S. C., Palazzo, L., and Concan-non, J. L., (1986), Length of the distal esophagus and competency of cardia. *Am. J. Surg.*, **15**: 25–36.

DeMeester, T. R., and Johnson, L. F., (1976), The evaluation of objective measurements of gastro-esophageal reflux and their contribution to patient management. *Surg. Clin. North Am.*, **56**: 39–53.

DeMeester, T. R., Wang, C. I., Wernly, J. A., Pelle-grini, C. A., Little, A. G., Klementschitsch, P., Bermudez, G., Johnson, L. F., and Skinner, D. B., (1980), Technique, indications and clinical use of 24-hour esophageal pH monitoring. *J. Thorac. Car-diovasc. Surg.*, **79**: 656–67.

Dent, J., Dodds, W. J., Friedman, R. H., Sekiguchi, T., Hogan, W. J., Arndorfer, R. C., and Petrie, C., (1980), Mechanism of gastroesophageal reflux in recumbent asymptomatic human subjects. *J. Clin. Invest.*, **65**: 256–70.

Helm, J. F., Dodds, W. J., Pelc, L. R., Palmer, D. W., Hogan, W. J., and Teeter, B. C., (1984), Effect of esophageal emptying and saliva on clearance of acid from the esophagus. *N. Engl. J. Med.*, **310**: 284–88.

Helm, J. F., Dodds, W. J., and Hogan, W. J., (1985), Esophageal clearance. In: *Gastroesophageal Reflux* (Eds. Castell, D. O., Wu, W. C., and Ott, D. J.), pp. 11–13, Futura Publishing, New York.

Johansson, K. E., and Tibbling, L., (1986), Gastric secretion and reflux pattern in reflux oesophagitis before and during Remetidine treatment. *Scand. J. Gastroenterol.*, **21**: 487–92.

Johnson, L. F., and DeMeester, T. R., (1986), Develop-ment of the 24-hour intraesophageal pH monitoring composite scoring system. *J. Clin. Gastroenterol.*, **8** (Suppl. 1): 52–8.

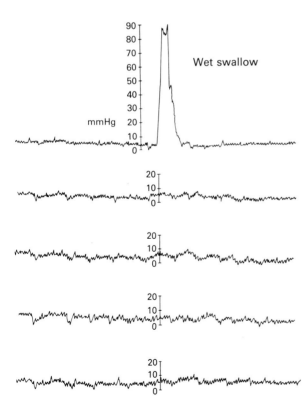

Figure 16. Oesophageal body motility in a patient with sclero-derma: the lack of any peristaltic contraction results in the patient's inability to clear refluxed gastric juice.

Johnson, L. W., and Harmony, J. W., (1986), Experimental esophagitis in a rabbit model. Clinical relevance. *J. Clin. Gastroenterol.*, **8** (Suppl. 1): 26–44.

Kaye, M. D., and Showalter, J. P., (1974), Pyloric incompetence in patients with symptomatic gastroesophageal reflux. *J. Lab. Clin. Med.*, **83:** 198–206.

Longhi, E. H., and Jordan, P. H., (1971), Simultaneous cimezadiographic and manometric analysis of incomplete emptying of the esophagus. *Am. J. Surg.*, **121:** 229–37.

Nebel, O. T., Foznes, M. F., and Castell, D. O., (1976), Symptomatic gastroesophageal reflux: incidence and precipitating factor. *Dig. Dis. Sci.*, **21:** 955–9.

Pellegrini, C. A., DeMeester, T. R., and Johnson, L. F., (1979), Gastroesophageal reflux and pulmonary aspiration: incidence, functional abnormality and results of surgical therapy. *Surgery*, **86:** 110–19.

Tibbling, L., (1982), Oesophageal dysfunction and angina pectoris in a Swedish population selected at random. *Acta. Med. Scand.*, **209** (Suppl. 644): 71–4.

Zaninotto, G., DeMeester, T. R., Schwizer, W., Johansson, K. E., Cheng, S. C., (1988), The lower esophageal sphincter in health and disease. *Am. J. Surg.*, **155:** 104–11.

25
STOMACH AND DUODENUM

Vincenzo Stanghellini, Roberto Corinaldesi

Institute of Clinical Medicine and Gastroenterology, University of Bologna, Bologna, Italy

Introduction

Numerous clinical syndromes may be related to motor abnormalities of the stomach and proximal portions of the small bowel. They range from the Pathophysiological digestive disorders accompanied by impaired gastric emptying, such as those experienced by most healthy people after ingestion of large over-rich meals, to dramatic, sometimes life-threatening, conditions of patients with severe gastroparesis and/or marked motor inco-ordination of the proximal small bowel.

Figure 1 depicts normal manometric findings during fasting and after ingestion of a meal with solid components in a healthy individual. The motor activities of the stomach and duodenum regulate the presence of contents in the two organs, as well as flux across the pyloric junction. Abnormalities of gastroduodenal motility therefore modify these parameters as indicated in Figure 2. Augmented tonic pressure of the gastric fundus and a decrease of the pyloric resistance lead to accelerated gastric emptying. Conversely, delayed gastric emptying may be determined by an increase in pyloric resistance, a decrease of antro-

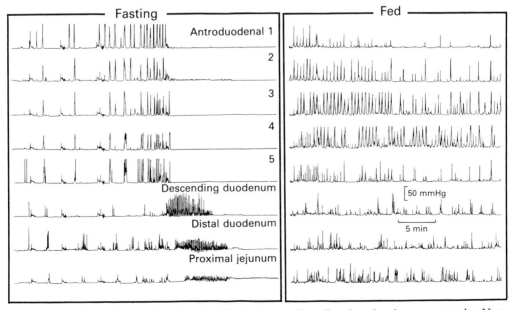

Figure 1. Normal gastrointestinal motility. Left (fasting): normal interdigestive migrating motor complex. Note the sequence of unco-ordinated motility (phase II), activity front (phase III) migrating from the stomach through the pyloric region into the duodenum, and motor quiescence (phase I). Right (fed): note the intense contractility of the distal antrum and the irregular motility following ingestion of a test meal with solid components.

$$F = \frac{\triangle P}{R}$$

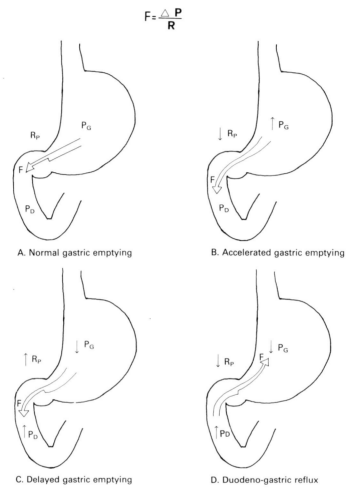

Figure 2. Main pathophysiological mechanism of transpyloric fluxes. F = transpyloric flux. $P = P_G - P_D$ = transpyloric pressure gradient. R_P = pyloric resistance.

duodenal co-ordination, and a decrease of the gastroduodenal pressure gradient. Inversion of the normally aborad pressure gradient existing between stomach and duodenum and insufficient pyloric resistance determine the reflux of intestinal contents into the stomach.

Table 1 lists the most typical clinical presentations of accelerated gastric emptying, delayed gastric emptying and abnormal duodenogastric reflux. Symptoms do not necessarily help to identify the underlying motor abnormality. However, diarrhoea, and postprandial symptoms of hypovolaemia and hypoglycaemia are more suggestive of accelerated gastric emptying, while early satiety, postprandial fullness, regurgitation and vomiting are more usually reported by patients with delayed gastric emptying. The presence of bile-stained vomiting signals an excessive enterogastric reflux. Nevertheless, one must keep in mind that abnormalities of gastrointestinal motility may be clinically silent (Kassander, 1958; Kalbasi et al, 1975) and also that symptomatic subjects may present motor patterns indistinguishable from those of healthy individuals (Corinaldesi et al, 1986; Malagelada and Stanghellini, 1985).

Table 1. Main pathophysiological mechanisms and possible clinical manifestations of abnormal gastric emptying and duodeno-gastric reflux.

Accelerated gastric emptying	
Pathophysiological mechanisms	Clinical manifestations
– Increased tonic pressure of the gastric fundus – Decreased pyloric resistance	– Epigastric pain and/or burning – Nausea – Abdominal cramps – Diarrhoea – Symptoms of hypovolaemia – Symptoms of hypoglycaemia
Delayed gastric emptying	
– Decreased tonic pressure of the gastric fundus – Decreased grinding of solids by the phasic contractions of the gastric antrum – Decreased gastro-duodenal co-ordination	– Epigastric pain and/or burning – Nausea – Early satiety – Vomiting – Postprandial fullness – Postprandial drowsiness – Belching – Regurgitation – Weight loss
Abnormal duodeno-gastric reflux	
– Reversed gastro-duodenal pressure gradient – Decreased pyloric resistance	– Epigastric pain and/or burning – Nausea – Heartburn – Regurgitation – Bilious vomiting

The main disorders presenting with abnormalities of the motility of the stomach and proximal small bowel are listed in Table 2.

Post-gastric Surgery States

Surgical procedures which directly or indirectly involve the stomach produce motor disturbances that may or may not be symptomatic (Kalbasi et al, 1975). Total and proximal gastric vagotomies induce a similar effect on the pattern of gastric emptying of a liquid meal, characterized by a shortening of half-times and a prolongation of complete emptying times (Clarke and Alexander-Williams, 1973) (Figure 3). If a pyloroplasty accompanies the vagotomies, half-emptying times of liquids remain accelerated, but total emptying times become normal.

Symptomatic gastric hypomotility may develop after surgical repair of a hiatal hernia by fundoplication. A manometric study demonstrated a marked reduction of antral phasic response to a solid meal in six of the patients shown in Figure 4 (Stanghellini and Malagelada, 1983).

Symptoms of gastric stasis in patients who underwent gastroenterostomy may also be related to abnormal motility in the efferent loop. In par-

Table 2. Main pathological conditions accompanied by abnormalities of motility of the stomach and of the proximal small bowel.

Postgastric surgery states

    Vagotomy
    Antrectomy
    Fundoplication
    Roux-en-Y diversion

Nonobstructive disorders

    Oesophageal disorders
    Gastroduodenal disorders
    Malabsorption syndromes

Abnormalities of myogenic and neurogenic control of gastointestinal motility

    Disorders of the smooth muscle
    Disorders of the intrinsic nervous system
    Disorders of the extrinsic nervous supplies
    Disorders of the central nervous system

Idiopathic motor abnormalities

---

ticular, a syndrome determined by unco-ordinated motility in the alimentary loop after Roux-en-Y anastomosis has been described (Mathias et al, 1985). Figure 5 depicts the manometric findings in one of these patients.

Non-obstructive Disorders

Oesophageal Disorders

Impaired gastric emptying may theoretically favour the reflux of gastric contents into the oesophagus.

Baldi et al (1981) observed a significant delay in gastric emptying of a caloric liquid meal in a group of patients who presented with oesophagitis and typical reflux symptoms, but with normal oesophageal motility and no evidence of hiatal hernia (Figure 6).

Gastroduodenal Disorders

Disturbances of gastrointestinal motor functions have been observed in different clinical conditions

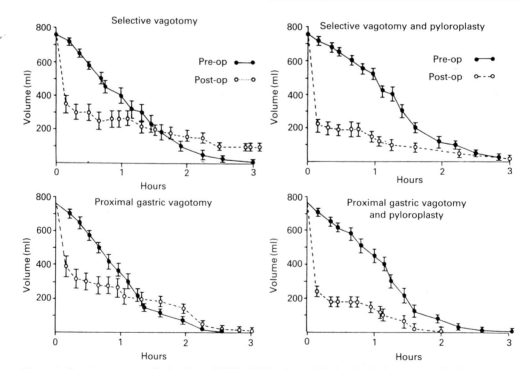

Figure 3. Gastric emptying of a liquid meal (750 ml 10% glucose) in duodenal ulcer patients, before and after surgery. From Clarke and Alexander-Williams (1973), with permission.

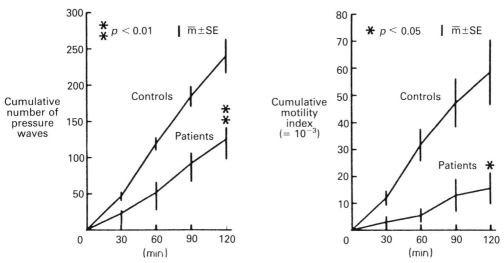

Figure 4. Postprandial cumulative antral motor activity in six patients who developed dyspeptic symptoms after fundoplication and in seven controls. Number of phasic contractions and motility index were pooled at 30-minute intervals.

characterized by abnormal gastric acid secretory rates. Patients with Zollinger-Ellison syndrome present an increased 'fractional emptying rate' (FER), which is the fraction of gastric contents emptied per minute (Malagelada, 1978, 1980). This phenomenon appears to be independent of both acid hypersecretion and hypergastrinaemia as it persists after treatment with the antagonists and it is not observed in healthy individuals receiving pentagastrin (Dubois et al, 1977).

Delayed gastric emptying of solids has been reported in atrophic gastritis patients with (Bromster, 1969; Frank et al, 1981) or without (Davies et al, 1971; Frank et al, 1981) pernicious anaemia (Figure 7).

Antral hypocontractility especially during phase II of the MMC cycle has been reported in gastric ulcer patients, both during fasting (Miranda et al, 1985) and after feeding (Miller et al, 1980). Figure 8 shows an example of phase III initiated in the proximal small bowel recorded in a patient with an ulcer in the body of the stomach. These motor abnormalities are accompanied by increased duodeno-gastric reflux which may play

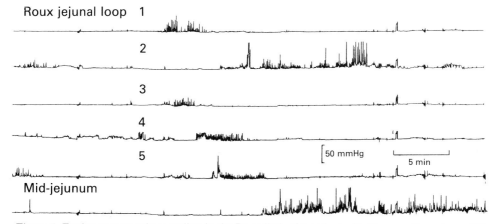

Figure 5. Fasting manometric recording in the Roux limb of a patient with Roux-en-Y syndrome (M, 49 yr). Note the abnormal aspect and propagation of a phase-III-like activity.

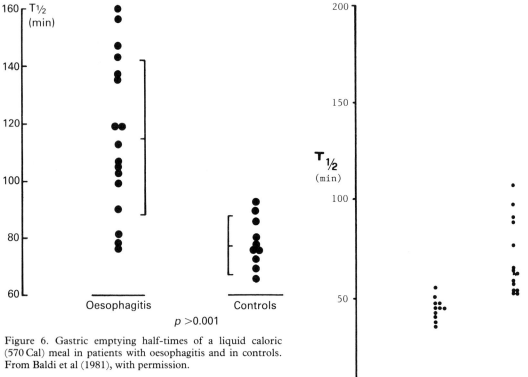

Figure 6. Gastric emptying half-times of a liquid caloric (570 Cal) meal in patients with oesophagitis and in controls. From Baldi et al (1981), with permission.

a role in the pathogenesis and maintenance of the mucosal lesion (Miranda et al, 1985). The reduced contractile response of the antrum to the ingestion of a meal with solid component (Figure 9) may be the cause of the selective delay of gastric emptying of solids observed in gastric ulcer patients (Miller et al, 1980).

Gastrointestinal motor defects may contribute to the pathogenesis of duodenal ulcer. Theoretically this may be due both to excessive emptying of acid from the stomach, and to reduced retrograde displacement of biliary and pancreatic secretions from the descending duodenum into the duodenal bulb (Rhodes and Prestwich, 1966). Patients with uncomplicated duodenal ulcer were found to have an abnormally prolonged secretory response to the meal and an excessive gastric emptying of unbuffered acid, especially in the late postprandial period (Malagelada et al, 1977; Faxen et al, 1978; Lam et al, 1982) (Figure 10). In contrast, Hunt (1957), Holt et al (1986), and Howlett et al (1976) have reported a bimodal distribution of gastric emptying results, suggesting the existence of two sub-populations

Figure 7. Gastric emptying half-times of a semi-solid meal in patients with atrophic gastritis and controls. From Davies et al (1971), with permission.

among duodenal ulcer patients: the first exhibiting accelerated gastric emptying, the second with gastric emptying times within normal limits.

Duodenal ulcer patients have been shown to have a reduced frequency of mixing waves in the proximal duodenum and an increased contractility in the distal duodenum (Monto et al, 1976). Borgström and Arborelius (1978), reported a decreased number of retrograde contractions in the duodenum of these patients, when compared to both healthy subjects and gastric ulcer patients.

Malabsorption Syndrome

Inhibitory intestinal feedback mechanisms tend to slow down gastric emptying. They are sensitive to pH and osmolality, as well as to specific elementary nutrients present in duodenal contents and are

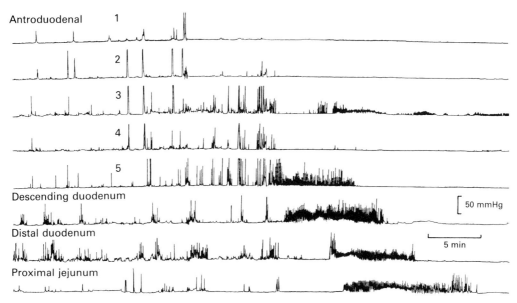

Figure 8. Gastrointestinal manometric recording during fasting in a patient (male, aged 50) with type I gastric ulcer. The activity front (phase III) is without gastric component. Note the apparently normal phase II activity in the distal antrum with irregular but intense contractions.

therefore triggered by the elementary components of food, rather than by macromolecules (Malagelada, 1981). Impaired digestion of food, such as that occurring in severe pancreatic insufficiency, may conceivably reduce the stimulation of duodenal receptors and determine an abnormally rapid gastric emptying. Indeed, results consistent with this hypothesis have been obtained in a study

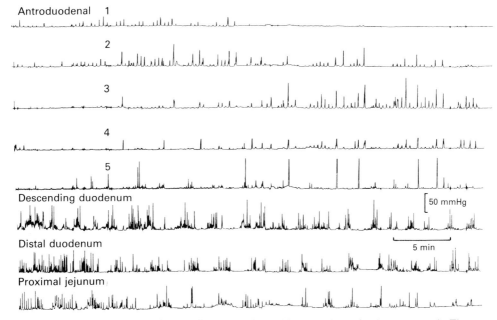

Figure 9. Postprandial manometric recording in a patient with a type I gastric ulcer (same as in Figure 8). Note the severe antral hypomotility (reduction of both frequency and intensity of phasic contractions). The patterns of duodenal and jejunal motility are apparently normal.

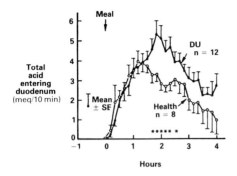

Figure 10. Gastric acid entering the duodenum in 12 duodenal ulcer patients (DU) and in 8 controls (Health), after feeding. From Malagelada et al (1977), with permission.

Abnormalities of Myogenic and Neurogenic Control of Gastrointestinal Motility

Smooth muscle cells and the intrinsic nervous system (INS) are so intimately related that many diseases affect them both simultaneously, and similar considerations apply to the intrinsic and extrinsic autonomic nervous supplies. Nevertheless, an attempt has been made to subdivide gastrointestinal motor abnormalities on the basis of the main regulatory mechanism disrupted.

Both myogenic and neurogenic disorders cause similar impairment of transit, although via opposite mechanisms. In myogenic diseases, the impairment of progression of intraluminal contents is due to a reduction of strength of muscle contractility, while neurogenic disturbances are characterized by powerful but inco-ordinated contractions which do not create the normal aborad pressure gradient. Examples of manometric recordings in patients with myogenic and neurogenic chronic intestinal pseudo-obstruction (CIP) are shown in Figures 12 and 13 respectively.

evaluating gastric emptying of fatty liquid meals by an intubation technique (Long and Weiss, 1974) (Figure 11). The accelerated gastric emptying of patients with pancreatic exocrine insufficiency returned to normal when active pancreatic enzymes were added to the test meal. In another study, gastric emptying of a mixed solid-liquid meal appeared similar in patients with pancreatic insufficiency and healthy controls (Regan et al, 1979).

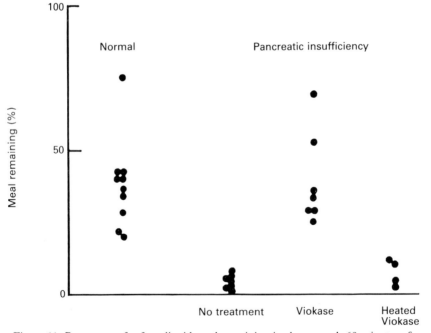

Figure 11. Percentage of a fatty liquid meal remaining in the stomach 60 minutes after ingestion, in patients with pancreatic insufficiency and controls. Patients received either no treatment, pancreatic enzymes (Viokase) or inactivated pancreatic enzymes (heated Viokase). From Long and Weiss (1974), with permission.

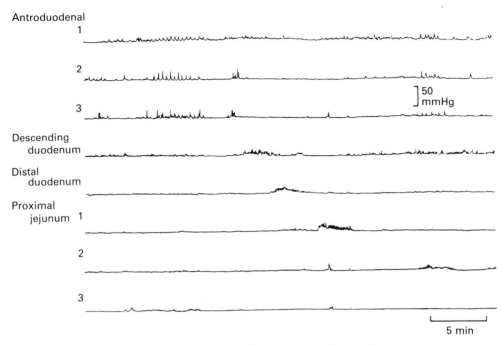

Figure 12. Fasting gastrointestinal manometric recording in a 71-year-old man affected by myogenic chronic intestinal pseudo-obstruction. Note the activity front with normal propagation, but severely reduced contractile force. From Malagelada et al (1986), with permission.

Disorders of the Smooth Muscle

Gastrointestinal smooth muscle may be affected as part of more generalized disease involving different muscle groups. Myotonic dystrophy and progressive muscular dystrophy are the most common diseases affecting both voluntary and smooth muscle cells. In myotonic dystrophy, gastrointestinal symptoms are frequent and may precede the appearance of the somatic disease by months or years (Kohn et al, 1964). Impairment of gastric emptying with formation of bezoar has been reported (Kuiper, 1971). In some instances, the visceral involvement is severe enough to cause a pseudo-obstructive syndrome (Harvey et al, 1965).

Fluid and electrolyte imbalances are frequent

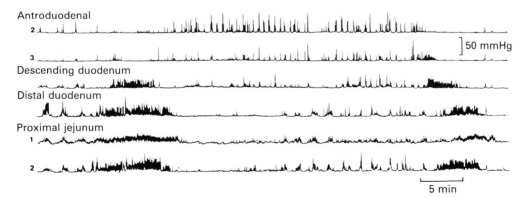

Figure 13. Abnormally propagated activity fronts in the duodenum and proximal small bowel of a 59-year-old man affected by neurogenic chronic intestinal pseudo-obstruction. From Malagelada et al (1986), with permission.

findings in patients with severe gastroparesis or other gastrointestinal motor abnormalities. They may represent both causes and consequences of the motor disorders. Intra- and extra-cellular ion concentrations regulate transmembrane fluxes responsible for myoelectrical events (Szurszewski, 1981); hypokalaemia and hypochloraemic alkalosis generally follow protracted vomiting (Malagelada and Camilleri, 1984).

Collagen vascular diseases, such as progressive systemic sclerosis (PSS or scleroderma), dermatomyositis, systemic lupus erythematosus and Ehlers–Danlos syndrome, may cause damage to smooth muscle as well as the INS. Di Marino et al in 1973 recorded myoelectrical events in patients affected by scleroderma. All the patients presented normal slow wave frequency, but a reduced number of action potentials in response to duodenal distension, suggesting abnormalities of the INS; furthermore, patients with longstanding disease also presented a reduced response to direct stimulation of smooth muscle by pentagastrin and secretin, suggesting a more diffuse gut involvement with impaired muscular contractility. An example of severe intestinal hypomotility is shown in Figure 14.

The motor abnormalities seen in collagen diseases may be secondary to ischaemia due to arteritis. *In vitro* studies, in fact, have shown that ischaemia may reduce slow wave frequency and impair coupling (Szurszewski and Steggerda, 1968).

Disorders of the Intrinsic Nervous System

Some diseases may selectively affect the INS. Hirschsprung's and Chagas' diseases are well-known causes of INS abnormalities and have been extensively investigated (Faulk et al, 1978). Other causes, however, have been identified and deserve mentioning. Viral infections responsible for flu-like episodes sometimes precede the acute onset of dyspeptic syndromes. Some viruses have been shown to induce motor abnormalities both in experimental animals (Burrows and Merritt, 1984) and in humans (Meeroff et al, 1980). In the latter study, healthy subjects voluntarily ingested parvovirus-like agents. Half of them became symp-

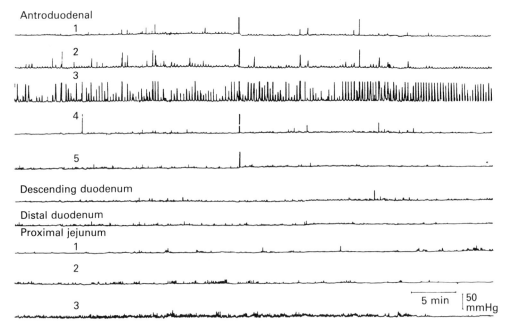

Figure 14. Postprandial antral dysmotility in a 53-year-old woman with a history of scleroderma and CREST syndrome of 3-year duration. Note the antral and duodenal hypomotility, with prominent pyloric motility. From Malagelada et al (1986), with permission.

tomatic and exhibited delayed gastric emptying. No change in gastric function was observed in those subjects who did not develop the illness (Figure 15). The authors concluded that nausea and vomiting induced by this viral infection 'may result from abnormal gastric motor function'.

As previously mentioned, the autonomic nervous supply of the gut exerts an overall inhibitory effect on intestinal motility and in fact diseases affecting the INS cause inco-ordinated hypercontractility (Figure 13). Distinct manometric abnormalities have been observed in patients with idiopathic CIP of neurogenic type (Stanghellini et al, 1987). These will be discussed in detail in Chapter 27B.

Disorders of the Extrinsic Nervous Supply

Effects of surgical vagotomy on gastric emptying have already been described. Neither vagotomy nor splanchnectomy, alone or in combination, substantially modify the intestinal motor patterns that seem to be regulated mainly at a local level (Sarna, 1985). Neural diseases affecting the extrinsic autonomic supply of the gut may severely affect the motor activity of the stomach as well as the small intestine. The gastroparesis observed in patients with insulin-dependent diabetes is commonly considered to be a consequence of impaired neural control. Delayed gastric emptying of both solids and liquids has been reported in diabetic patients (Campbell et al, 1977), but since only limited groups of patients have been investigated, the prevalence of this form of gastroparesis is not known. It may also be found in asymptomatic patients (Kassander, 1958) and tends to follow a cyclical course of remission and recurrence, concomitant with fluctuating conditions of the underlying metabolic disorders. Antral hypocontractility, observed in these patients, both during fasting and after feeding, may account for retention of indigestible and digestible solids respectively (Malagelada et al, 1980). An example of postprandial antral hypomotility in a patient with insulin-dependent diabetes is shown in Figure 16. More recent manometric studies have demonstrated that the motor abnormalities may not be limited to the gastric antrum. Some diabetic patients with symptomatic gastroparesis exhibit normal antral motility, but inco-ordinated hypercontractility of the proximal small bowel that may create a decrease of the gastro-duodenal pressure

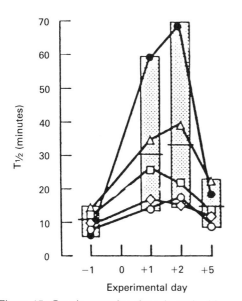
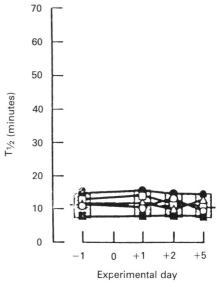

Figure 15. Gastric emptying times in 10 healthy volunteers before and after virus inoculation ($\Diamond$, $\triangle$, $\square$, Norwalk virus; $\bullet$ Hawaii virus). Each subject is indicated by a separate symbol. Left: Results in five volunteers who developed gastroenteritis. Right: Results in five volunteers who did not develop gastroenteritis. From Meeroff et al (1980), with permission.

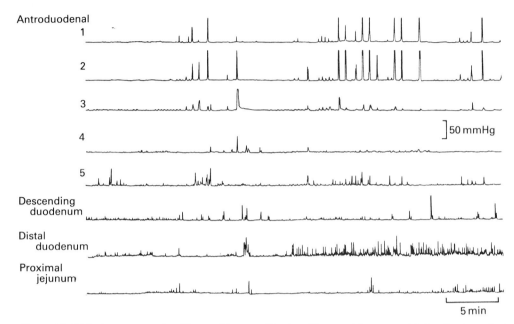

Figure 16. Diabetic gastroparesis with antral hypomotility in a 27-year-old woman with insulin-dependent diabetes. Antral waves that are visible are of normal amplitude, but they are separated by prolonged periods of motor quiescence. From Malagelada et al (1986), with permission.

gradient responsible for the gastroparesis (Figure 17). The latter abnormal motor pattern is indistinguishable from that recorded in patients with diseases affecting the sympathetic system, thus suggesting that abnormalities of these pathways may also occur as a consequence of the metabolic disorder.

Several neurological disorders affecting the autonomic nervous pathways may induce severe abnormalities of gastrointestinal motility (Malagelada et al, 1986). Figures 18 and 19 show examples of severe dysmotility recorded in the stomach and proximal small bowel of patients affected by idiopathic orthostatic hypotension and pandysautonomy respectively. Manometric abnormalities of intestinal motility are similar to those described in neurogenic CIP, with abnormal MMCs, bursts, and sustained inco-ordinated hypercontractility. None of the above-described abnormal motor patterns has been recorded in subjects who had undergone traumatic spinal cord transection (Fealey et al, 1984), but bursts of non-propagated spike potentials have been observed in the small bowel of dogs after coeliac and superior

mesenteric ganglionectomy, or after complete ablation of sympathetic supply (Heppel et al, 1983). These results suggest that gastrointestinal motor abnormalities may be induced by post- (but not pre-) ganglionic denervation. Post-ganglionic denervation conceivably also affects the INS, but the respective roles of the disturbed extrinsic and intrinsic neural controls inducing gastrointestinal motor abnormalities have not been identified.

Diseases of the Central Nervous System

Gastrointestinal motor abnormalities have been described both in psychogenic disorders and in organic diseases involving the CNS. In healthy individuals, acute stressful stimuli acting on the CNS have been shown to delay gastric emptying (Thompson et al, 1982) and to modify the normal postprandial motor patterns, inhibiting antral phasic motility and stimulating, in some instances, the appearance of a complex-like activity in the duodenum (Thompson et al, 1982; Stanghellini et al, 1983) (Figure 20). These motor abnormalities are, at least partially, mediated via adrenergic and

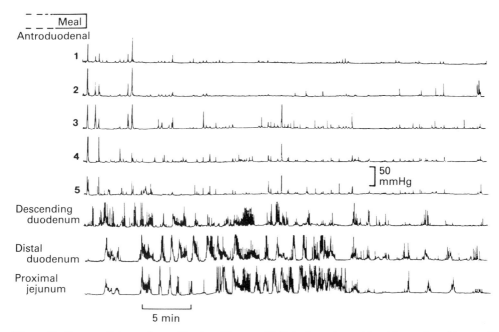

Figure 17. Postprandial gut dysmotility in a 71-year-old diabetic patient with a 10-year long history of episodic vomiting. Note the severe antral hypomotility and the bursts of phasic contractions superimposed upon tonic elevations of the baseline. From Malagelada et al (1986), with permission.

opioid pathways. Firstly, a significant increase in circulating levels of norepinephrine and beta-endorphin has been detected concomitant to the motor abnormalities (Stanghellini et al, 1983). Secondly, both opiate (naloxone) and adrenergic (phentolamine + propanolol) blockers prevent the stress-induced inhibition of antral contractility (Stanghellini et al, 1984). Finally, infusion of exogenous endorphins mimics the effect of stressful stimuli on duodenal motility (Camilleri et al, 1986). Recent electrogastrography studies in healthy subjects have shown that experimentally

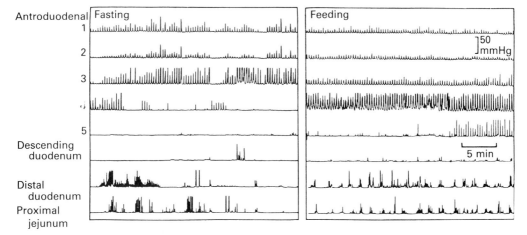

Figure 18. Uninterrupted intense antral contractility in a 63-year-old woman presenting with dyspeptic symptoms and idiopathic orthostatic hypotension. From Malagelada et al (1986), with permission.

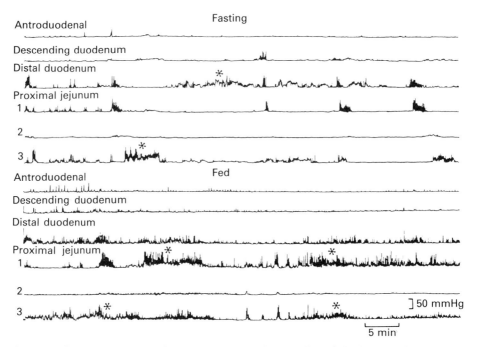

Figure 19. Severe hypomotility of the distal antrum and inco-ordinated phasic and tonic (*) pressure activities of the proximal small bowel in a 46-year-old woman with pandysautonomia. From Malagelada et al (1986), with permission.

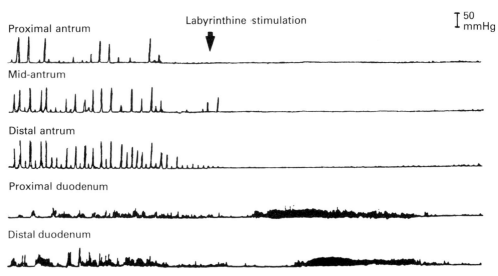

Figure 20. Effect of an acute centrally acting stressful stimulus (vertigo) on fed gastrointestinal motility. Note the marked inhibition of antral contractility and the appearance, in the duodenum, of a phase-III-like activity. From Stanghellini et al (1983), with permission.

induced motion sickness is accompanied by tachygastria (Stern et al, 1987). Abnormalities of myoelectrical control may represent the cause of the antral hypocontractility induced by centrally acting stimuli.

Primary anorexia nervosa (PAN) is a psychiatric disease affecting primarily young females. It is characterized by gastrointestinal symptoms such as inability to eat a normal meal, postprandial fullness, nausea, vomiting, epigastric pain, abdominal bloating and distension. The syndrome may be extremely severe and mortality rates ranging from 7 to 21% have been reported (Dubois et al, 1979). Both gastric acid secretion and gastric emptying rates were found reduced by an intubation technique employing a liquid meal (Dubois et al, 1979). Simultaneous evaluation of gastric emptying of the solid and liquid components of a test meal was obtained in PAN patients by a dual marker radio-isotopic method (McCallum et al, 1985). Liquid emptying was normal but 80% of the patients presented delayed emptying of solids (Figure 21). Delayed gastric

emptying only partially improves following weight gain (Dubois et al, 1979) and the cause and effect relationship between abnormal gastric emptying and decrease in body weight remains to be clarified.

Severe motor disturbances have also been reported in patients with organic diseases of the CNS. Sudden onset of pseudo-obstructive syndromes may occur after vascular accidents involving the CNS (Reynolds and Eliasson, 1977). Inco-ordinated hypermotility of the proximal small bowel similar to that seen in neurogenic CIP has also been recorded in a patient affected by a brain stem tumour (Wood et al, 1985).

Idiopathic Motor Abnormalities

'Functional' syndromes are the most frequent diagnoses in gastroenterological practice (Switz, 1976), but, rather surprisingly only a few studies have systematically investigated the possible pathogenic mechanisms involved. These syn-

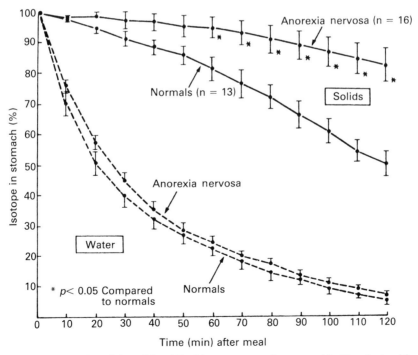

Figure 21. Gastric emptying of the solid and liquid components of a test meal in 16 patients with anorexia nervosa and in 13 controls. From McCallum et al (1985), with permission.

dromes are commonly believed to represent the expression of a gut motility disorder (Cohen, 1983). In particular, functional dyspepsia is thought to be related to motor abnormalities of the proximal part of the digestive tract. We have recently evaluated gastric emptying of solids in 47 patients complaining of dyspeptic symptoms in the absence of any recognizable underlying disease; in 29 of them we have also evaluated basal and pentagastrin-stimulated gastric acid secretion, and in seven gastric emptying of a homogenized meal (Corinaldesi et al, 1986; Stanghellini et al, 1986). No significant difference was found in basal and stimulated acid secretion between dyspeptic patients and healthy controls. Dyspeptic patients exhibited a significant delay of gastric emptying of solids (about 50% of the patients had abnormally prolonged gastric emptying), but not of the homogenized meal. This selective abnormal gastric emptying of solids confirms previous reports (Rees et al, 1980) and is suggestive of a motor disorder confined to the antrum. Indeed, abnormalities of antral myo-electrical activity have been detected, by *in vivo* and *in vitro* techniques, in patients with unexplained dyspepsia (Telander et al, 1978; You et al, 1980). The patients were found to have ectopic antral pacemakers firing at higher than normal rates (> 5 cycles/minute) with regular (tachygastria), or irregular (tachyarrhythmia) frequencies (Figure 22). Abnormal slow waves may be driven by the ectopic pacemaker both aborally and in anterograde direction.

A systematic manometric study showed the existence of recognizable abnormal motor patterns in the stomach and/or proximal small bowel of the majority of a large group of dyspeptic patients (Malagelada and Stanghellini, 1985). Over 40% of the patients had antral hypomotility alone (Figure 23), while about 30% presented both gastric hypomotility and intestinal motor inco-ordination. The exact mechanism of gastrointestinal dysmotility was not elucidated in this study and warrants further investigation.

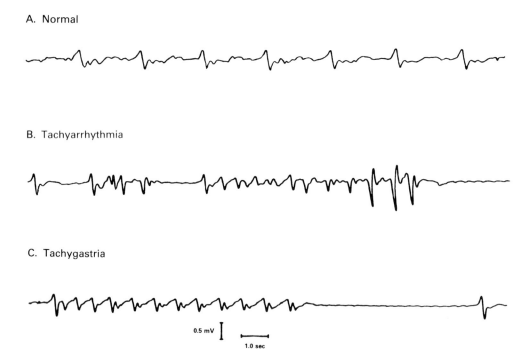

A. Normal

B. Tachyarrhythmia

C. Tachygastria

0.5 mV

1.0 sec

Figure 22. *In vivo* recordings of antral myoelectrical activity in an asymptomatic control and in patients with functional upper gut symptoms. From You et al (1980), with permission.

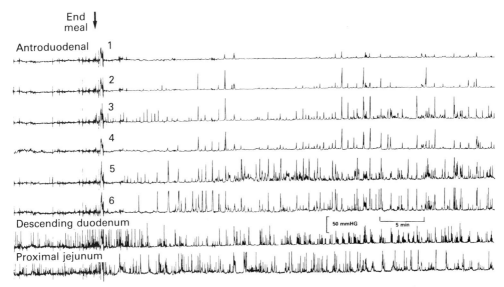

Figure 23. Postprandial antral hypomotility (reduced frequency and intensity of antral contractions) in a 44-year-old woman complaining of dyspeptic symptoms (early satiety, postprandial fullness, nausea).

References

Baldi, F., Corinaldesi, R., Ferrarini, F., Stanghellini, V., Miglioli, M., and Barbara, L., (1981), Gastric secretion and emptying of liquids in reflux esophagitis. *Dig. Dis. Sci.*, 26:886–9.

Borgström, S., and Arborelius, M. Jr., (1978), Duodenal motility pattern in duodenal ulcer disease. *Scand. J. Gastroenterol.*, 13:349–52.

Brömster, D. (1969), Gastric emptying rate in gastric and duodenal ulceration. *Scand. J. Gastroenterol.*, 4:193–201.

Burrows, C. F., and Merritt, A. M., (1984), Influence of corona virus (transmissible gastroenteritis) infection on jejunal myoelectrical activity on the neonatal pig. *Gastroenterology*, 87:386–91.

Camilleri, M., Malagelada, J. R., Stanghellini, V., Zinsmeister, A. R., Kao, P. C., and Li, C. H., (1986), Dose-related effects of synthetic human beta-endorphin and naloxone on fed gastrointestinal motility. *Am. J. Physiol.*, 251:G147–54.

Campbell, I. W., Heading, R. C., Tothill, P., Buist, T. A. S., Ewing, D. J., and Clarke, B. F., (1977), Gastric emptying in diabetic autonomic neuropathy. *Gut*, 18:462–7.

Clarke, R. J., and Alexander-Williams, J., (1973), The effect of preserving antral innervation and of a pyloroplasty on gastric emptying after vagotomy in man. *Gut*, 14:300–7.

Cohen, S., (1983), Neuromuscular disorders of the gastrointestinal tract. *Hosp. Pract.*, 18:121–4, 130–1.

Corinaldesi, R., Stanghellini, V., Raiti, C., Rea, E., Salgemini, R., Paternicó, A., Paparo, G. F., and Barbara, L., (1986), Gastric acid secretion and gastric emptying (GE) of solids in patients with chronic idiopathic dyspepsia (CID). *Dig. Dis. Sci.*, 31 (10 Suppl): 343 (abstr).

Davies, W. T., Kirkpatrick, J. R., Owen, G. M., and Shields, R., (1971), Gastric emptying in atrophic gastritis and carcinoma of the stomach. *Scand. J. Gastroenterol.*, 6:297–301.

Di Marino, A. J., Carlson, G., Myers, A., Schumacher, R., and Cohen, S., (1973), Duodenal myoelectric activity in scleroderma: abnormal responses to mechanical and hormonal stimuli. *New Engl. J. Med.*, 2:1220–3.

Dubois, A., Gross, H. A., Ebert, M. H., and Castell, D. O., (1979), Altered gastric emptying and secretion in primary anorexia nervosa. *Gastroenterology*, 77:319–23.

Dubois, A., Van Eerdewegh, P., and Gardner, J. D., (1977), Gastric emptying and secretion in Zollinger-Ellison syndromes. *J. Clin. Invest.*, 59:255–63.

Faxen, A., Kewenter, J., and Kock, N. G., (1978), Gastric emptying of a liquid meal in health and duodenal ulcer disease. *Scand. J. Gastroenterol.*, 13:735–40.

Faulk, D. L., Anuras, S., and Christensen, J., (1978), Chronic intestinal pseudoobstruction. *Gastroenterology*, 74:922–31.

Fealey, R. D., Szurszewski, J. H., Merritt, J. L., and Di Magno, E. P., (1984), Effect of traumatic spinal cord transection on human upper gastrointestinal motility and gastric emptying. *Gastroenterology*, **87**:69–75.

Frank, E. B., Lange, R. C., and McCallum, R. W., (1981), Abnormal gastric emptying in patients with atrophic gastritis with or without pernicious anaemia. *Gastroenterology*, **80**:1151 (abstr).

Harvey, J. C., Sherbourne, D. H., and Siegel, C. I., (1965), Smooth muscle involvement in myotonic dystrophy. *Am. J. Med.*, **39**:81–90.

Heppel, J., Kelly, K. A., and Sarr, M. G., (1983), Neural control of canine small intestine interdigestive complexes. *Am. J. Physiol.*, **244**:G95–100.

Holt, F., Heading, R. C., Taylor, T. V., Forrest, J. A., and Tothill, P., (1986), Is gastric emptying abnormal in duodenal ulcer? *Dig. Dis. Sci.*, **31**:685–92.

Howlett, P. J., Sheiner, H. J., Barber, D. C., Ward, A. S., Perez-Avila, C. A., and Duthie, H. L., (1976), Gastric emptying in control subjects and patients with duodenal ulcer before and after vagotomy. *Gut*, **17**:542–50.

Hunt, J. N., (1957), Influence of hydrochloric acid on gastric secretion and emptying in patients with duodenal ulcer. *Br. Med. J.*, **1**:681–4.

Kalbasi, H., Hudson, F. R., Herring, A., Moss, S., Glass, H. I., and Spencer, J., (1975), Gastric emptying following vagotomy and antrectomy and proximal gastric vagotomy. *Gut*, **16**:509–13.

Kassander, P., (1958), Asymptomatic gastric retention in diabetes (gastroparesis diabeticorum). *Ann. Int. Med.*, **48**:797–812.

Kohn, N. N., Faires, J. F., and Rodman, T., (1964), Unusual manifestations due to involvement of involuntary muscle in dystrophia myotonica. *New. Engl. J. Med.*, **271**:1179–83.

Kuiper, D. H., (1971), Gastric bezoar in a patient with myotonic dystrophy. *Am. J. Dig. Dis.*, **16**:529–34.

Lam, F. K., Isenberg, J. I., Grossman, M. I., Lane, W. H., and Hogan, D. L., (1982), Rapid gastric emptying in duodenal ulcer patients. *Dig. Dis. Sci.*, **27**:598–604.

Long, W. B., and Weiss, J. B., (1974), Rapid gastric emptying of fatty meals in pancreatic insufficiency. *Gastroenterology*, **67**:920–5.

Malagelada, J. R., (1978), Pathophysiological response to meal in the Zollinger-Ellison syndrome. 1. Paradoxical postprandial inhibition of gastric secretion. *Gut*, **19**:284–9.

Malagelada, J. R., (1980), Pathophysiological responses to meal in the Zollinger-Ellison syndrome. 2. Gastric emptying and its effect on duodenal function. *Gut*, **21**:98–104.

Malagelada, J. R., (1981), Gastric, pancreatic and biliary responses to a meal. In: *Physiology of the Gastrointestinal Tract* (Ed. Johnson, L. R.), pp. 893–924, Raven Press, New York.

Malagelada, J. R., and Camilleri, M., (1984), Unex-

plained vomiting: a diagnostic challenge. *Ann. Int. Med.*, **101**:211–18.

Malagelada, J. R., Camilleri, M., and Stanghellini, V., (1986), *Manometric Diagnosis of Gastrointestinal Motility Disorders*, Georg Thieme Verlag, Stuttgart, New York.

Malagelada, J. R., Longstreth, G. F., Deering, T. B., Summerskill, W. H. J., and Go, V. L. W., (1977), Gastric secretion and emptying after ordinary meals in duodenal ulcer. *Gastroenterology*, **73**:989–94.

Malagelada, J. R., Rees, W. D. W., Mazzotta, L. J., and Go, V. L. W., (1980), Gastric motor abnormalities in diabetic and postvagotomy gastroparesis: effect of metoclopramide and bethanechol. *Gastroenterology*, **78**:286–93.

Malagelada, J. R., and Stanghellini, V., (1985), Manometric evaluation of functional upper gut symptoms. *Gastroenterology*, **88**:1223–31.

Mathias, J. R., Fernandez, A., Sninsky, C. A., Clench, M. H., and Davis, R. H., (1985), Nausea, vomiting, and abdominal pain after Roux-en-Y anastomosis: motility of the jejunal limb. *Gastroenterology*, **88**:101–7.

McCallum, R. W., Grill, B. B., Lange, R., Planky, M., Glass, E. E., and Greenfeld, D. G., (1985), Definition of a gastric emptying abnormality in patients with anorexia nervosa. *Dig. Dis. Sci.*, **30**:713–22.

Meeroff, J. C., Schreiber, D. S., Trier, J. S., and Blacklow, N. R., (1980), Abnormal gastric motor function in viral gastroenteritis. *Ann. Int. Med.*, **92**:370–3.

Miller, L. J., Malagelada, J. R., Longstreth, G. F., and Go, V. L. W., (1980), Dysfunctions of the stomach with gastric ulceration. *Dig. Dis. Sci.*, **25**:857–64.

Miranda, M., Defilippi, C., and Valenzuela, J. E., (1985), Abnormalities of interdigestive motility complex and increased duodenogastric reflux in gastric ulcer patients. *Dig. Dis. Sci.*, **30**:16–21.

Monto, G. L., Ashworth, W. D., Malecki, M., Thompson, A. B., and Englert, E., (1976), Duodenal contraction wave patterns in patients with and without ulcer. *Am. J. Gastroenterol.*, **65**:52–6.

Rees, W. D. W., Miller, L. J., and Malagelada, J. R., (1980), Dyspepsia, antral motor dysfunction, and gastric stasis of solids. *Gastroenterology*, **78**:360–5.

Regan, P. T., Malagelada, J. R., Di Magno, E. P., and Go, V. L. W., (1979), Postprandial gastric function in pancreatic insufficiency. *Gut*, **20**:249–54.

Reynolds, B. J., and Eliasson, F. G., (1977), Colonic pseudo-obstruction in patient's stroke. *Ann. Neurol.*, **1**,305.

Rhodes, J., and Prestwich, C. J., (1966), Acidity at different sites in the proximal duodenum of normal subjects and patients with duodenal ulcer. *Gut*, **7**:509–14.

Sarna, S. H., (1985), Cyclic motor activity: migrating motor complex. *Gastroenterology*, **89**:894–913.

Stanghellini, V., Camilleri, M., and Malagelada, J. R., (1987), Chronic idiopathic intestinal pseudo-obstruction: clinical and intestinal manometric findings. *Gut*, **28**:5–12.

Stanghellini, V., Corinaldesi, R., Monetti, N., Raiti, C., Rea, E., Salgemini, R., Corbelli, C., and Barbara, L., (1986), Gastric emptying of solids and homogenized meals in patients with chronic idiopathic dyspepsia. *Dig. Dis. Sci.*, **31** (10 Suppl): 178S (abstr).

Stanghellini, V., and Malagelada, J. R., (1983), Gastric manometric abnormalities in patients with dyspeptic symptoms after fundoplication. *Gut*, **24**:790–7.

Stanghellini, V., Malagelada, J. R., Zinsmeister, A. R., Go, V. L. W., and Kao, P. C., (1983), Stress-induced gastroduodenal motor disturbances in human: possible humoral mechanisms. *Gastroenterology*, **85**:83–91.

Stanghellini, V., Malagelada, J. R., Zinsmeister, A. R., Go, V. L. W., and Kao, P. C., (1984), Effect of opiate and adrenergic blockers on the gut motor response to centrally-acting stimuli. *Gastroenterology*, **87**:1104–13.

Stern, R. M., Koch, K. L., Stewart, W. R., and Lindblad, I. M., (1987), Spectral analysis of tachygastria recorded during motion sickness. *Gastroenterology*, **92**:92–7.

Switz, D. M., (1976), What the gastroenterologist does all day. A survey of a state society's practice. *Gastroenterology*, **70**:1048–50.

Szurszewski, J. H., (1981), Electrical basis of gastrointestinal motility. In: *Physiology of the Gastrointestinal Tract* (Ed. Johnson, L. R.), pp. 1435–66, Raven Press, New York.

Szurszewski, J. H., and Steggerda, F. R., (1968), The effect of hypoxia on the electrical slow wave on the canine small intestine. *Am. J. Dig. Dis.*, **13**:168–74.

Telander, R. L., Morgan, K. G., Kreulen, D. L., Schmalz, P. F., Kelly, K. A., and Szurszewski, J. H., (1978), Human gastric atony with tachygastria and gastric retention. *Gastroenterology*, **75**:497–501.

Thompson, D. G., Richelson, E., and Malagelada, J. R., (1982), Perturbation of gastric emptying and duodenal motility through the central nervous system. *Gastroenterology*, **83**:1200–6.

Wood, J. R., Camilleri, M., Low, P. A., and Malagelada, J. R., (1985), Brain stem tumor presenting as an upper gut motility disorder. *Gastroenterology*, **89**:1411–14.

You, C. H., Lee, K. Y., Chey, W. Y., and Menguy, R., (1980), Electrogastrographic study of patients with unexplained nausea, bloating, and vomiting. *Gastroenterology*, **79**:311–14.

26
BILIARY TRACT

Aldo Torsoli, Enrico Corazziari
Università 'La Sapienza', Rome, Italy

Biliary motor disorders may affect the gall-bladder, the cholecystocystic junction and the sphincter of Oddi. The scheme of classification shown below will be followed in this chapter.

Gall-bladder
    Atonic gall-bladder
    Hyperkinetic gall-bladder
Cholecystocystic junction
    Functional obstruction of the cholecystocystic junction
Sphincter of Oddi (SO)
    SO dysfunction
    SO stenosis and dyskinesia
    SO incompetence

Motor abnormalities of the extrahepatic biliary tree may occur in the presence or absence of local organic disorders. The term dyskinesia usually refers to the latter. In clinical terms, however, the exact nature of such abnormalities is ill-defined because:

(1) Biliary motor activity cannot be easily assessed and quantified in man;
(2) The exclusion of local organic disorders is usually based on standard radiological and/or echographic examination.
(3) The causal relationship between symptoms and motor abnormalities can only be ascertained in some cases.

Atonic Gall-bladder

Atony of the gall-bladder is suggested by the radiological finding of an elongated, flaccid viscus which may be easily compressed by the adjacent organs. In some patients the viscus does not contract after either a standard fatty meal or exogenous cholecystokinin (CCK) administration; in others, the lack of contraction after a fatty meal contrasts with the regular contraction after exogenous CCK administration (Figure 1) (Torsoli et al, 1961). This suggests that the abnormality may be the result of either a primary smooth muscle disorder or secondary to an altered release of endogenous CCK or an abnormal response to the neuro-hormonal stimulus. Gall-bladder atony secondary to insufficient release of endogenous CCK has in fact been observed after Billroth II gastric resection, after vagotomy, in coeliac disease and in patients with delayed gastric emptying (Maton et al, 1985; Johnson and Boyden, 1952; Malagelada et al, 1974). In patients with somatostinoma the cholecystokinetic effect of CCK is blocked by the high blood levels of somatostatin (Fisher et al, 1987). Atony may also be the consequence of a long-standing obstruction to gall-bladder evacuation as may occur in inflammatory strictures and/or stones at the cholecystocystic junction. In this case, however, the primary cause of the gall-bladder disorder is organic.

Atony of the gall-bladder is often an incidental finding in either asymptomatic or dyspeptic patients with no apparent relationship between the motor abnormality and symptomatology. The clinical relevance of an atonic gall-bladder remains to be established but it is probable that it facilitates bile stasis within the gall-bladder, thus predisposing to cholelithiasis.

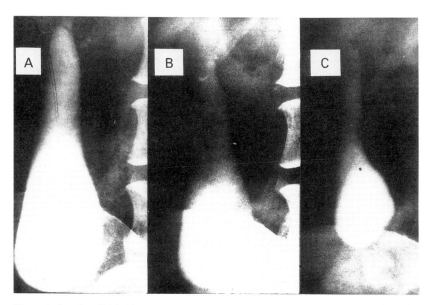

Figure 1. Atonic gall-bladder showing partial gall-bladder emptying after a fatty meal and normal response to CCK (75 IDU in 3 min), indicating absence of organic alterations at the cholecystocystic junction. Cholecystography: A. Preliminary X-ray film. B. 30 min after fatty meal. C. In a second examination 5 days later, 15 min after CCK. From Torsoli et al (1973) with permission.

Hyperkinetic Gall-bladder

Complete gall-bladder emptying within 30 minutes after a fatty meal has been considered by radiologists as evidence of a hyperkinetic gall-bladder, but the clinical relevance of this finding is not clear (Torsoli, 1964). Gall-bladder hypermotility is often associated with adenomyomatosis (Figure 2).

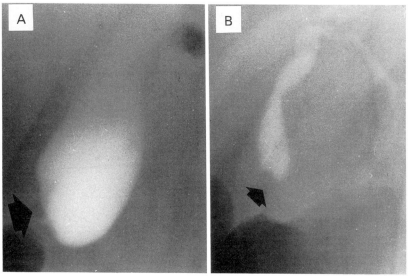

Figure 2. Hyperkinetic gall-bladder. Cholecystography. Gall-bladder in basal conditions (A) and 30 min after a standard fatty meal (B). Arrow indicates the presence of adenomyomatosis.

Functional Obstruction of the Cholecystocystic Junction

The sudden occlusion of the cholecystocystic junction causes a rapid intra-gall-bladder pressure increment which appears to be the pathogenetic factor underlying the colicky pain (Torsoli, 1964). Although the occlusion of the cholecystocystic junction is usually secondary to gallstone(s), it may occur due to inflammatory oedema, torsion of the gall-bladder and smooth muscle spasm. In patients with biliary colic and no evidence of organic disease, functional obstruction has occasionally been reproduced with high dose CCK administration (Torsoli, 1964). At radiology, the gall-bladder is tonically distended with no passage of contrast medium through the cholecystocystic junction but flow can be re-established by administration of nitrates (Figure 3). The functional nature of the obstruction cannot be ascertained by non-invasive techniques such as radiology and echography; sometimes the presence of microlithiasis has been found after cholecystectomy.

Sphincter of Oddi Dysfunction

Obstruction to flow through the sphincter of Oddi (SO) may induce retention of bile and/or pancreatic juice in the common bile and pancreatic duct respectively. Bile stasis may present clinically with elevated values of gamma-GT, alkaline phosphatase and direct bilirubin; rapid increment in the choledochal pressure may cause the typical biliary colic. Sudden occlusion of the pancreatic SO may induce episodes of acute pancreatitis or hyperamylasaemia.

SO Stenosis and SO Dyskinesia

The most frequent obstruction to flow at the level of the sphincter of Oddi is caused by stones or structural stenosis of the sphincter region. SO motor disorders (dyskinesia) may also cause functional obstruction of the sphincter. The obstruction to flow secondary to functional disorders is intermittent and may be reversed by administering

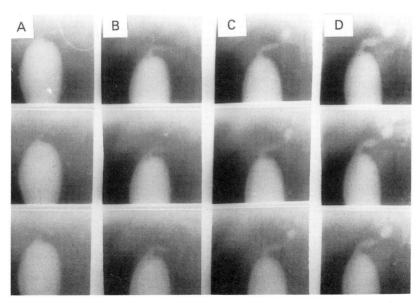

Figure 3. Functional obstruction of the cholecystocystic junction. Effect of amyl nitrate on blockage of the cholecystocystic junction, produced by a high dose of CCK (75 IDU in 30 sec). Cholecystography in a subject with apparently normal gall-bladder. A. Blockage of the junction. B, C and D. Relaxing effect of amyl nitrate. From Torsoli et al (1961) with permission.

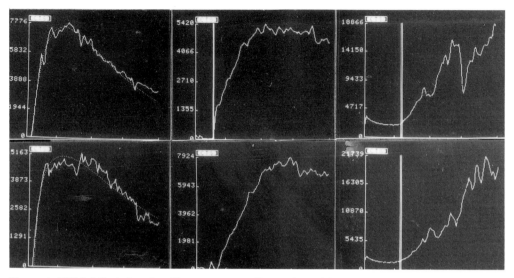

Figure 4. EIDA biliscintigraphy. Two separate studies performed in the same subject following chole-cystectomy. Time-activity curves show radionuclide uptake by the liver (left), arrival into the main bile ducts (middle) and arrival into the duodenum (vertical bar in the right images). The time interval from radionuclide i.v. administration to first appearance in the duodenum did not exceed 16 minutes in a group of healthy cholecystectomized subjects.

suitable drugs having spasmolytic effect on the sphincteric smooth muscle. Ruggero Oddi first hypothesized that, in some instances, jaundice could be the consequence of a 'spasm' of the sphincter (Oddi, 1887).

^{99m}Tc IDA can be used to evaluate biliary excretion by computer assisted cholescintigraphy. This method may detect any obstruction to flow at the level of the choledochoduodenal junction and, at least in cholecystectomized subjects, appears to offer reproducible data (personal unpublished data) (Figure 4), which are com-parable with those derived from endoscopic retro-grade cholangiography (Pace et al., 1983; Shaffer et al, 1986; Zeman et al, 1985). Since chole-scintigraphy is non-invasive and free of risk it might become the test of choice for screening patients with postcholecystectomy syndrome (Figure 5).

The most recent advances in the study of the SO and in the diagnosis of SO dysfunction orig-inate from the cannulation of the papilla by means of subminiaturized manometry catheters via the perendoscopic route (Csendes et al, 1979; Geenen et al, 1980; Carr-Locke and Gregg, 1981; Toouli et al, 1982a; De Masi et al, 1982). An elevated

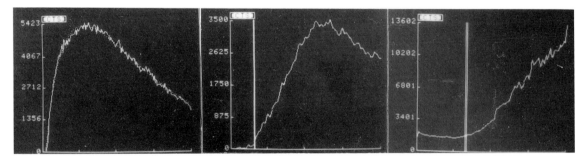

Figure 5. EIDA biliscintigraphy in a patient with biliary like pain after cholecystectomy in the absence of recurrent chole-docholithiasis. Time-activity curves show normal radionuclide uptake by the liver (left), normal excretion in the bile ducts (middle) and delayed bile entrance into the duodenum (20 min after i.v. administration) in the presence of Oddian stenosis.

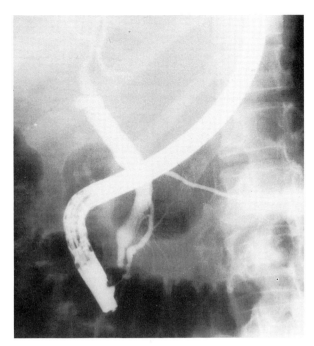

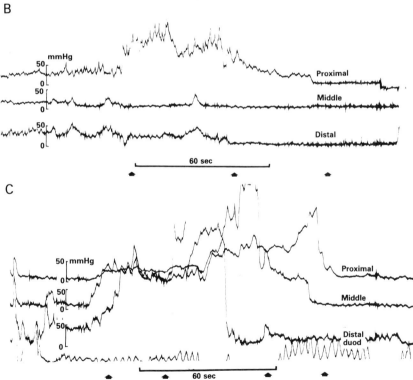

Figure 6. Endoscopic retrograde cholangiopancreatography is suggestive of stenosis of the distal common bile duct and duct of Wirsung (A). Perendoscopic manometry of the sphincter of Oddi performed by means of three recording side-holes (proximal, middle, distal) shows a 2 mm long hypertonic zone of the choledochal sphincter located between 4 and 2 mm above the papillary orifice (B) and a full length hypertonic pancreatic sphincter (C). Manometric indication of a partial stenosis of the proximal part of the choledochal sphincter and of the entire pancreatic sphincter was confirmed at operation. Arrows indicate a 2 mm step withdrawal of the catheter from bile or pancreatic ducts into the duodenum. Duod, duodenal recording.

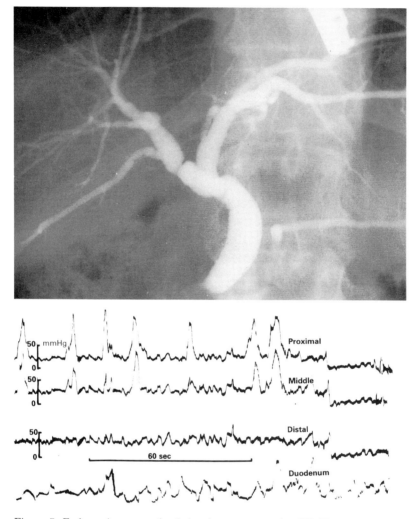

Figure 7. Endoscopic retrograde cholangiopancreatography (ERCP) suggestive of an Oddian stenosis. Perendoscopic manometry of the sphincter of Oddi performed by means of three recording side-holes (proximal, middle, distal) shows normal resting and phasic motor activities. Duodenum = duodenal recording.

basal SO pressure together with an increased choledochoduodenal pressure gradient is diagnostic of either an organic stenosis or functional hypertonicity of the sphincter (Bar-Meir et al, 1979; Funch-Jensen et al, 1982; Meshkinpour et al, 1984; Toouli et al, 1985) (Figures 6, 7 and 8). In functional hypertonicity, SO pressure decreases following administration of smooth muscle relaxants (amyl nitrate, nitroglyerin) (Staritz et al,

1984), CCK (Toouli et al, 1982b) or caerulein (Corazziari et al, 1982).

A paradoxical motor response with marked elevation of the SO resting pressure following CCK or caerulein i.v. administration may occur in patients with unexplained biliary colic (Hogan et al, 1983; Toouli, 1986; Rolny et al, 1986). Since a similar response to CCK or caerulein has been described in the denervated feline SO (Behar and

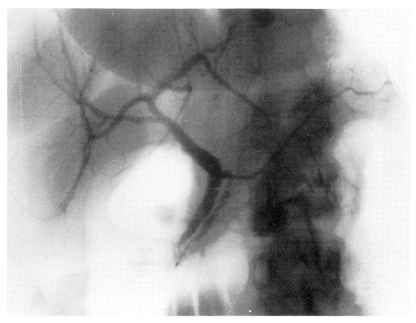

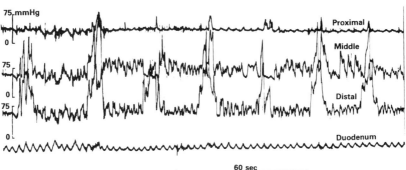

Figure 8. ERCP showing a normal biliary tree in a patient with recurrent biliary colic after cholecystectomy. Perendoscopic manometry of the sphincter of Oddi performed by means of three recording side-holes (proximal, middle, distal) shows abnormally elevated resting pressure.

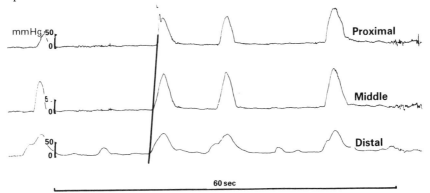

Figure 9. Retrograde contractions seen on perendoscopic manometry of the sphincter of Oddi, performed by means of three recording side-holes (proximal, middle, distal).

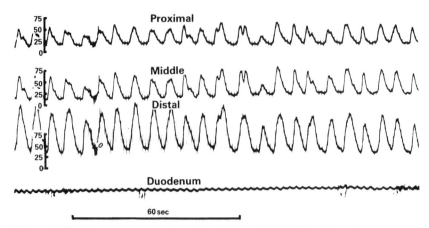

Figure 10. High frequency contraction of the sphincter of Oddi. Perendoscopic manometry of the sphincter of Oddi, performed by means of three recording side-holes (proximal, middle, distal) showing phasic contractions (12 c/min) unaccompanied by duodenal motor activity.

Biancani, 1980) and in the lower oesophageal sphincter of achalasic patients (Dodds et al, 1981), this paradoxical contraction is likely to be due to a defect in the inhibitory innervation of the SO. Predominance of retrograde propagating waves (Figure 9) and high frequency contractions (Figure 10) are two additional manometric findings which have been repeatedly reported to occur in patients with post-cholecystectomy pain or recurrent idiopathic pancreatitis (Hogan et al, 1984; Toouli et al, 1984).

Although SO dysfunction appears to be a relatively frequent occurrence in well-selected, thoroughly investigated post-cholecystectomy patients with recurrent biliary colic and/or biochemical signs of cholestasis in the absence of organic abnormality, the prevalence of SO abnor- malities is not well known. SO motor dysfunction was found in less than 1% of a large series of cholecystecytomized subjects and in 14% of a small group of patients complaining of post-cholecystectomy syndrome (Bar-Meir et al, 1984). In personal unpublished data an elevated SO resting pressure was detected in 15% of patients with choledocholithiasis and in 33% of patients with radiological evidence of stenosis of the distal common bile duct. Clinical relevance of SO dysfunction is poorly understood; in a double blind controlled clinical study, symptom relief has been reported after sphincterotomy in patients with elevated SO resting pressure (Geenen et al, 1984). No data from controlled studies are available concerning patients with SO abnormalities other than elevated resting sphincter pressure.

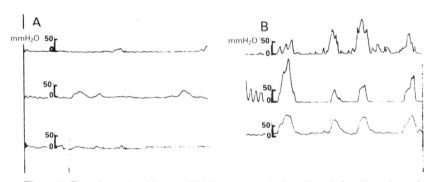

Figure 11. Perendoscopic sphincter of Oddi manometry before (B) and after (A) endoscopic sphincterotomy. Note the absence of resting and phasic contraction after sphincterotomy.

Incompetence of the Sphincter of Oddi

Division of the sphincter of Oddi is followed by the disappearance of phasic contractions and the choledochoduodenal pressure gradient (Figure 11). Air and/or duodenal contents may reflux into the biliary tree and cause inflammation of the ducts. Transient SO incompetence may occur after the passage of calculi migrating from the common bile duct into the duodenum.

References

Bar-Meir, S., Geenen, J. E., Hogan, W. J., Dodds, W. J., Stewart, E. T., and Arndorfer, R. C., (1979), Biliary and pancreatic duct pressures measured by ERCP manometry in patients with suspected papillary stenosis. *Dig. Dis. Sci.*, **24**:209–13.

Bar-Meir, S., Halpern, Z., Bardan, E., and Gilat, T., (1984), Frequency of papillary dysfunction among cholecystectomized patients. *Hepatology*, **4**:328–30.

Behar, J., and Biancani, P., (1980), Effect of cholecystokinin and the octapeptide of cholecystokinin on the feline sphincter of Oddi and gallbladder. Mechanism of action. *J. Clin. Invest.*, **66**:1231–9.

Carr-Locke, D. L., and Gregg, J. A., (1981), Endoscopic manometry of pancreatic and biliary sphincter zones in man: basal results in healthy volunteers. *Dig. Dis. Sci.*, **26**:7–15.

Corazziari, E., De Masi, E., Gatti, V., Habib, F. I., De Simoni, A., Primerano, L., Torsoli, A., and Fegiz, G., (1982), Caerulein and sphincter of Oddi pressure activity. *Ital. J. Gastroenterol.*, **14**:238–41.

Csendes, A., Kruse, A., Funch-Jensen, P., Oster, M. J., Ornsholt, J., and Amdrup, E., (1979), Pressure measurements in the biliary and pancreatic duct systems in controls and in patients with gallstones, previous cholecystectomy or common bile duct stones. *Gastroenterology*, **77**:1203–10.

De Masi, E., Corazziari, E., Habib, F. I., Fontana, B., Gatti, V., Fegiz, G. F., and Torsoli, A., (1982), Manometric study of the sphincter of Oddi in patients with and without common bile duct stones. *Gut*, **25**:275–8.

Dodds, W. J., Dent, J., Hogan, W. J., Patel, G. K., Toouli, J., and Arndorfer, R. C., (1981), Paradoxical lower oesophageal sphincter contraction induced by cholecystokinin-octapeptide in patients with achalasia. *Gastroenterology*, **80**:327–33.

Fisher, R. S., Rock, E., Levin, G., and Malmud, L., (1987), Effect of somatostatin on gallbladder emptying. *Gastroenterology*, **92**:885–90.

Funch-Jensen, P., Kruse, A., Csendes, A., Oster, M. J.,

and Amdrup, E., (1982), Biliary manometry in patients with post-cholecystectomy syndrome. *Acta Chir. Scand.*, **148**:267–8.

Geenen, J. E., Hogan, W. J., Dodds, W. J., Stewart, E. T., and Arndorfer, R. C., (1980), Intraluminal pressure recordings from the human sphincter of Oddi. *Gastroenterology*, **78**:317–24.

Geenen, J. E., Hogan, W. J., Toouli, J., Dodds, W. J., and Venu, R., (1984), A prospective randomized study of the efficacy of endoscopic sphincterotomy for patients with presumptive sphincter of Oddi dysfunction. *Gastroenterology*, **86**:1086.

Hogan, W. J., Geenen, J. E., Dodds, W. J., Toouli, J., Venu, R., and Helm, J., (1983), Paradoxical motor response to cholecystokinin (CCK-OP) in patients with suspected sphincter of Oddi dysfunction. *Gastroenterology*, **82**:1085.

Hogan, W. J., Geenen, J. E., Venu, R., Dodds, W. J., Helm, J., and Toouli, J., (1984), Abnormally rapid contractions of the human sphincter of Oddi (tachyoddia). *Gastroenterology*, **84**:1289.

Johnson, F. E., and Boyden, E. A., (1952), The effect of double vagotomy on the motor activity of the human gallbladder. *Surgery*, **32**:591–601.

Malagelada, J. R., Go, V. L. W., and Summerskill, W. H. J., (1974), Altered pancreatic and biliary function after vagotomy and pyloroplasty. *Gastroenterology*, **66**:22–7.

Maton, P. N., Selden, A. C., Fitzpatrick, M. L., and Chadwick, V. S., (1985), Defective gallbladder emptying and cholecystokinin release in celiac disease. *Gastroenterology*, **88**:391–6.

Meshkinpour, H., Mollot, M., Eckerling, G. B., and Bookman, L., (1984), Bile duct dyskinesia. *Gastroenterology*, **87**:759–62.

Oddi, R., (1887), D'une disposition á sphincter speciale de l'ouverture du canal choledoque. *Arch. It. Biol.*, **8**:317–22.

Pace, R. F., Chamberlain, M. J., and Bassi, R. B., (1983), Diagnosing papillary stenosis by technetium-99m HIDA scanning. *Can. J. Surg.*, **26**:191-3.

Rolny, P., Arleback, A., Funch-Jensen, P., Kruse, A., Ravnsbaeck, J. and Jarnerot, G., (1986), Paradoxical response of sphincter of Oddi to i.v. injection of cholecystokinin or ceruletide. Manometric findings and results of treatment in biliary dyskinesia. *Gut*, **27**:1507–11.

Shaffer, E. A., Hershfield, N. B., Logan, K., and Kloiber, R., (1986), Cholescintigraphic detection of functional obstruction of the sphincter of Oddi. *Gastroenterology*, **90**:728–33.

Staritz, M., Poralla, T., and Meyer zum Buschenfelds, K. H., (1984), Effects of nitroglycerin on the SO motility and baseline pressure. *Gut*, **26**:A1312.

Toouli, J., Geenen, J. E., Hogan, W. J., Dodds, W. J., and Arndorfer, R. C., (1982a), Sphincter of Oddi motor activity: a comparison between patients with common bile duct stones and controls. *Gastroenterology*, **82**:111–17.

Toouli, J., Hogan, W. J., Geenen, J. E., Dodds, W. J., and Arndorfer, R. C., (1982b), Action of cholecystokinin-octapeptide on sphincter of Oddi basal pressure and phasic activity in humans. *Surgery*, **92**:497–503.

Toouli, J., Roberts-Thompson, I., and Dent, J., (1984), Sphincter of Oddi (SO) manometric profile in patients with idiopathic relapsing pancreatitis. *Gastroenterology*, **86**:1283.

Toouli, J., Roberts-Thomson, I. C., Dent, J. and Lee, J., (1985), Manometric disorders in patients with suspected sphincter of Oddi dysfunction. *Gastroenterology*, **88**:1243–50.

Toouli, J., (1986), Motor abnormalities of the sphincter of Oddi. *Ital. J. Gastroenterol.*, **18**:105–7.

Torsoli, A., Ramorino, M. L., Colagrande, C., and De Maio, G. P., (1961), Experiments with cholecystokinin. *Acta Radiol.*, **55**:193.

Torsoli, A., (1964), Studi sull'attivitá motoria biliare. *Il Fegato*, **10**:133–221.

Torsoli, A., Ramorino, M. L., and Carratu, R., (1973), On the use of CCK in roentgenologic examination of the extrahepatic biliary tract and intestines. In: *Handbook of Experimental Pharmacology*, **34**:247–60, Springer Verlag, Heidelberg.

Zeman, R. K., Burrell, M. I., Dobbins, J., Jaffe, M. H., and Choyke, P. L., (1985), Postcholecystectomy syndrome: evaluation using biliary scintigraphy and endoscopic retrograde cholangiopancreatography. *Radiology*, **156**:787–92.

27
SMALL AND LARGE INTESTINE

A.
MECHANICAL GASTROINTESTINAL OBSTRUCTION AND PARALYTIC ILEUS

Andre Dubois

Uniformed Services University of Health Sciences, Bethesda, Maryland, USA

In this review, I will focus mainly on mechanical obstruction of the small intestine and colon, and abnormalities encountered throughout the gastrointestinal tract during paralytic ileus.

Mechanical Obstruction

Causes of Obstruction

Since the intestine is a tube floating freely in a cavity, obstruction of this tube may result from obstacles occurring within the lumen, e.g. foreign bodies, bezoars, gallstones, intussusception (Figure 1), polyps, and tumours. Obstructions may also arise from abnormalities of the wall of the intestine, e.g. neoplasms, congenital atresia, and strictures due to inflammation, chemical irritation, or vascular insufficiency. Finally, mechanical obstruction may be due to extra-intestinal causes such as adhesions, internal or external hernias, volvulus (Figure 2), abscesses, the superior mesenteric artery syndrome, or congenital bands.

Pathophysiology

As discussed by Wangensteen (1955), conflicting results have been reported regarding abnor-

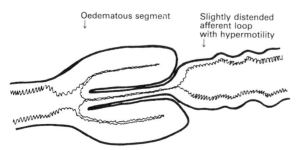

Figure 1. Illustration of mechanical obstruction due to intussusception.

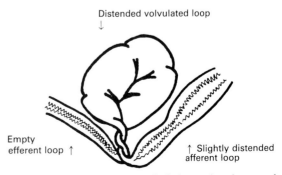

Figure 2. Illustration of mechanical obstruction due to volvulus.

malities of gastrointestinal motility during mechanical obstructions. Using intra-abdominal balloons, Carlson and Wangensteen (1930) observed that contractile activity of the small intestine appeared qualitatively normal several days after the establishment of mechanical obstruction in dogs. There was no difference between motility above and below the site of obstruction (Carlson and Wangensteen, 1930) and barium moved in an aboral direction both above and below intestinal block (Wangensteen and Lynch, 1930), suggesting the presence of normal peristaltic activity. For example, a barium meal injected into the stomach reached the site of the ileal obstruction in 20 hours (Wangensteen and Lynch, 1930). Using a window placed in the abdominal wall of rabbits with small intestinal obstruction, Brandberg (1939) demonstrated that ileal contractility was initially increased above the site of the block; at a later stage, however, paralytic ileus and distension were observed. Using implanted bipolar electrodes in the oppossum, Coelho et al (1986) found that cyclic phase III of migrating myoelectric complexes was abolished following 80% and total ileal obstruction. These propagated activities were replaced by episodes of intense spike burst activity, which were initially localized in the vicinity of the site of the total obstruction. At a later stage, this increased activity was more frequent in the stomach and jejunum. In contrast, Dahlgren and Thorén (1967) observed normal intestinal motility above and below experimental mechanical obstructions in rabbits and dogs equipped with implanted endoradiosondes. This discrepancy may be related to insufficient sensitivity of the endoradiosonde and should be re-evaluated using an implanted extraluminal strain gauge.

In conclusion, the classical concept of bursts of increased intestinal motility during mechanical obstructions was experimentally supported or at least not excluded by the more recent studies. Unfortunately, none of these experimental studies included a sham operated group. Therefore, one cannot assess the possible participation of post-operative ileus in the abnormalities observed immediately after the creation of mechanical obstruction.

Aetiology

The mechanism of the abnormal motility induced by intestinal obstruction is at present unknown. Both neural and hormonal factors may be involved; since motilin is closely associated with phase III of the MMC, it would be particularly interesting to determine plasma levels of this peptide in conjunction with measurements of MMC during clinical or experimental mechanical obstruction.

Treatment

The treatment of intestinal obstruction is obvious and the only difficulty resides in making the correct diagnosis pre-operatively and in choosing the best time for intervening (Sarr et al, 1983).

Paralytic Ileus

Non-mechanical obstruction may be caused by one or several of the following abnormalities (Figure 3):

(1) Increased activity of extrinsic or intrinsic inhibitory neurones.
(2) Decreased activity of extrinsic or intrinsic excitatory neurones.
(3) Increased levels of inhibitory hormones.

Causes of functional obstruction

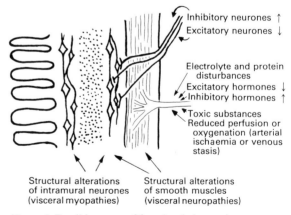

Figure 3. Possible causes of functional obstructions.

(4) Decreased levels of excitatory hormones.

(5) Electrolyte imbalance.

(6) Endogenous or exogenous toxins.

(7) Reduced perfusion or oxygenation (arterial ischaemia or venous stasis).

(8) Structural alterations of intrinsic neurons (visceral neuropathies).

(9) Structural alterations of intestinal smooth muscles (visceral myopathies).

Chronic idiopathic intestinal obstruction (see Chapter 27B) is caused by the last two abnormalities. In contrast, paralytic ileus may be produced by any of the first seven abnormalities, alone or in combination. Reflex ileus may be observed after any stress of psychological or physical nature (trauma, burns, etc.), but the most common type of paralytic ileus is the state observed after surgery, i.e. postoperative ileus.

Postoperative Ileus

Definition

In 1899 Bayliss and Starling demonstrated that spontaneous and stimulated movements of the gastrointestinal tract could be inhibited by the opening of the peritoneal cavity and by manipulations of the intestines (Bayliss and Starling, 1899). Cannon and Murphy (1906) expanded these observations and pointed out that ileus may be observed after extra-abdominal operations. Since that time, many studies have confirmed this observation and recent studies using modern techniques have been sufficiently precise to quantitate the extent and duration of the motor abnormalities induced by abdominal surgery in man (see pathophysiology, below).

Clinically, postoperative ileus is usually defined as the time period during which the patient does not pass flatus or stools. Since gastric ileus appears to resolve earlier than colonic ileus (Wakim and Mann, 1943; Goodall, 1964; Rothnie et al, 1953; Devine, 1946–47; Wells et al, 1964), oral administration of fluids may be attempted at an early stage. In fact, colonic motility could be promoted by early oral feedings, because of the stimulatory effect of the gastrocolic reflex induced by moderate

gastric distension. Finally, since the motility of the small intestine is believed to be normalized within a few hours of the completion of surgery, it is usually assumed that the jejunum and ileum do not participate in postoperative ileus. However, this latter concept may have to be revised in the light of recent observations.

Gastrointestinal motility is a vague term that may have a different meaning according to the technique used to measure it. For example, the frequency of electrical or mechanical events may be normalized long before the gut is able to fulfil its propulsive function. Therefore, each postoperative abnormality of gastrointestinal activity has to be considered in the light of the restoration of the co-ordinated motility of the digestive tract.

Pathophysiology

Stomach. The frequency of gastric slow waves (electrical control activity, ECA) is slightly decreased three to four hours after a laparotomy in dogs (Figure 4; Smith et al, 1977) and has

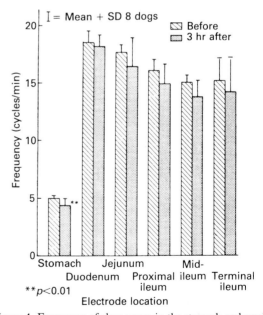

Figure 4. Frequency of slow waves in the stomach and small intestine of the dog postoperatively and 3 hours after abdominal surgery. Note that the frequency of gastric slow wave is decreased 3 hours after operations, whereas no significant difference is observed in the small intestine. From Smith et al (1977), with permission.

returned to normal at 24 hours. In monkeys with implanted strain gauges, a similar initial brady-gastria has been observed at 2 hours, followed by episodes of tachygastria lasting through the first postoperative day (Woods et al, 1978). In man, gastric contractions measured by intragastric telemetric capsules had a decreased frequency up to 14 hours after a cholecystectomy (Goodall, 1964).

The strength of gastric contractions has not yet been evaluated but the spike bursts (electrical response activity, ERA) were abolished or greatly diminished for at least 24 hours after surgery in dogs (Figures 5 and 6; Smith et al, 1977), sug-gesting that gastric mechanical contractions were either suppressed or decreased. Two days after surgery, phase III activity was still absent in the dog stomach (Figure 7).

Aboral propagation of bursts of ERA and phase III contractions sweeping through the stomach

were suppressed during the first 24 hours after surgery in dogs (Figure 6), and gastric emptying of non-digestible spheres required a mean of 65 hours compared to a normal of 1 hour (Smith et al, 1977). Similarly, gastric emptying of liquids was delayed in dogs (Figure 8; Dubois et al, 1973a) and in rats (Figures 9 and 10; Dubois et al, 1973b) during the first postoperative day. In chole-cystectomized patients, gastric and intestinal slow waves and spike bursts were observed during post-operative ileus, but their frequencies were irregu-lar and/or increased, and they were markedly disorganized and unphase-locked (Sarna et al, 1973; Dauchel et al, 1976).

Small intestine. Slow wave frequency was normal in the small intestine 3–4 hours after surgery in dogs (Figure 4; Smith et al, 1977). However, the frequency of mechanical contractions was decreased for up to 5 hours after laparotomy in

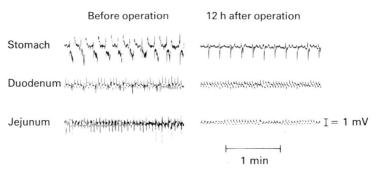

Figure 5. Electrical recordings obtained before (left tracings) and 12 hours after (right tracings) abdominal surgery in dogs. Note the absence of spike bursts in the postoperative tracings, while normal slow waves are present. From Smith et al (1977), with permission.

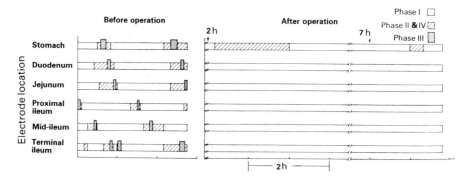

Figure 6. Immediate effect of surgery on MMC in dogs on the first postoperative day. Phase III activity is absent throughout the gastrointestinal tract. From Smith et al (1977), with permission.

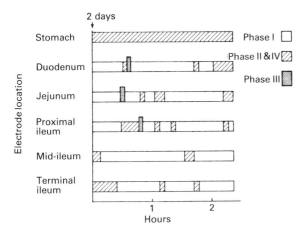

Figure 7. Late effect of surgery on gastrointestinal electrical activity 2 days after surgery. No phase III activity is visible in the stomach and phase III activity appearing in the small intestine failed to migrate aborally. From Smith et al (1977), with permission.

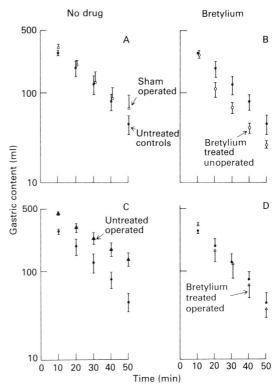

Figure 8. Postprandial intragastric volumes 24 hours after abdominal surgery (handling, exteriorization, but no resection) in dogs. A. No significant difference between controls and sham operated animals. B. Bretylium treatment in the control state significantly decreases gastric volume. C. In the absence of medication, gastric volume is significantly increased by surgery compared to controls. D. Following surgery, bretylium restores normal intragastric volumes. From Dubois et al (1973a), with permission.

monkeys (Woods et al, 1978), and phase III activities failed to appear (Figure 6) and/or to migrate aborally (Figure 7) for up to 3–7 days in dogs (Smith et al, 1977; Bueno et al, 1978). However, a transient phase of normal activity was observed 3–6 hours after surgery in dogs, but not in sheep (Bueno et al, 1978).

In dogs, transit of non-digestible spheres from the duodenum to the colon required a mean of 23 hours compared to a normal of about 2 hours (Smith et al, 1977). Similarly, intestinal transit of a barium meal or of a non-absorbable marker is suppressed for 12 hours (Figure 10B) to one day after surgery (Noer, 1968; Dubois et al, 1973b). In the small intestine, the duration of ileus depended on the type of surgery (Figure 11; Bueno et al, 1978).

Colon. It has long been recognized that motility is inhibited for a longer period in the colon than in the stomach and small intestine (Devine, 1946, 1947; Rothnie et al, 1963; Wells et al, 1964). Using radiotelemetry capsules, Wilson (1975) observed that colonic contractions were inhibited during the first two postoperative days. In monkeys, Woods et al (1978) used implanted electrodes and strain gauges to demonstrate that motility was inhibited for 24 hours in the right colon and for 72 hours in the sigmoid colon: Recently, Condon

et al (1986) extended these observations to human subjects using bipolar electrodes sutured to the ascending and descending colon during laparotomy. They observed that the dominant slow wave frequency in the right colon tended to decrease from 11/min on postoperative day 3 to 3/min on postoperative day 6 (Figure 12). In contrast, slow wave frequency in the left colon remained at about 11/min throughout the recovery period. Initially, spike bursts were composed of low amplitude, disorganized single bursts which became progressively more complex, of higher amplitude, and lasted for a longer time (Figure 13). Initially, some of these bursts propagated very slowly both in an oral and an aboral direction. At the time of the resolution of the ileus, however,

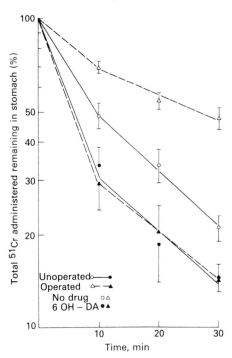

Figure 9. Percentage of gastric marker remaining in the stomach over time in rats. Gastric emptying is significantly delayed 12 hours after surgery (△) in untreated rats. Following 6-OH-dopamine treatment, however, surgery does not modify gastric emptying significantly (▲) compared to unoperated 6-OH-dopamine-treated controls (●). From Dubois et al (1973b), with permission.

propagation became very rapid and only in an aboral direction, which coincided with passage of flatus and stools (Figures 14 and 15).

Stimulus Initiating Postoperative Ileus

Surgical trauma. Handling of the intestines, of the other abdominal organs, and of the retroperitoneal space appears to be the main cause of postoperative ileus (Cannon and Murphy, 1906). Traction, handling or section of abdominal organs produce incomplete and short-lasting inhibition of gastrointestinal motility (Bisgard and Johnson, 1939; Tinckler, 1965; Schamaun, 1966), and the duration of gastrointestinal ileus appears related to the type of operation both in dogs and sheep (Bueno et al, 1978). In addition, laparotomy alone, without handling of the intestine, does not cause postoperative ileus in rats and dogs (Figure 8) (Dubois et al, 1973a and 1973b). However, other factors must play a role, since the pattern and timing of

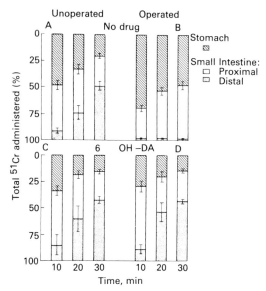

Figure 10. Percentage of marker present in stomach, and proximal and distal small bowel. A. Controls; note that the marker progresses along the proximal small intestine without accumulation. B. Twelve hours after surgery, none of the marker emptied from the stomach had reached the distal bowel. C and D. In 6-OH-dopamine-treated animals, gastric emptying and intestinal propulsion are not significantly modified 12 hours after surgery. From Dubois et al (1973b), with permission.

recovery of the clinical ileus, as well as of normal colonic motility does not appear to be related to the magnitude and length of surgical procedures (Wilson, 1975; Woods et al, 1978; Graber et al, 1980 and 1982; Condon et al, 1986). Inhibition of digestive motility in turn produces intra-abdominal accumulation of gases and fluids, dilatation of the gastrointestinal tract, and further activation of visceral sensory nerves, which may initiate a vicious circle (Devine, 1946–47), and, in addition, collection of fluids or blood within the parietal or visceral peritoneum as well as subclinical peritonitis ileus (Lindquist, 1968). Thus, a number of factors produced by the 'brutal invasion of the abdominal cavity' (Wakim and Mann, 1943) could induce a reflex ileus similar to the one observed after spinal cord injury or intraperitoneal irritation (Landman and Longmire, 1967; Lindquist, 1968; Mishra et al, 1975).

Pharmaceutical agents. Pre-operative administration of anticholinergic agents is likely to inhibit gastrointestinal motility, but this possi-

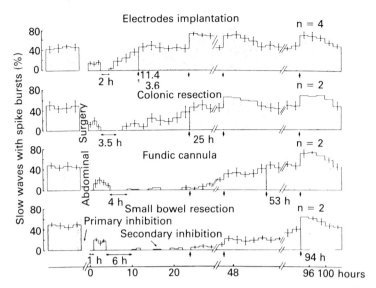

Figure 11. Effect of different surgical procedures on the electrical correlate of jejunal motility. The percentage of slow waves on which spike bursts were superimposed is illustrated for four types of operation. Note the dramatic difference between the effects of the various operations on jejunal activity. From Bueno et al (1978), with permission.

bility has not yet been evaluated experimentally. Various anaesthetic agents have been shown to disrupt gastrointestinal motility for only a very brief period of time (Figure 16) (Smith et al, 1977; Woods et al, 1978). Postoperative administration of analgesics could conceivably modify the course of ileus. In dogs, intravenous or intramuscular morphine produces non-peristaltic contractions of the small intestine and colon resulting in an arrest of transit (Dubois and Bremer, 1968). When given two days or more after surgery, i.v. or i.m. morphine produced a similar response in the human colon (Figure 17), whereas no consistent response was observed when morphine was given on the first postoperative day (Condon et al, 1986). However, morphine never induced either passage

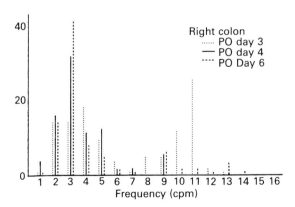

Figure 12. Fast Fourier transform of slow wave in the right colon in man 3, 4 and 6 days after electrode implantation. Note the disappearance of the 11/min frequency and the progressive increase of the 3/min frequency. From Condon et al (1986), with permission.

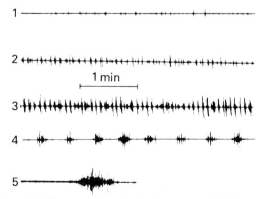

Figure 13. Five examples of spike bursts recorded after operation. 1. Postoperation, day 1, random single bursts of short duration; 2. day 2, short spike bursts; 3. day 3, long spike bursts; 4. day 3 and 4, spike bursts longer than the slow wave cycle; 5. day 4 afterwards, very long spike bursts. From Condon et al (1986), with permission.

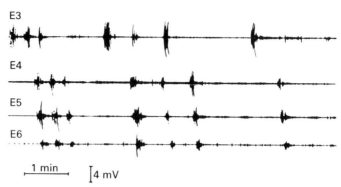

E3

E4

E5

E6

1 min   4 mV

Figure 14. Short spike bursts propagating in the human colon. These bursts propagated from the right colon (E3) to the left colon (E4–E6) and coincide with both the recovery from ileus and the passage of flatus. From Condon et al (1986), with permission.

of flatus or defecation or a significant shortening of the time to clinical recovery from ileus (Condon et al, 1986). In man, postcholecystectomy inhibition of gastric emptying was mostly related to administration of opiates (Ingram and Sheiner, 1981). Although it has not yet been documented, the possible role of other postoperative analgesic agents should always be taken into account when clinical studies are performed.

Epidural or peridural morphine had no significant effect on colonic motility in man (Condon et al, 1986). In contrast, spinal anaesthesia appears to shorten the duration of postoperative ileus (Duval, 1927; Markowitz and Campbell, 1927),

although the efficacy of this treatment is not established (Davis and Hansen, 1945). In dogs and sheep, splanchnicectomy and paravertebral anaesthesia almost completely prevented postoperative ileus (Figures 18 and 19; Bueno et al, 1978).

Mediator(s) Responsible for Postoperative Ileus

Surgical trauma induces a number of neural and hormonal responses which are apparently

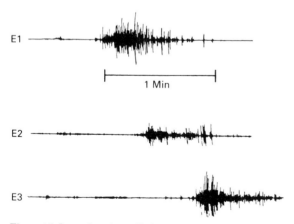

E1

E2

E3

1 Min

Figure 15. Long duration spike bursts propagating aborally in the human colon. Although this was more common on the left side, it was observed in the entire colon, and coincided with both the recovery from ileus and the passage of stools. From Condon et al (1986), with permission.

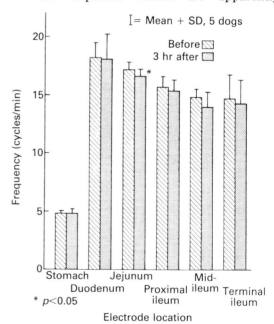

Figure 16. Frequency of gastrointestinal slow waves 3 hours after halothane anaesthesia. Only jejunal frequency is slightly decreased. From Smith et al (1977), with permission.

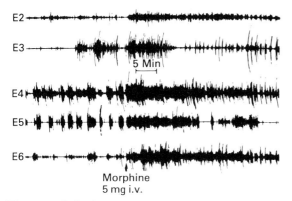

E2

E3

5 Min

E4

E5

E6

Morphine
5 mg i.v.

Figure 17. Spike burst response to i.v. morphine given at postoperation day 2. The strong non-propagated activity is of longer duration in the left colon. From Condon et al (1986), with permission.

intended to restore normal homeostasis. One or several of these responses is probably responsible for the postoperative inhibition of gastrointestinal motility.

Circulating catecholamines. Elevated plasma concentrations of epinephrine and norepinephrine (NE) have been found following general anaesthesia (Roizen et al, 1974) and postoperatively (Figure 20) (Moore, 1959; Dubois et al, 1975; Smith et al, 1976). However, adrenalectomy or

adrenal demedullation did not prevent postoperative ileus (Figures 21 and 22) (Douglas and Mann, 1941; Dubois et al, 1975), although a partial improvement was reported by others (Öhrn, 1976). The cause of this discrepancy is unclear especially since baseline gastrointestinal propulsion was not modified by demedullation in one study (Dubois et al, 1975) whereas it was significantly increased by both demedullation and adrenalectomy in the other (Öhrn, 1976).

Sympathetic nervous activity. In order to understand the experiments used to evaluate the role of noradrenergic nerves in postoperative ileus, it is necessary first to review the metabolism of NE in sympathetic nerve endings. Under normal circumstances, NE released by sympathetic terminals upon nerve stimulation is constantly replaced to maintain a steady state level (Figure 23). Circulating tyrosine is taken up by nerve endings and hydroxilated into DOPA through tyrosine hydroxylase (TH), a rate-limiting enzyme). DOPA is then transformed to dopamine by DOPA-decarboxylase and then into NE by dopamine-beta-hydroxylase (two non-rate-limiting enzymes). In addition, endocytosis permits the re-uptake of a large fraction of the released NE.

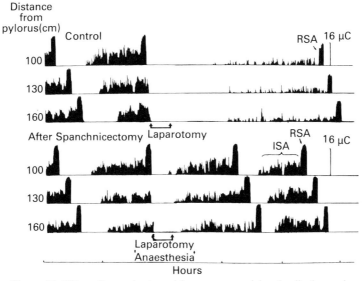

Figure 18. Effect of anaesthesia and laparotomy on jejunal spike bursts in dogs. Splanchnicectomy does not prevent inhibition of jejunal activity during laparotomy, but it permits restoration of jejunal MMC immediately after completion of anaesthesia. From Bueno et al (1978), with permission.

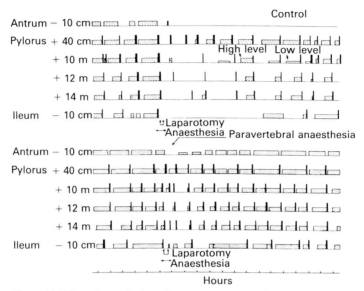

Figure 19. Effect of anaesthesia and laparotomy on gastrointestinal spike bursts in sheep. Bipolar electrodes were placed on the antrum 10 cm proximal to the pylorus, on the jejuno-ileum 40 cm, 10 m, 12 m and 14 m from the pylorus, and on the ileum 10 cm from the ileo-caecal valve. Black columns represent phases of regular spike bursts and shaded areas illustrate phases of irregular spike bursts. Laparotomy caused only slight modifications of spike bursts in the proximal jejunum and marked exhibition of spike bursts in the antrum and the distal small bowel. Paravertebral anaesthesia inhibited these changes almost completely. From Bueno et al (1978), with permission.

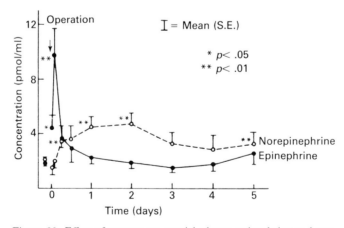

Figure 20. Effect of surgery on arterial plasma epinephrine and norepinephrine in dogs. The significant increase of epinephrine lasts only for a few hours and could reflect adrenal discharge. In contrast, the rise of norepinephrine lasts for 2 days and appears to reflect increased release by both the adrenals and the sympathetic nerve endings. From Smith et al (1977), with permission.

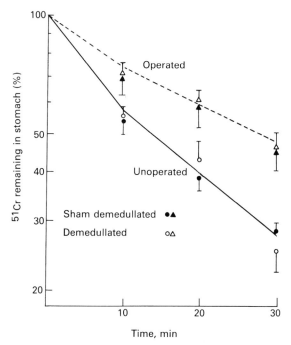

Figure 21. Effect of surgery on gastric emptying 12 hours after operation in the rat. Both sham demedullated and adrenal demedullated animals have delayed gastric emptying. From Dubois et al (1975), with permission.

As stated above, the rate of NE synthesis from tyrosine is regulated by the activity of TH, which in turn depends on the NE concentration in sympathetic nerve endings. When noradrenergic nerves are stimulated, NE concentration decreases, TH activity increases and more tyrosine is transformed into NE. Therefore, simple measurement of NE levels in a given tissue does not provide information regarding sympathetic nervous activity. In contrast, this evaluation may be performed by measuring NE turnover in this tissue and using two different methods. Firstly, one can administer ^{14}C-tyrosine intravenously and measure either the amount or the specific activity of ^{14}C-NE in the tissues one hour later (Sedvall et al, 1968). Secondly, one can inhibit TH activity by administering alpha-methyl-para-tyrosine and measure the progressive decline of NE in the tissue, either histochemically (Falck et al, 1962; Dubois et al, 1974) or biochemically (Sedvall et al, 1968; Costa and Neff, 1970; Dubois et al, 1973b). Sympathetic nervous activity is directly proportional to the specific activity of ^{14}C-NE in the first case, and inversely proportional to the tissue levels of NE in the second case. These methods

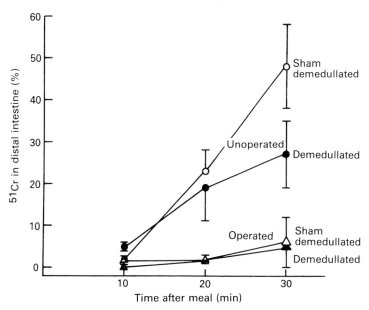

Figure 22. Effect of surgery on intestinal propulsion in the rat. In the control state, intestinal propulsion is not significantly modified by adrenal demedullation. Twelve hours after surgery, intestinal propulsion is suppressed in both demedullated and sham demedullated animals. From Dubois et al (1975), with permission.

Sympathetic nerve ending

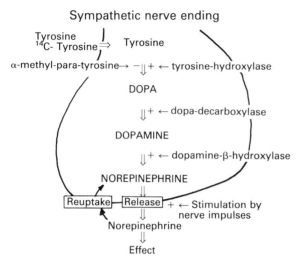

Figure 23. Schematic representation of a sympathetic nerve ending. See explanation in text.

permitted the demonstration of a stimulation of the sympathetic nervous system 12 hours after a laparotomy with intestinal manipulation (Figures 24–26) (Dubois et al, 1973b and 1974). This stimulation coincided with a decreased propulsion of the gastrointestinal contents (Figures 9 and 10) and occurred in the stomach, small intestine and colon, but not in the heart.

Parasympathetic activity. A decrease of cholinergic activity could account for postoperative ileus, although this hypothesis has not yet been tested. Direct damage to the intramural cholinergic nerves could be due to handling and/or anoxaemia of the gastrointestinal tract (Davison, 1979; Malone, 1987). In addition, depression of cholinergic stimulation could result from a postoperative deficit of pantothenic acid, because this vitamin plays an important role in the synthesis of coenzyme A, which, in turn, is involved in the synthesis of acetylcholine (Jacques, 1951). Treatment of postoperative ileus with pantothenic acid was successful in one series (Jacques, 1951), but no other study has tried to replicate these results.

Non-adrenergic, non-cholinergic nerves. Gastric relaxation induced by vagal stimulation is not suppressed by a combination of cholinergic and adrenergic blockade. (Abrahamsson, 1973, Jahnberg et al, 1977). The nature of the mediator(s) involved is unknown but a release of ATP (purinergic) (Burnstock, 1972), of VIP, or of another neuropeptide could be responsible for this effect. A similar gastric relaxation has been noted during a few hours after laparotomy or gastroduodenal

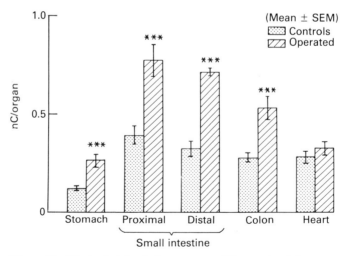

Figure 24. Effect of abdominal surgery on ^{14}C-norepinephrine synthetized from ^{14}C-tyrosine 12 hours after operation. Norepinephrine synthesis is increased throughout the gastrointestinal tract but not in the heart. From Dubois et al (1973b), with permission.

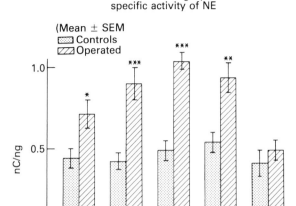

Influence of surgery on specific activity of NE

(Mean ± SEM
Controls
Operated)

Figure 25. Effect of abdominal surgery on the specific activity of ^{14}C-norepinephrine 12 hours after surgery. This figure indicates changes that are almost identical to those shown in Figure 18, illustrating that norepinephrine levels were not modified after surgery in animals which were not receiving any medication. From Dubois et al (1973b), with permission.

nociceptive stimulation (Abrahamsson et al, 1979), which suggests that these peptidergic mechanisms could mediate, at least in part, postoperative inhibition of gastrointestinal motility.

Hypoproteinaemia. Hypoproteinaemia and hypoalbuminaemia are not unusual after extensive surgery. Plasma transudation and oedema of the gut muscularis and myenteric plexus could impair gastrointestinal motility, as is suggested by the resolution of some cases of postoperative ileus following intravenous administration of plasma (Devine, 1946–47). In addition, protein synthesis appears to be decreased following abdominal surgery (O'Keefe and Sender, 1974).

Ionic imbalance. The complex equilibrium between intracellular and extracellular fluids and ions is modified after surgical trauma (Moore, 1959). However, routine measurement of serum concentration of Na^+, K^+ and Cl^- provides only a very incomplete picture of this imbalance. Hypokalaemia was shown to induce a marked inhibition of intestinal motility (Streeten and Vaughan Williams, 1952), but it is unclear whether the alterations of hydro-ionic balance induced by surgery are sufficient to produce an ileus. However, intravenous hypertonic saline appeared to be successful in the treatment of some cases of postoperative ileus (Wangensteen, 1955).

Motilin. Plasma motilin levels were suppressed pre- and postoperatively in man after cholecystectomy and hernia repair, and return of normal gastrointestinal transit appeared to correlate with a rise of plasma motilin above basal concentrations (Rennie et al, 1980). However, given the well-known cycling of plasma motilin levels in relation with migrating motor complexes, these results deserve re-evaluation.

Corticosteroids. The elevation of plasma corticosterone that was observed postoperatively in the rat (Dubois et al, 1975) probably reflects a stimulation of the hypothalamo-pituitary axis. In man, plasma corticosteroids are also elevated postoperatively (Kreuzer and Wenze, 1970). However, no elevation of corticosterone was observed postoperatively in demedullated rats, whereas a normal ileus was present (Dubois, 1977). Therefore, corticosteroids may not play an important role in postoperative ileus.

Treatment. Postoperative ileus remains a major problem during the period that follows any surgical procedure, and it is of particular importance after extensive abdominal surgery. Simple conservative measures such as gastric suction and intravenous rehydration usually allow uneventful course and spontaneous restoration of normal transit after 2–4 days. However, an effective and safe treatment of ileus would be extremely useful when other complications do occur or when the patient is in a poor general condition.

As stated before, spinal or peridural anaesthesia was already tried half a century ago (Duval, 1927; Markowitz and Campbell, 1927), and experimental studies have confirmed these observations (Bueno et al, 1978). However, the application of this treatment is often difficult in a clinical setting and the results are frequently disappointing (Davis and Hansen, 1945).

Experimentally, postoperative ileus was mark-

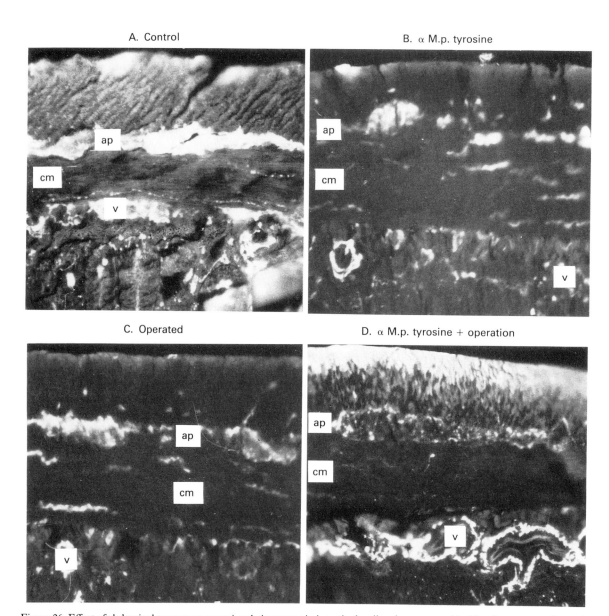

Figure 26. Effect of abdominal surgery on norepinephrine stores in intestinal wall as demonstrated by histofluorescence. Intensity of norepinephrine fluorescence in the myenteric and submucosal plexus is not modified by either surgery or alpha-methyl-para-tyrosine (B) or surgery (C) alone. In contrast treatment with alpha-methyl-para-tyrosine before surgery (D) markedly reduced histofluorescence in the plexus, but not around blood vessels. This observation illustrates that the turnover of norepinephrine is increased 12 hours after surgery in the small intestine but not around the blood vessels. From Dubois et al (1974), with permission.

edly improved or completely prevented by the blockade of NE release in the dog (Dubois et al, 1973a). Similarly, destruction of sympathetic nerve endings with 6-OH-dopamine 2 days before surgery (Bloom et al, 1969; Kostrzewa and Jacobowitz, 1974) (Figure 27) produced normal gastrointestinal propulsion 5 and 12 hours after laparotomy (Dubois et al, 1973b; Ruwart et al, 1980). In contrast, pretreatment with 6-OH-dopamine did not prevent ileus 15 hours after laparotomy in another study in rats, although direct experimental evidence of complete sym-

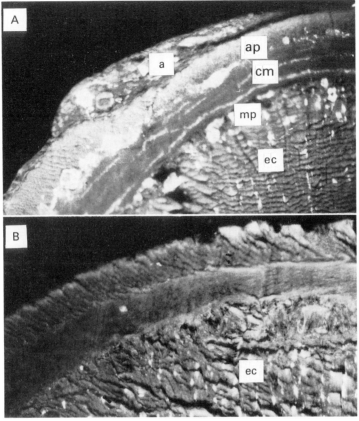

Figure 27. Histochemical evidence of complete chemical sympathectomy 2 days after treatment with 150 mg/kg 6-OH-dopamine (B) compared to control (A). Complete sympathectomy is observed in the Auerbach plexus (ap), the Meissner plexus (mp), the circular muscle (cm) and around blood vessels (a). Only enterochromaffine cells (ec) retain their fluorescence. From Dubois et al (1973a), with permission.

phathectomy was not provided (Öhrn, 1976). The apparent discrepancy is similar to that previously quoted concerning the effect of demedullation or adrenalectomy, and may be due to insufficient sympathectomy in the latter study or to differences in either experimental design, time of study or rat strain. Alpha-adrenergic blockade produced marked improvement in the rat (Ruwart et al, 1980) but not in the dog (Smith et al, 1977), while beta-adrenergic blockade was ineffective in both species. In man, inhibition of sympathetic nervous activity using adrenergic blocking drugs (Catchpole, 1969) or neuroleptics (Petri et al, 1971) provided good results in the hands of their proponents, but a double blind study did not confirm these results (Heimbach and Crout, 1971). In contrast, another sympatholytic agent (dihydroergotamine) (Schutze et al, 1980) proved to be effective in a double blind study (Altaparmakov et al, 1984).

Cholinergic agents alone (Abel, 1933; Carmichael et al, 1934; Harger and Wilkey, 1938; Marsden and Williamson, 1939; Ruwart et al, 1980) or in combination with a sympatholytic (Catchpole, 1969; Neely and Catchpole, 1971; Petri et al, 1971; Ruwart et al, 1980) produced significant improvement experimentally and clinically, although some authors have not confirmed such a beneficial effect (Heimbach and Crout, 1971).

Many other treatments have been proposed, suggesting that neither is entirely satisfactory.

Pituitary extracts (Devine, 1946–47; Dauchel et al, 1975), and pantothenic acid (Jacques, 1951) were effective in some studies. Electrical pacing of the stomach (Kelly and Laforce, 1972) or of the small intestine (Babin et al, 1968; Wenzel, 1976) holds promise when and if disorders of the gastric and intestinal pacemaker are identified in post-operative ileus.

Reflex Ileus

Inhibition of gastrointestinal motility may be induced by any kind of physical or psychological stress (Bennett and Venables, 1920; Wolff, 1951; Landman and Longmire, 1967; Lindquist, 1968; Appert and Howard, 1972; Thompson et al, 1982; Stanghellini et al, 1983). Since postoperative ileus is a special case of reflex ileus, and since reflex ileus is responsible in part for postoperative ileus, most statements made earlier are valid in this condition.

Acknowledgements

I thank Drs L. Bueno, R. E. Condon and K. Kelly for kindly allowing the reproduction of figures from their original articles.

References

Abel, A. L., (1983), Acetylcholine in paralytic ileus. *Lancet*, **ii**:1247–51.

Abrahamsson, H., (1973), Studies on the inhibitory nervous control of gastric motility. *Acta Physiol. Scand.*, **390**:1–38.

Abrahamsson, H., Glise, H., and Glise, K. (1979), Reflex suppression of gastric motility during laparotomy and gastroduodenal nociceptive stimulation. *Scand. J. Gastroenterol.*, **14**:101–6.

Altaparmakov, I., Erckenbrecht, J. F., and Wienbeck, M., (1984), Modulation of the adrenergic system in the treatment of postoperative bowel atonia. *Scand. J. Gastroenterol.*, **19**:1104–6.

Appert, H. E., and Howard, J. M., (1972), Autonomic inhibition of intestinal motility in dogs associated with intra-abdominal injury. *Ann. Surg.*, **176**:19–24.

Babin, S., Arantes, W. L., Lampert, M., et al, (1968), Utilization of a gastrointestinal pace-maker in surgery. *Hospital* (*Rio de J.*), **74**:779–85.

Bayliss, W. M., and Starling, E. H., (1899), The movements and innervation of the small intestine. *J. Physiol.*, **24**:99–143.

Bennet, T. I., and Venables, J. F., (1920), The effect of the emotions on gastric secretion and motility in the human being. *Br. Med. J.*, **2**:662–3.

Bisgard, J. D., and Johnson, E. K., (1939), The influence of certain drugs and anesthetics on gastrointestinal tone and motility. *Ann. Surg.*, **110**:802–22.

Bloom, F. E., Algeri, S., Groppetti, A., Revuelta, A., and Costa, E., (1969). Lesions of central norepinephrine terminals with 6-OH-dopamine: Biochemistry and fine structure. *Science*, **166**:1284–6.

Brandberg, R., (1939), An experimental study of intestinal motility in mechanical ileus. *Acta Chir.*, **83**:287–92.

Bueno, L., Fioramonti, J., and Ruckebusch, Y., (1978), Postoperative intestinal motility in dogs and sheep. *Dig. Dis. Sci.*, **23**:682–9.

Burnstock, G., (1972), Purinergic nerves. *Pharmacol. Rev.*, **24**:509–81.

Carlson, H. A. and Wangensteen, O. H., (1930), Motor activity of the distal bowel in intestinal obstruction: Comparison with the obstructed and normal. *Proc. Soc. Exp. Biol. Med.*, **27**:676–8.

Cannon, W. B., and Murphy, F. T., (1906), The movements of the stomach and intestines in some surgical conditions. *Ann. Surg.*, **43**:512–36.

Carmichael, E. A., Fraser, F. R., McKelvey, D., and Wilkie, D. P., (1934), The therapeutic action of prostigmine. *Lancet*, **i**:942.

Catchpole, B. N., (1969), Ileus: use of the sympathetic blocking agents in its treatment. *Surgery*, **66**:811–20.

Coelho, J. C., Gouma, D. J., Moody, F. G., Li, Y. F., and Senninger, N., (1986), Gastrointestinal motility following small bowel obstruction in the opossum. *J. Surg. Res.*, **41**:274–8.

Condon, R. E., Cowles, V. E., Schulte, W. J., Frantzides, C. T., Mahoney, J. L., and Sarna, S. K. (1986), Resolution of postoperative ileus in humans. *Ann. Surg.*, **203**:574–81.

Costa, E., and Neff, N. H., (1970), Estimation of turn-over rates to study the metabolic regulation of the steady-state level of neuronal monoamines. In: *Handbook of Neurochemistry*, Vol. 4, Chapter 3, Plenum Press, New York.

Dahlgren, S., and Thóren, L., (1967), Intestinal motility in low small bowel obstruction. *Acta Chir. Scand.*, **133**:417–22.

Dauchel, J., Schang, J. C., Kachelhoffer, J., and Eloy, R., (1976), Gastrointestinal myoelectrical activity during the postoperative period in man. *Digestion*, **14**:293–303.

Dauchel, J., Schang, J. C., Pousse, A., Hiatt, R. B., and Grenier, J. F., (1975), Electromyographic study of the effects of coherin, a posterior pituitary extract, on the intestinal motility in man. *Proc. 5th Int. Symp.*

GI Motility (Ed. Vantrappen, G.) Typoff-Press Herentals, Belgium.

Davis, H. H., and Hansen, T. M., (1945), Investigation of the cause and prevention of gas pains following abdominal operation. Surgery, 17:492–7.

Davison, J. S., (1979), Selective damage to cholinergic nerves: Possible cause of postoperative ileus. Lancet, i (8129):1288.

Devine, J., (1946–47), A concept of paralytic ileus: A clinical study. Br. J. Surg., 34:158–79.

Douglas, D. M., and Mann, F. C., (1941), The effect of peritoneal irritation on the activity of the intestine. Br. Med. J., 1:227–31.

Dubois, A., (1977), Etudes physiologiques de l'ileus postoperatoire. Acta Chir. Belg., 76:141–66.

Dubois, A., and Bremer, A., (1968), Aspects de l'activite propulsive d'une anse de Thiry-Vella colique chez le chien eveille. Arch. Int. Physiol. Bioch. 76:893–912.

Dubois, A., Henry, D. P., and Kopin, I. J., (1975), Plasma catecholamines and postoperative gastrointestinal propulsion in the rat. Gastroenterology, 68:466–9.

Dubois, A., Kopin, I. J., Pettigrew, K., and Jacobowitz, D. M., (1974), Chemical and histochemical studies of postoperative sympathetic activity in the digestive tract. Gastroenterology, 66:403–7.

Dubois, A., Watanabe, A., and Kopin, I. J., (1973a), Postoperative gastric retention in the dog. Amer. J. Dig. Dis., 18:39–42.

Dubois, A., Weise, V. K., and Kopin, I. J., (1973b), Postoperative ileus in the rat: physiopathology, etiology and treatment. Ann. Surg., 178:781–6.

Duval, R. (1927), La rachianesthesie dans l'ileus aigu. Bull. Soc. Chir., Paris, 53:596–610.

Falck, B., Hillarp, N. A., Thieme, G., and Torp, A., (1962), Fluorescence of catecholamines and related compounds condensed with formaldehyde. J. Histochem. Cytochem., 10:348–54.

Goodall, P., (1964), Early gastroduodenal motility following operation. Br. J. Surg., 51:864–7.

Graber, J. N., Schulte, W. J., Condon, R. E., and Cowles, V. E., (1980), Duration of postoperative ileus related to the extent and site of operative dissection. Surgical Forum, 31:141–4.

Graber, J. N., Schulte, W. J., Condon, R. E., and Cowles, V. E. (1982), Relationship of duration of postoperative ileus to extent and site of operative dissection. Surgery, 92:87–92.

Harger, J. R., and Wilkey, J. L., (1938), Management of post-operative distension and ileus. JAMA, 10:1165–9.

Heimbach, D. M., and Crout, J. R., (1971), Treatment of paralytic ileus with adrenergic neuronal blocking drugs. Surgery, 69:582–7.

Ingram, D. M., and Sheiner, H. J., (1981), Postoperative gastric emptying. Br. J. Surg., 68:572–6.

Jacques, J. E., (1951), Pantothenic acid in paralytic ileus. Lancet, ii:861–2.

Jahnberg, T., Abrahamsson, H., Jansson, G., and Martinson, J., (1977), Vagal gastric relaxation in the dog. Scand. J. Gastroenterol., 12:221–4.

Kelly, K. A., and Laforce, R. C., (1972), Pacing the canine stomach with electric stimulation. Amer. J. Physiol., 222: 588–94.

Kostrzewa, R. M., and Jacobowitz, M., (1974), Pharmacological actions of 6-hydroxydopamine. Pharmacol. Rev., 26:199–288.

Kreuzer, von W., and Wenze, G., (1970), Untersuchung der postoperativen Darmmotilitatsstorung. Zbl. Chir., 95:41–6.

Landman, M. D., and Longmire, W. P. Jr., (1967), Neural and hormonal influence of peritonitis on paralytic ileus. Amer. Surgeon, 33:756–62.

Lindquist, B., (1968), Propulsive gastrointestinal motility related to retroperitoneal irritation. An experimental study in the rat. Acta Chir. Scand., 384:3–53.

Malone, P. C., (1987), The physiology of intestinal oxygenation and the pathophysiology of intestinal ileus. Medical Hypotheses, 22:111–57.

Marsden, P. A., and Williamson, E. G., (1939), The use of prostigmine methylsulfate in the prevention of post-operative intestinal atony and urinary bladder retention. Surg. Gynecol. Obstet., 69:61.

Markowitz, J., and Campbell, W. R., (1927), The relief of experimental ileus by spinal anesthesia. Amer. J. Physiol., 81:101–6.

Mishra, N. K., Appert, H. E., and Howard, J. M., (1975), Studies of paralytic ileus. Effect of intraperitoneal injury on motility of the canine small intestine. Amer. J. Surg., 129:559–63.

Moore, F. D., (1959), The Metabolic Care of the Surgical Patient, W. B. Saunders, Philadelphia/London.

Neely, J., and Catchpole, B., (1971), The restoration of alimentary tract motility by pharmacological means. Br. J. Surg., 58:21–8.

Noer, T., (1968), Roentgenological transit time through the small intestine in the immediate postoperative period. Acta Chir. Scand., 134:577–80.

Öhrn, P. G., (1976), Postoperative gastrointestinal propulsion. Acta Chir. Scand., 5 (Supplement 461):1–76.

O'Keefe, S. J., and Sender, P. M., (1974), 'Catabolic' loss of body nitrogen in response to surgery. Lancet, ii:1035–8.

Petri, G., Szenohradszky, J., and Poszasz-Gibiszer, K., (1971), Sympatholytic treatment of 'paralytic' ileus. Surgery, 70:359–67.

Rennie, J. A., Christofides, N. D., Mitchenere, D., Fletcher, D., Stockley-Leathard, H. L., Bloom, S. R., Johnson, A. G., and Rains, A. J., (1980), Neural and humoral factors in postoperative ileus. Br. J. Surg., 67:694–8.

Roizen, M. F., Moss, J., Henry, D. P., and Kopin, I. J., (1974), Effect of halothane on plasma catecholamines. *Anesthesiology*, **41**:432–9.

Rothnie, N. G., Kemp Harper, R. A., and Catchpole, B. N., (1963), Early postoperative gastrointestinal activity. *Lancet*, **ii**:64–7.

Ruwart, M. J., Klepper, M. S., and Rush, B. S., (1980), Adrenergic and cholinergic contributions to decreased gastric emptying, small intestinal transit, and colonic transit in the postoperative ileus rat. *J. Surg. Res.*, **29**:126–34.

Sarna, S. K., Bowes, K. L., and Daniel, E. E., (1973), Postoperative gastric electrical control activity in man. In: *Proc. IVth Int. Symp. on Gastrointestinal Motility*. pp. 73–84. Mitchell Press Limited, Vancouver, Canada.

Sarr, M. G., Bulkley, G. B., and Zuidema, G. D., (1983), Preoperative recognition of intestinal strangulation obstruction: a prospective evaluation of diagnostic capability. *Am. J. Surg.*, **145**:176–82.

Schamaun, M., (1966), Experimentelle elektromyographisches Untersuchungen zur Pathophysiologie der Dunndarmmotorik bei chirurgischen Krankheitsbildern', *Zbl. Ges. Exp. Med.*, **141**:89–162.

Schutze, U., Ruf, W., Terwey, B., Wiedemann, K., and Clausen, C., (1980), Dihydroergotamine—stimulation of intestinal peristalsis. An experimental and clinical study. *Hepato-Gastroenterology*, **27**:317–21.

Sedvall, G. C., Weise, V. K., and Kopin, I. J., (1968), The rate of norepinephrine synthesis measured in vivo during short intervals: influence of adrenergic nerve impulse activity. *J. Pharmacol. Exp. Ther.*, **159**:274–82.

Smith, J., Kelly, K. A., and Weinshilboum, R. M., (1977), Pathophysiology of postoperative ileus. *Arch. Surg.*, **112**:203–9.

Stanghellini, V., Malagelada, J.-R., Zinsmeister, A. R., Go, V. L. W., and Kao, P. C., (1983), Stress-induced gastroduodenal disturbances in humans: possible humoral mechanisms. *Gastroenterology*, **85**: 83–91.

Streeten, D. H. P., and Vaughan Williams, E. M., (1952), Loss of cellular potassium as a cause of intestinal paralysis in dogs. *J. Physiol.*, **118**:149–70.

Thompson, D. G., Richelson, E., and Malagelada, J.-R., (1982), Perturbation of gastric emptying and duodenal motility via the central nervous system. *Gastroenterology*, **83**:1200–6.

Tinckler, L. F., (1965), Surgery and intestinal motility. *Br. J. Surg.*, **52**:140–50.

Wakim, K., and Mann, F. C., (1943), The effects of some intra-abdominal operative procedures on intestinal activity. *Gastroenterology*, **1**:513–17.

Wangensteen, O. H., (1955), The effects of distension. In: *Intestinal Obstruction* (Ed. Wangensteen, O. H.) 3rd edition, Charles C. Thomas, Springfield, Illinois.

Wangensteen, O. H., and Lynch, F. W., (1930), Evaluation of X-ray evidence as criteria of intestinal obstruction. *Proc. Soc. Exp. Biol. Med.*, **27**:674–80.

Wells, C., Tinckler, L., Rawlinson, K., Jones, H., and Saunders, J., (1964), Postoperative gastrointestinal motility. *Lancet*, **i**:4–10.

Wenzel, M., (1976), A new treatment principle in the therapy of postoperative paralytic ileus. *Deutsch. Med. J.*, **18**:702–3.

Wilson, J. P., (1975), Postoperative motility of the large intestine in man. *Gut*, **16**:689–92.

Wolff, H. G., (1951), The mechanism and significance of the cold pressor response. *Q. J. Med.*, **20**:261–73.

Woods, J. H., Erickson, L. W., Condon, R. E., Schulte, W. J., and Sillin, L. F., (1978), Postoperative ileus: a colonic problem? *Surgery*, **84**:527–33.

27B.

CHRONIC IDIOPATHIC INTESTINAL PSEUDO-OBSTRUCTION

Michael D. Schuffler

Seattle Public Health Hospital, Seattle, Washington, USA

Intestinal pseudo-obstruction is a syndrome characterized by symptoms and signs of intestinal obstruction in the absence of mechanical blockage (Faulk et al, 1978a; Schuffler, 1981). It is caused by abnormal neuromuscular function of the small intestine, the colon, or both, resulting in ineffective intestinal propulsion. *Acute* intestinal pseudo-obstruction is synonymous with acute ileus, and is usually secondary to self-limited illnesses such as acute pancreatitis, myocardial infarction, renal colic, etc. Acute intestinal pseudo-obstruction limited to the colon is also known as Ogilvie's syndrome, named after the British surgeon who described two cases of colonic ileus associated with metastatic cancer (Ogilvie, 1948).

Chronic intestinal pseudo-obstruction is a syndrome of months to years' duration which is usually associated with pathological abnormalities of the intestinal smooth muscle or myenteric plexus. Chronic intestinal pseudo-obstruction may be secondary to well-known systemic disorders, such as progressive systemic sclerosis, myotonic dystrophy, or amyloidosis, or it may be a primary disorder of the gastrointestinal tract, not associated with well-known systemic disorders. In this case, it is known as chronic *idiopathic* intestinal pseudo-obstruction (CIIP).

The manifestations of CIIP may not be limited to the gastrointestinal tract. Abnormalities of intestinal smooth muscle, e.g. *visceral myopathies*, may be accompanied by abnormalities of smooth muscle elsewhere, as in the bladder, ureters, and irises. Abnormalities of the myenteric plexus, e.g. *visceral neuropathies*, may be confined to the plexus or accompanied by abnormalities of the extra-intestinal nervous system, e.g. in the brain, spinal cord, autonomic, and/or peripheral nervous systems. Thus, patients may have CIIP associated with mental retardation, autonomic nervous system dysfunction, parkinsonian signs and symptoms, ataxia, etc.

The small intestine is usually the major site of involvement in CIIP, but almost always, this is accompanied by colonic involvement. Occasionally, the colon is the major site of involvement. Some patients have only colonic pseudo-obstruction, whereas others have only small bowel involvement. Quite often, CIIP involves all or almost all areas of the gut, so that motor dysfunction may exist in the oesophagus and stomach as well as the small bowel and/or colon.

Structural abnormalities of the smooth muscle or myenteric plexus not only produce chronic intestinal pseudo-obstruction; they also produce other motor disorders characteristic of particular sites of involvement. Thus, achalasia and diffuse spasm may result from involvement of the oesophageal myenteric plexus, and gastroparesis may result from involvement of either the gastric smooth muscle or myenteric plexus. Structural abnormalities of the smooth muscle or myenteric plexus may also have a variety of anatomical consequences, such as mega-oesophagus, megaduodenum, megacolon, and diffuse diverticulosis of the small intestine and occasionally the colon.

Classification

Chronic intestinal pseudo-obstruction is a heterogeneous syndrome caused by a variety of abnormalities of either the smooth muscle or myenteric plexus (Krishnamurthy and Schuffler, 1987). The disorders of the myenteric plexus are more frequent than the disorders of smooth muscle. Either type can be familial or sporadic, and the familial types are either autosomal dominant or autosomal recessive.

The disorders of the myenteric plexus can be further subdivided into those which are degenerative (visceral neuropathies) and those which are problems of development in utero. The degenerative disorders are either inflammatory or non-inflammatory. Those which are inflammatory may be idiopathic or secondary to Chagas' disease or small cell carcinoma of the lung, i.e. paraneoplastic visceral neuropathy.

The disorders of smooth muscle can be divided into those which are characterized by muscle cell degeneration, dropout, and fibrosis (visceral myopathies); those which are characterized by fibrosis in the absence of muscle cell degeneration and dropout; and those which are characterized by diffuse lymphoid infiltration of the muscle in the absence of muscle cell degeneration and dropout.

A classification of these disorders is presented in Table 1. This table includes both primary and secondary causes of chronic intestinal pseudo-obstruction.

Diagnostic Techniques

Radiography

The most commonly used and available diagnostic technique is radiography (Schuffler et al, 1976; Rohrmann et al, 1984). It is indispensable for accurate diagnosis. Findings on plain films may include a picture of paralytic ileus or one which mimics true mechanical obstruction (Figures 1 and 2). Approximately 15–20% of patients have normal findings, the abnormality of motor function being apparent only on barium studies. Additional findings on plain films may include pneumatosis intestinalis and benign pneumo-peritoneum.

Barium contrast studies of the entire gastro-intestinal tract are important in defining the distribution of abnormalities and excluding mechanical obstruction. In many cases, CIIP manifests as a diffuse disorder, with abnormalities of motility and structure throughout the gastrointestinal tract. The more sites of involvement, the greater

Table 1

I. Disorders of the Myenteric Plexus
  A. Familial visceral neuropathies
    1. Recessive, with intranuclear inclusions
    2. Recessive, with mental retardation and calcification of the basal ganglia
    3. Dominant, with neither of above
  B. Sporadic visceral neuropathies
    1. Degenerative, non-inflammatory
    2. Degenerative, inflammatory
      a. Paraneoplastic
      b. Non-paraneoplastic (Chagas', cytomegalovirus, idiopathic)
      c. Isolated axonopathy
  C. Developmental abnormalities
    1. Hirschsprung's disease
    2. Total colonic aganglionosis (sometimes with small intestinal aganglionosis)
    3. Maturational arrest
      a. With mental retardation
      b. With other neurological abnormalities
      c. Isolated to myenteric plexus, without the above
    4. Neuronal intestinal dysplasia
      a. With neurofibromatosis
      b. With MEA II
      c. Isolated to intestine, without above
  D. Severe, idiopathic constipation
  E. Drug induced/toxic damage
II. Disorders of the Smooth Muscle
  A. Primary
    1. Familial visceral myopathies
      a. Autosomal dominant
      b. Autosomal recessive (with ptosis and external ophthalmoplegia)
      c. Autosomal recessive with total GI tract dilatation.
    2. Sporadic visceral myopathies
  B. Secondary
    1. Progressive systemic sclerosis/polymyositis
    2. Myotonic dystrophy
    3. Progressive muscular dystrophy
    4. Amyloidosis
    5. Ceroidosis?
  C. Diffuse lymphoid infiltration
III. Small Intestinal Diverticulosis
    1. With muscle resembling visceral myopathy
    2. With muscle resembling progressive systemic sclerosis
    3. With visceral neuropathy and neuronal intranuclear inclusions
    4. Secondary to Fabry's disease

the probability of CIIP. In contrast, abnormalities limited to the small bowel, while not excluding

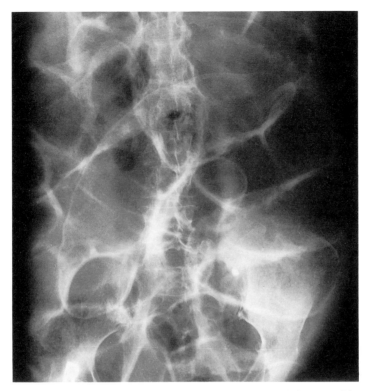

Figure 1. Supine film showing markedly distended bowel and close apposition of dilated loops producing appearance resembling obstruction and extramural free air. From Schuffler et al (1976), with permission.

a diagnosis of CIIP, raise the possibility of real mechanical obstruction, so that careful study is necessary to exclude an area of true obstruction.

In general, disorders of the smooth muscle produce hypocontractility, dilatation, and, in the colon, loss of haustration (Rohrmann et al., 1984). The most common muscle disorders are visceral myopathy and progressive systemic sclerosis. Although these two disorders cannot always be differentiated by barium contrast studies, there are clues to the correct diagnosis in many cases. For instance, the oesophagus in progressive systemic sclerosis is characterized by weak or absent contractions, dilatation, reflux, and stricture. Visceral myopathy is also characterized by oesophageal hypocontractility and dilatation, but reflux is less common and strictures have not been reported (Figure 3). These differences can be explained by their differences in pathology. Progressive systemic sclerosis is more likely to affect

the circular muscle, while visceral myopathy is more likely to affect the longitudinal muscle (Schuffler and Beegle, 1979; Mitros et al, 1982). A fibrotic circular muscle will not produce an effective lower oesophageal sphincter pressure, thus allowing reflux and stricture formation. In visceral myopathy, the circular muscle may remain intact and thus maintain an adequate lower oesophageal sphincter pressure, preventing significant reflux and stricture formation.

In contrast to the myopathies, the oesophagus in visceral neuropathies may mimic achalasia or diffuse oesophageal spasm (Figure 4). There may be aperistalsis, oesophageal dilatation, and retarded flow through the gastro-oesophageal junction. Oesophageal contractions are sometimes hypercontractile and disorganized.

In all types of chronic intestinal pseudo-obstruction, the stomach may be enlarged and have slow emptying. However, the stomach is

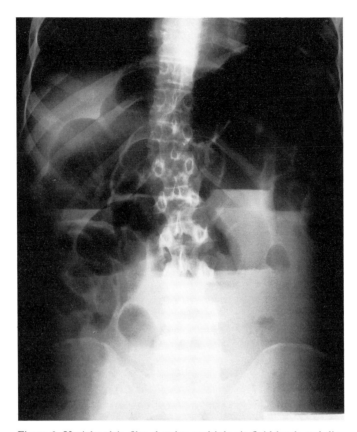

Figure 2. Upright plain film showing multiple air-fluid levels and distended bowel mimicking mechanical obstruction.

usually unaffected in the autosomal dominant type of visceral myopathy.

The small intestine in visceral myopathy may have a variety of findings. In the autosomal dominant familial type, the duodenum is markedly widened ('megaduodenum') whereas the rest of the small intestine may or may not be widened and hypocontractile (Figure 5) (Faulk et al, 1978b). In the recessive form associated with ptosis and external ophthalmoplegia, the entire small bowel is mildly dilated and contains multiple diverticula (Anuras et al, 1983). In a third familial type, with probable autosomal recessive transmission but without ptosis and ophthalmoplegia, the entire small bowel is moderately dilated, but without diverticula (Anuras et al, 1986).

The small intestine in progressive systemic sclerosis may also show a megaduodenum and widening of the intestine. In contrast to visceral myopathy, it may show valvular packing (close

pleating of the folds) and wide-mouthed diverticula or sacculations (Figure 6) (Rohrmann et al, 1984). Valvular packing probably results from the predominance of circular muscle fibrosis relative to longitudinal muscle fibrosis. Thus, if the longitudinal muscle is more intact and better able to contract in the relative absence of circular muscle contraction, shortening of the small intestine could cause the pleated pattern of valvular packing. Because of the greater amount of longitudinal muscle degeneration and fibrosis in visceral myopathy, it is almost impossible for valvular packing to occur. The wide-mouthed diverticula and sacculations result from the occurrence of abrupt, focal, and severe fibrosis of both muscle layers, a characteristic of progressive systemic sclerosis, but not of visceral myopathy.

The small intestine in visceral neuropathies may show a variety of abnormalities depending on the type of pathology and its location within the small

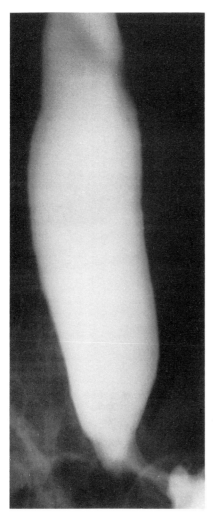

Figure 3. Dilated, atonic oesophagus, mimicking achalasia. From Schuffler et al (1976), with permission.

bowel. In familial visceral neuropathy associated with neuronal intranuclear inclusions, the duodenum and jejunum are mildly dilated and fluoroscopy reveals a hypercontracting, uncoordinated bowel (Figure 7) (Rohrmann et al, 1984). The head of the barium column may reach the caecum within a normal time, but the small bowel may not empty all its barium for one or more days. In a second type of familial visceral neuropathy, of autosomal dominant transmission, the duodenum is normal, but the jejunum and ileum are moderately dilated (Mayer et al, 1986). In one sporadic form of visceral neuropathy, the

small bowel between the ligament of Treitz and the terminal two feet of ileum was massively dilated and had few contractions, very prolonged transport, and dilution of barium from excessive fluid (Figure 8) (Schuffler et al, 1985). In paraneoplastic visceral neuropathy, the small intestine can be moderately dilated and fluoroscopy may reveal a hypercontracting small intestine, with retrograde propulsion of barium and some areas undergoing spasm severe enough to mimic true obstruction (Schuffler et al, 1983). Transport through the small intestine can be delayed for days. Chagas involvement of the small intestine, although less common than its involvement of the oesophagus or colon, can produce a megaduodenum or megajejunum. Finally, both visceral neuropathies and visceral myopathies can be associated with diffuse small bowel diverticulosis (Figure 9) (Krishnamurthy et al, 1983).

The colon in progressive systemic sclerosis usually has a normal width, but there may be loss of the haustral pattern and the presence of colonic sacculations (Rohrmann et al, 1984). The colon in visceral myopathy is more often widened and lacks haustrations and sacculations (Figure 10). It may result in megacolon.

The colon in visceral neruopathies may have a variety of abnormalities, including diffuse and extensive diverticular disease, as in the autosomal recessive form of familial visceral neuropathy with neuronal intranuclear inclusions (Figure 11); widening, but with normal length and haustral pattern; elongation and redundancy; and frank megacolon and megarectum (Schuffler et al, 1978a; Schuffler and Jonak, 1982; Rohrmann et al, 1984).

In visceral myopathy, intravenous pyelograms may reveal massive enlargement of the bladder, ureters, and calyces, i.e. megacystis and megaloureters, and the bladder may fail to empty adequately on voiding (Schuffler et al, 1977; Faulk et al, 1978b). It is not yet certain whether histologically confirmed cases of visceral neuropathy are associated with such urological abnormalities, although urological dysfunction can occur.

Barium, rather than gastrografin, should be used to study these cases. Gastrografin becomes too diluted in the small bowel, so that detail is lost

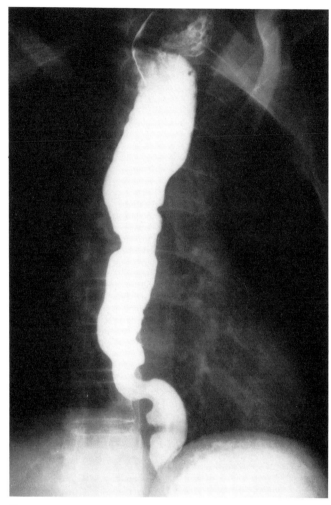

Figure 4. Oesophagogram showing mildly dilated upper oesophagus and irregular oesophageal lumen produced by multiple non-peristaltic contractions. This may also mimic achalasia. From Schuffler et al (1976), with permission.

and it becomes difficult to differentiate mechanical obstruction from pseudo-obstruction. Should a real small bowel obstruction be present, the excess fluid in the small bowel will prevent drying and inspissation of the barium.

Oesophageal Manometry

Approximately 75% of patients with CIIP have abnormalities of oesophageal peristalsis (Schuffler, 1981; Schuffler et al, 1981). Thus, the finding of abnormal peristalsis helps to support a diagnosis of CIIP, whereas the finding of normal peristalsis does not exclude it. Visceral myopathy is characterized by low amplitude, simultaneous waves, or absence of contractions, and the lower oesophageal sphincter pressure varies from borderline low to high (Figure 12). In contrast, progressive systemic sclerosis is characterized by low amplitude but peristaltic contractions, or in more severe disease, absence of contractions (Figure 13). The lower oesophageal sphincter pressure is usually below the normal range, and reflux is common.

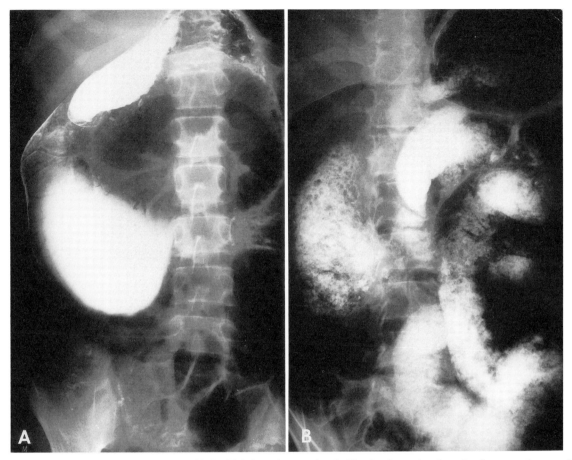

Figure 5. Small bowel series in a patient with familial visceral myopathy. A. The duodenum is enlarged and appears obstructed on the early X-ray. B. On follow-up radiography two days later, the barium has moved to the distal jejunum. The small bowel loops are distended with fluid and particulate material. From Schuffler et al (1977), with permission.

Several patterns of abnormal motility may occur in the visceral neuropathy syndromes. In the autosomal recessive form of visceral neuropathy with neuronal intranuclear inclusions, peristalsis is absent and there are repetitive simultaneous and non-simultaneous waves both spontaneously and in response to swallows (Figure 14). Sphincter pressure is normal to high and there is poor relaxation with swallows. Other types of visceral neuropathy may have patterns indistinguishable from achalasia or diffuse oesophageal spasm, or they may have low amplitude, simultaneous waves in response to swallows, much like the patients with visceral myopathy.

Gastric/Small Bowel Manometry

Abnormalities of the migrating motor complex (MMC) occur in both visceral myopathies and visceral neuropathies (Summers et al, 1983; Stanghellini et al, 1987). In visceral myopathies, the phasic pressure waves of the MMC are of low amplitude, or in severe disease there are no pressure waves whatsoever. In visceral neuropathy, four abnormal patterns of contractions may occur, either singly, or in various combinations. According to Stanghellini et al, these consist of (1) abnormal propagation or configuration of the MMCs; (2) uncoordinated bursts of phasic pressure activity; (3) sustained (>30 minutes) unco-

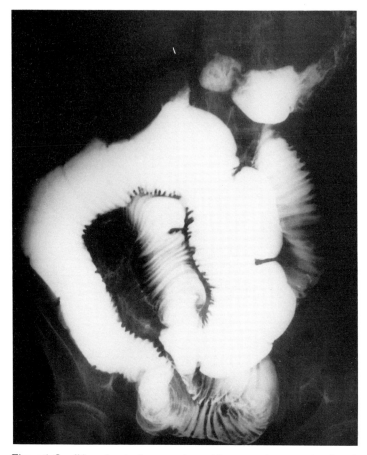

Figure 6. Small bowel series from a patient with progressive systemic sclerosis showing valvular packing and sacculations of the jejunum. From Rohrmann et al (1984), with permission.

ordinated intestinal pressure activity; and (4) failure of a meal to induce a fed pattern (Figure 15) (Stanghellini et al, 1987).

To date, gastric and small bowel manometry have mainly been utilized by a small number of investigators in scattered research centres. It is still unavailable in many communities. In contrast to oesophageal manometry, which takes about 1 hour to perform, gastric and small bowel manometry requires about 6 hours of recording time once the manometry assembly is in place. Of course, getting it in place takes additional time. Because oesophageal manometry is widely available and no longer experimental, it is of greater value as a diagnostic tool. As gastric and small bowel manometry become more widely used in a larger number of patients, both with and without CIIP, we will gradually learn how sensitive and specific it is for the diagnosis of this syndrome.

Pathology

Because space does not permit a comprehensive review of the pathology of chronic intestinal pseudo-obstruction, the reader is referred to a recent review of the pathology of neuromuscular disorders of the small intestine and colon (Krishnamurthy and Schuffler, 1987). These disorders are classified in Table 1.

Visceral myopathy is characterized by vacuolar degeneration and fibrosis of one or both layers of the smooth muscle (Schuffler and Pope, 1977;

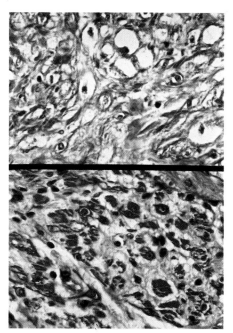

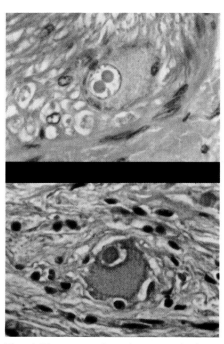

Plate 1. Smooth muscle layers of the small intestine from a patient with sporadic visceral myopathy. The circular muscle (cm) is normal whereas the outer, longitudinal muscle has vacuolar degeneration (arrows) and blue-staining collagen.

Plate 2. Top: higher magnification of vacuolar degeneration and blue-staining collagen from a patient with familial visceral myopathy. Faintly-staining degenerating muscle cells are seen within some of the spaces. Bottom: fibrosis of smooth muscle from the small intestine of a patient with progressive systemic sclerosis. There is blue-staining collagen intermixed with scarlet-staining muscle cells which are either normal in size or smaller than normal, but there is no vacuolar degeneration.

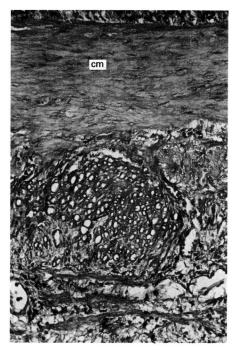

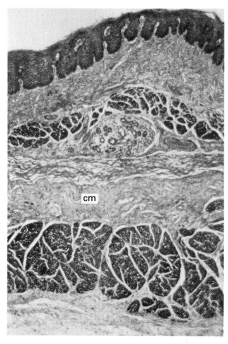

Plate 3. Postmortem specimen of the oesophagus from a patient with progressive systemic sclerosis. The circular muscle (cm) is replaced by collagen, yet the adjacent longitudinal muscle is normal.

Plate 4. Top: neuron from the myenteric plexus of a 63 year old woman with familial visceral neuropathy which contains two intranuclear inclusions. Bottom: neuron from the patient's 64 year old brother, which contains a single intranuclear inclusion.

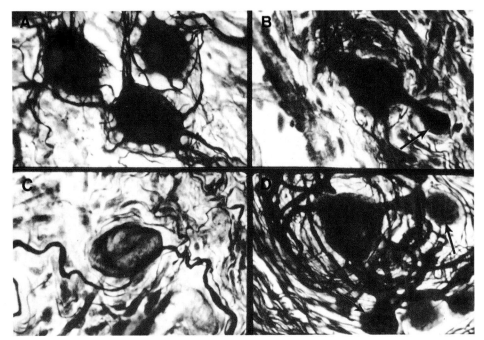

Plate 5. A. Normal oesophageal neurons from a control case. B. Degenerated neuron with one clubbed dendrite (arrow) and paucity of nerve processes from a patient with familial visceral neuropathy and intranuclear inclusions. C. Degenerated neuron. D. Neuron with multiple clubbed dendrites (arrows) from the same patient.

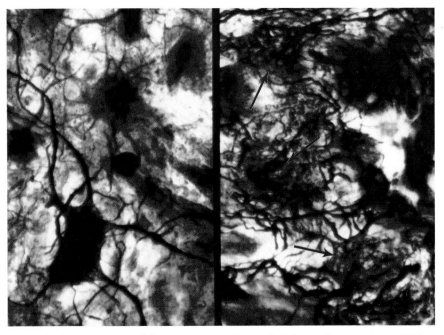

Plate 6. Left: normal argyrophilic neurons from the terminal ileum of a control case. Right: three degenerated neurons (arrows) from a patient with sporadic visceral neuropathy. The neurons are indistinct and have a very irregular uptake of silver.

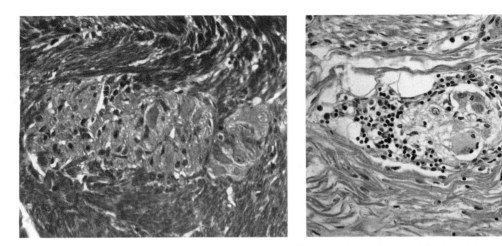

Plate 7. Left: myenteric plexus from a normal control case. Neuron bodies and small glial cell nuclei are visible, but there are no inflammatory cells. Right: myenteric plexus from a patient with paraneoplastic visceral neuropathy. There is a round cell infiltrate in the plexus.

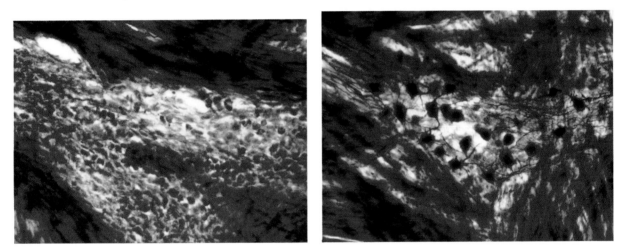

Plate 8. Left, part of the colonic myenteric plexus from a normal control case. Right: part of the colonic myenteric plexus from a patient with paraneoplastic visceral neuropathy. The plexus is replaced with a proliferation of cells containing small nuclei, which probably represents the nuclei of inflammatory and glial cells. Neurons and axons are absent.

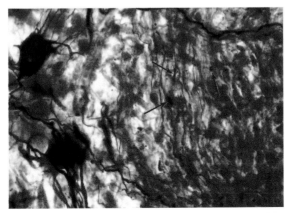

Plate 9. Area of the ileal myenteric plexus from a patient with inflammatory axonopathy. Two normal argyrophilic neurons are seen on the left. A number of dark-staining axons are seen, but their numbers are greatly reduced. Argyrophilic fragments of axons can be seen (arrows) indicating axonal degeneration.

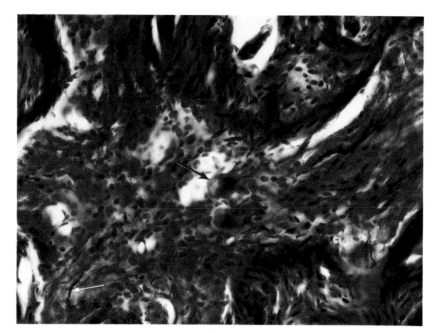

Plate 10. Myenteric plexus from an infant with pseudo-obstruction. Only one argyrophilic neuron with processes is seen (arrow). The rest of the plexus is filled with a multitude of small nuclei which probably represent glial cells and immature neurons. Part of one axon can be seen (white arrow).

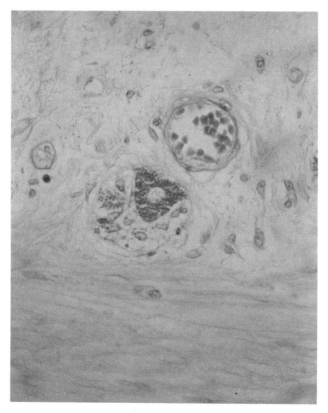

Plate 11. Luxol blue-PAS stain of a cross section of the myenteric plexus from a patient with Fabry's disease. A prominent neuron is seen which is filled with multiple blue-staining granules. The smaller collections of blue granules are located within axons. The blue-staining material is ceramide trihexoside.

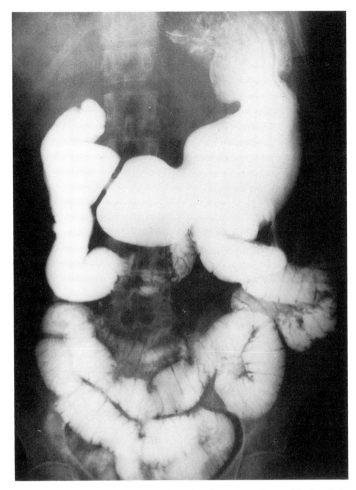

Figure 7. Upper gastrointestinal series from a patient with familial visceral neuropathy associated with intranuclear inclusions. The stomach is large; the proximal small intestine is wide; and the barium is diluted by excessive small bowel fluid. The fluoroscopy revealed hyperactive and uncoordinated contractions. From Schuffler et al (1976), with permission.

Schuffler and Beegle, 1979; Mitros et al, 1982). The longitudinal muscle is usually more involved than the circular and the severity of involvement may vary from one area to another (Plates 1 and 2). Diverticulosis of the small intestine can occur as the result of focal fibrosis of both muscle layers, resulting in weak spots in the wall which then protrude (Krishnamurthy et al, 1983; Anuras et al, 1983).

Progressive systemic sclerosis is characterized by fibrosis of one or both muscle layers, but in the absence of vacuolar degeneration (Schuffler and Beegle, 1979; Mitros et al, 1982). The remaining

muscle cells vary from normal to tiny in size. The circular muscle is usually more affected than the longitudinal, and the involvement can be abrupt and focal, with severely fibrotic muscle being immediately adjacent to perfectly normal muscle (Plate 3). Such severe, focal involvement of both muscle layers can result in diffuse diverticulosis and/or sacculations of the small bowel and colon.

Visceral neuropathy is characterized by a variety of abnormalities of the myenteric plexus, consisting of degeneration and dropout of neurons, with or without inflammation (Krishnamurthy

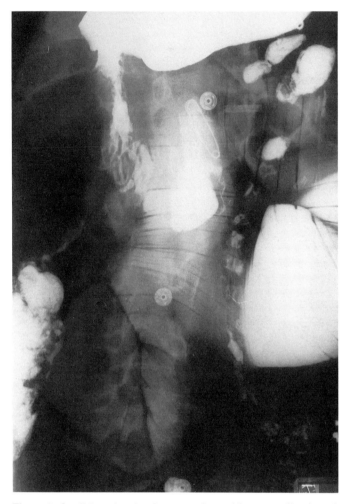

Figure 8. Small bowel series from a patient with a sporadic visceral neuropathy. The jejunum is massively dilated and the barium is diluted by excessive fluid, whereas the duodenum appears unaffected. Contractions were ineffective.

and Schuffler, 1987). Depending on the particular syndrome, the neuronal degeneration may take several forms. There can be:

(1) Swollen neurons, which may have clubbed dendrites and a decreased number of processes, associated with intranuclear inclusions (familial visceral neuropathy, autosomal recessive) (Plates 4 and 5) (Schuffler et al, 1978a);

(2) Swollen and fragmented argyrophilic and argyrophobic neurons, fragmented axons, and glial cell proliferation which may replace parts of the plexus (one type of sporadic visceral neuropathy) (Plate 6) (Schuffler and Jonak, 1982);

(3) Vacuolated neurons which look like signet ring cells (second type of sporadic visceral neuropathy) (Schuffler et al, 1985);

(4) Fragmented and vacuolated neurons, fragmented axons, and marked neuron dropout, associated with chronic inflammatory cell infiltration and glial cell replacement of parts of the plexus (paraneoplastic visceral neuropathy, Chagas' disease, and idiopathic (Plates 7 and 8) (Schuffler et al, 1983);

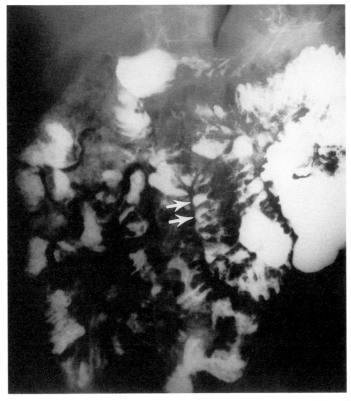

Figure 9. Multiple small-mouthed diverticula (arrows) in a patient with small intestinal diverticulosis. From Schuffler (1981), with permission.

(5) Axon degeneration and dropout associated with a chronic inflammatory cell infiltrate in the plexus, but with normal neurons (inflammatory axonopathy) (Plate 9) (Krishnamurthy et al, 1986);

(6) Fewer than normal numbers of argyrophilic neurons and axons, associated with increased numbers of nuclei in the ganglia and nerve tracts (incomplete maturation of the plexus) (Plate 10) (unpublished data);

(7) Large, hyperplastic plexus with neurons and axons in abnormal locations, such as the lamina propria and within the substance of the smooth muscle, along with large, bizarre-appearing neurons and disorganized axons (neuronal intestinal dysplasia) (Feinstat et al, 1984; Achem et al, 1987); and

(8) Enlarged neurons positive for Luxol blue (Fabry's disease, with involvement of the enteric nervous system) (Plate 11) (Friedman et al, 1984).

What role does pathology play in the diagnosis of CIIP and when should a tissue diagnosis be sought? In the majority of cases, the diagnosis of CIIP can be made by utilizing a combination of history, physical findings, radiography, and manometry. In such cases, exploratory laparotomy should be avoided, primarily to decrease the possibility of adhesion formation and subsequent confusion as to whether recurrent symptoms represent pseudo-obstruction or mechanical obstruction from adhesions. However, when the above tests do not provide certainty of diagnosis, exploratory laparotomy should be undertaken to exclude mechanical obstruction and to obtain full thickness biopsies of the small intestine. The biopsies should be large enough to study the

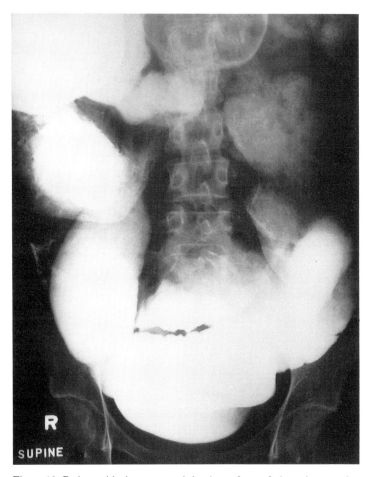

Figure 10. Patient with the autosomal dominant form of visceral myopathy. The colon is redundant, enlarged and without haustra. Barium had been given three days earlier when the stomach was examined. Despite numerous enemas and cathartics, it was 14 days before the colon emptied. From Schuffler et al (1976), with permission.

myenteric plexus by Smith's technique (Smith, 1972; Schuffler and Jonak, 1982). Because this usually means an opened piece of intestine measuring about 2×2 cm, a small resection is optimal for tissue diagnosis. In fact, because of the patchy distribution of some lesions, I recommend taking two samples from the small intestine.

Laparotomy is sometimes undertaken for palliation, as in the case of side-to-side duodenojejunostomy for megaduodenum or subtotal colectomy for megacolon. In such cases, plentiful tissue is available for study and accurate pathological diagnosis. Accurate diagnosis is important

because these patients have long-term chronic problems that can be expressed in other parts of the gut after resection. An understanding of the pathology will make subsequent diagnosis of new symptoms that much easier.

Exploratory laparotomy, with tissue diagnosis, is almost always required in infants and young children in order to exclude congenital abnormalities and to produce certainty of diagnosis to guide the paediatrician and parents as to prognosis and long-term management, which may require a commitment to home parenteral nutrition.

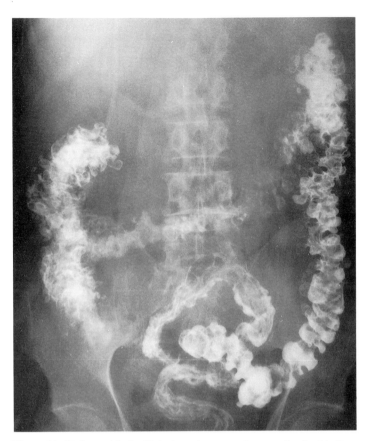

Figure 11. Patient with familial visceral neuropathy associated with intranuclear inclusions. There is extensive diverticular disease involving the entire colon. From Schuffler et al (1976), with permission.

Management

All management is palliative, because no specific treatment is of proven value for any of the disorders producing chronic intestinal pseudo-obstruction. Prokinetic drugs, such as metoclopramide and domperidone, have not been successful in the few cases reported (Lipton and Knauer, 1977). There is hope that cisapride may be effective in some cases. A recent study demonstrated that it could speed transport through the small bowel in a limited number of patients studied acutely (Camilleri et al, 1986). No long-term studies of cisapride have yet been reported.

Broad-spectrum antibiotics directed against coliforms and anaerobes are useful in treating the small bowel bacterial overgrowth syndrome which occurs in some of these patients (Schuffler et al,

1978b, 1981). Liquid formula diets may be of some value for short periods of time, although they do not seem to alter outcome. Palliative surgery, in extreme situations and directed at specific problems, may be of value in selected patients (Anuras et al, 1979; Schuffler and Deitch, 1980; Schuffler et al, 1981; Pitt et al, 1985). Depending on the problem treated, such surgery may consist of subtotal gastrectomy with Roux-en-Y anastomosis, duodenojejunostomy with or without duodenoplasty, limited or extended small bowel resections, subtotal colectomy, and decompressive gastrostomy. Should the patient be unable to maintain nutrition despite the above measures, home parenteral nutrition will be necessary for an indefinite period of time (Pitt et al, 1985; Warner and Jeejeebhoy, 1985).

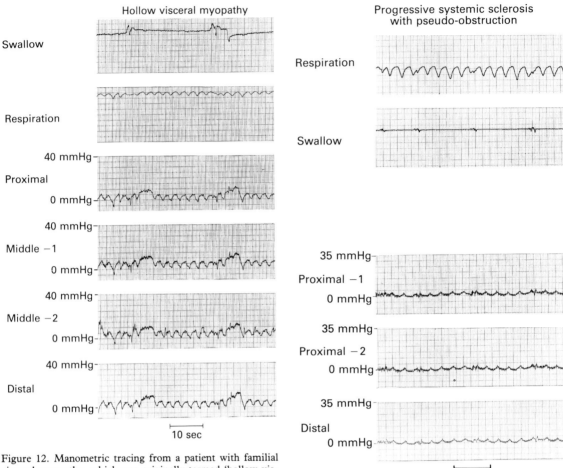

Figure 12. Manometric tracing from a patient with familial visceral myopathy, which was originally termed 'hollow visceral myopathy'. Swallows produce low amplitude simultaneous contractions in the proximal, middle and distal catheters. From Schuffler (1981), with permission.

Figure 13. Manometric tracing from a patient with progressive systemic sclerosis with pseudo-obstruction. No contractile activity of any sort is present in the body of the oesophagus. The fluctuations of the baseline recorded from the proximal and distal catheters are due to respirations. From Schuffler (1981), with permission.

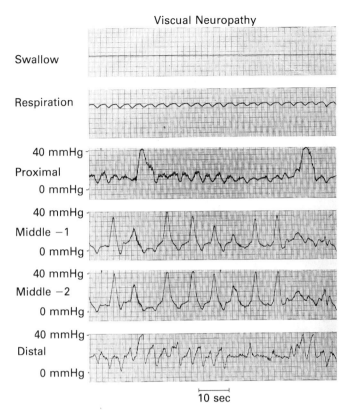

Figure 14. Manometric tracing in familial visceral neuropathy. Although no swallows are occurring, the body of the oesophagus demonstrates repetitive, spontaneous contractions. From Schuffler and Pope (1977), with permission.

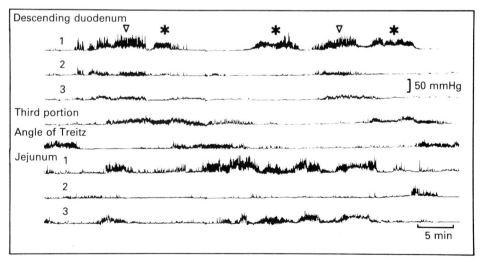

Figure 15. Bursts of propagated (▽) and non-propagated (*) pressure activity in the intestine in a patient with CIIP presumably caused by a visceral neuropathy. Non-propagated bursts are greater than two minutes duration. From Stanghellini et al (1987), with permission.

References

Achem, S. R., Owyang, C., Schuffler, M. D., and Dobbins, W. O., III, (1987), Neuronal dysplasia and chronic idiopathic intestinal pseudo-obstruction: rectal biopsy as an aid to diagnosis. *Gastroenterology*, **92**:805–9.

Anuras, S., Mitros, F. A., Milano, A., Kuminsky, R., Decanio, R., and Green, J. B., (1986), A familial visceral myopathy with dilatation of the entire gastrointestinal tract. *Gastroenterology*, **90**:385–90.

Anuras, S., Mitros, F. A., Nowak, T. V., Ionasescu, V. V., Gurll, N. J., Christensen, J., and Green, J. B., (1983), A familial visceral myopathy with external ophthalmoplegia and autosomal recessive transmission. *Gastroenterology*, **84**:346–53.

Anuras, S., Shirazi, S., Faulk, D. L., Gardner, G. D., and Christensen, J., (1979), Surgical treatment in familial visceral myopathy. *Ann. Surg.*, **189**:306–10.

Camilleri, M., Brown, M. L., and Malagelada, J.-R., (1986), Impaired transit of chyme in chronic intestinal pseudo-obstruction. Correction by cisapride. *Gastroenterology*, **91**:619–26.

Faulk, D. L., Anuras, S., and Christensen, J., (1978a), Chronic intestinal pseudo-obstruction. *Gastroenterology*, **74**:922–31.

Faulk, D. L., Anuras, S., Gardner, G. D., Mitros, F. A., Summers, R. W., and Christensen, J., (1978b), A familial visceral myopathy. *Ann. Intern. Med.*, **89**:600–6.

Feinstat, T., Tesluk, H., Schuffler, M. D., Krishnamurthy, S., Verlenden, L., Gilles, W., Frey, C., and Trudeau, W., (1984), Megacolon and neurofibromatosis: a neuronal intestinal dysplasia. Case report and review of the literature. *Gastroenterology*, **86**:1573–9.

Friedman, L. S., Platika, D., Thistlethwaite, J. R., Kirkham, S. E., Kolodny, E. H., and Schuffler, M. D., (1984), Jejunal diverticulosis with perforation as a complication of Fabry's disease. *Gastroenterology*, **86**:558–63.

Krishnamurthy, S., Kelly, M. M., Rohrmann, C. A., and Schuffler, M. D., (1983), Jejunal diverticulosis: a heterogeneous disorder caused by a variety of abnormalities of smooth muscle or myenteric plexus. *Gastroenterology*, **85**:538–47.

Krishnamurthy, S., and Schuffler, M. D., (1987), Pathology of neuromuscular disorders of the small intestine and colon. *Gastroenterology*, in press.

Krishnamurthy, S., Schuffler, M. D., Belic, L., and Schweid, A., (1986), An inflammatory axonopathy of the myenteric plexus causing rapidly progressive intestinal pseudo-obstruction. *Gastroenterology*, **90**:754–8.

Lipton, A. B., and Knauer, C. M., (1977), Pseudo-obstruction of the bowel. Therapeutic trial of metoclopramide. *Am. J. Dig. Dis.*, **22**:263–5.

Mayer, E. A., Schuffler, M. D., Rotter, J. I., and Hanna, P., (1986), A familial visceral neuropathy with autosomal dominant transmission. *Gastroenterology*, **91**:1528–35.

Mitros, F., Schuffler, M. D., Teja, K., and Anuras, S., (1982), Pathology of familial visceral myopathy. *Human Pathol.*, **13**:825–33.

Ogilvie, H., (1948), Large intestine colic due to sympathetic deprivation. *Br. Med. J.*, **2**:671–3.

Pitt, H. A., Mann, L. L., Berquist, W. E., Ament, M. E., Fonkalsrud, E. W., and DenBesten, L., (1985), Chronic intestinal pseudo-obstruction. Management with total parenteral nutrition and a venting enterostomy. *Arch. Surg.*, **120**: 614–18.

Rohrmann, C. A., Ricci, M. T., Krishnamurthy, S., and Schuffler, M. D., (1984), Radiologic and histologic differentiation of neuromuscular disorders of the gastrointestinal tract: visceral myopathies, visceral neuropathies, and progressive systemic sclerosis. *Am. J. Roentg.*, **143**:933–41.

Schuffler, M. D., (1981), Chronic intestinal pseudo-obstruction syndromes. *Med. Clins. N. Am.*, **65**:1331–58.

Schuffler, M. D., Baird, H. W., Fleming, C. R., Bell, C. E., Bouldin, T. W., Malagelada, J.-R., McGill, D. G., Le Bauer, S. M., Abrams, M., and Lowe, J., (1983), Intestinal pseudo-obstruction as the presenting manifestation of small cell carcinoma of the lung: a paraneoplastic neuropathy of the gastrointestinal tract. *Ann. Intern. med.*, **98**:129–34.

Schuffler, M. D., and Beegle, R. G., (1979), Progressive systemic sclerosis of the gastrointestinal tract and hereditary hollow visceral myopathy: two distinguishable disorders of intestinal smooth muscle. *Gastroenterology*, **77**:664–71.

Schuffler, M. D., Bird, T. D., Sumi, S. M., and Cook, A., (1978a), A familial neuronal disease presenting as intestinal pseudo-obstruction. *Gastroenterology*, **75**:889–98.

Schuffler, M. D., and Deitch, E. A., (1980), Chronic intestinal pseudo-obstruction: a surgical approach. *Ann. Surg.*, **192**:752–61.

Schuffler, M. D., and Jonak, Z., (1982), Chronic idiopathic intestinal pseudo-obstruction caused by a degenerative disorder of the myenteric plexus: the use of Smith's method to define the neuropathology. *Gastroenterology*, **82**:476–86.

Schuffler, M. D., Kaplan, L. R., and Johnson, L. (1978b). Small intestinal mucosa in pseudo-obstruction syndromes, *Digestive Diseases*, **23**:821–8.

Schuffler, M. D., Leon, S. H., and Krishnamurthy, S., (1985), Intestinal pseudo-obstruction caused by a new form of visceral neuropathy: palliation by radical small bowel resection. *Gastroenterology*, **89**:1152–6.

Schuffler, M. D., Lowe, M. C., and Bill, A. H., (1977), Studies of idiopathic intestinal pseudo-obstruction.

I. Hereditary hollow visceral myopathy: Clinical and pathological studies. *Gastroenterology*, **73**:327–38.

Schuffler, M. D., and Pope, C. E., II, (1977), Studies of idiopathic intestinal pseudo-obstruction. II. Hereditary hollow visceral myopathy: Family studies. *Gastroenterology*, **73**: 339–44.

Schuffler, M. D., Rohrmann, C. A., Chaffee, R. G., Brand, D. L., Delaney, J. H., and Young, J. H., (1981), Chronic intestinal pseudo-obstruction: A report of 27 cases and review of the literature. *Medicine*, **60**:173–96.

Schuffler, M. D., Rohrmann, C. A., and Templeton, F. E., (1976), The radiologic manifestations of idiopathic intestinal pseudo-obstruction. *Am. J. Roentg.*, **127**:729–36.

Smith, B., (1972), *The Neuropathology of the Alimentary Tract*, Edward Arnold, London.

Stanghellini, V., Camilleri, M., and Malagelada, J.-R., (1987), Chronic idiopathic intestinal pseudo-obstruction: clinical and intestinal manometric findings. *Gut*, **28**:5–12.

Summers, R. W., Anuras, S., and Green, J., (1983), Jejunal manometry patterns in health, partial intestinal obstruction and pseudo-obstruction. *Gastroenterology*, **88**:1290–300.

Warner, E., and Jeejeebhoy, K. N., (1985), Successful management of chronic intestinal pseudo-obstruction with home parenteral nutrition. *J. Parent. Ent. Nutr.*, **9**:173–8.

27C.

IRRITABLE BOWEL SYNDROME

Devinder Kumar, David L. Wingate
London Hospital Medical College, London, UK

Irritable bowel syndrome is probably one of the commonest gastrointestinal disorders, yet it has proved to be one of the most difficult conditions to diagnose and manage. Of patients attending gastroenterology clinics 20–50% suffer from functional gastrointestinal symptoms (Switz, 1976). Thompson and Heaton (1980), from a survey of 327 patients, concluded that clinically distinct functional bowel disorders existed in approximately one-third of the subjects studied (Figure 1). In the past there has been a paucity of studies of this disorder because of difficulties in patient selection, choice of appropriate marker to be tested and, above all, the correlation of findings with the clinical presentation. Furthermore, the prevalence of psychiatric disease in irritable bowel syndrome (IBS) is high (Liss et al, 1973); this makes patient selection even more difficult. This difficulty is borne out by the comments of a contemporary psychiatrist '... the label of psychiatric disease or IBS is determined by whether the patient sees a psychiatrist or gastroenterologist first' (J. Pfeffer).

Definition

Irritable bowel syndrome has generally been defined on the basis of exclusion criteria; that is,

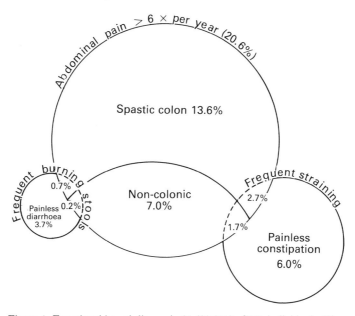

Figure 1. Functional bowel disease in 91 (30.2%) of 301 individuals. The large circle indicates the 62 who have abdominal pain more than six times per year. It is divided to show 41 with IBS and 21 with non-colonic pain. The small circles represent 14 with diarrhoea and 31 with constipation. Overlap of these by the large circle indicates that some with diarrhoea and constipation also have abdominal pain. From Manning et al (1978), with permission.

by what it is not, or in more simple terms that it is not organic disease. In the absence of a pathophysiological marker, a more rational approach would be to define it by its symptoms. The most commonly accepted definition based on symptomatology is that of Manning et al (1978). They have defined IBS as a homogeneous syndrome which consists of abdominal pain or discomfort usually related to defecation, constipation or diarrhoea, passage of mucus and a feeling of incomplete evacuation. In our experience, the single most common symptom in patients with IBS is a feeling of incomplete evacuation associated with frequency of defecation; the latter being common to both constipation and diarrhoea sub-groups. In addition, abdominal pain and discomfort and/or passage of mucus but not blood with stools, seem to form the rest of the symptom complex in this syndrome. A proportion of patients give a strong history of stress-related or stress-evoked symptoms. A clear and precise definition of IBS or the so-called 'functional gut syndromes' is of utmost importance in the understanding of psychopathophysiological markers in this group of disorders.

Pathophysiology

The exact aetiology of IBS is unknown. Psychological abnormalities, secretory/absorptive disturbances, food intolerance, laxative abuse and hormonal imbalances have all been implicated in the pathophysiology of IBS. Figure 2 shows a schematic illustration of various factors involved in the pathogenesis of IBS. Stress is yet another factor which remains to be substantiated in its aetiopathogenesis. Under experimental conditions, acute stress has been shown to alter gastrointestinal secretory and motor activity. Comparable investigations on the effect of chronic stress are lacking. This is mainly due to the lack of methodology for quantification of the effect of stress on life events and more importantly their relationship to clinical manifestations.

It is plausible that psychological factors lead to perturbation of the CNS resulting in anxiety states associated with symptoms (Figure 3). Whether anxiety states are the cause or effect of IBS symptoms is not known. The other factor which is important here is the individual's perception of life events or stress in general. This factor alone

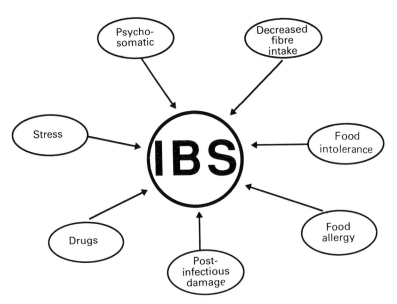

Figure 2. Schematic representation of various factors involved in the aetiology of irritable bowel syndrome (IBS).

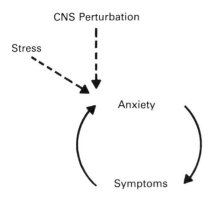

Figure 3. An illustration of anxiety-symptom loop caused by stress/CNS perturbation.

may determine what brings an IBS patient to see a doctor in the first place.

Several workers have looked for a satisfactory marker of IBS. Figure 4 lists the possible markers which could prove of significance in the diagnosis of IBS. Several hormones such as cholecystokinin, motilin and adrenal medullary activity have been suggested as possible markers of IBS (Harvey and Read, 1973; Vantrappen et al, 1979; Esler and Goulston, 1973).

Evidence of abnormal gastrointestinal motor activity in patients with IBS is being reported consistently, giving weight to the hypothesis that functional bowel disorders are caused by, or at

least related to, motor abnormalities in the gut. Most of the earlier studies focused on colonic motor activity in IBS because it was generally believed to be a disorder of the colon. More recently, motor abnormalities in other parts of the gastrointestinal tract have been reported in IBS. In this review we will discuss the role of a motility marker in various parts of the gastrointestinal tract.

Oesophageal Motility in the IBS

Motor activity of the oesophagus in IBS has been studied on the assumption that it may be a more diffuse disorder than was previously supposed. Whorwell et al (1981) studied oesophageal manometry in 30 patients with IBS and focused mainly on lower oesophageal sphincter pressures in their analysis. They showed (Figure 5) that patients with the IBS have a significantly reduced oesophageal sphincter pressure. There was also a significantly higher incidence of spontaneous activity, variable amplitude waves, simultaneous waves and repetitive contractions in patients with IBS. Interestingly, all these abnormalities were seen only in the smooth muscled part of the oesophagus and no abnormalities were found in the striated upper oesophageal sphincter.

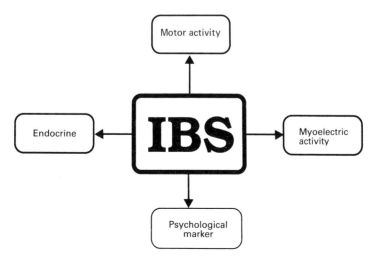

Figure 4. A schematic representation of possible markers of irritable basel syndrome (IBS).

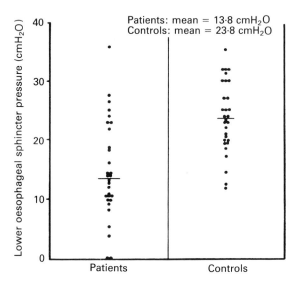

Figure 5. Lower oesophageal sphincter pressures in patients with irritable bowel syndrome and matched controls. From Whorwell et al (1981), with permission.

Gastric Motility

Abnormalities of gastric motor function, either in terms of transit or contractile activity, have not been reported in patients with IBS. Cann et al (1983) studied gastric emptying in 61 patients diagnosed to have irritable bowel syndrome. They found no significant differences in gastric emptying ($T\frac{1}{2}$) between controls and IBS patients. However, Malagelada and Stanghellini (1985), in another study on 104 patients with functional dyspepsia, reported manometric abnormalities both in the fasting as well as the postprandial state in the stomach. They argued that there was a significant overlap between functional dyspepsia and patients with IBS, thereby suggesting that some of these abnormalities could well represent gastric motor abnormality in IBS. In our view, with a careful history and assessment, patients with IBS can be separated from a large group of functional dyspepsia patients; therefore avoiding a possible overlap and more importantly confusion in interpretation of manometric data.

Upper Small Bowel Motility

Due to its easy accessibility, and backed up by well-established motor patterns in normal sub-

jects, upper small bowel has become the main region of study in patients with IBS (Kumar and Wingate, 1985; Thompson et al, 1979; Kellow and Phillips, 1987). Motor abnormalities in the upper small bowel in patients with IBS have been reported since as early as 1962 (Horowitz and Farrar, 1962). Thompson et al (1979) reported abnormal contractile activity in one IBS patient studied for 36 hours using radiotelemetry capsules. However, Kingham et al (1984) in their study of six IBS patients found the frequency of migrating motor complexes to be normal and also failed to record any abnormal contractions in their patients. They, however, pointed out that their technique '... did not allow accurate quantitation of phase I and phase II activities'. We have studied

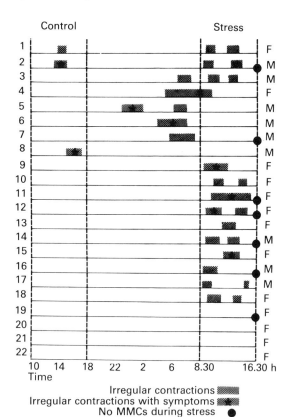

Figure 6. Frequency of contractile activity in 22 IBS patients. Each line summarizes the findings in an individual patient study. In patients 1–8 there were spontaneous episodes of abnormal irregular contractions, in patients 9–19 abnormalities occurred only during stress, while patients 20–22 showed no abnormality. From Kumar and Wingate (1985), with permission.

22 patients diagnosed to have IBS and have shown one of three motor abnormalities in 19 of these patients (Figure 6). The motor abnormalities seen were complete abolition of motor complexes, spontaneous irregular contractions and stress evoked irregular contractile activity (Figure 7). The important conclusion from this study was the fact that these patients need to be studied for a prolonged period of time if any abnormality is to be detected. If these 22 patients were studied for a period of only 8 hours, only three showed abnormal motor activity (Figure 8). However, if the study time was prolonged to 24 hours, another five

Stress-evoked irregular contractile activity in an IBS patient

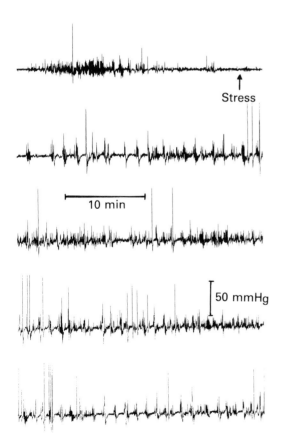

Figure 7. Irregular contractile activity under stress in an IBS patient. A continuous record of motility recorded at one sensor is shown. Stress-induced irregular contractions are present for two hours. Transient pressure rises of more than 50 mmHg are due to rises in intra-abdominal pressure. Negative deflections indicate brief episodes of signal loss.

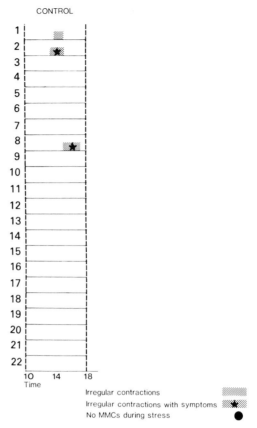

Figure 8. Incidence of irregular contractile activity in the first 8 hours of study in 22 IBS patients. Each line represents a patient. Hatched areas indicate the occurrence and duration of irregular activity; episodes which were accompanied by symptoms are starred.

patients were added to the diagnostic yield (Figure 9). When the study was extended to 36 hours and also a period of stress was included, 19 of the 22 patients studied showed one of the three abnormalities described. This study, we believe, highlights the value of prolonged intestinal manometry in the diagnosis of IBS. Another important finding is that these abnormalities are intermittent and paroxysmal. This is consistent with a syndrome which is characterized by intermittent symptoms. Kellow and Phillips (1987) in their study of 16 patients with IBS have confirmed the presence of spontaneous clustered contractions in the jejunum of patients with IBS (Figure 10). Similar prolonged duodenojejunal clustered contractions have been reported in ambulant studies on IBS

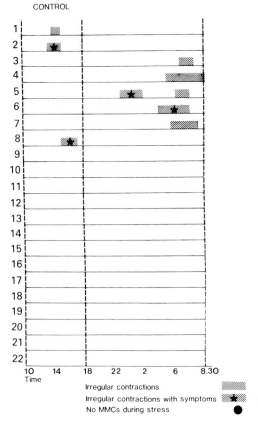

Figure 9. Incidence of irregular contractile activity in the first 22 hours of study in 22 IBS patients (see Figure 8 for key).

patients (Kellow et al, 1987). They have also shown that the MMC periodicity is significantly reduced in both diarrhoea and constipation-pre-

dominant patients with IBS. In their study there was no difference in the distribution of MMCs along the small bowel in IBS. An interesting feature of their study (as well as ours) was the association of abdominal symptoms with abnormal motor activity, suggesting that the central nervous system influences subjective perception. It is indeed possible that IBS is represented by a group of people who have exaggerated physiological responses or are more aware of intestinal motor events (Whitehead and Schuster, 1981).

In addition to abnormalities of motor activity, small bowel transit has been reported as abnormal in IBS patients. Cann et al (1983) have shown that small bowel transit is shorter in patients who complain of diarrhoea and longer in patients with constipation (Figure 11).

Ileal Motor Activity in IBS

Kellow and Phillips in 1987 studied ileal motor activity in 16 patients with IBS and have shown the presence of prolonged propagated contractions (Figure 12) in 12 patients and also in six controls in the fasting state. There was no qualitative difference in the characteristics of these pressure waves in the two groups. They also recorded discrete clustered contractions in 15 IBS patients and nine controls. The maximal pressures generated by discrete clustered contractions were greater in IBS patients than in controls. Trotman and Price (1985) studied ileal transit in patients with IBS

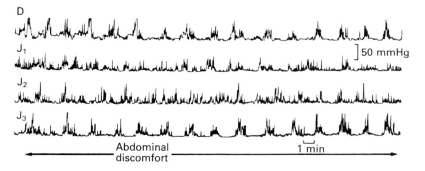

Figure 10. Recording of intraluminal pressure from jejunum of a patient with IBS showing 30 minutes of discrete clustered contractions. Sensors were in the duodenum (D) and at three jejunal sites (J1–J3). This pattern was associated with abdominal symptoms. From Kellow and Phillips (1987), with permission.

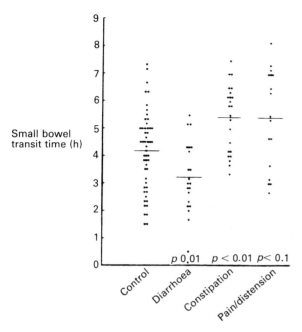

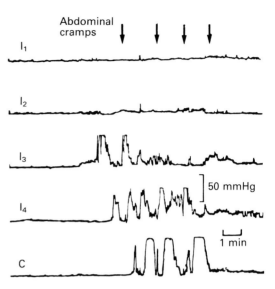

Figure 11. Small bowel transit times in control subjects and patient subgroups. Group means are shown with probability figures indicating significance of differences from control group. From Cann et al (1983), with permission.

Figure 12. Recording of intraluminal pressure from the ileum and proximal colon of a patient with IBS. Sensors were at four ileal sites and in the caecum. High pressure, propagated pressure waves were recorded in association with complaints of abdominal pain (arrows). From Kellow and Phillips (1987), with permission.

using scintigraphic techniques (bran scan) and showed that ileal transit in patients with IBS was slower than in normal controls (Figure 13), again suggesting abnormality of ileal motor function in IBS.

Colonic Motility

Motor Activity

Due to the symptoms of diarrhoea and constipation, the colon has been the main site of investigation in IBS. Since normal patterns of colonic motility in man have not been fully established,

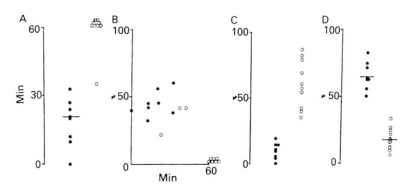

Figure 13. (a) Ileal half-emptying time, (b) peak percentage counts in caecum, (c) percentage counts in ileum at 60 minutes, and (d) ileocaecal clearance at 60 minutes. Filled circles represent controls and open circles represent irritable bowel syndrome. From Trotman and Price (1986), with permission.

abnormalities are difficult to pick up and therefore have to be interpreted with caution. Sigmoid tone has been reported to be decreased in diarrhoea and increased in constipation-predominant patients (Connell, 1962). Whitehead et al (1980) reported more frequent fast contractions in diarrhoea-predominant than constipation-dominant IBS patients. Similarly, during constipation, increased intraluminal segmented activity has been noted in the sigmoid (Holdstock et al, 1969; Connell et al, 1965). During periods of diarrhoea, reduced segmental activity has also been recorded (Waller and Misiewicz, 1972). Swarbrick et al (1980) were recently able to reproduce the pain of IBS by inflating balloons at various points throughout the colon in 29 of 48 IBS patients studied.

Myoelectric Activity

Electrical activity in the smooth muscle of human rectosigmoid has two basic intermittent slow wave rhythms; one approximately 3 cycles per minute (cpm) and the other 6–12 cpm. Snape et al (1976, 1977) found that the proportion of 3 cpm activity was greater in IBS patients than controls, and that this was associated with increased 3 cpm motor activity (Figure 14). Similar findings were also reported by Taylor et al (1978) but the concept remains controversial, since Latimer et al (1981)

found no difference in the slow wave frequency and colonic contractions in controls, IBS patients with pain, and psychoneurotic patients with no bowel symptoms. In the postprandial state, IBS patients show a prolonged increase in both colonic spike and motor activity (Figure 15) (Sullivan et al, 1978).

It is not yet known how abnormal slow wave activity can account for clinical features of IBS. More research is necessary before it will be possible to accept abnormal myoelectrical activity of the colon as a marker of IBS.

Therapy

In the absence of a well-defined pathophysiology, the management of IBS remains largely symptomatic. However, we believe that a positive approach to the whole problem, rather than a diagnosis of exclusion, goes a long way in managing patients with this ill-defined disorder. Patients who know what is wrong with them as opposed to those who know 'what is not wrong with them' are much more compliant and yield favourable results to therapy.

Since a fibre-deficient diet is said to be one of the causes of IBS, various people have tried a fibre-rich diet with conflicting results. Manning et al (1977) reported significant improvement in

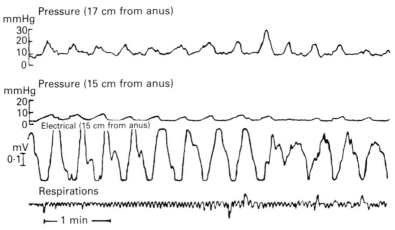

Figure 14. Simultaneous recordings of colonic myoelectrical activity and intraluminal pressure obtained in the distal colon of a patient with the irritable bowel syndrome after cholecystokinin administration. The frequency of slow waves and the colonic contractions are both 2.9 cpm. Respirations are shown below. Reproduced from Snape et al (1977), with permission.

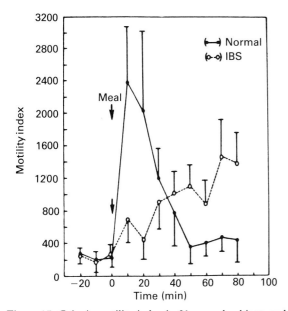

Figure 15. Colonic motility index in 21 normal subjects and 10 patients with IBS, measured for three 10-minute periods before and for 80 minutes after a 1000 calorie meal. The patients showed a prolonged increase in colonic motor activity as compared to the normal subjects. All values are shown as means ± SEM. Reproduced from Sullivan et al (1978), with permission.

symptoms from a six-week course of high-fibre diet. In contrast, Cann et al (1984) found no benefit from wheat bran in their patients. In our experience only a small proportion of patients, mainly constipation predominant, are helped by a fibre-rich diet. Again, fibre supplements such as psyllium and lactulose are helpful in the management of the constipation-predominant group of patients. The patients should be warned that these agents, as well as a fibre-rich diet, can aggravate flatulence and bloating.

Abdominal pain is traditionally treated with antispasmodics or anticholinergics. Psychological aspects of IBS may require supportive measures which under selected circumstances may have to be combined with an anxiolytic agent.

References

Cann, P. A., Read, N. W., Brown, C., Hobson, N. and Holdsworth, C. D., (1983), Irritable bowel syndrome: relationship of disorder in the transit of a single solid meal to symptom patterns. *Gut*, 24:405–11.

Cann, P. A., Read, N. W. and Holdsworth, C. D., (1984), What is the benefit of coarse wheat bran in patients with irritable bowel syndrome? *Gut*, 25:168–73.

Connell, A. M., (1962), The motility of the pelvic colon II. Paradoxical motility in diarrhoea and constipation. *Gut*, 3:342–8.

Connell, A. M., Jones, F. A. and Rowlands, E. N., (1965), Motility of the pelvic colon IV. Abdominal pain associated with colonic hypermotility after meals. *Gut*, 6:105–12.

Esler, M. D. and Goulston, K. J. (1973), Levels of anxiety in colonic disorders. *N. Engl. J. Med.*, 288:16–20.

Harvey, R. F. and Read, A. E. (1973). Effect of cholecystokinin on colonic motility and symptoms in patients with the irritable bowel syndrome. *Lancet*, i:1–3.

Holdstock, D. J., Misiewicz, J. J. and Waller, S. L. (1969), Observations on the mechanism of abdominal pain. *Gut*, 10:19–31.

Horowitz, L. and Farrar, J. T., (1962), Intraluminal small intestinal pressures in normal patients and in patients with functional gastrointestinal disorders. *Gastroenterology*, 42:455–64.

Kingham, J. G. C., Brown, R., Colson, R. and Clark, M. L. (1984). Jejunal motility in patients with functional abdominal pain. *Gut*, 25:375–80.

Kellow, J., Gill, R. C. and Wingate, D. L. (1987), Proximal gut motor activity in irritable bowel syndrome (IBS). Patients at home and at work. *Gastroenterology*, 92:1463.

Kellow, J. E. and Phillips, S. F. (1987), Altered small bowel motility in irritable bowel syndrome is correlated with symptoms. *Gastroenterology*, 92:1885–93.

Kumar, D. and Wingate, D. L. (1985), The irritable bowel syndrome. A paroxysmal motor disorder. *Lancet*, ii:973–7.

Latimer, P., Sarna, S., Campbell, D., Latimer, M., Waterfall, W., and Daniel, E. E., (1981), Colonic motor and myoelectrical activity: a comparative study of normal subjects, psychoneurotic patients and patients with the irritable bowel syndrome. *Gastroenterology*, 80:893–901.

Liss, J. L., Alpers, D. and Woodruff, R. A., (1973), The irritable colon syndrome and psychiatric illness. *Dis. Nerv. System*, 34:151–7.

Malagelada, J.-R. and Stanghellini, V., (1985), Manometric evaluation of functional upper gut symptoms. *Gastroenterology*, 88:1223–31.

Manning, A. P., Heaton, K. W. and Harvey, R. F., (1977), Wheat fibre and irritable bowel syndrome. *Lancet*, ii:417–18.

Manning, A. P., Thompson, W. G., Heaton, K. W. and

Morris, A. F. (1978), Towards positive diagnosis of the irritable bowel. *Br. Med. J.*, **2**:653–4.

Snape, W. J., Carlson, G. M. and Cohen, S. (1976), Colonic myoelectric activity in the irritable bowel syndrome. *Gastroenterology*, **72**:383–7.

Snape, W. J., Carlson, G. M., Matarazzo, S. A. and Cohen, S., (1977), Evidence that abnormal myoelectric activity produces colonic motor dysfunction in the irritable bowel syndrome. *Gastroenterology*, **72**:383–7.

Sullivan, M. A., Cohen, S. and Snape, W. J., (1978), Colonic myoelectrical activity in irritable bowel syndrome—effect of eating and anticholinergics. *N. Engl. J. Med.*, **298**:878–83.

Swarbrick, E. T., Hegarty, J. E., Bat, L., Williams, C. B. and Dawson, A. M., (1980), Site of pain from the irritable bowel. *Lancet*, **ii**:443–6.

Switz, D. M., (1976), What the gastroenterologist does all day. *Gastroenterology*, **70**:1048–50.

Taylor, I., Darby, C. and Hammond, P., (1978), Comparison of recto-sigmoid myoelectrical activity in the irritable colon syndrome during relapses and remissions. *Gut*, **19**:923–9.

Thompson, D. G., Laidlaw, J. M. and Wingate, D. L., (1979), Abnormal small bowel motility demonstrated by radio-telemetry in a patient with irritable colon. *Lancet*, **ii**:321–323.

Thompson, W. G. and Heaton, K. W., (1980), Functional bowel disorders in apparently healthy people. *Gastronenterology*, **79**:283–8.

Trotman, I. F. and Price, C. F. (1986), Bloated irritable bowel syndrome defined by dynamic ^{99m}Tc bran scan. *Lancet*, **ii**:364–6.

Vantrappen, F., Janssens, J., Peeters, T. L., Bloom, S. R., Christofides, N. D. and Hellemans, J., (1979), Motilin and the interdigestive migrating motor complex in man. *Dig. Dis. Sci.*, **24**:97–500.

Waller, S. L. and Misiewicz, J. J., (1972), Colonic motility in constipation or diarrhoea. *Scand. J. Gastroenterol.*, **7**:93–6.

Whitehead, W. E., Engel, B. T. and Schuster, M. M., (1980), Irritable bowel syndrome. Physiological and psychological differences between diarrhoea predominant and constipation predominant patients. *Dig. Dis. Sci.*, **25**:404–13.

Whitehead, W. E. and Schuster, M. M., (1981), Behavioral approaches to the treatment of gastrointestinal motility disorders. *Med. Clin. North. Am.*, **65**:1397–411.

Whorwell, P. J., Prior, A. and Faragher, E. B., (1984), Controlled trial of hypnotherapy in the treatment of severe refractory irritable bowel syndrome. *Lancet*, **ii**:1232.

Whorwell, P. J., Clouter, C. and Smith, C. L., (1981), Oesophageal motility in the irritable bowel syndrome. *Br. Med. J.*, **282**:1101–2.

27D.

CONSTIPATION

Ghislain Devroede
University of Sherbrooke, Quebec, Canada

The Nature of Constipation

A thorough review of constipation is beyond the scope of this publication, and has been published elsewhere (Devroede, 1988). In this chapter, I shall thus limit myself to those data about constipation which generate relatively little controversy, and can be applied directly to clinical situations.

Constipation is a symptom. It is not a disease. It is not a sign. As a symptom, constipation may be indicative of many diseases. Clinicians should make a differential diagnosis just as well as they would do, for instance, for abdominal pain. There are dozens of causes of constipation. Organic disease should be eliminated before a diagnosis of chronic idiopathic constipation is made. On occasions, constipation is caused by highly infrequent congenital or acquired abnormalities. It would then be a major disservice to the patient to focus on functional abnormalities and forget potentially curable lesions.

The approach to a sign and a symptom is different. The scientific method relies upon observations and measurements, and is only applicable to the sign. A symptom, however, is the experience of this sign by a patient. Not only is the subjective appreciation of this system highly variable, but previous unpleasant experiences of the same nature, both physical and emotional, interfere with the perception of the present experience. Thus, it is not surprising to see a lot of misunderstanding between physicians and the general public about what constitutes 'constipation'. Physicians tend to rely upon observable variables, in particular stool frequency (Figure 1). Outside of the medical profession, however, there is more emphasis on the associated subjective symptoms of constipation (Figure 2) (Sandler and Drossman, 1988). Dismissing the symptom as unimportant

as compared to the sign, dismissing the associated emotions as marginally relevant, is bound to lead to an oversimplified approach to constipation.

Constipation has different meanings for different patients. The term may imply that the stools are too small, too hard, too difficult to expel, or too infrequent, or that patients have a feeling of incomplete evacuation after defecation. These symptoms are difficulty to quantify.

Size cannot be recorded accurately because of the deformity imposed upon stools by the anorectal structures and by gravity during the act of defecation. Normal stool weight has a wide range (35–225 g per stool) (Rentorff and Kashgarian, 1967). If a patient passes lighter stools, this suggests constipation, although stool weight does not necessarily correlate well with stool size and deformability, factors which are probably also important. There are, however, marked geographic variations in stool weight and this parameter of constipation is probably not very practical in a clinical situation.

Stool frequency is the easiest parameter of constipation to quantify. To avoid potential exaggeration of the problem (Manning et al, 1976), stools should be counted prospectively over a number of weeks. A recent study (Verduron et al, 1988) on patients with constipation and a megarectum has shown that the difference between recalled and recorded stool frequency may vary according to diagnosis (Figure 3). Four uncontrolled studies of stool frequency show that normal subjects pass at least three stools per week but recent studies suggest it should be five (Sandler and Drossman, 1988; Martelli et al, 1978). Proportionally more women have few stools. Whites also defecate more often than blacks (Sandler and Drossman, 1988). In Senegal, people usually defecate in the morning and in the evening and con-

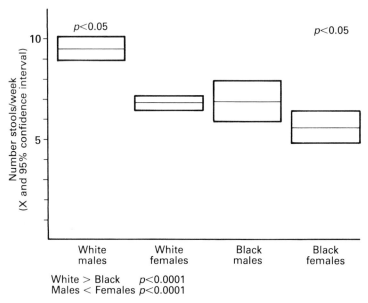

Figure 1. Normal bowel habits of healthy young adults (Sandler and Drossman, 1988). On the basis of this study, physicians concluded that people who have more than five stools per week are not constipated.

sider themselves constipated if they have only one stool per day; while over three stools per day is considered abnormal in the west, it is considered quite normal for many of these people (Epelboin, 1982). One should, therefore, never forget ethnic considerations in studies of 'normality'. The epidemiological range expresses what most people do at a given time of history. It may change quickly and vary with culture, and thus does not totally coincide with an intrinsic physiological 'normality'.

The transit time of food from mouth to anus is markedly influenced by dietary fibre. Thus vegetarians have shorter transit time than non-vegetarians (Gear et al, 1981) (Figure 4). The individual differences in stool output and response to dietary fibre are as much related to the personality as they are to the diet: this recent finding is of paramount importance and has largely been ignored in all studies of diet and bowel habit relationship (Tucker et al, 1981).

The recent interest in constipation has also neglected its relationship with the irritable bowel syndrome. The advantage of focusing on constipation is that this approach is amenable to scientific measurements, in contrast to what happens in making a diagnosis of irritable bowel syndrome, which is largely clinical and by exclusion. Many more symptoms are associated to constipation than to diarrhoea (Thompson and Heaton, 1980) (Figure 5). Thus many of the data obtained from patients with the irritable bowel syndrome may be relevant to a study of constipation. Pain has always been recognized as one of the key symptoms of the irritable bowel syndrome. Thus it is of interest to note that patients with chronic idiopathic constipation and abdominal pain have a faster transit through the large bowel than those who do not (Figure 6). This is true for all sites in the large bowel (Figure 7) (Lafranchi et al, 1984). Abdominal pain seems to be a good prognostic indicator in children who are brought for consultation because of constipation (Figure 8) (Abrahamian and Lloyd-Still, 1984).

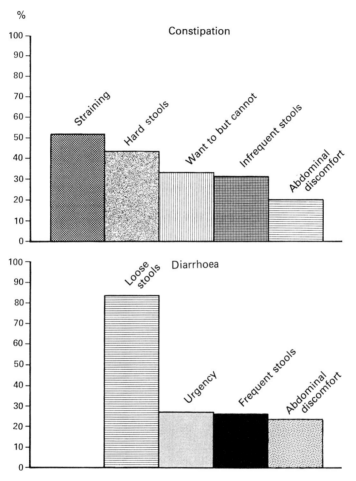

Figure 2. Straining, hard stools and impossibility to defecate at will are more worrisome to ordinary people than a number of stools less than a predetermined epidemiological range (Sandler and Drossman, 1988).

Faecal incontinence (leakage of stools of a different consistency from those in the rectum, and often liquid) and encopresis (involuntary passage of a normal stool) may be presenting symptoms of constipation, particularly in children (Levine, 1975). Thus, patients with these symptoms should be evaluated for constipation first. There is no good study at present that distinguishes incontinence and encopresis with regards to a relationship with constipation.

Because studies differ in terms of definition of constipation, and because there has never been an epidemiological survey of a random sample of a healthy population, it is impossible at this stage to conclude on the exact incidence or prevalence of constipation. What is very intriguing is that constipation seems to be a problem of little boys and of adult women: nothing is known about the age at which the sex ratio reverses, nor why (Figures 9 and 10). The sex difference is even more striking when constipation is defined and when a motor disorder is used as selection criterion. For instance, patients who have delayed transit in the ascending colon are largely females (Watier, 1983), and those with delayed colonic transit and a normal sized large bowel on barium enema are all

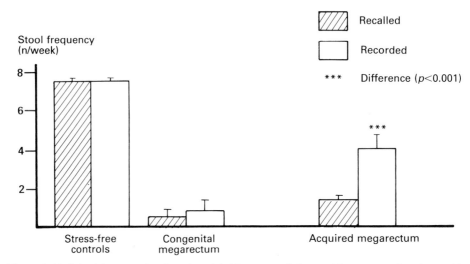

Figure 3. Both healthy controls whose bowel habits are not influenced by stress and patients with megarectum and constipation from birth produce as many stools as they claimed they did when first interviewed. However, those patients with megarectum, who became constipated somewhat later in life, defecate more often when they record their stool frequency on a diary, than what they claimed at entry into the study (Verduron et al, 1988).

female (Preston and Lennard-Jones, 1986). Similarly more constipated women have a normotonic anal canal and the proportion decreases in groups of subjects with a tight anal canal (Ducrotte, 1985).

In summary, a patient who complains of constipation should never be dismissed as 'not sick' on the basis of quantitative studies. The merits of these lie principally in the opportunity to 'take care' of the patient in a positive fashion (rather than simply making an exclusion diagnosis), and to give some objective weight to the symptom.

The Nuisance of Constipation

The economic aspects of constipation are staggering (Devroede, 1988) presumably because people do not like to be constipated and are determined to have frequent and satisfying defecation. However, constipation is not necessarily innocuous.

Urinary tract infections are often associated with constipation and may disappear when bowel habit is restored to normal (O'Regan, 1985). It should be remembered, however, that association

is not causation and that the pelvic floor is one unit, traversed by the urinary, genital and intestinal tract (Meier, 1977). Maybe those subjects who have both constipation and urinary tract disorders are those where the motor function of pelvic floor is not normal.

Obese subjects tend to be more often constipated (Figure 11) (Percora, 1981). Whether this is modulated via a motor disorder of the upper part of the gastrointestinal tract is not known.

Stercoral perforation of the colon may complicate prolonged storage of hard faeces in the same bowel segment but it is a rare complication (Gekas and Schuster, 1981). However, four controlled studies have determined that constipated subjects are at risk for large bowel cancer (Devroede, 1988; Vobecky et al, 1983).

Constipated patients are at high risk of unnecessary surgery. Few of them present with acute abdominal pain, but a history of long-standing constipation in a patient presenting to the emergency room with such a complaint should caution against surgery. Similarly, chronic pain exposes to unnecessary surgery, often of exploratory nature. This is particularly evident in those with slow

Total gastrointestinal transit time

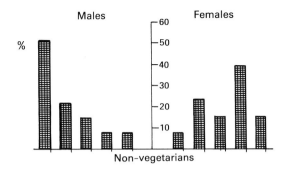

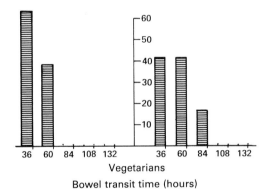

Figure 4. The transit time from mouth to anus is faster among vegetarians as compared to non-vegetarians. Several variables may be at work because life-styles may be different. However, the sex difference remains identical in both groups, females having a slower transit (Gear et al, 1981).

transit constipation, who are all women, and have, as compared to controls, an increased incidence of ovarian cystectomy and hysterectomy (Preston and Lennard-Jones, 1986) (Figure 12). Similarly women with megarectum who are not constipated from birth but somewhat later in life also often undergo hysterectomy but the specimen is normal (Verduron, 1988).

The Mechanisms of Constipation

It is possible to learn about the mechanisms of constipation by examining the pathophysiological derangements that are present in patients with specific diseases and injuries. Unfortunately such studies are scarce.

Constipation Secondary to Disease

Normally, meals increase the motor activity of the sigmoid colon (Figure 13) (Frexinos et al, 1985; Schang et al, 1986). This does not occur in diabetic patients who complain of severe constipation, presumably because of autonomic neuropathy (Battle et al, 1980). Diabetic patients with mild constipation have a delayed postprandial increase in colonic motility, but those with severe constipation have no response.

That the integrity of the nervous system is important for normal defecation and for the increase in motor activity of the sigmoid colon after a meal is also shown in studies performed on patients with traumatic transection of the spinal cord above the level of the first lumbar vertebra (Glick et al, 1984). There is no colonic response to a meal (Figure 14), but the response to Prostigmin indicates that the muscle itself is normal (Figure 15). The tone of the large bowel is also increased: colonic compliance and tolerance to fluid filling is markedly reduced (Figure 16) (Glick et al, 1984). The reverse occurs in patients with lower lesions of the spinal cord and destruction of the cauda equina. Pressure volume curves within the colon are flat during filling and the compliance is markedly enhanced (White et al, 1940; Scott and Cantrell, 1949).

The parasympathetic innervation is essential for normal function; resection of the nervi erigentes leads to obstipation, loss of rectal sensation and delayed transit through the large bowel. Bypass of the hindgut leads to resumption of transit suggesting that sacral parasympathetic outflow exerts no influence on the ascending colon (Devroede and Lamarche, 1974). Patients who sustain trauma to the cauda equina, even in the absence of paraplegia, may become constipated (Devroede et al, 1979). The recto-anal inhibitory reflex persists after trauma of this nature (Gunterberg et al, 1976; Devroede et al, 1979); but its amplitude is maximal for minimal levels of rectal distension, and the normal relationship (Martelli et al, 1978) between an increasing relaxation of the internal sphincter and an increasing distension of the rectum disappears. Coexistent with this, the rectoanal contractile reflex of the external anal sphincter is much

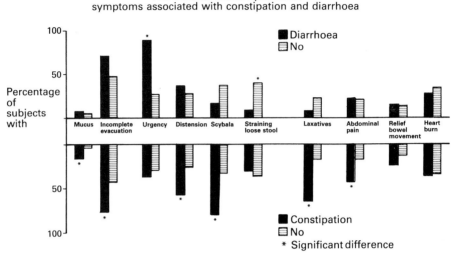

Figure 5. In patients with irritable bowel syndrome and constipation, there are many associated symptoms, including abdominal pain, but this is not so in those with diarrhoea (Thompson and Heaton, 1980).

weaker than normal. This combination is of course conducive to faecal incontinence if laxatives or enemas are used to overcome constipation. Rectal sensation is also lost and rectal capacity to distension increased after bilateral but not unilateral sacrifice of sacral nerves (Gunterberg et al, 1976). The loss of rectal sensation may be neurogenic, through damage to the afferent nerves, but conceivably could simply be due to the loss of rectal muscle tone.

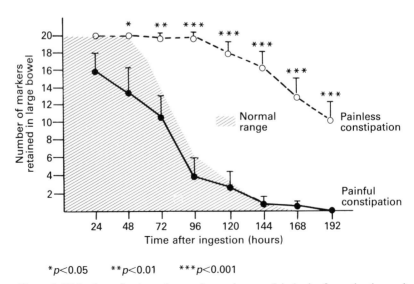

*p<0.05   **p<0.01   ***p<0.001

Figure 6. Eight days after ingestion, patients who complain both of constipation and abdominal pain have fewer markers retained in their large bowel than those who do not have pain (Lanfranchi et al, 1984).

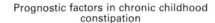

Figure 7. Patients with painless constipation have a greater motor derangement of the large bowel than those who complain of abdominal pain (Lanfranchi et al, 1984).

Segmental Constipation

On the basis of radio-opaque marker studies (Martelli et al, 1978; Arhan et al, 1981), patients with constipation may be divided into three different groups (Schang, 1985) (Figure 17). The first group has delayed transit in the colon (Watier et al, 1983; Martelli et al, 1978b). There are relatively few such subjects. The second group has normal transit but has abnormally long storage of stools in the rectum (Verduron et al, 1988; Martelli et al, 1978b). In the third, transit time of the radio-opaque markers is normal (Schang, 1985). This is important to recognize: it occurs in one-third of patients (Wald, 1986). Such subjects should not be dismissed as 'not constipated'.

Colonic Constipation

In patients with colonic inertia (Watier et al, 1983), markers stagnate along the entire large intestine because the bowel musculature is ineffective. However, delayed transit in the

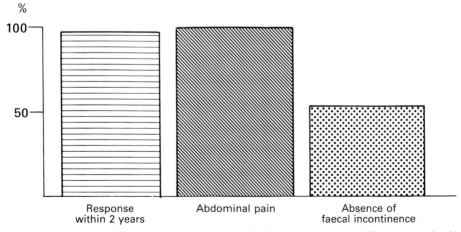

Figure 8. Constipated children with abdominal pain will all eventually be cured. The response should be expected in a reasonably short period of time. In contrast, it is more difficult to help constipated children who are also faecally incontinent: faecal incontinence is present in 53% of children who will be cured from their constipation, while it is present in 89% of those who will not (Abrahamian and Lloyd-Still, 1984).

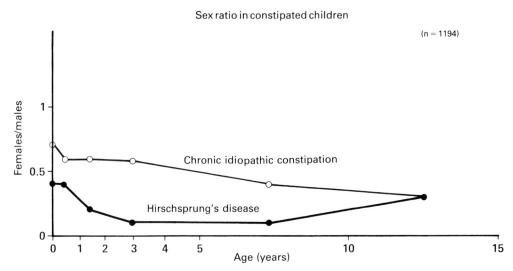

Figure 9. These 1194 constipated underwent anorectal manometry because of chronic idiopathic consti-pation. More little boys are present in the sample, not only among those diagnosed as suffering from Hirschsprung's disease but also in the group labelled as having chronic idiopathic constipation.

ascending colon may also be due to a distal obstacle which counteracts an effective colonic muscu-lature in the ascending colon (Likongo et al, 1986). The term constipation by delayed colonic transit has been proposed for this situation, where markers can be seen to move back and forth from right to left colon, and do not progress in an expon-ential fashion. Patients with normal size large bowel have also been labelled to suffer from slow transit constipation (Preston and Lennard-Jones, 1986): when markers are retained in the colo-rectum.

Slow transit constipation and colonic inertia are found almost exclusively in women. This is

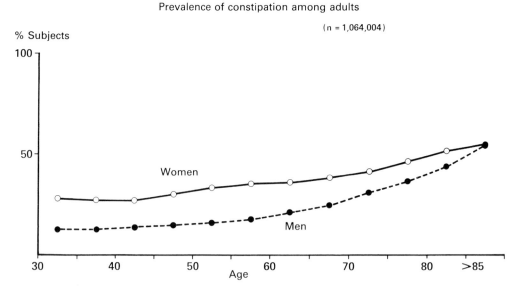

Figure 10. In contrast to what is shown in Figure 9, more adult women complain of constipation than men. In this sample over one million people, constipation was what the subjects labelled as such. Of note, sex differences are abolished with advancing age (Hammond, 1964).

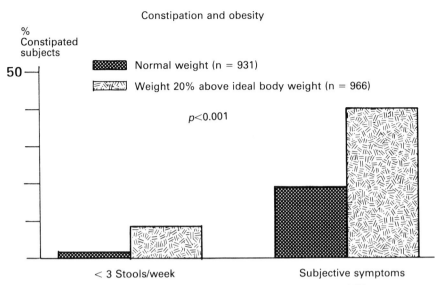

Figure 11. Obese subjects are often constipated (Percova, 1981).

important, since they have other complaints exclusive to the female sex (Figure 18).

Colonic motility, as measured with miniature balloons, does not differ in patients with slow transit constipation and controls, but bisacodyl does not induce peristaltic waves (Preston and Lennard-Jones, 1985) (Figure 19). In some constipated subjects, motor activity of the sigmoid colon after a meal increases to an abnormal degree, suggesting spasticity. In other constipated

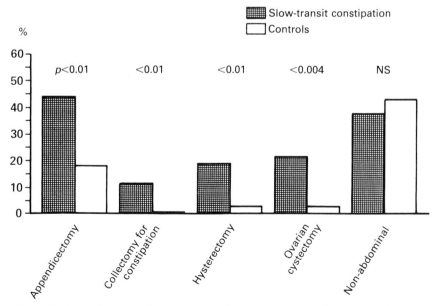

Figure 12. Appendicectomy, hysterectomy and oophorectomy are often performed in constipated women who have a normal-sized large bowel and delayed transit, and more so than in controls who are not constipated (Preston and Lennard-Jones, 1986).

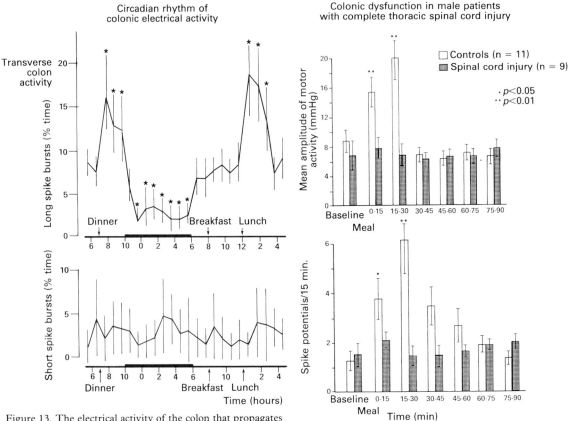

Figure 13. The electrical activity of the colon that propagates along a long segment varies according to a circadian rhythm (Frexinos et al, 1985). At night, the bowel goes at rest. Conversely, substantial meals increase the amount of electrical activity, and the increase in pressure which is its counterpart has been demonstrated by other authors (Schang et al, 1986). This study does not show any effect of breakfast, but it was performed in France, where bacon and eggs are not standard at that time. Carbohydrates do not trigger a postprandial colic response.

Figure 14. In male patients with complete thoracic spinal cord injury, the ingestion of a meal does not increase the number of spike potentials in the large bowel. The intraluminal pressure, accordingly, does not change either (Glick et al, 1984).

patients, it is the reverse, and hypomotility is observed postprandially. This suggests the existence of three families of constipated subjects (Figure 20) (Meunier et al 1979). Myoelectric spiking activity can be recorded in the descending and sigmoid colon. As compared to both control subjects and constipated patients with outlet obstruction, the number of propagating potentials is significantly decreased in fasting conditions and does not increase after a meal (Schang, 1985) (Figure 21). Similarly, no postprandial increase in long spike bursts occurs in patients with the irritable bowel syndrome who have fewer than

three stools per week (Figure 22) (Dapoigny et al, 1985).

Dysphagia and gastro-oesophageal reflux are associated with hypertonicity of the pharyngo-oesophageal sphincter and a weak gastro-oesophageal sphincter in patients with colonic inertia. There is also a high incidence of simultaneous contractions of the oesophagus (tertiary contractions) together with a hypersensitivity of the bladder to urecholine (Watier et al, 1983). There is a high incidence of urinary problems in patients with slow transit constipation (Preston and Lennard-Jones, 1986). Finally, there is a high incidence of galactorrhoea and of orthostatic hypotension in these two groups of constipated women (Watier et al, 1983). This points to a systemic disease or disorder.

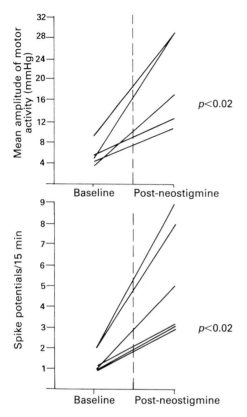

Figure 15. In contrast to what is seen in Figure 14, neostigmine evokes a normal response of the large bowel in male patients with complete thoracic spinal cord injury. Thus, the muscle itself is normal and the lack of response to a meal means that the response is modulated by extrinsic innervation (Glick et al, 1984).

Outlet Obstruction

In constipated patients with outlet obstruction, the rectum serves as an elective site of storage (Figure 17) and there is an increased number of retrograde, orally moving propagating electrical potentials (Figure 23) (Schang et al, 1985).

Several mechanisms are possible for outlet obstruction.

A zone of complex wave activity has been described in the rectosigmoid area of severely constipated subjects, but it is also found in patients with diarrhoea (Figure 24) (Dinoso et al, 1983).

The association of megarectum and constipation has long been known. In these patients, the rectal wall is very inelastic, and thus the rectum can accommodate large volumes of material, faeces, or fluid within a balloon (Figure 25), particularly when constipation begins at birth (Verduron et al, 1988). In the latter condition, colonic motility is more normal so that stasis is essentially in the rectosigmoid area: thus this is one of the mechanisms of outlet obstruction (Figure 26). Faecal incontinence is more common among males (Figure 27) and those patients who have a huge rectal capacity (Figure 28). Although impaired rectal sensation has been reported in these patients (Meunier et al, 1976), and related to the incidence of incontinence (Figure 29) (Meunier et al, 1979a), the level of pressure at which it occurs is the same regardless of rectal volume, and this suggests that there is no impaired sensation but inelasticity of the musculature: a greater stretch is needed before sufficient tension occurs and sensation begins (Verduron et al, 1988). The rectoanal inhibitory reflex is impaired, since it is triggered by rectal stretch and accommodation (Arhan et al, 1979). Amplitude is less than normal and the reflex may even be absent: this should not lead to a diagnosis of Hirschsprung's disease. Elderly patients also seem to have decreased rectal elasticity, when they are found to have faecal impaction, and thus they are likely to have a megarectum (Figure 30) (Read et al, 1985).

Resting pressure in the anal canal of patients with chronic idiopathic constipation has been found to be increased, normal, or decreased. These differences probably reflect differences in patient selection. For instance, the mere association of pain with constipation is accompanied by marked differences in pathophysiology (Lafranchi et al, 1984). In painful constipation, colonic transit time is faster (Figures 6 and 7), the rectum is more elastic and thus its capacity is decreased (Figure 31), the anus has greater tonicity (Figure 32) and the amplitude of the recto-anal inhibitory reflex is greater (Figure 33). Unstable pressure is another abnormality that has been recognized (Martelli et al, 1978b; Ducrotte et al, 1985). These ultra slow waves may or may not be associated to a higher than normal level of pressure.

When the rectum is briefly distended, the

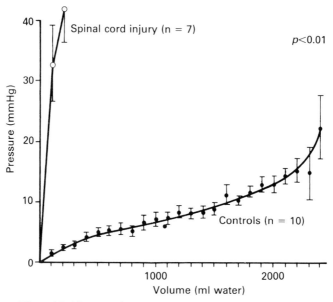

Figure 16. After complete transection of the thoracic spinal cord, the colorectal compliance is severely reduced (Glick et al, 1984).

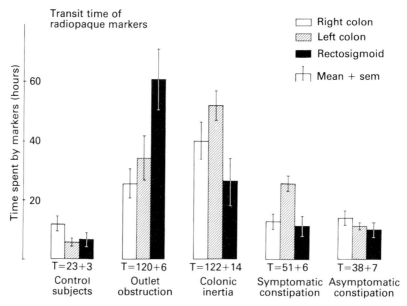

Figure 17. Constipated patients, where no known organic aetiology can be recognized, may be divided into three different groups according to transit times of radio-opaque markers. In outlet obstruction, stasis is distal. In colonic inertia, it is proximal in the colon. Patients with 'normal' transit may (symptomatic) or may not (asymptomatic) still complain of constipation, even when reassured about the innocuity of their condition (Schang, 1985).

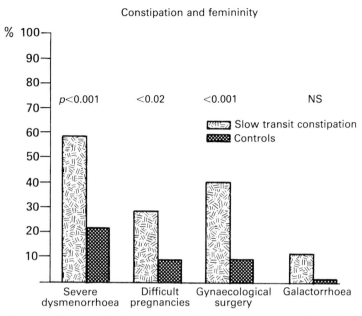

Figure 18. Women with slow transit constipation have other complaints related to the fact of being female (Preston and Lennard-Jones, 1986).

internal anal sphincter normally relaxes. In constipation, the recto-anal inhibitory reflex may be present and normal, absent, or present but abnormal (Martelli et al, 1978a; Ducrotte et al, 1985). Its absence is a hallmark of Hirschsprung's disease (Schuster et al, 1968; Faverdin et al, 1981) but a differential diagnosis still remains to be done since it may be absent in patients with megarectum (Barnes et al, 1986; Verduron et al, 1988), chronic rectal ischaemia and systemic sclerosis (Devroede et al, 1982), and may disappear after low anterior resection or anorectal myectomy. Faecal impaction also creates a technical artefact (Devroede et al, 1985).

Rectosphincteric dyssynergia (Meunier, 1985) is a recently identified mechanism of outlet obstruction, and also labelled as 'anismus' (Preston and Lennard-Jones, 1985), 'spastic pelvic floor' syndrome (Kuijpers and Bleijenberg, 1985) or 'sphincteric disobedience' syndrome (Hero et al, 1985). Normally during defecation, the pelvic floor, which at rest is in a state of constant activity and contraction, relaxes completely (Parks et al, 1962; Fry et al, 1966; Rutter, 1974). Some constipated patients, in contrast, contract the external

anal sphincter during straining in an effort to defecate. Records of electromyographic activity may show a transient increase in activity at the onset and end of straining, or a highly increased level of activity during the entire duration of the act of defecation (Figure 34) (Preston and Lennard-Jones, 1985b). A few subjects exhibit bursts of repetitive tetanic-like grouped action potentials succeeding each other in a fast (8/sec) rhythm, and completely different to those recorded during voluntary contraction of the perianal musculature (Kerremans, 1969). The term anismus is quite appropriate because of its analogy with vaginismus, where a spasm of the pelvic floor muscles also occurs, the difference of course being that vaginismus is resistance to penetration and anismus to expulsion. Vesico-urethral dyssynergia is probably part of the full syndrome and conducive to bladder retention and infection: patients contract the external urethral sphincter when they try to void. Chronic pelvic tensions have been said to result from psychological conflicts during childhood and lead to urinary control problems and orgasmic responses (Lowen, 1967; Reich, 1943), and indeed the contractile strength of the

Rectosigmoid pressure in constipation

Normal transit constipation

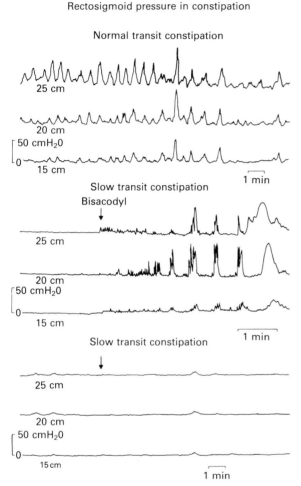

Figure 19. Bisacodyl, in some women with slow transit constipation, does not modify colonic motility (Preston and Lennard-Jones, 1985).

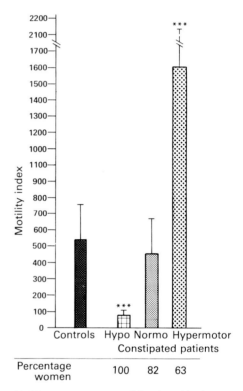

Figure 20. The motor response of the sigmoid colon to a meal makes it possible to distinguish different types of constipation (Meuniêr et al, 1979).

pelvic floor muscles is related to both urinary control and orgasmic response (Meier, 1977). The relationship between rectosphincteric dyssynergia and large bowel transit time is not clear, because not all patients are constipated (Kuijpers et al, 1986; Kuijpers and Bleijenberg, 1985).

In some constipated patients, the perineum descends during straining and the level of descent can be measured by defecography (Bartolo et al, 1985). Anismus may be associated with this (Rutter, 1974; Kuijpers et al, 1986), but in about one-half of the patients, prolonged inhibition of the pelvic floor muscles occurs on defecation straining (Bartolo et al, 1985; Rutter, 1974). Mean

motor unit potential duration may be prolonged in the puborectalis and external anal sphincter muscles of patients and this indicates neuropathic changes (Bartolo et al, 1985). The descending perineum syndrome is possibly the long-term consequence of anismus, but this has not been studied longitudinally to discover the natural history of anismus and the descending perineum syndrome, and their respective contribution to the development of constipation. Similarly megarectum possibly results from rectosphincteric dyssynergia but this remains unproven.

In patients with severe intractable obstructed defecation, defecography may demonstrate occlusion of the anal canal and variants of recto-

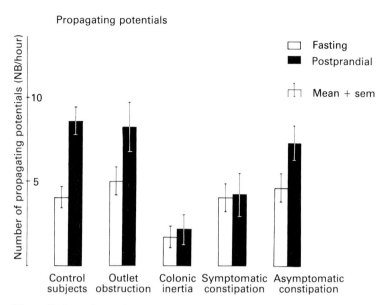

Figure 21. In patients with colonic inertia (defined as having a delayed transit of radio-opaque markers in the ascending colon), there is little propagating electrical activity in the colon, and no response to a meal. Compare to Figure 17: in the other groups of subjects with chronic idiopathic constipation, there is no marked difference from controls (Schang, 1985).

rectal intussusception, which are appealing as an explanation for the symptomatology (Bartolo et al, 1985). It is difficult to diagnose an internal rectal prolapse at endoscopy and defecography: often there is a subtle progression from simple closure of the rectal lumen, to descent of the anterior rectal mucosa, to true rectal prolapse to the level of the dentate line. Moreover, not enough studies have been performed in healthy subjects to formally incriminate these radiological findings in the genesis of constipation.

Constipation with Normal Transit Times

A large proportion of constipated patients have normal transit time of radio-opaque markers (Verduron et al, 1988; Kuijpers et al, 1986; Schang, 1984; Wald, 1986). They often take psychotropic agents, particularly antidepressants, receive psychiatric counselling or are involved in medical or non-medical litigation (Wald, 1986). Colonic motor activity in these patients may be excessive (Preston and Lennard-Jones, 1985b), and there is an increase in the number of rhythmical and stationary potentials, particularly after meals (Schang, 1984).

Some of these patients clearly deny that they defecate: markers are disappearing from plain films of the abdomen, while they fail to report any stool (Lennard-Jones, 1985; Hinton and Lennard-Jones, 1968). There is no way to recognize this unless marker studies are performed. Follow-up studies show that almost all patients with outlet obstruction improve clinically during follow-up, two-thirds improve when transit is normal and only 25% when there is delayed transit in the ascending colon (Wald, 1986). An appealing hypothesis, in view of the psychosocial disturbances in patients with normal transit, would then be that the more distal the mechanism of constipation, the more mentalized the patient (Devroede, 1985; Bonfils et al, 1982): emotional conflicts are more amenable to resolution than constipation. An exception to this hypothesis would be the patient who denies any bowel movement and defecates markers.

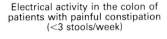

Electrical activity in the colon of
patients with painful constipation
(<3 stools/week)

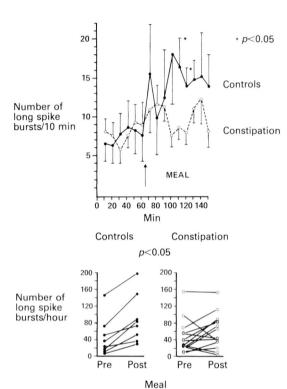

Figure 22. This figure provides the same information as Figure 21. However, in the previous figure, patients were selected on the basis of radio-opaque markers studies, while in this, they were diagnosed as suffering from the irritable bowel syndrome, with a second selection criterion of having less than three stools per week (Dapoigny et al, 1985).

Can Chronic Idiopathic Constipation be Ascribed to a Single Pathophysiological Mechanism?

It is highly unlikely that a single mechanism is responsible for chronic idiopathic constipation, and at least one motor abnormality is found in almost all patients (Meunier et al, 1979b; Shouler and Keighley, 1986) (Figure 35). Common abnormal mechanisms are found in apparently very different groups of constipated patients. For instance, patients have difficulties in expelling rectal balloons whether they have slow transit constipation, normal transit constipation, or megarectum (Barnes and Lennard-Jones, 1985).

Psychological Relationships

The relationship between emotions, the psyche, and bowel habits is very poorly known. The personality profile of healthy subjects correlates to stool weight and frequency (Tucker et al, 1981). Individuals who display a greater degree of self-esteem and who are more outgoing tend to produce more frequent and heavier stools. Megacolon may be found in psychotic patients (Ehrentheil and Wells, 1955), and a close relationship exists between levels of anxiety and transit time in the ascending colon, in patients where constipation is caused by delayed colonic transit (Figure 36) (Devroede et al, 1988). This is a rich field for research.

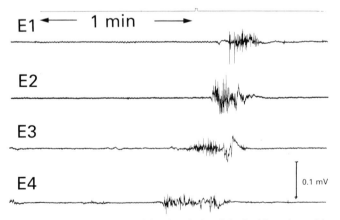

Figure 23. The propagation of the electrical activity in this patient with outlet obstruction is in a retrograde fashion: electrode E1 is proximal in the colon to electrode E4 (Schang et al, 1985).

Motility of the rectosigmoid junction

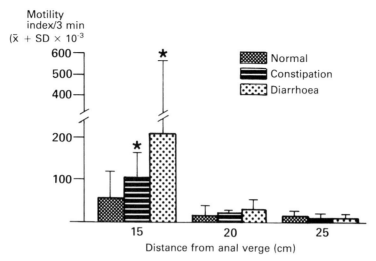

Figure 24. There is a hyperactive rectosigmoid segment both in patients with constipation and in those with diarrhoea. Dinoso et al, 1983.

Maximum tolerable volume in megarectum

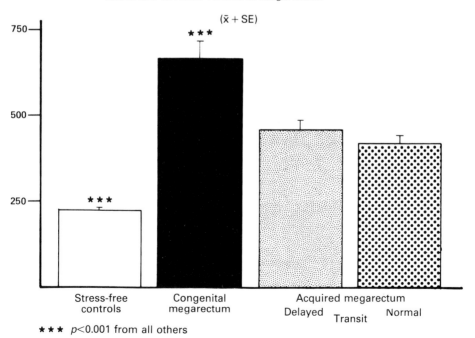

★★★ p<0.001 from all others

Figure 25. Patients with megarectum have an abnormally large rectal capacity. There are three groups of such patients: those with onset of the constipation at birth (congenital megarectum) and those with a late onset of constipation; the latter group is compared to two subgroups according to the 'normality' of colorectal transit times (Verduron et al, 1988).

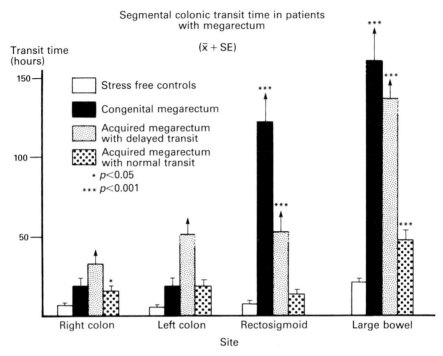

Figure 26. In patients with megarectum who were constipated at birth, colonic transit is near normal and thus there is outlet obstruction (Verduron et al, 1988).

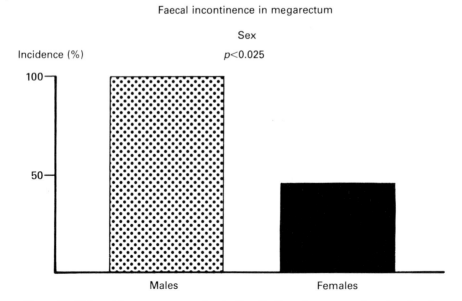

Figure 27. Males with megarectum tend to be faecally incontinent more often than females (Verduron et al, 1988).

Faecal incontinence in megarectum
maximum tolerable volume in the rectum

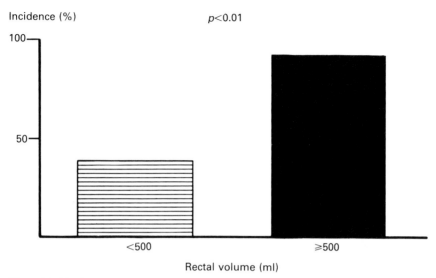

Figure 28. The larger the rectal capacity, the greater the risk of faecal incontinence (Verduron et al, 1988).

Faecal incontinence in chronically constipated
(<3 stools/week) children
(% subjects with abnormality)

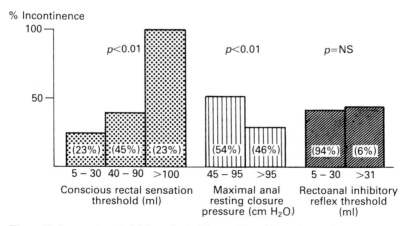

Figure 29. In constipated children, the incidence of faecal incontinence increases when rectal sensation is impaired. To some extent, this is counteracted if the anal canal is hypertonic (Meunier et al, 1979a).

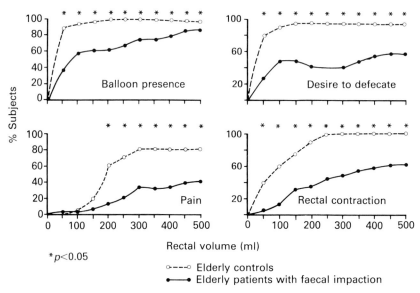

Figure 30. Elderly patients with faecal impaction have a relative rectal anaesthesia, and do not feel normally balloon distension of the rectum. This triggers little pain and the rectal wall does not contract normally on the balloon (Read et al, 1985).

The Approach to a Constipated Patient

The evaluation of constipated patients follows from the understanding of the mechanisms and the knowledge of various aetiologies. It should be a three-stage process.

Organic Evaluation

The morphological evaluation is essentially a search for an organic cause.

The key question to ask at the first visit is about the onset of constipation. Most patients who have a congenital cause of constipation, such as Hirschsprung's disease or meningocele, have had difficulties with their bowel habits from birth. When constipation occurs later in life, the presenting symptom may be of chronic or recent origin. Constipation of recent onset is frequently suggestive of significant pathology. The disease

that is most important to diagnose in this situation is, of course, colonic malignancy.

A meticulous clinical evaluation of the patient will then help to sort out its causes.

Endoscopy is one of the most useful techniques in the investigation of constipation. A search for lesions is of course important but local anorectal reflexes can also be appreciated.

Cutaneous sensations around the anus and cutaneous sphincteric contractile reflexes may be absent in patients with neurogenic disorders; this may indicate the level and side of the abnormality. A reliable sign of disordered innervation of the anus is the gaping of the canal when the puborectalis muscle is grasped by the examining finger and pulled posteriorly. In some patients, anal tone is normal but does not resist traction. In some others, a return to the resting position is very slow. Medullary dysfunction is present if these abnormalities are demonstrated. In cervical transection, the anus remains closed and a balloon can

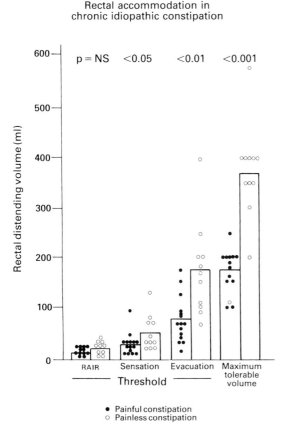

Rectal accommodation in
chronic idiopathic constipation

Figure 31. In patients with painful constipation, the rectum is more sensitive and less stretchable (Lanfranchi et al, 1984).

be retained in the rectum, whereas in low, flaccid lesions of the medulla, the anus is patulous and unable to contract to prevent extrusion of the balloon (Connell, 1963). Finally, in Hirschsprung's disease, after rectal examination a profuse faecal discharge occurs. Recto-anal dyssynergia may be recognized during the rectal examination by simply asking the patient to strain while maintaining the finger in the rectum: patients with anismus will squeeze, instead of relaxing as is normal. Descent of the perineum will also be recognized during this examination step. It is often associated with the presence of a rectocele: curbing the finger through the anterior rectal wall makes it appear in the vagina, on the other side of the perineal body. Posteriorly, pain can be triggered by pulling the levator ani. This

has been labelled the puborectalis syndrome (Wasserman, 1964) and is akin to anismus.

Endoscopy is usually performed with flexible instruments, but the rigid instrument is superior to demonstrate the presence of internal rectal prolapse and anterior mucosal prolapse. In melanosis coli, the colorectal mucosa has a brown-black spotty coloration because of deposits of lipofuscin, both free and in macrophages in the lamina propria. This is indicative of laxative abuse, particularly those of the anthraquinone family. The distal rectum may be spared by the melanosis; this suggests that the colon functions normally to the junction between melanotic and amelanotic bowel and that the abnormality lies in the distal bowel, free from melanosis.

In constipation of recent origin, a barium enema is mandatory in order to determine whether obstruction due to organic narrowing, particularly carcinoma, underlies the change in bowel habit. In chronic constipation, the size of the distal bowel is greater than normal, but on a single examination the radiologist is unable to distinguish constipated from non-constipated patients, and the change in bowel size after treatment does not correlate well with its outcome (Patriquin et al, 1978). The lack of value of barium enema to evaluate chronic idiopathic constipation is confirmed by another study which demonstrates that there is no correlation between rectal size as determined radiologically and rectal elastic properties, as determined by manometric studies (Meunier et al, 1984). Nevertheless, a useful measure to remember is 6.5 cm, as upper limit of rectosigmoid width on lateral view at the pelvic brim (Preston et al, 1985). This can be used to recognize quickly the presence of megarectum. In patients with long-segment Hirschsprung's disease, a narrow rectum can be demonstrated at barium enema, and in children with this problem it is thus not necessary to complete the investigation to the caecum. However, barium enema is useless in short-segment Hirschsprung's disease, because there is no narrow segment.

In the infant, the absence of neurons in a rectal suction biopsy specimen, taken at least 25 mm above the distal edge of the internal sphincter is suggestive of Hirschsprung's disease. Rectal

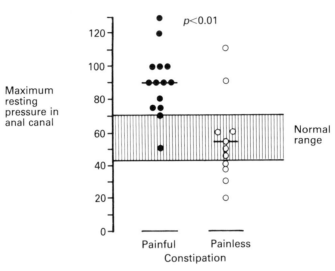

Figure 32. The pressure in the anal canal is greater in patients who have constipation and pain than in those who are pain-free (Lanfranchi et al, 1984).

Functional Evaluation

Studies of Colonic Transit Times

The major step in the evaluation of patients with chronic idiopathic constipation is to measure colonic transit times of radio-opaque markers. To distinguish between different types of constipation the progression of these markers along the colon should be followed by taking successive films of the abdomen (Martelli et al, 1978a; Arhan et al, 1981; Hinton et al, 1969). Markers are counted in the right and left colon and the rectosigmoid area by using bony landmarks. Segmental transit time is probably the most practical measure to obtain. A simplified formula can be obtained if the patient swallows   markers and a film is taken every 24 hours. Markers are counted in each site each day until disappearance: these numbers are added and the sum multiplied by 1.2 (Arhan et al, 1981).

biopsies should not be used to evaluate adult patients who complain of long-standing idiopathic constipation.

Normal published values have been used as standard (Wald, 1986), but this practice is dangerous when evaluating subjects complaining of minor constipation. The transit times of controls whose bowels are not influenced by stress are shorter; the longest transit time through the large bowel is only 34 hours (instead of 93), and segmental transit times in the ascending, descending colon and rectosigmoid are a maximum of 18, 13 and 20 hours respectively instead of 38, 37 and 34 (Verduron et al, 1988). More studies on normality are needed.

Colorectal Motility Studies

There are many technical difficulties in studying colorectal motility. Pressure studies have little value in clinical practice and are still used exclusively in research situations. Recording the electrical activity of the intestinal smooth muscle begins to be both interesting, because spike bursts are the electrical counterpart of smooth muscle contraction, and useful. Intraluminal tubes can be

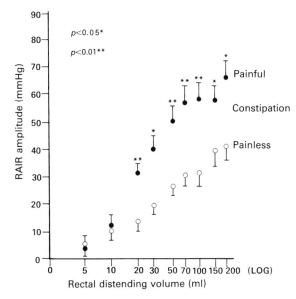

Rectoanal inhibitory reflex
in chronic idiopathic constipation

Figure 33. As in health (Martelli et al, 1978a), the amplitude of the recto-anal inhibitory reflex increases with increasing rectal distension in patients with chronic idiopathic constipation. The slope of this relationship differs, however, if patients have pain, where it is steeper than when they have no pain (Lanfranchi et al, 1984).

equipped with ring electrodes that can pick up the signals by simple contact with the bowel wall (Schang and Devroede, 1984; Fioramonti et al, 1980; Fleckenstein, 1978) and introduced by flexible colonoscopy in the left colon. The colonic myoelectric spike bursts consist basically of two types. The first type, 'rhythmic and stationary bursts', are of short duration and generally occur in sequences lasting for several minutes. These bursts have been described as 'short spike bursts' (Bueno et al, 1980) or as 'discrete electrical response activity' (Sarna et al, 1982). They seem to represent a rather localized activity, although it is not known whether these bursts may propagate over very short distances. In healthy subjects, they occur at a rhythm of 11–80 per hour, but may go beyond 100 in constipated patients who complain of pain. The second type, the 'sporadic bursts', consists of bursts with more variable duration, ranging from 5 to 120 sec. These bursts have been described as 'long spike bursts' (Bueno et al, 1980)

and also as 'continuous electrical response activity' (Sarna et al, 1982). These sporadic spike bursts can in turn be divided into two subgroups: some of the bursts show evidence of propagation as they can be observed to move from one recording site to another over long distances (Schang and Devroede, 1984) or even over the whole length of the colon (Bueno et al, 1980); the others do not seem to propagate so far since they are seen at only one or two electrode sites located a few centimetres apart (Figure 37).

Anorectal Pressure Studies

There are three kinds of anorectal pressure studies and these are complementary.

A pressure profile from rectum to anal margin can be recorded by withdrawing an open-tipped recording catheter, but this type of measurement has little practical diagnostic value.

The most commonly performed type of anorectal manometry investigates resting tones in the anal canal and recto-anal reflexes. Several probes are available for this purpose (Figure 38). Essential differences are the use of balloons or of water perfusion systems. It must be remembered that measurements in a sphincter do not reflect pressure but resistance to distension. Balloons have the advantage that the deformation is standardized, particularly when water is used instead of air. Each laboratory should have its own controls if it does not use a standard published balloon size, because the bigger the balloon, the higher the pressure. Water perfusion systems are probably less reliable. Pressure is measured in fact in a dynamic cavity: water accumulates into the sphincteric area and creates a space, until it leaks into the rectum and at the anal margin. It is the pressure within this space which is recorded. It is easy to conceive that anal leakage of fluid will, consciously or unconsciously, trigger reflex activity of the external anal sphincter and puborectalis muscles. Thus, if both a balloon system and a perfused system are used in the same individual, on occasion, the recto-anal inhibitory reflex—so essential to detect in pathological states—may be found only with the balloon system.

Visco-elastic properties of the rectum differ in

Anismus

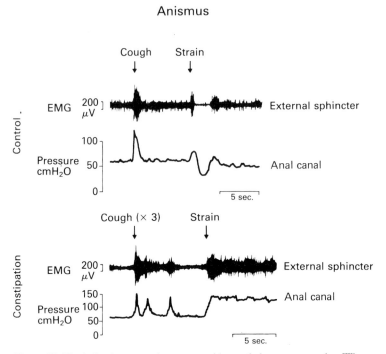

Figure 34. Typical anismus, as demonstrated by anal electromyography. When the constipated patient (bottom) strains, electromyographic recordings increase and so does anal canal pressure (Preston and Lennard-Jones, 1985b).

health and disease (Ahran et al, 1976, 1978; Colin et al, 1979; Farthing and Lennard-Jones, 1978; Ihre, 1974) and should be studied to distinguish outlet obstruction induced by a hypo- or hypertonic rectum from simple anal achalasia. These types of studies (Figure 39), investigating the accommodation properties of the rectum to rapid (with air) and slow (with water) distension, complement the simple study of anal tone and rectoanal reflexes. Viscous properties reflect accommodation of the rectum to distension, and elastic properties the residual tension after accommodation.

Dynamic Evaluation of Defecation

Balloon defecation is a new method to investigate the recto-anal dynamics during defecation. Impairment of expulsion has to be correlated to the mechanisms of constipation (Barnes and Lennard-Jones, 1985; Loening-Baucke and Cruikshank, 1986).

The balloon proctogram permits the evaluation

of the anorectal angle and its relationship with the pubococcygeal level (Preston et al, 1984; Lahr et al, 1986).

Defecography is another way to investigate anorectal morphology and dynamics during defecation. The most popular technique is easy to use and reliable because the barium paste which is used mimics stool consistency (Mahieu et al, 1984a, 1984b).

Third Level of Investigation: the Colon is within a Person

Most physicians are accustomed to a scientific clinical practice. They are not familiar with the notion that the unconscious representation of the body is not anatomical but imaginary. Constipation is not only the passage of hard and infrequent stools via different investigable mechanisms, but what this does to the patient, who relates a symptom, and not a sign. Forgetting this essential subjective element is bound to lead to a therapeutic failure. With some humour one could

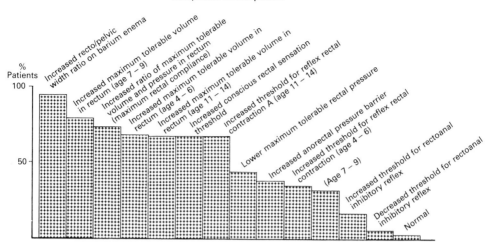

Figure 35. If extensive functional evaluation is made of patients with chronic idiopathic constipation, only a negligible proportion of them is found to be 'normal' (Meunier et al, 1984).

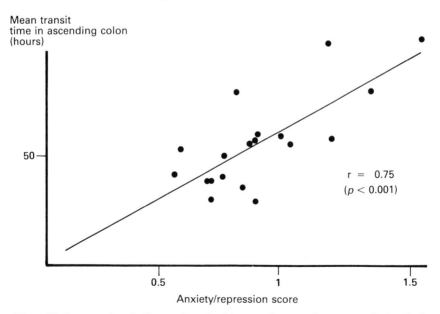

Figure 36. In some chronically constipated subjects anxiety correlates to transit time in the ascending colon. The scores of anxiety and repression were measured with the Minnesota Multiphasic Personality Inventory (Devroede et al, 1988).

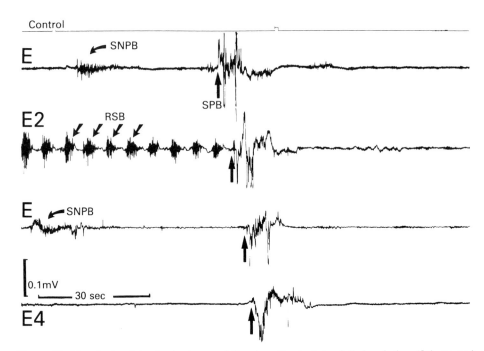

Figure 37. Electrical activity in the human left colon. See text for full description (Schang and Devroede, 1984).

say that constipated patients may constipate physicians. The anxiety of being rendered 'impotent' is probably the cause of unnecessary surgery and of breaks in the therapeutic relationship.

Functional disorders are not synonymous with absence of disorders. Too often, the patient leaves the clinician with a high level of frustration, after having been told there was nothing wrong with him/her. Making a positive diagnosis that there *is* something wrong, and relating the findings of the functional evaluation of constipation serves an important purpose to establish a therapeutic alliance with the patient. When trust is present, it becomes easier to relate the message that the basis for the functional abnormality is not necessarily organic.

An interview reviewing in depth the life experience of the patient may be used to explore the subjective elements of constipation. This may trigger marked emotional responses, which the physician must be ready to handle. Working on self becomes essential for physicians interested not only in taking care of the patient but caring for them. A simpler approach is to use the Minnesota Multiphasic Personality Inventory and relating to the patient the findings and the profile interpretation usually provided by it. Some patients resent even the idea of having a psychological problem and caution must be exerted in this regard for fear of seeing the patient go shopping for another doctor (Wald, 1986).

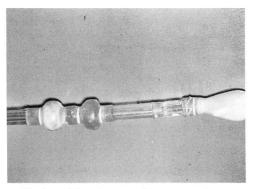

Figure 38. A useful probe to perform anorectal manometry (Martelli et al, 1978a).

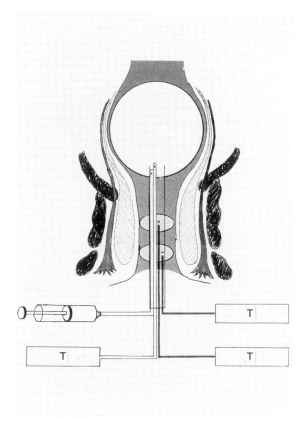

Figure 39. To study rectal accommodation, a balloon is distended in the rectum while the intraballoon pressure is recorded. This is done *in vivo* and *in vitro*. The *in vitro* values are subtracted from the *in vivo* values to provide true rectal wall contribution to pressure. Pressure can be converted to tension by using Laplace's law and the elasticity coefficient calculated as the angle of the slope expressing the relationship between rectal wall tension and rectal balloon radius. Pressure can also be recorded in the upper anal canal (mainly internal anal sphincter) and lower anal canal (mainly external anal sphincter), to evaluate the rectoanal inhibitory and contractile reflex (Ahran et al, 1976).

Treatment

The only word that applies to the treatment of chronic idiopathic constipation is 'controversy'.

The non-specificity of all therapeutic approaches to constipation is exemplified in a report describing the effects of staying in a spa station on colonic transit time: immediately after the stay in the resort, transit is accelerated, but the effect is short-lived. Of course drinking water is not the only variable and leading a peaceful life is probably just as important (Figure 40) (Nisard et al, 1982). Studies of the treatment of constipation are never randomized, because there is no gold standard. Caution is in order and the old dictum 'primum est non nocere' is a useful guideline.

Ideally, treatment of constipation should be curative. Palliation, for instance with laxatives, is not of this nature; yet this is what we have to accept when no definitive treatment is effective. It must be remembered that, even if the patient remains clinically improved, functional disorders may persist over long periods of time (Figure 41) (Loening-Baucke, 1984; Denis et al, 1981).

Management begins when the patient walks into the consultation room for the first time. Many have cool clammy hands, a clear sign of anxiety. A lot of attention must be directed to non-verbal communication. Transference and counter-transference are there and should come eventually to consciousness.

If a specific cause of constipation is found, it should be dealt with. If a diagnosis of chronic idiopathic constipation is made, the least harmful approaches to treatment are dietary manipulations, biofeedback exercises and psychotherapy.

Dietary Trial

Dietary fibre increases stool output and a high-fibre trial should be performed in all patients with constipation of unknown origin.

Most subjects who complain of constipation simply do not eat enough residue. Adequate amounts (30 g of dietary fibre) should be taken daily. It is expected this will increase stool weight and frequency and decrease stool consistency, but it must be remembered there is a strong placebo effect in diet and that transit time through the large bowel is not influenced by fibre (Ornstein et al, 1981). Similarly, pain, sensation of incomplete emptying, flatus, need for laxatives and abdominal distension are susceptible to a placebo effect (Ornstein et al, 1981; Søltoft et al, 1976).

The patient should keep a diary of stool frequency, daily, for at least a month, and stop taking laxatives and non-essential drugs (particularly those for pain), and not use enemas. Some effort is required to make this regimen acceptable to

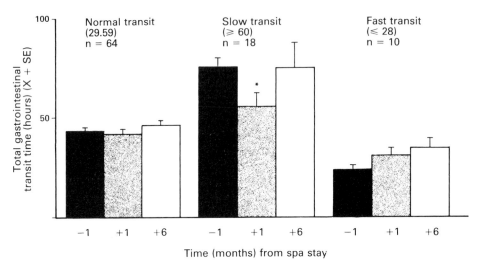

Figure 40. Holidays improve constipation (Nisaird et al, 1982).

patients. A useful approach is to stress its therapeutic advantage.

A difference in stool frequency should be expected between recalled data and recorded data: many subjects defecate more often than they say. Apart from the effect of diet, two elements should be kept in mind. The patient may have unconsciously or consciously exaggerated the problem initially, or simply taking care of him/her has already modified bowel function. The use of a diary is important because quite often the constipation is worse or less at times and patients may be taught to look for coincidences or associations with events in their life; although just understanding a link will not change behaviour and bowel function (Devroede, 1985b).

Patients with large bowel pseudo-obstruction may pass watery, at time colourless, stools, and patients with short-segment Hirschsprung's disease sometimes suffer from 'overflow' incontinence.

Dietary fibre is no panacea for treating constipation, and may even increase the symptoms of patients with slow transit constipation (Preston and Lennard-Jones, 1986). Patient satisfaction and not stool frequency should be the end point of results from the dietary trial.

The patient should be seen at regular intervals and encouraged with empathy. If the need is evident, psychiatric help should be offered but caution needs to be exerted because this may end the medical relationship. Conversely, a good doctor–patient relationship is a partnership enterprise; it is useful, when organic lesions have been ruled out, to let the patient determine the rhythm of encounters and surrender all power so that end of therapy is determined not by the doctor but by a patient who has become autonomous.

Biofeedback Approach

The spastic pelvic floor syndrome is amenable to biofeedback treatment. In a group of patients with a long history of constipation, impossibility to defecate without enemas or laxatives, sporadic or absent defecation urge, difficult and painful defecation once every 4–14 days biofeedback therapy cured eight out of 10 patients (Bleijenberg and Kuijpers, 1988). An anal-plug electrode is inserted to record the elctromyographic activity of the

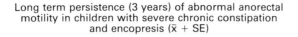

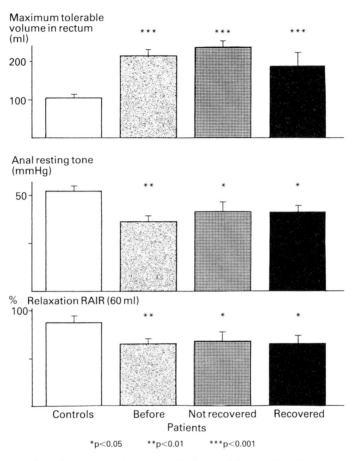

Figure 41. Anorectal motility may remain persistently abnormal despite clinical improvement (Loening-Baucke, 1984).

external anal sphincter. A visual arithmetic anal drawing feedback is produced to the patient. The patient is asked to strain, and this, in recto-anal dyssynergia, increases muscular activity. The patient has to learn that straining must be carried out in a different manner, without pelvic floor contraction.

Psychological Approaches

This area is undergoing major developments. Several studies have demonstrated the advantages of a psychological approach to patients with con-

stipation and the irritable bowel syndrome. Several key points remain unclear, namely the selection modalities of patients and the type of therapy to be used.

In a preliminary study of a highly selected group of patients, colonic transit time has been shown to become faster during psychotherapy (Devroede, 1985b, 1985c). Bowel function improves during psychotherapy more (Svedlund, 1981) or as much (Bennet and Wilkinson, 1985) than with a purely organic approach (Figure 42), and even better during hypnotherapy (Whorwell et al, 1984) (Figure 43), but these results apply to patients

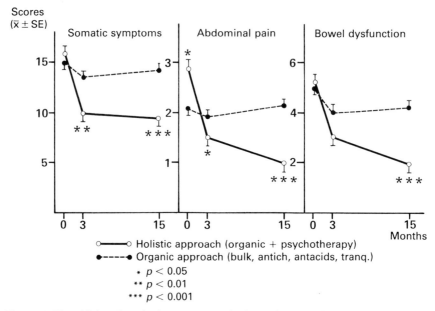

Figure 42. The addition of psychotherapy to a standard organic approach to patients with irritable bowel syndrome is superior in terms of bowel dysfunction (Svedlund, 1981).

selected on the basis of a diagnosis of irritable bowel syndrome. Similar studies should be performed on patients with well-defined mechanisms of chronic idiopathic constipation.

Behavioural Approach

Bowel training in terms of spending time on the toilet at regular intervals is seldom prescribed solely as treatment. Its value is thus debatable. Asking the patient to go to the bathroom after each breakfast and spend a stated period of time, is usually accompanied by other procedures. This has been used mainly in children.

The initial and probably very important step is to evacuate the bowel completely. This can be done with multiple oil or saline enemas (Sarahan et al, 1982, Davidson et al, 1963). It takes generally one week to completely clean the colon and rectum and eliminate faecal soiling. Thereafter, the patient is asked to take milk of magnesia (0.5–1 ml/kg/day), mineral oil (0.5 ml/kg/day) or colace (3–5 mg/kg/day), enough to produce one to three stools per day. It is also acceptable to rely solely upon enemas, daily for a month and with decreasing frequency afterwards. The objective is to create an artificial regularity. Simultaneously, the patient is placed on a high-fibre diet, and one may consider the addition of bran cereal or a bulk laxative such as metamucil. A request is made to go to the toilet for 5–15 minutes after breakfast, each day. Thereafter, it has been shown that negative reinforcement is useful (Rolider and Van Houten, 1985). Spending increasingly longer periods of time in the toilet deprives a child of constantly increasing periods of play time. Conversely, if the child defecates (s)he is left in peace the next day. The successful outcome suggests that attending the bathroom *per se* may have some value. The effect of ageing and natural history on treatment is not known. Above all, the medical approach should not be a fight to force a child to behave, and the office should never become a battleground between parents and child: the battle will be lost.

No good data are available to support the usefulness of a behavioural approach in adults.

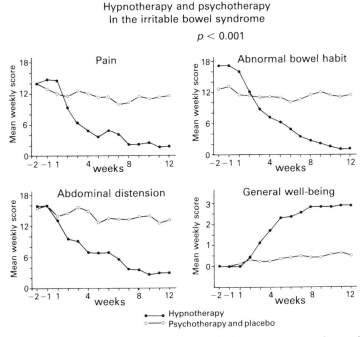

Figure 43. Hypnotherapy is superior to psychotherapy to correct abnormal bowel habits of patients with irritable bowel syndrome (Whorwell et al, 1984).

Surgical Approach

Surgery should be abandoned if rectosphincteric dyssynergia has been demonstrated, because both posterior division of the puborectalis muscle (Barnes et al, 1985) and subtotal colectomy (Barnes et al, 1985; Jennings, 1967; Kuijpers et al, 1986) have been tried without success, and because we now know that biofeedback therapy offers some hope (Bleijenberg and Kuijpers, 1988; Denis et al, 1981).

Surgery is of course the treatment of choice in Hirschsprung's disease, but its role and usefulness in the field of chronic idiopathic constipation are the subject of research and debate. Anorectal myectomy, rectal bypass and total colectomy with ileorectal anastomosis have all been used with some success in some situations (Devroede, 1988). In my opinion and with some experience, I do not envisage a major impact of surgery in the future to cure patients with chronic idiopathic constipation.

References

Abrahamian, F.P., and Lloyd-Still, J.D., (1984), Chronic constipation in childhood: a longitudinal study of 186 patients. *J. Ped. Gastr. Nutr.*, 3:460–7.

Arhan, P., Faverdin, C., Persoz, B., Devroede, G., Dubois, F., Dornic, C., and Pellerin, D., (1976), Relationship between viscoelastic properties of the rectum and anal pressure in man. *J. Appl. Physiol.*, 41:677.

Arhan, P., Devroede, G., Danis, K., Dornic, C., Faverdin, C., Persoz, B., and Pellerin, D., (1978), Viscoelastic properties of the rectal wall in Hirschsprung's disease. *J. Clin. Invest.*, 62:82.

Arhan, P., Devroede, G., Persoz, B., Faverdin, C., Dornic, C., and Pellerin, D., (1979), Response of the anal canal to repeated distension of the rectum. *Clin. Invest. Med.*, 2:83.

Arhan, P., Devroede, G., Jehannin, B., Lanza, M., Faverdin, C., Dornic, C., Persoz, B., Tetreault, L., Perey, B., and Pellerin, D., (1981), Segmental colonic transit time. *Dis. Colon Rectum*, 24:625.

Barnes, P.R.H., Hawley, P.R., Preston, D.M., and Lennard-Jones, J.E., (1985), Experience of posterior division of the puborectalis muscle in the management of chronic constipation. *Br. J. Surg.*, **72**:475.

Barnes, P. R. H., and Lennard-Jones, J. E., (1985), Balloon expulsion from the rectum in constipation of different types. *Gut*, **26**:1049.

Barnes, P. R. H., Lennard-Jones, J. E., Hawley, P. R., and Todd, I. P., (1986), Hirschsprung's disease and idiopathic megacolon in adults and adolescents. *Gut*, **27**:534.

Bartolo, D. C. C., Roe, A. M., Virjee, J., and Mortensen, N. J. McC., (1985), Evacuation proctography in obstructed defaecation and rectal intussuception. *Br. J. Surg.*, **72**:S111.

Battle, W. M., Snape, W. J. Jr., Alair, A., Cohen, S., and Braunstein, S., (1980), Colonic dysfunction in diabetes mellitus. *Gastroenterology*, **79**:1217.

Bennett, P., and Wilkinson, S., (1985), A comparison of psychological and medical treatment of the irritable bowel syndrome. *Br. J. Clin. Psychol.*, **24**:215.

Bleijenberg, G., and Kuijpers, H. C., (1988), Treatment of the spastic pelvic floor syndrome with biofeedback. *Dis. Col. Rect.* (in press).

Bonfils, S., Hachette, J. C., and Danne, O., (1982), *L'abord Psychosomatique en Gastroentérologie*. Masson, Paris, New York, Barcelona, Milan, Mexico, Rio de Janeiro.

Bueno, L., Fioramonti, J., Ruckebusch, Y., Frexinos, J., and Coulom, P., (1980), Evaluation of colonic myoelectric activity in health and functional disorders. *Gut*, **21**:480.

Colin, D. R., Galmiche, J. P., Geoffroy, Y., Hecketsweiler, P. H., Denis, P. H., Lefrançois, R., and Pasquis, P., (1979), Elastic properties of the rectal wall in normal adults and patients with ulcerative colitis. *Gastroenterology*, **77**:45.

Connell, A. M., Frankel, H., and Guttman, L., (1963), The motility of the pelvic colon following complete lesions of the spinal cord. *Paraplegia*, **1**:98.

Dapoigny, M., Tournut, D., Trolese, J. F., Bommelaer, G., and Tournut, R., (1985), Activité myoélectrique colique à jeûn et en période post-prandiale chez le sujet sain et chez le colopathe. *Gastroenterol. Clin. Biol.*, **9**:223.

Davidson, M., Kugler, M. M., and Bauer, C. H., (1963), Diagnosis and management in children with severe and protracted constipation and obstipation. *J. Pediatr.*, **62**:261–75.

Denis, P., Cayran, G., and Galmiche, J. P., (1981), Biofeedback: the light at the end of the tunnel? Maybe for constipation. *Gastroenterology*, **80**:1089.

Devroede, G., and Lamarche, J., (1974), Functional importance of extrinsic parasympathetic innervation to the distal colon and rectum in man. *Gastroenterology*, **66**:273.

Devroede, G., Arhan, P., Duguay, C., Tetreault, L., Akoury, H., and Perey, B., (1979), Traumatic constipation. *Gastroenterology*, **77**:1258.

Devroede, G., Vobecky, S., Masse, S., Arhan, P.,

Leger, C., Duguay, C., and Hemond, M., (1982), Ischemic fecal incontinence and rectal angina. *Gastroenterology*, **83(5)**:970.

Devroede, G., Arhan, P., Schang, J. C., and Heppell, J., (1985), Orderly and disorderly fecal incontinence. In: *Colon, Rectal and Anal Surgery: Current Techniques and Controversies*. (Eds. Kodner, I. J., Fry, R. D., and Roe, J. P.) pp. 40–62. C. V. Mosby Company, St Louis, Toronto, Princeton.

Devroede, G., (1985a), La constipation: du symptôme vers la personne (éditorial). *Gastroenterol. Clin. Biol.*, **9**:3–6.

Devroede, G., (1985b) La constipation: du symptôme à la personne. *Psychologie Médicale*, **17(10)**:1515.

Devroede, G., (1985c), The irritable bowel syndrome: clinical and therapeutical aspects. In: *Proceedings of the First International Symposium on Small Intestinal and Colonic Motility* (Ed. Poitras, P.) pp. 129–39, Centre de recherches cliniques, Hôpital Saint-Luc and Jouveinal, Montreal, Canada.

Devroede, G. (1988), Constipation. In: *Gastrointestinal Disease* (Eds. Sleisenger, M. H., and Fordtran, J. S.) Holt Saunders (in press).

Devroede, G., Roy, T., Bouchoucha, M., Pinard, G., Camerlain, M., Girard, G., Black, R., Schang, J. C., and Arhan, P., (1988), Women with idiopathic colonic dysfunction have a distinct personality and their constipation may reflect anxiety. *Dig. Dis. Sci.* (submitted).

Dinoso, V. P. Jr., Murphy, S. N. S., Goldstein, J., and Rosner, B., (1983), Basal motor activity of the distal colon: a reappraisal. *Gastroenterology*, **85**:637.

Ducrotte, P., Denis, P., Galmiche, J. P., Hellot, M. F., Desechalliers, J. P., Colin, R., Pasquis, P., and Hecketsweiler, P., (1985), Motricité anorectale dans la constipation idiopathique. Etude de 200 patients consécutifs. *Gastroenterol. Clin. Biol.*, **9**:10.

Ehrentheil, O. F., and Wells, E. P., (1955), Megacolon in psychotic patients. A clinical entity. *Gastroenterology*, **29**:285.

Epelboin, A., (1981–82), Selles et urines chez les Fulbe Bande du Sénégal Oriental. Un aspect particulier de l'ethnomédicine. *Cah. O.R.S.T.O.M.*, *Ser. Sci. Hum.*, **184**:515–30.

Farthing, M. J. G., and Lennard-Jones, J. E., (1978), Sensibility of the rectum to distension and the anorectal reflex in ulcerative colitis. *Gut*, **19**:64.

Faverdin, C., Dornic, C., Arhan, P., Devroede, G., Jehannin, B., Revillon, Y., and Pellerin, D., (1981), Quantitative analysis of anorectal pressures in Hirschsprung's disease. *Dis. Colon Rectum*, **24**:422.

Fioramonti, J., Bueno, L., and Frexinos, J., (1980), Sonde endoluminale pour l'exploration électromyographique de la motricité colique chez l'homme. *Gastroentérol. Clin. Biol.*, **4**: 546.

Fleckenstein, P., (1978), A probe for intraluminal recording of myoelectric activity from multiple sites in the human small intestine. *Scand. J. Gastro-enterol.*, **73**:767.

Frexinos, J., Bueno, L., and Fioramonti, J., (1985), Diurnal changes in myoelectric spiking activity of the human colon. *Gastroenterology*, **88**:1104.

Fry, I. K., Griffiths, J. D., and Smart, P. J. G., (1966), Some observations on the movement of the pelvic floor and rectum with special reference to rectal prolapse. *Br. J. Surg.*, **53**:784.

Gear, J. S. S., Brodribb, A. J. M., Ware, A., and Mann, J. I., (1981), Fibre and bowel transit times. *Br. J. Nutr.*, **45**:77.

Gekas, P., and Schuster, M. M., (1981), Stercoral perforation of the colon: case report and review of the literature. *Gastroenterology*, **80**:1054.

Glick, M. E., Meshkinpour, H., Haldeman, S., Hoehler, F., Downey, N., and Bradley, W. E., (1984), Colonic dysfunction in patients with thoracic spinal cord injury. *Gastroenterology*, **86**:287.

Gunterberg, B., Kewenter, J., Petersen, I., and Stener, B., (1976), Anorectal function after major resection of the sacrum with bilateral or unilateral sacrifice of sacral nerves. *Br. J. Surg.*, **63**:546.

Hammond, E. C., (1964), Some preliminary findings on physical complaints from a prospective study of 1,054,004 men and women. *Am. J. Public Health*, **54**:11.

Hero, M., Arhan, P., Devroede, G., Jehannin, B., Faverdin, C., Babin, C., and Pellerin, D., (1985), Measuring the anorectal angle. *J. Biomed. Eng.*, **7**:321.

Hinton, J. M., and Lennard-Jones, J. E., (1968), Constipation: definition and classification. *Postgrad. Med. J.*, **44**:720.

Hinton, J. M., Lennard-Jones, J. E., and Young, A. C., (1969), A new method for studying gut transit times using radiopaque markers. *Gut*, **10**:842.

Ihre, T., (1974), Studies on anal function in continent and incontinent patients. *Scand. J. Gastroenterol.*, **9**(Suppl 25):1.

Jennings, P. J., (1967), Megarectum and megacolon in adolescents and young adults: result of treatment at St Marks's Hospital. *Proc. R. Soc. Med.*, **60**:805.

Kerremans, R., (1969), *Morphological and Physiological Aspects of Anal Continence and Defecation*. Editions Arscia SA, Bruxelles, Presses Académiques Européenes, Bruxelles.

Kuijpers, H. C., and Bleijenberg, G., (1985), The spastic pelvic floor syndrome. A cause of constipation. *Dis. Col. Rect.*, **28**:669.

Kuijpers, H. C., Bleijenberg, G., and De Morree, H., (1986), The spastic pelvic floor syndrome. Large bowel outlet obstruction caused by pelvic floor dysfunction: a radiological study. *Int. J. Colorect. Dis.*, **1**:44.

Lafranchi, G. A., Bazzoichi, G., Brignola, C., Campieri, M., and Labo, G., (1984), Different patterns of intes-tinal transit time and anorectal motility in painful and painless chronic constipation. *Gut*, **25**:1352–7.

Lahr, C. J., Rothenberger, D. A., Jensen, L. L., and Goldberg, S. M., (1986), Balloon topography. A simple method of evaluating anal function. *Dis. Col. Rect.*, **29**:1.

Lennard-Jones, J. E., (1985), Constipation: pathophysiology, clinical features and treatment. In: *Coloproctology and the Pelvic Floor. Pathophysiology and Management* (Eds. Henry, M. M., and Swash, M.) pp. 350–75. Butterworths, London, Boston, Durban, Singapore, Sydney, Toronto, Wellington.

Levine, M. D., (1975), Children with encopresis: a descriptive analysis. *Pediatrics*, **56**:412–16.

Likongo, Y., Devroede, G., Schang, J. C., Arhan, P., Vobecky, S., Navert, H., Carmel, M., Lamoureux, G., Strom, B., and Duguay, C., (1986), Hindgut dysgenesis as a cause of constipation with delayed colonic transit. *Dig. Dis. Sci.*, **31**(9):993.

Loening-Baucke, V. A., (1984), Abnormal rectoanal function in children recovered from chronic constipation and encopresis. *Gastroenterology*, **87**:1299.

Loening-Baucke, V. A., and Cruikshank, B. M., (1986), Abnormal defecation dynamics in chronically constipated children with encopresis. *J. Pediatr.*, **108**(4):562.

Lowen, A., (1967), *Love and Orgasm*, New York, New American Library.

Mahieu, P., Pringot, J., and Bodart, P., (1984a), Defecography: I. description of a new procedure and results in normal patients. *Gastrointest. Radiol.*, **9**:247.

Mahieu, P., Pringot, J., and Bodart, P., (1984b), Defecography: II. contribution to the diagnosis of defecation disorders. *Gastrointest. Radiol.*, **9**:253.

Manning, A. P., Wyman, J. B., and Heaton, K. W., (1976), How trustworthy are bowel histories? Comparison of recalled and recorded information. *Br. Med. J.*, **2**:213.

Martelli, H., Duguay, C., Devroede, G., Arhan, P., Dornic, C., and Faverdin, C., (1978a), Some parameters of large bowel function in normal man. *Gastroenterology*, **75**:612.

Martelli, H., Devroede, G., Arhan, P., and Duguay, C., (1978b), Mechanisms of idiopathic constipation: Outlet obstruction. *Gastroenterology*, **75**:623.

Meier, E., (1977), *Pubococcygeal Strength: Relationship to Urinary Control Problems and to Female Orgasmic Response*. PhD thesis, California School of Professional Psychology, published by University Microfilms International, Ann Arbor, Michigan, USA; London, England.

Meunier, P. (1985), Rectoanal dyssynergia in constipated children. *Dig. Dis. Sci.*, **30**(8):784 (abstr.).

Meunier, P., Mollard, P., and Marechal, J.-M., (1976), Physiopathology of megarectum: the association of megarectum with encopresis. *Gut*, **17**:224.

Meunier, P., Rochas, A., and Lambert, R., (1979a), Motor activity of the sigmoid colon in chronic constipation: comparative study with normal subjects. *Gut*, **20**:1095.

Meunier, P., Marechal, J.-M., and Jaubert de Beaujeu, M., (1979b), Rectoanal pressures and rectal sensitivity studies in chronic childhood constipation. *Gastroenterology*, **77**:330.

Meunier, P., Louis, D., and Jaubert de Beaujeu, M., (1984), Physiologic investigation of primary chronic constipation in children: comparison with the barium enema study. *Gastroenterology*, **87**:1351.

Nisard, A., Jian, R., Chevalier, J., and Lefrant, L., (1982), Effet d'une cure thermale à Châtel-Guyon sur le temps de transit intestinal total de patients atteints de colopathie fonctionnelle. *Rev. Fr. De Gastroentérologie*, **175**:5.

O'Regan, S., Yazbeck, S., and Shick, E., (1985), Constipation, bladder instability, urinary tract infection syndrome. *Clinical Nephrology*, **23**:152.

Ornstein, M.H., Littlewood, E.R., Baird, I.M., Fowler, J., North, W.R.S., and Cox, A.G., (1981), Are fibre supplements really necessary in diverticular disease of the colon? A controlled clinical trial. *Br. Med. J.*, **282**:1353.

Parks, A.G., Porter, N.H., and Melzack, J., (1962), Experimental study of the reflex mechanism controlling the muscles of the pelvic floor. *Dis. Col. Rect.*, **5**:407.

Patriquin, H., Martelli, H., and Devroede, G., (1978), Barium enema in chronic constipation: is it meaningful? *Gastroenterology*, **75**:619.

Percora, P., Suraci, C., Antonelli, M., De Maria, S., and Marrocco, W., (1981), Constipation and obesity: a statistical analysis. *Bull. Soc. It. Biol. Sper.*, **57**:2384.

Preston, D.M., Lennard-Jones, J.E., and Thomas, B.M., (1984), The balloon proctogram. *Br. J. Surg.*, **71**:29.

Preston, D.M., and Lennard-Jones, J.E., (1985a), Pelvic motility and response to intraluminal bisacodyl in slow-transit constipation. *Dig. Dis Sci.*, **30**:289.

Preston, D.M., and Lennard-Jones, J.E., (1985b), Anismus in chronic constipation. *Dig. Dis. Sci.*, **30**:413.

Preston, D.M., Lennard-Jones, J.E., and Thomas, B.M., (1985), Towards a radiologic definition of idiopathic megacolon. *Gastrointest. Radiol.*, **10**:167.

Preston, D.M., and Lennard-Jones, J.E., (1986), Severe chronic constipation in young women: idiopathic slow transit constipation. *Gut*, **27**:41–8.

Read, N.W., Abouzekry, L., Read, M.G., Howell, P., Ottewell, D., and Donnelly, T.C., (1985), Anorectal function in elderly patients with fecal impaction. *Gastroenterology*, **89**:959–66.

Reich, W., (1943), *The Function of the Orgasm: Sex-economic Problems of Biological Energy*. New York: Farrar, Straub and Giroux.

Rendtorff, R.C., and Kashgarian, M., (1967), Stool patterns of healthy adult males. *Dis. Colon Rectum*, **10**:222.

Rolider, A., and Van Houten, R., (1985), Treatment of constipation-caused encopresis by a negative reinforcement procedure. *J. Behav. Ther. Exp. Psychiatr.*, **16**:67.

Rutter, K.R.P., (1974), Electromyographic changes in certain pelvic floor abnormalities. *Proc. R. Soc. Med.*, **67**:53.

Sandler, R.S., and Drossman, D.A., (1988), Bowel habits in apparently healthy young adults. *Dig. Dis. Sci.* (in press).

Sarahan, T., Weintraub, W.H., Coran, A.G., and Wesley, J.R., (1982), The successful management of chronic constipation in infants and children. *J. Ped. Surg.*, **17**:171.

Sarna, S.K., Latimer, P., Campbell, D., and Waterfall, W.E., (1982), Electrical and contractile activities of the human rectosigmoid. *Gut*, **23**:698.

Schang, J.C., and Devroede, G., (1984), Fasting and postprandial myoelectric spiking activity in the human sigmoid colon. *Gastroenterology*, **85**:1048.

Schang, J.C., (1985), Colonic motility in subgroups of patients with the irritable bowel syndrome. *Proceedings of the First International Symposium on Small Intestinal and Colonic Motility*. (Ed. Poitras, P.) pp. 101–12, Centre de Recherches Cliniques, Hôpital Saint-Luc, and Jouveinal Laboratoires/Laboratories Inc., Montreal, Canada.

Schang, J.C., Devroede, G., Duguay, C., Hemond, M., and Hebert, M., (1985), Constipation par inertie colique et obstruction distale: étude électro-myographique. *Gastroenterol. Clin. Biol.*, **9**:480.

Schang, J.C., Hemond, M., Hebert, M., and Pilote, M., (1986), Myoelectrical activity and intraluminal flow in human sigmoid colon. *Dig. Dis. Sci.*, **31**:1331.

Schuster, M.M., Tobon, F., Reid, N.C.R.W., and Talbert, J.L., (1968), Nonsurgical test for the diagnosis of Hirschsprung's disease. *N. Engl. J. Med.*, **278**:188.

Scott, H.W. Jr., and Cantrell, J.R., (1949), Colonmetrographic studies of the effects of section of the parasympathetic nerves of the colon. *Bull. Johns Hopkins Hospital*, **85**:310.

Shouler, P., and Keighley, M.R.B., (1986), Changes in colorectal function in severe idiopathic chronic constipation. *Gastroenterology*, **90**:414.

Søltoft, J., Gudman-Høyes, E., Krag, B., Kristensen, E., and Wulfe, M.R., (1976), A double-blind trial of the effect of wheat bran on symptoms of irritable bowel syndrome. *Lancet*, **i**:270.

Svedlund, J., (1981), Psychotherapy in irritable bowel syndrome: a controlled outcome study. *Acta Psychiatrica Scand.*, **306**:67.

Thompson, W. S., and Heaton, K. W., (1980), Functional bowel disorders in apparently healthy people. *Gastroenterology*, **79**:283.

Tucker, D. M., Sandstead, H. H., Logan, G. M. Jr., Klevay, L. M., Mahalko, J., Johnson, L. K., Inman, L., and Inglett, G. E., (1981), Dietary fiber and personality factors as determinants of stool output. *Gastroenterology*, **81**:879.

Verduron, A., Devroede, G., Bouchoucha, M., Arhan, P., Schang, J. C., Poisson, J., Hemond, M., and Hebert, M., (1988), Megarectum. *Dig. Dis. Sci.* (in press).

Vobecky, J., Caro, H., and Devroede, G., (1983), A case control study of risk factors for large bowel carcinoma. *Cancer*, **51**:1958.

Wald, A., (1986), Colonic transit and anorectal manometry in chronic idiopathic constipation. *Arch. Int. Med.*, **146**:1713.

Wasserman, I. F., (1964), Puborectalis syndrome (rectal stenosis due to anorectal spasm). *Dis. Col. Rect.*, **7**:87.

Watier, A., Devroede, G., Duranceau, A., Abdel-Rahman, M., Duguay, C., Forand, M., Tetreault, L., Arhan, P., Lamarche, J., and Elhilali, M., (1983), Constipation with colonic inertia. A manifestation of systemic disease? *Dig. Dis. Sci.*, **28(11)**:1025.

White, J. C., Verlot, M. G., and Ehrentheil, O., (1940), Neurogenic disturbances of the colon and their investigation by the colonmetrogram. *Ann. Surg.*, **112**:1042.

Whorwell, P. J., Prior, A., and Faragher, E. B., (1984), Controlled trial of hypnotherapy in the treatment of severe refractory irritable-bowel syndrome. *Lancet*, **ii**:1232.

28
ABNORMALITIES OF ANORECTAL FUNCTION

Michael Swash, Susan Mathers

St Mark's Hospital and The London Hospital, London, UK

Anorectal function reflects the interaction of the smooth muscle of the anorectum and its internal anal sphincter with the striated muscle of the external anal sphincter ring, and of the voluntary pelvic floor sphincters and diaphragm. Disorders of the pelvic floor (Henry and Swash, 1985) are common and cause much disability. These disorders form a group of functional disorders of the pelvic floor that cause anorectal, urinary and gynaecological problems (Table 1). In this chapter only the anorectal aspects of these problems will be described.

These 'pelvic floor' or 'anorectal' disorders have interrelated (Table 1) underlying causative mechanisms (Swash et al, 1985). The underlying functional disturbance can be assessed clinically,

pathologically and electrophysiologically (Beersiek et al, 1979; Kiff and Swash, 1984; Snooks et al, 1984a, 1985a, 1985b).

Anatomy of the Pelvic Floor

The pelvic floor consists of the levator ani diaphragm, a muscle that stretches across the pelvis at its outlet and that is perforated by the urethra, the vagina in women, and by the anorectum. Specialized striated muscular sphincters surround the urethra and the anorectum. These muscles provide precise voluntary control of urinary and faecal continence and of micturition and defecation. The functional interactions of the involuntary and voluntary components of these sphincter mechanisms remain controversial and ill-understood (Lubowski et al, 1987).

Faecal continence is maintained by the tonic contraction of the external anal sphincter muscle and the pull of the puborectalis muscle. The latter is a sling of striated muscle arising from the posterior part of the pubis, that passes posteriorly to envelop the posterior part of the anorectum at the anorectal angle (Figure 1). The anorectal angle forms an anteroposterior kink at the junction of the rectum and the anal canal that apposes the anterior and posterior walls of the anorectum so that downward pressure of the abdominal contents ensures that the anorectum is maintained closed, by a flap-valve action (Parks, 1975). Only when this angle is opened by relaxation of the puborec-

Table 1. Pelvic floor disorders

Anorectal incontinence
Urinary incontinence (genuine stress incontinence)
Double incontinence
Anorectal prolapse
Genital prolapse
Pelvic pain syndromes
Intractable constipation
Solitary rectal ulcer syndrome
Complications of childbirth
   sphincter injuries
   vaginal and uterine prolapse
   incontinence
   delayed complications
   e.g. altered bowel habit
      incontinence of urine or faeces

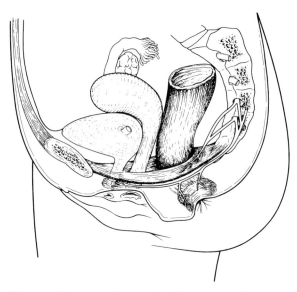

Figure 1. Drawing of the pelvic floor in sagittal section, showing the puborectalis and external sphincter muscles in relation to the anorectum. The external anal sphincter and periurethral striated sphincter muscles are innervated by branches of the pudendal nerves; the puborectalis is innervated by direct pelvic branches of the sacral plexus.

talis muscle can faeces pass through the anorectum; relaxation of this muscle is thus an essential part of the process of defecation (Preston and Lennard-Jones, 1985).

The muscles of the pelvic floor are innervated (Figure 1) by branches of the sacral plexus that originate from the Onuf nucleus of somatic motoneurons in the S2, S3 and S4 spinal segments (Schroder, 1980). These nerves enter the levator ani and puborectalis muscles (Percy et al, 1981; Snooks and Swash, 1986) from their peritoneal surface. The external anal sphincter and peri-urethral striated sphincter muscles, forming the somatic, striated component of the anorectal and urinary sphincters, receive their innervation from the paired pudendal nerves. Inferior rectal branches of these nerves innervate the two sides of the external anal sphincter, and perineal branches innervate the peri-urethral sphincter muscle. Thus, the latter nerves are slightly longer than the former.

The internal anal sphincter, itself formed from the circular smooth muscle component of the anorectal wall, receives modulatory innervation from

the sympathetic nervous system that causes relaxation of this muscle (Lubowski et al, 1987), and the smooth muscle of the rectum is innervated through Meisner's and Auerbach's plexuses by VIPergic nerve fibres; the parasympathetic and sympathetic innervation of the gut modulates ganglion cells in Auerbach's plexus.

Continence

The external anal sphincter and puborectalis muscles are in a state of continuous, tonic, background contraction (Floyd and Walls, 1953; Taverner and Smiddy, 1959). This background activity supplements tonic contraction of the internal anal sphincter in maintaining a region of pressure in the anorectum at the sphincter zone. Puborectalis activity sustains the anorectal angle so that the flap-valve mechanism is continuously operative. The peri-urethral striated sphincter of the urethra, the abductor muscles of the larynx and the cricopharyngeus muscles also exhibit this functional characteristic, needed to maintain urinary continence, the patency of the laryngeal airway, and closure of the pharyngeal sphincter respectively. These muscles contain one or more muscle spindles (Winckler, 1958; Swash, 1982), but the factors responsible for maintaining this continuous contraction have not so far been elucidated.

As would be expected of muscles in a state of tonic contraction the external anal sphincter and puborectalis muscles contain a predominance of type 1, tonically active muscle fibres; these are larger in diameter than the type 2 fibres in these muscles. In these respects these muscles differ from other human striated skeletal muscles, and from the other muscles of the pelvic floor (Beersiek et al, 1979; Wunderlich and Swash, 1983).

Pathology of Pelvic Floor Disorders

In idiopathic anorectal incontinence, the common variety of faecal incontinence that principally affects middle-aged women, there is extensive damage to the external anal sphincter and puborectalis muscles and, to a lesser extent, to the lowermost fibres of the levator ani muscle. This consists of loss of muscle fibres, fibrosis and fat replacement, together with fibre type grouping consistent with a neurogenic process (Swash and Schwartz, 1984). In the most severely affected cases virtually nothing remains of the external anal sphincter and puborectalis muscles (Parks et al, 1977; Beersiek et al, 1979; Swash, 1982). In other pelvic floor disorders, for example, in intractable constipation and in patients with weakness of the pelvic floor muscles not accompanied by faecal incontinence there is less marked denervation and destruction of these muscles (Henry et al, 1982). Detailed anatomical studies of the smooth muscle of the anorectum and internal anal sphincter in incontinence and related disorders are lacking.

Tests of Anorectal Motility

The anorectum functions as a reservoir and as an organ for the orderly evacuation of faeces and flatus. Normal anorectal function depends on smooth muscle in the gut wall and in the internal anal sphincter, and also on the integrity of the perineal muscle diaphragm and of the striated pelvic sphincter muscles. The competence of the anorectum in maintaining continence and in defecation can be tested by anorectal manometry. Electrical activity in the smooth muscle of the anorectum and internal anal sphincter can be assessed electrophysiologically but, as yet, this has no clinical relevance.

Anorectal Manometry

Several methods are available for recording pressure in the anal canal and rectum. The simplest utilizes a latex balloon of high compliance and low elastic resistance that can gradually be filled with air or water (Denny-Brown and Robertson, 1935; Henry et al, 1985). The pressure in the system is measured continuously by a transducer attached to a stiff-walled polyethylene tube, using DC amplifiers. The subject lies in the left lateral position and the balloon is inserted into the anal canal and passed into the rectum. Pressures are recorded

according to a station/pull-through protocol at 1 cm intervals, both at rest and during maximum voluntary contraction (squeeze pressure) of the anal sphincter, using the anal verge as a reference point. The station technique allows the pressure in the anal canal and rectum to be compared with that in the sphincter zone (Henry et al, 1985) (Figure 2).

The balloon method can also be used to study the volume/pressure relationship at which the first sensation of rectal filling is perceived, and the maximum tolerable rectal volume/pressure before involuntary evacuation (defecation) of the balloon occurs. These observations give a crude measure of sensory function in the anorectum.

Anorectal manometry can also be carried out using open-tipped, perfused catheter recording techniques. The pressure in the catheter lumen (or lumens) is dependent on the resistance to flow out of the catheter at the outlet. During perfusion the pressure increases, and suddenly yields when fluid escapes beneath the anorectal mucosa. This 'yield pressure' represents the pressure exerted by the anorectal wall or sphincter (Harris et al, 1966). Rectal pressure profiles can be recorded with complex multilumen perfusion systems or with a microtransducer (Varma and Smith, 1984).

Resting pressure

The anal sphincter zone is 3–5 cm in length. The pressure recorded in this zone (Figure 2) is largely (about 80%) dependent on internal anal sphincter tone (Frenckner and Von Euler, 1975). Continuous recordings in this region reveal two types of quasi-rhythmic fluctuation in resting pressure. Slow waves are cyclic pressure waves of frequency 10–20/min, and amplitude 5–25 cm water. Larger amplitude, ultra-slow waves of frequency <3/min and amplitude 30–100 cm water are superimposed on the slow waves when the resting pressure is high. There is a slight anal-oral gradient in frequency of slow waves in the anal canal suggesting that these smooth muscle contractions are concerned with keeping the anal canal empty in the continent state (Kerremans, 1969; Haynes and Read, 1982).

Resting anal sphincter zone pressure is in-

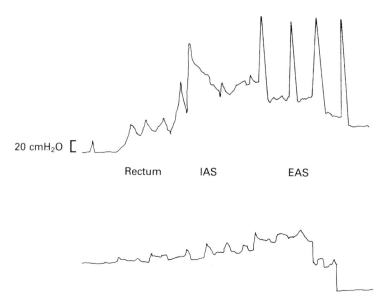

Figure 2. Anorectal manometry; the anal sphincter zone is shown by a region of resting pressure generated by the internal anal sphincter muscle. Voluntary squeeze pressures and cough-induced reflex contractions indicate the functional capacity of the external anal sphincter. The rectal pressure is much lower than that in the anal sphincter region. The upper recording is from a normal subject. The lower, from a patient with neurogenic anorectal incontinence, shows a poor squeeze pressure, and a less well-marked zone of resting pressure.

creased by the erect posture, by coughing, and by voluntary contraction of the external anal sphincter (squeeze pressure). During straining, as in defecation, the resting pressure often decreases. The resting pressure is lower than normal in many patients with anorectal incontinence (Figure 2), and in women who have borne children. It is also lower in the elderly (Taylor et al, 1984; Poos et al, 1986). In haemorrhoids the resting pressure may be increased. In diabetes mellitus there may be a sensory deficit in the anal canal resulting in disturbed pressure/volume relationships. The patient is unable to perceive the rectal balloon until it is relatively fully inflated.

Squeeze Pressure

The maximum squeeze pressure is a crude estimation of the functional capability of the external anal sphincter. Unfortunately this measurement is more dependent on patient compliance than on changes in functional capacity due to disease. The cough pressure usually approximates the maximal squeeze pressure (Figure 2).

Rectal Pressure

The resting pressure in the rectum is lower than that in the anal canal, about 5 cm water. Contractile activity in the rectal smooth muscle occurs at slow (<5/min) and faster (<10/min) rates, but this activity is only rarely propagated through the rectum towards the anal canal.

Effects of Rectal Distension

Inflation of the balloon causes a slight initial increase in rectal pressure, followed by a fall in pressure to the baseline, representing accommodation of the rectum to the change in volume of its contents. This is a normal response of the rectum representing its storage function.

If a distensible balloon is placed in the rectum and a recording balloon in the anal sphincter zone

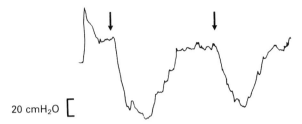

20 cmH₂O [

Figure 3. Anorectal manometry. When a balloon is expanded in the rectum there is a reflex decrease in pressure in the anal sphincter region, due to relaxation of the internal anal sphincter muscle. This anorectal reflex is mediated by intra-mural neural pathways. This is part of the normal response to rectal filling that precedes defecatory activity.

the effect of rectal distension on the anal sphincter pressure can be studied. Rectal distension causes an initial rise in anal pressure, caused by contraction of the external anal sphincter. This response is mediated by stretch receptors in the pelvis through a spinal reflex. This transient rise in pressure is followed by a briefly sustained fall in anal pressure due to relaxation of the internal anal sphincter; the recto-anal reflex (Figure 3). This is an intramural reflex, that is abolished by a circular incision in the muscular coat of the rectum (Lubowski et al, 1987). It is absent in Hirschsprung's disease, and has become a test of major diagnostic importance in this condition (Meunier et al, 1978). Frequently, the recto-anal relaxation response to rectal distension is followed by a brisk and sustained contraction of the external anal sphincter, representing an attempt to maintain continence and to inhibit defecation. If rectal distension is increased further, relaxation of the internal and external anal sphincters is accompanied by relaxation of the puborectalis muscles, and defecation may occur with the onset of rhythmic contractions of abdominal and respiratory muscles, and of rectal contraction (Kerremans, 1969).

In patients with anorectal incontinence the normal recto-anal relaxation response of the internal anal sphincter to rectal distension may be impaired, indicating an abnormality in internal anal sphincter function.

Perineal Descent

Perineal descent consists of descent of the pelvic floor towards the examiner during simulated defecatory straining. It is best demonstrated by asking the patient to cough during inspection of the perineum, when the perineum will be seen to bulge briefly downward. Perineal descent is important because it is associated with a more obtuse anorectal angle, and thus anorectal incontinence.

The extent of perineal descent can be measured in relation to the plane of the ischial tuberosities using the St Mark's perineometer (Figure 4), an instrument in which a movable graduated pillar rests on the perineum while two fixed legs rest on the ischial tuberosities (Henry et al, 1982). More

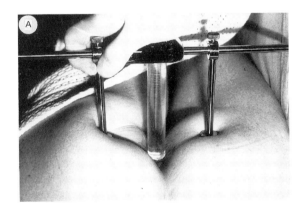

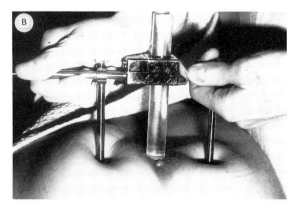

Figure 4. Measurement of perineal plane. The position of the perineal plane at rest (A) and during a defecatory strain (B) is shown in relation to the plane of the ischial tuberosities. The latter corresponds to the plane of the anorectal angle in defecating proctograms.

accurate measurements can be made of the plane of the anorectal angle in relation to the pelvis from lateral radiographs taken with contrast in the anorectum, as in defecating proctography (see Chapter 19).

Electrophysiological Investigations of the Pelvic Floor

Two types of investigation are available. Electromyography (EMG) is used to examine the extent of reinnervation in the external anal sphincter and puborectalis muscles. The amount of denervation cannot be directly quantified electrophysiologically; histological studies are required to evaluate denervation. However, electrophysiological measurements of the terminal motor latencies in the innervations of these muscles directly evaluate the extent and site of any abnormality.

Electromyography

Concentric needle EMG (Bartolo et al, 1983), with motor unit potential analysis, can be used to study the external anal sphincter and puborectalis muscles (Figure 5) but this technique is tedious and, unless backed up by computer analysis of the motor unit potentials, is subject to observer error. Measurement of the fibre density with the single

A

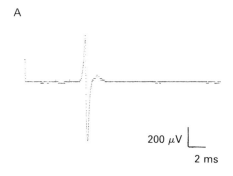

200 μV

2 ms

B

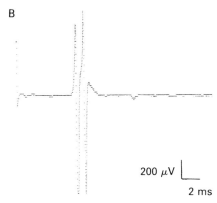

200 μV

2 ms

C.

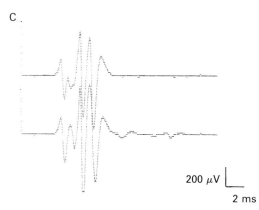

200 μV

2 ms

Figure 6. Single fibre EMG. In the normal external anal sphincter single or double potentials are found (A and B). The mean number of potentials in 20 separate recordings is called the fibre density. In reinnervated muscles there is an increase in the fibre density so that individual motor unit recordings tend to show multiple components (C).

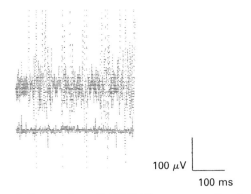

100 μV

100 ms

Figure 5. Concentric needle EMG. The upper recording shows tonic resting activity in the puborectalis muscle. During a simulated defecatory effort, in the lower trace, there is relaxation of the puborectalis muscle, thus allowing the anorectal flap-valve sphincter to open preparatory to defecation.

fibre EMG technique is a relatively robust measure that shows concordance between different examiners and in serial investigations. Further, it is a good index of reinnervation in a muscle (Stalberg and Trontelj, 1979; Swash and

Schwartz, 1988). The method consists of calculating the mean of the number of spike potentials, linked to the triggering potential, in 20 different motor units recorded at different sites in the muscle. Each component represents an action potential of a single muscle fibre (Figure 6). The fibre density in the external anal sphincter and puborectalis muscles in a group of 20 normal subjects was 1.5 (SD 0.1) (Neill and Swash, 1980; Henry and Swash, 1985). In reinnervated muscles the fibre density is increased (Figure 6, Table 2).

Pudendal and Perineal Nerve Terminal Motor Latencies

The terminal motor latency in the pudendal and perineal nerves (PNTML and PerNTML

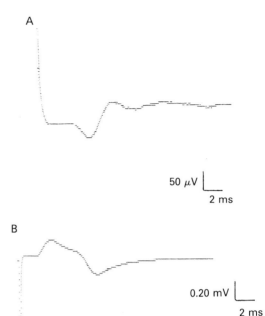

Figure 8. Perineal nerve terminal motor latency (PerNTML). The latency to the peri-urethral striated sphincter muscle is measured, using the same pudendal nerve stimulator and catheter-mounted recording electrodes. (A) Normal latency, (B) increased latency.

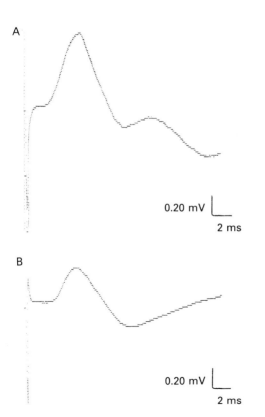

Figure 7. Pudendal nerve terminal motor latency (PNTML). In a normal subject (A) the stimulus is followed, about 2 ms later, by an evoked compound muscle action potential in the external anal sphincter muscle. The latency of this response is measured and is called the PNTML. In a patient with neurogenic anorectal incontinence (B) the PNTML is increased.

respectively) can be used to assess function in the distal parts of the innervations of the external anal sphincter (Figure 7) and peri-urethral striated sphincter muscles (Figure 8). The latency of the evoked muscle action responses in these muscles is recorded after stimulation of the pudendal nerves in the pelvis (Kiff and Swash, 1984; Snooks and Swash, 1984a, 1984b; Snooks et al, 1984a, Snooks et al, 1985a, 1985b). This is accomplished by using a finger-mounted array of recording and stimulating electrodes (Figure 9), with fixed inter-electrode distances (3.5 cm). The two stimulating electrodes are mounted at the tip of the finger, with the cathode arranged distally, and the recording electrodes are mounted side by side at the base of the finger so as to be in a suitable position to pick up the response in the external anal sphincter muscle. Stimulation of the pudendal nerves is achieved on either side of the pelvis by directing the exploring finger in the rectum towards the lateral rim of the pelvis, i.e. towards the ischial spine. The onset of the stimulus is used to trigger the oscilloscope. Stimuli of square wave type,

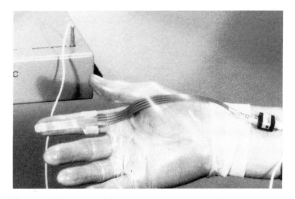

Figure 9. The pudendal nerve electrode array is disposable, and mounted with a self-adhesive backing to an ordinary surgical glove. A ground electrode is applied to the patient's thigh.

lating the spinal column overlying the cauda equina, thus allowing a motor latency to these muscles to be measured (Kiff and Swash, 1984; Snooks et al, 1984a, 1984b).

The patient is placed in the left lateral position and a separate ground electrode is connected from the upper thigh to the preamplifier of the EMG apparatus. Single shocks of 500 to a maximum of 1500 V, of 0.5 msec duration, decaying with a time constant of $50\,\mu$sec (Digitimer D180 stimulator), are delivered through two 1 cm diameter, saline-soaked gauze electrode pads, arranged 5 cm apart,

0.1 msec duration and of about 50 V, but always supramaximal, are used to find the shortest latency, measured from the onset of the stimulus artefact to the onset of the response in the external anal sphincter muscle. The latter can be felt through the examiner's gloved finger. The electrode array used for this method is now commercially available (Dantec Electronics).

The perineal nerve terminal motor latency can be measured using a similar stimulation technique. The response evoked in the peri-urethral striated sphincter muscle is recorded (Figure 8) using a pair of catheter-mounted recording electrodes in the urethra (Dantec 21L11). The mean PNTML in a group of 31 normal subjects was 2.0 msec (SD 0.2 msec), and the mean PerNTML in this group of normal subjects was 2.4 msec (SD 0.2 msec) (Snooks et al, 1984a).

The puborectalis muscle is not innervated by the pudendal nerves. Investigation of the integrity of its innervation therefore requires a different technique.

Transcutaneous Spinal Stimulation

Since the innervation of the puborectalis is derived from pelvic branches of the sacral plexus its innervation is not accessible to intra-rectal electrical stimulation techniques. The nerves innervating this muscle, and other muscles of the perineum or legs, can be excited transcutaneously by stimu-

A

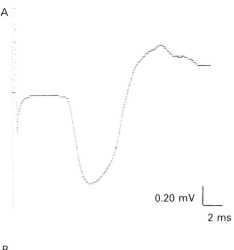

0.20 mV

2 ms

B

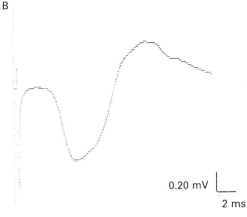

0.20 mV

2 ms

Figure 10. Spinal stimulation. The motor latencies to the external anal sphincter muscle can be measured from transcutaneous stimulation of the cauda equina nerve roots at the L1 and L4 vertebral levels. Because of the longer distance the latency from L1 (A) is slightly longer than that from L4 (B). Similar responses can be obtained from the puborectalis and peri-urethral striated sphincter muscles.

and placed with the cathode at the level of the 1st or 4th lumbar vertebra respectively. The anode is directed cranially. An initial 500 V stimulus is applied, and increased by 200 V increments until the amplitude and latency of the evoked response recorded in the pelvic sphincter muscles does not change with further stimulus increments, thus indicating that the response is supramaximal (Figure 10). Three consecutive responses recorded at stimulus voltages 20% greater than this level are used for measurement of the latency of the response. The muscle responses in the external anal sphincter muscle are recorded using the electrode array designed for PNTML measurements, or with an anal plug electrode. The puborectalis response is recorded with a similar glove-mounted electrode array as that used for the PNTML measurements consisting of two metal plates mounted 1 cm apart on the tip of the gloved index finger. The finger bearing this device is inserted into the rectum so that the electrode array is in contact with the puborectalis muscle, i.e. the

recording surfaces face posteriorly (Henry et al, 1985). Normal values are given in Table 2.

Stimulation at the L1 and L4 vertebral levels activates the conus medullaris and the lumbosacral nerve roots of the cauda equina respectively. It is not possible to stimulate these nerve roots consistently at a more caudal vertebral level, presumably because the current is attenuated by the bony mass of the sacrum.

The stimulus electrodes, situated on the skin overlying the cauda equina, are several centimetres distant from the underlying excitable nervous tissue, so that the precise site of stimulation of the nerve roots is not necessarily represented by the surface marking of the cathode. However, this error is probably similar at the two points of stimulation. Measurement of the length of the cauda equina between the two stimulation points is also likely to be inaccurate because of the distance of the nerve roots from their surface markings (Kiff and Swash, 1984; Swash and Snooks, 1986). We have therefore preferred to base interpretations of the meaning of differences between control subjects and patients with suspected cauda equina lesions on the latency measurements themselves rather than on calculated conduction velocities.

Table 2. Normal values (mean and 1 SD)

Anorectal Manometry:	
Resting pressure	60 ± 20 cm water
Squeeze pressure	100 ± 30 cm water
Perineal plane:	
Resting position	2.5 ± 0.6 cm
Straining position	0.9 ± 1.0 cm
Single fibre EMG:	
Fibre density	1.5 ± 0.16
Concentric needle EMG:	
Motor unit potential duration	5.5 ± 0.2 msec
PNTML	2.0 ± 0.2 msec
PerNTML	2.4 ± 0.2 msec

Spinal Latencies:

	L1 (msec)	L4 (msec)	SLR
EAS	5.5 ± 0.4	4.3 ± 0.4	1.33 ± 0.1
PR	4.8 ± 0.4	4.0 ± 0.3	1.3 ± 0.1
USSM	4.8 ± 0.3	4.1 ± 0.3	—

Spinal Latency Ratio

The difference in motor latency in the responses in the external anal sphincter or puborectalis muscles from stimulation at the L1 and L4 levels represents the conduction time in the S2, S3 and S4 cauda equina nerve roots between these vertebral levels (Figure 10). We have found it useful to express this as a ratio of the two latencies, since the absolute values of the latencies from L1 and L4 stimulation are modified not only by damage to these nerve roots but also by variations in height, pelvic size and other morphometric features. The spinal latency ratio (SLR) obviates these difficulties without introducing error from measurements of the inter-electrode distance (Snooks and Swash, 1984b).

The SLR is represented by:

$$SLR = \frac{\text{Latency to puborectalis after stimulation at L1}}{\text{Latency to puborectalis after stimulation at L4}}$$

In the presence of distal conduction delay both L1 and L4 motor latencies will be increased, since the abnormal zone of nerve conduction is contained within both measurements; the SLR will therefore become slightly smaller. However, in the case of proximal conduction delay, due to a lesion situated within the cauda equina between the L1 and L4 vertebral levels, the L1 motor latency will be increased compared to the L4 motor latency and, consequently, the SLR will be increased. Stimulation at these two vertebral sites can thus be used to determine whether there is conduction delay within or distal to the L1/L4 portion of the cauda equina.

The SLR is also increased in patients in whom there is slowed motor conduction both proximally and distally since the increased proximal (terminal) motor latency is then contained only in the measurement from the L1 stimulus (see Swash and Snooks, 1986).

The variance of the SLR between normal subjects is relatively small. In 20 female control subjects the SLR to the puborectalis from L1 and L4 stimulation was 1.3 (SD 0.1), and in 12 male control subjects it was 1.35 (SD 0.09). The motor conduction velocity in the motor nerve roots of the cauda equina derived from these latency measurements is 58 m/sec (SD 10 m/sec). The SLR to the external anal sphincter muscle from stimulation at the same vertebral sites is comparable with the SLR to the puborectalis muscle. The SLR to the peri-urethral striated sphincter

muscle from these two vertebral levels in 21 control female subjects was 1.3 (SD 0.1) (Snooks and Swash, 1984a, 1984b; Swash and Snooks, 1986).

Cortical Stimulation

It has recently become possible to stimulate the sphincter area in the motor cortex using an electrical or magnetic stimulator, and to record the latency to the response of the sphincter muscles (Figure 11). This new technique offers the possibility of quantitatively investigating disorders of continence resulting from disease of the central nervous system, such as multiple sclerosis and stroke, in which the motor latency from cortical stimulation may be increased. The sensory pathway to the cerebral cortex can be investigated using evoked response techniques with computer averaging.

Clinical Applications

Anorectal Incontinence

Anorectal manometry is chiefly useful in quantifying the extent of functional weakness of the pelvic floor sphincters, but it also gives information about resting tone in the anal canal. The latter is currently the best method for assessment of internal anal sphincter function. Manometry has been used in recent years in the assessment of patients with defecatory disorders other than incontinence,

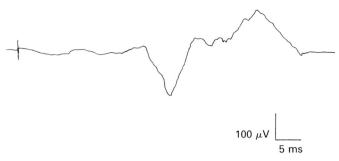

100 μV

5 ms

Figure 11. Cortical stimulation. The response in the external anal sphincter from transcutaneous electrical stimulation of the motor cortex. The latency of the response is a measure of conduction time in the corticospinal pathway to this sphincter muscle, and is useful in the investigation of patients with neurological disorders causing sphincter dysfunction.

especially in constipation. Its use in the diagnosis of Hirschsprung's disease is discussed above.

Electrophysiological investigation of the pelvic floor and striated sphincter muscles is useful in the assessment of patients with incontinence, and related pelvic floor disorders (Henry and Swash, 1985; Henry et al, 1985). These investigations enable quantitative assessment (Table 2) to be made of distal motor conduction in the pudendal innervation of the external anal sphincter muscle, in the perineal innervation of the peri-urethral striated sphincter muscle, and of proximal motor conduction in the motor nerve roots of the cauda equina that innervate the external anal sphincter, puborectalis and peri-urethral striated sphincter muscles. Single fibre EMG fibre density or concentric needle EMG studies can be used as an index of reinnervation in these muscles.

The fibre density in the external anal sphincter muscle was slightly increased (> 1 SD greater than the control group) in 93% of patients with anorectal incontinence (Snooks et al, 1985b) and in 70% of these patients it was increased more than 2 SD compared with the control value. In 75% of these patients the SLR from L1 and L4 spinal stimulation suggested a distal lesion, and in 23% a proximal lesion. These findings thus indicate that in the majority of patients with idiopathic anorectal incontinence there is a distal lesion in the sphincter innervation causing denervation of the sphincter musculature (see Womack et al, 1986). We have previously provided evidence from retrospective and prospective studies that this results from stretch injury to these nerves during perineal descent associated with prolonged and repeated defecation straining, often initiated by a difficult labour but sometimes associated with intractable constipation, or with a history of direct injury to the sphincter musculature (Beersiek et al, 1979; Snooks et al, 1984b, 1985b; Lubowski et al, 1987).

In most patients with incontinence in whom there were electrophysiological features of cauda equina lesion, shown by the increased L1 latency and SLR, there were no clinical signs of cauda equina disease (Snooks et al, 1985c). However, the anal reflex is often absent in patients with anorectal incontinence and this may be evidence of a spinal lesion in some such patients. Most patients presenting with anorectal incontinence in whom the SLR is increased also have an increased pudendal nerve terminal motor latency (Snooks et al, 1985b), indicating the coexistence of lesions at both proximal and distal sites, and surgical repair of the incontinence is probably the most appropriate management for these patients, rather than extensive neurological investigation, which would include myelography. The latter is only indicated in the presence of clinical features supporting the presence of surgically remediable cauda equina disease.

In idiopathic, genuine stress urinary incontinence the perineal nerve terminal motor latency is markedly increased, but the PNTML is normal, or only slightly increased (Snooks et al, 1984a, 1985b). The SLR to the peri-urethral striated sphincter muscle is normal. About 10% of patients with anorectal incontinence also have stress incontinence of urine. These results suggest that genuine stress urinary incontinence, like anorectal incontinence, is usually due to neurogenic weakness of the perineal musculature (see Snooks et al, 1985c).

In other pelvic floor disorders, for example, in solitary rectal ulcer syndrome, intractable constipation, sphincter injuries and urogenital prolapse, less severe abnormalities are found in the electrophysiological tests. Thus the fibre density in the external anal sphincter muscle is less than

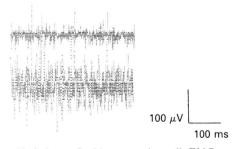

100 μV

100 ms

Figure 12. Anismus. In this concentric needle EMG recording of activity in the puborectalis muscle normal resting activity is present (upper trace). However, during attempted defecation straining there is a paradoxical increase in activity in this muscle, perhaps interfering with the normal relaxation of this muscle during attempted defecation. This abnormal response is found in some patients with severe constipation, but it also occurs in some apparently normal subjects.

1.8 and the PNTML is less than 2.5 ms; more marked abnormalities in these tests are commonly associated with anorectal incontinence (Swash et al, 1985b). In anorectal prolapse without incontinence there is no abnormality in the electrophysiological investigations indicating that the innervation of the pelvic floor sphincter muscles is normal. In some patients with constipation there is inappropriate contraction of the puborectalis muscle during attempted defecation straining (Figure 12), suggesting that the pelvic outlet is functionally obstructed by failure to release the flap-valve (Preston and Lennard-Jones, 1985). However, a similar abnormality is sometimes found in patients investigated for other reasons, for example, for anal pain, and the specificity of this observation is thus uncertain at present.

Cauda Equina Disease

In these patients comparison of distal motor conduction in the pudendal innervation of the external anal sphincter muscle, and of proximal motor conduction in the motor nerve roots that innervate this muscle and the puborectalis, is particularly useful (Swash and Snooks, 1986). Single fibre EMG studies of the fibre density in these two muscles can be used as an index of reinnervation. The SLR, calculated from the L1/L4 motor latency ratio, measured to the puborectalis (Figure 10) or external anal sphincter muscle is increased, and the PNTML and PerNTML are normal. These findings should prompt referral for neurological assessment.

References

Bartolo, D. C. C., Jarratt, J. A., and Read, N. W. (1983), The use of conventional EMG to assess external anal sphincter neuropathy in man. *J. Neurol. Neurosurg. Psychiatry*, **46**:1115–18.

Beersiek, F., Parks, A. G., and Swash, M., (1979), Pathogenesis of idiopathic anorectal incontinence; a histometric study of the anal sphincter musculature. *J. Neurol. Sci.*, **42**:111–27.

Denny-Brown, D., and Robertson, E. G., (1935), An investigation of the nervous control of defecation. *Brain*, **58**:256–310.

Floyd, W. F., and Walls, E. W., (1953), Electromyography of the sphincter ani externus in man. *J. Physiol.*, **122**:599–609.

Frenckner, B., and von Euler, C., (1975), Influence of pudendal block on the function of the anal sphincter. *Gut*, **16**:482–9.

Harris, L. D., and Winnans Pope, C. E., (1966), Determination of yield pressures; a method for measuring anal sphincter competence. *J. Clin. Invest.*, **43**:2272–8.

Haynes, W. G., and Read, N. W., (1982), Anorectal activity in man during rectal infusion of saline; a dynamic assessment of the anal sphincter mechanism. *J. Physiol.*, **330**:45–56.

Henry, M. M., and Swash, M., (1985), *Coloproctology and the Pelvic Floor*. Butterworth, London.

Henry, M. M., Parks, A. G., and Swash, M., (1982), The pelvic floor musculature in the descending perineum syndrome. *Br. J. Surg.*, **69**:470–2.

Henry, M. M., Snooks, S. J., Barnes, P. R. H., and Swash, M., (1985), Investigation of disorders of the anorectum and colon. *Ann. Roy. Coll. Surg. (Engl.)*, **67**:355–60.

Kerremans, R., (1969), *Morphological and Physiological Aspects of Anal Continence and Defecation*. Editions Arscia, Brussels.

Kiff, E. S., and Swash, M., (1984), Normal proximal and delayed distal conduction in the pudendal nerves of patients with idiopathic (anorectal) incontinence. *J. Neurol. Neurosurg. Psychiatry*, **47**:820–3.

Lubowski, D. Z., Nicholls, R. J., Swash, M., and Jordan, M. J., (1987), Neural control of internal anal sphincter function. *Br. J. Surg.*, **74**, 668–70.

Meunier, P., Marechal, J. M., and Mollard, P., (1978), Accuracy of the manometric diagnosis of Hirschsprung's disease. *J. Paediat. Surg.*, **13**:411–15.

Neill, M. E., and Swash, M., (1980), Increased motor unit fibre density in the external anal sphincter muscle in anorectal incontinence; a single fibre EMG study. *J. Neurol. Neurosurg. Psychiatry*, **43**:343–7.

Parks, A. G., (1975), Anorectal incontinence. *Proc. Roy. Soc. Med.*, **68**:681–90.

Parks, A. G., Swash, M., and Urich, H., (1977), Sphincter denervation in anorectal incontinence and rectal prolapse. *Gut*, **18**:656–65.

Percy, J. P., Neill, M. E., Swash, M., and Parks, A. G., (1981), Electrophysiological study of motor nerve supply of pelvic floor. *Lancet*, **i**:16–17.

Poos, R. J., Frank, J., Bittner, R., and Beger, H. G., (1986), Influence of age and sex on anal sphincters; manometric evaluation of anorectal continence. *Eur. Surg. Res.*, **18**:343–8.

Preston, D. M., and Lennard-Jones, J. E., (1985), Anismus in chronic constipation. *Digest. Dis. Sci.*, **30**:413–18.

Schroder, H. D., (1980), Organisation of the motor neurones innervating the pelvic muscles of the male rat. *J. Comp. Neurol.*, **192**:567–87.

Snooks, S. J., and Swash, M. (1984a), Abnormalities of the innervation of the urethral striated sphincter musculature in incontinence. *Br. J. Urol.*, **56**:401–5.

Snooks, S. J., and Swash, M., (1984b), Perineal nerve and transcutaneous spinal stimulation; new methods for the investigation of the urethral striated sphincter musculature. *Br. J. Urol.*, **56**:406–9.

Snooks, S. J., and Swash, M., (1986), The innervation of the muscles of continence. *Ann. Roy. Coll. Surg. (Engl.)*, **68**:45–9.

Snooks, S. J., Badenoch, D., Tiptaft, R., and Swash, M., (1985a), Perineal nerve damage in genuine stress urinary incontinence. *Br. J. Urol.*, **57**:422–6.

Snooks, S. J., Barnes, P. R. H., and Swash, M., (1984a), Damage to the innervation of the voluntary anal and periurethral striated sphincter musculature in incontinence; an electrophysiological study. *J. Neurol. Neurosurg. Psychiatry*, **47**:1269–73.

Snooks, S. J., Barnes, P. R. H., Swash, M., and Henry, M. M., (1985b), Damage to the innervation of the pelvic floor musculature in chronic constipation. *Gastroenterol.*, **89**:971–81.

Snooks, S. J., Swash, M., Setchell, M. and Henry, M. M., (1984b), Injury to innervation of pelvic floor sphincter musculature in childbirth. *Lancet*, **ii**:546–50.

Snooks, S. J., Swash, M., and Henry, M. M., (1985c), Abnormalities in peripheral and central nerve conduction in anorectal incontinence. *J. Roy. Soc. Med.*, **78**:294–300.

Stalberg, E., and Trontelj, J., (1979), *Single Fibre Electromyography*. Mirvalle Press, Old Woking.

Swash, M., (1982), The neuropathology of idiopathic anorectal incontinence. In: *Recent Advance in Neuropathology*, Vol 2 (Ed. Thomas Smith, W., and Cavanagh, J. B.), pp. 243–70, Churchill-Livingstone, Edinburgh.

Swash, M., (1985), Histopathology of the pelvic floor.

In: *Coloproctology and the Pelvic Floor* (Eds Henry, M. M. and Swash, M.), pp. 129–50, Butterworth, London.

Swash, M., and Schwartz, M. S., (1984), *Biopsy Pathology of Muscle*. p. 206, Chapman and Hall, London.

Swash, M., and Schwartz, M. S., (1988), *Neuromuscular Disorders: a Practical Approach to Diagnosis and Management*. 2nd edition. Springer-Verlag, London. In press.

Swash, M., and Snooks, S. J., (1986), Slowed motor conduction in lumbosacral nerve roots in cauda equina lesions; a new diagnostic technique. *J. Neurol. Neurosurg. Psychiatry*, **49**:808–16.

Swash, M., Snooks, S. J., and Henry, M. M., (1985), A unifying concept of pelvic floor disorders and incontinence. *J. Roy. Soc. Med.*, **78**:906–11.

Taverner, D., and Smiddy, J., (1959), An electromyographic study of the normal function of the external anal sphincter and pelvic diaphragm. *Dis. Colon Rectum*, **2**:153–60.

Taylor, B. M., Beart, R. W. Jr., and Phillips, S. F., (1984), Longitudinal and radial variations of pressure in the human anal sphincter. *Gastroenterology*, **86**:693–7.

Varma, J. S., and Smith, A. N., (1984), Anorectal profilometry with the microtransducer. *Br. J. Surg.*, **71**:867–9.

Winckler, G., (1958), Remarques sur la morphologie et l'innervation du M releveur de l'anus. *Arch. Anat. Histol. Embryol. (Strasbourg)*, **41**:77–95.

Womack, N. R., Morrison, J. F. B., and Williams, N. S., (1986), The role of pelvic floor denervation in the aetiology of idiopathic faecal incontinence. *Br. J. Surg.*, **73**:404–7.

Wunderlich, M., and Swash, M. (1983), The overlapping innervation of the two sides of the external anal sphincter by the pudendal nerves. *J. Neurol. Sci.*, **59**:97–109.

INDEX

This publication was made possible
by a grant from the
Janssen Research Foundation